Diagnostic Interviewing
Third Edition

Diagnostic Interviewing

Third Edition

Edited by

Michel Hersen

Pacific University
Forest Grove, Oregon

and

Samuel M. Turner

University of Maryland
College Park, Maryland

Kluwer Academic/Plenum Publishers

New York • Boston • Dordrecht • London • Moscow

Library of Congress Cataloging-in-Publication Data

Diagnostic interviewing / edited by Michel Hersen and Samuel M. Turner.—3rd ed.
    p. cm.
    Includes bibliographical references and index.
    ISBN 0–306–47760–2
    1. Interviewing in psychiatry. 2. Mental illness—Diagnosis. I. Hersen, Michel. II. Turner,
Samuel M., 1944–
    [DNLM: 1. Interview, Psychological. 2. Mental Disorders—diagnosis. WM 141 D53664 2003]
RC480.7.D5 2003
616.89′075—dc21   2003051335

ISBN: 0-306-47760-2
© 2003 Kluwer Academic Publishers
233 Spring Street, New York, New York 10013

http://www.wkap.nl

10 9 8 7 6 5 4 3 2 1

A C.I.P. Catalogue record for this book is available from the Library of Congress

Permissions for books published in Europe: permissions@wkap.nl
Permissions for books published in the United States of America:
permissions@wkap.com

Printed in the United States of America

Contributors

Ron Acierno, National Crime Victims Research and Treatment Center, Medical University of South Carolina, Charleston, South Carolina 29425

Jennifer Antick, School of Professional Psychology, Pacific University, Forest Grove, Oregon 97116

Deborah C. Beidel, Department of Psychology, University of Maryland, College Park, Maryland 20742

Gary Birchler, Department of Veterans Affairs, San Diego Healthcare System, San Diego, California 92108

Michelle Bobowick, Dialectical Behavior Therapy Program, Portland, Oregon 97202

Koren M. Boggs, Department of Psychology, University of Mississippi, University, Mississippi, 38677

Kimberly Carsia, Department of Psychiatry and Philadelphia Veterans Affairs Medical Center, University of Pennsylvania Health Systems, Philadelphia, Pennsylvania 19104

Carrie J. Crider, School of Professional Psychology, Pacific University, Forest Grove, Oregon 97116

Judith A. Cohen, Department of Psychiatry, Allegheny General Hospital, Pittsburgh, Pennsylvania 15212

Michael S. Daniel, School of Professional Psychology, Pacific University, Forest Grove, Oregon 97116

Katherine M. Diskin, University of Calgary, Addiction Center, Foothills Hospital, Calgary, Alberta, Canada T2N 1N4

Barry Edelstein, Department of Psychology, West Virginia University, Morgantown, West Virginia 26506

Jon D. Elhai, Psychological Services, Veterans Affairs Medical Center, Charleston, South Carolina 29401

William Fals-Stewart, Research Institute on Addictions, State University of New York at Buffalo, Buffalo, New York

John P. Foreyt, Nutrition Research Clinic, Baylor College of Medicine, Houston, Texas 77030

DAVID M. FREED, Department of Human Resources, Oregon State Hospital, Salem, Oregon 97310

B. CHRISTOPHER FRUEH, Psychological Services, Veterans Affairs Medical Center, Charleston, South Carolina 29401

K. M. GOODALE, School of Professional Psychology, Pacific University, Forest Grove, Oregon 97116

G. KEN GOODRICK, Department of Family and Community Medicine, Baylor College of Medicine, Houston, Texas 77030

REBECCA S. GRIFFIN, Department of Psychology, University of Mississippi, University, Mississippi 38677

ALAN M. GROSS, Department of Psychology, University of Mississippi, University, Mississippi 38677

MARK B. HAMNER, Psychological Services, Veterans Affairs Medical Center, Charleston, South Carolina 29401

NANCY HEISER, Department of Psychology, University of Maryland, College Park, Mary land 20742

MICHEL HERSEN, School of Professional Psychology, Pacific University, Forest Grove, Oregon 97116

DAVID C. HODGINS, University of Calgary, Addiction Center, Foothills Hospital, Calgary, Alberta, Canada T2N 1N4

SOONIE A. KIM, Dialectical Behavior Therapy Program, Portland, Oregon 97202

LESLEY KOVEN, Department of Psychology, West Virginia University, Morgantown, West Virginia 26506

CRISTINA MAGANA, Department of Veterans Affairs, San Diego Healthcare System, San Diego, California 92108

ANTHONY P. MANNARINO, Department of Psychiatry, Allegheny General Hospital, Pittsburgh, Pennsylvania 15212

JILLAYNE Z. MCCLANAHAN, Portland Dialectical Behavioral Therapy Program, Portland, Oregon 97237

NATHANIEL MCCONAGHY, School of Psychiatry, University of New South Wales, Paddington, N.S.W. 2021, Australia

CATHERINE MILLER, School of Professional Psychology, Pacific University, Forest Grove, Oregon 97116

KIM T. MUESER, NH-Dartmouth Psychology Center, Concord, New Hampshire 03301

WILLIAM T. NAY, Department of Psychology, University of Maryland, College Park, Maryland 20742

WALKER S. C. POSTON, Department of Psychology, University of Missouri-Kansas City, Kansas City, Missouri 64110

ALYSSA A. RHEINGOLD, National Crime Victims Research and Treatment Center, Medical University of South Carolina, Charleston, South Carolina 29425

STEVEN L. SAYERS, Department of Psychiatry and Philadelphia Veterans Affairs Medical Center, University of Pennsylvania Health System, Philadelphia, Pennsylvania, 19104

LISA SELTHON, Counseling Psychology Program, Pacific University, Portland, Oregon 97205

ANDREA SHREVE-NEIGER, Department of Psychology, West Virginia University, Morgantown, West Virginia, 26506

ADAM SPRIA, Department of Psychology, West Virginia University, Morgantown, West Virginia, 26506

RISA STEIN, Department of Psychology, Rockhurst University, Kansas City, Missouri 64110

SHANI STEWART, Department of Psychology, University of Missouri-Kansas City, Kansas City, Missouri 64110

ELLIE T. STURGIS, Counseling Association of Southwest Virginia, Blacksburg, Virginia 24060

PAULA TRUAX, Counseling Psychology Program, Pacific University, Portland, Oregon 97205

SAMUEL M. TURNER, Department of Psychology, University of Maryland, College Park, Maryland 20742

Preface

Perhaps the most difficult milestone in a young clinician's career is the completion of the first interview. For the typical trainee, the endeavor is fraught with apprehension and with some degree of dread. If the interview goes well, there is considerable rejoicing; if it goes badly, much consternation results. Irrespective of the amount of preparation that has taken place before the interview, the neophyte will justifiably remain nervous about this endeavor. Thus, the first edition of *Diagnostic Interviewing* was devoted to providing a clear outline for the student in tackling a large variety of patients in the interview setting.

In consideration of the positive response to the first edition of *Diagnostic Interviewing*, published in 1985 and the second in 1994, we, and our editor at Plenum Press, Sharon Panulla, decided that it was time to update the material. However, the basic premise that a book of this nature needs to encompass theoretical rationale, clinical description, and the pragmatics of "how to" once again has been followed. As in the case of the first and second editions, this third edition does not represent the cat's being skinned in yet another way. Quite to the contrary, we still believe that our students truly need to read the material covered herein with considerable care, and once again the book is dedicated to them. We are particularly concerned that in the clinical education of our graduate students, interviewing continues to be given short shrift. Considering that good interviewing leads to appropriate clinical and research targets, we can only underscore the critical importance of the area.

Almost two decades have passed since publication of the first edition, and many developments in the field have taken place, including the various revisions of the DSM. However, the basic structure of the new edition remains identical to that of the first and second editions, in that Part I deals with General Issues, Part II with Specific Disorders, and Part III with Special Populations. In some instances, the contributors are identical; in others, co-authors have been changed; in still others, we have entirely new contributors. However, all the material is either updated or completely new. Part III now contains chapters on interviewing strategies for marital dyads, children, sexually and physically abused children, and older adults.

Chapters in Parts II and III generally follow the outline below:

Description of the Disorders or Special Populations
Procedures for Gathering Information
Case Illustrations
Standardized Interview Formats

Of the nineteen chapters in the book, four are completely new (Chapters 3, 4, 14, and 15). Nine chapters have been totally updated (Chapters 1, 5, 7, 10, 11, 12, 16, 17, and 18). In the third edition, six chapters that originally appeared in the second edition have been written by different authors (Chapters 2, 6, 8, 9, 13, and 19).

Many individuals have contributed to the development and production of this book. First, we thank our contributors for sharing with us their clinical and research expertise. Second, we thank Carole Londerée, Alex Duncan, and Angelina Marchand for their technical assistance and help with the preparation of the index. Finally, we thank Sharon Panulla for her appreciation of the need for this third revision.

MICHEL HERSEN
SAMUEL M. TURNER

Contents

PART III. SPECIAL POPULATIONS

I

General Issues

The Interviewing Process

SAMUEL M. TURNER, MICHEL HERSEN, AND
NANCY HEISER

INTRODUCTION

The interview is the foundation for all clinical enterprises. During the interview, the clinician learns about the patient's difficulties and establishes the rapport needed for a productive relationship. Also, during the course of the interview, the clinician obtains the critical information needed to make decisions regarding diagnosis and, in some cases, disposition. One cannot be a good diagnostician or clinician without proper interviewing skills. Indeed, a clinician with poor interviewing skills who makes critical decisions about a patient's needs represents a threat to the health of those being served.

In our experience from many years of working with psychology graduate students, interns, and other mental health trainees, not enough attention is focused on the interviewing enterprise in our training programs. Indeed, some offer little or no formal or practical training in interviewing. Being a good interviewer requires a broad knowledge of psychopathology and the current diagnostic schema to properly evaluate the information obtained, as well as the basic social skills and sensitivity needed to garner the cooperation and trust of patients.

The first diagnostic interview is perhaps the most difficult milestone in a young trainee's career, and no amount of preparation can completely abolish the apprehension associated with this task. However, having some practical guidelines to follow can alleviate some of the anxiety and further the likelihood that the initial interviewing experience will be a positive one. One of the purposes of this chapter is to elucidate some of the factors that can facilitate the interviewing process for the novice as well as the more experienced clinician.

SAMUEL M. TURNER AND NANCY HEISER • Department of Psychology, University of Maryland, College Park, Maryland 20742. MICHEL HERSEN • School of Professional Psychology, Pacific University, Forest Grove, Oregon 97116.

We will address a number of issues that confront the clinician in the interview setting. These issues include the type of setting and its influence on the interview, confidentiality, issues pertaining to interviewing ethnic minorities, methods of gathering information, the impact of therapist behavior on the interview, and challenges posed by specific diagnostic groups. It is our intent to discuss these issues in a clinical fashion, supporting our discussion with information from our own clinical experience as well as findings from the empirical literature.

CLINICAL ISSUES IN THE INTERVIEW SETTING

The nature of the interview varies depending on the setting in which it is conducted. The interview may take place in a variety of settings, including an emergency room of a psychiatric or general hospital, an outpatient clinic, or a private consulting office. The setting dictates how a patient should be approached, what types of questions need to be asked, and what degree of cooperation might be expected. For example, interviewing a patient in an emergency room requires a different approach from interviewing a regularly scheduled patient in a private practice office. Similarly, interviewing a patient on a medicine unit in a general hospital requires a different approach from interviewing a person in a psychiatric unit. The reason for these differences is that the circumstances of how each patient comes to be interviewed are different, and each no doubt brings a different set of expectations. To address the issue of the interview setting more fully, we discuss interviewing in emergency and crisis settings, outpatient and private consulting settings, and medical settings.

Emergency Diagnostic Centers and Crisis Settings

Emergency diagnosis takes place in general hospital emergency rooms, diagnostic centers within psychiatric facilities, intake centers in comprehensive mental health clinics, and crisis centers via telephone or actual contact in the community. Emergency and crisis settings frequently serve as the first mental health contact for persons who decide on their own to seek mental health services; those who are hospitalized for related and unrelated medical disorders; those who are brought for evaluation by law enforcement or emergency medical personnel; those who are persuaded to seek help by relatives or friends; those who are remanded by the judiciary through involuntary commitment proceedings; and those who are encountered in volatile crisis situations. In any of these emergency settings, a wide variety of mental disorders will be confronted, including psychotic disturbances (e.g., schizophrenia, bipolar affective illness); organic brain syndromes caused by substance abuse, disease, and injury; drug and alcohol problems; other affective (e.g., major depression) and anxiety (e.g., panic disorder) disorders; and a host of personality and adjustment difficulties.

In one recent study, characteristics of over 2,000 psychiatric emergency visits to a large public hospital over a 7-month period were examined. About one third of the patients were self-referred, about one third were referred by police, and

TABLE 1. Primary Diagnosis of Patients who Visited
a Crisis Triage Unit of a Large Public Hospital

Primary diagnosis	Number	Percent
Unipolar depression	662	30
Functional psychosis	576	26
Substance use disorder	442	20
Bipolar disorder	322	14
Adjustment disorder	99	4
Anxiety disorder	75	3
Dementia	33	2
Other	27	1

Source: Based on Wingerson et al. (2001), p. 1497.

the remaining one third were referred by family or friends or other sources (Wingerson, Russo, Ries, Dagadakis, & Roy-Byrne, 2001). The primary diagnosis of these patients is presented in Table 1. A significant proportion was diagnosed with affective disorders, substance use disorders, or functional psychosis. In addition, it was not uncommon for patients to be either currently intoxicated or in a state of substance withdrawal upon presentation. Although most of the patients (68%) were not hospitalized as a result of their visit, 19% were voluntarily hospitalized and 13% were involuntarily hospitalized.

The level of cooperation expected from the patient as well as other important factors such as presenting disturbance may be influenced by the reason for admission and the referral source. For example, the clinician might expect more cooperation from a person who was self-referred compared to someone who was referred by the police. Similarly, patients who are actively psychotic or intoxicated most likely require a different approach from that for those with affective disorders.

In emergency settings, clinicians must be aware that patients are often frightened by their perceptions and feelings, as well as by the surroundings in which they find themselves. Hence, they may not be lucid enough or they may be too frightened to provide detailed histories. The goal in such situations should be to gain enough information to make a reasonable diagnostic decision in order to arrange for a proper disposition. Thus, in an emergency situation, it would be sufficient to determine that a person is psychotic and in need of hospitalization without being certain of the exact nature or cause of the psychosis. Similarly, it might be sufficient to determine that a patient is suffering anxiety symptoms as a result of situational stress and that the individual could best be served on an outpatient basis without obtaining a detailed history.

It is particularly important in interviews conducted in emergency settings to make a careful examination of mental status rather than take a detailed social history or undertake an evaluation with formal psychological tests. As noted above, the clinician needs to understand that patients in emergency settings are frequently frightened by their symptoms as well as by the situation in which they find themselves. Such pronounced apprehension is often a particularly acute problem with those who are psychotic. Inexperienced clinicians are frequently surprised to learn that even the most psychotic individuals are concerned and frightened by the unusual thoughts and perceptual experiences that they are encountering. Although actively psychotic, they are often keenly perceptive and sensitive to interpersonal interactions. A calm and understanding attitude on the clinician's part can serve to mitigate fear in such persons and increase their comfort level enough to allow the interviewer to obtain a reasonable sense of the nature of the problem. Thus, an interview in an emergency setting requires the clinician to be calm, empathic, flexible, and focused, while addressing the psychological emergency.

At times, it may be necessary to supplement information from the patient with comments from family members, the police, court records, or other mental health professionals who have treated the patient. They may provide critical information about factors that precipitated the emergency and about medical, psychological, and family history. Such information particularly is important when the patient is uncooperative, disorganized, or psychotic, or if the information obtained from the patient is suspect. Finally, an important source of information is observation of the patient's behavior prior to and during the interview. In fact, patient behavior frequently is the single most important source of information in the emergency room.

Crisis situations might altogether supersede concern about a diagnosis. Frequently, the goal is to prevent an impending tragedy, and thus the interview is devoted to that end. In such cases, the interview focuses on assessing the risk of suicide or violence toward others and formulating an appropriate response. For example, a trainee under supervision by one of us (Turner) received a call from a patient who had been seen only once previously. This patient expressed a desire to die and articulated a specific plan by which she might commit suicide. Because she had access to several firearms, the clinician's immediate task was to get her to move the weapons to a place where she could not easily get at them on impulse. A second strategy was to engage the patient in conversation while the police were sent to take her to an emergency room. Of course, another crisis situation might dictate a different course of action.

Clinicians are likely to encounter persons with suicidal or homicidal intent both in emergency and other settings; therefore, they should be competent in conducting risk assessments and making decisions about disposition and knowledgeable about procedures for managing such individuals. In addition, because people who present in emergency settings may be intoxicated or in a state of withdrawal, clinicians need to be able to recognize the need for and obtain medical attention as indicated. As noted above, in all of these situations, it is of utmost importance that one remain calm, flexible, empathic, and attentive while at the same time obtaining the information necessary to make critical decisions about mental status and disposition. By being knowledgeable about the types of crises that may arise and procedures and strategies to handle them, both the clinician's and patient's anxiety can be reduced, further facilitating the interview process. For further discussion about conducting a clinical interview in an emergency setting and related issues to emergency psychiatric care, see Kleespies (1998).

Outpatient Settings and the Private Consulting Office

Because patients seen regularly in outpatient settings and private offices are likely to be somewhat less acute as well as less severe than those seen in emergency and crisis settings, the nature of the interview in outpatient settings will be considerably different. Similarly, the goal of the interview will also be different. Although the mental status remains an important issue, and diagnosis is still an objective, disposition normally is not a major concern because the person already is in a setting in which ongoing treatment can be provided. Therefore, the patient can be approached in a more inquiring manner and there should be sufficient time for detailed questioning. The objective is to learn as much about the patient's emotional functioning as possible and to ascertain the reasons for seeking consultation.

Of course, the nature of any interview is governed by what is perceived to be tolerable for each individual. Thus, one would choose not to pressure a patient with paranoid features about his or her sexual behavior in an initial interview because paranoid patients are known to be exquisitely sensitive in this area. In general, interviews conducted in these settings should allow ample time for establishing rapport and laying the groundwork for a fruitful therapeutic relationship.

Many patients seen in these settings are inquisitive about the causes of their disorders as well as treatments that might be available. They typically bring a medical model conception to the initial interview. When one goes to the doctor, it is expected that the doctor will tell you what is wrong and provide treatment. Although diagnosis and prescription of treatment typically cannot be accomplished on the basis of the initial psychological interview, clinicians still should provide some information to patients regarding their condition at the end of the first interview. Also, it might be appropriate to discuss the best possible treatment options, or at least what is believed to be the best course of action to follow.

Thus, in outpatient and private consulting office settings, the clinician will have to engage in much more of an information exchange process than is typical in emergency or crisis situations. For example, it is not uncommon for many patients with anxiety disorders to engage the clinician in protracted discussions concerning their distress, why they rather than someone else developed the symptoms, what types of treatments can be used, what the "cure" for their condition is, how many people have problems identical to theirs, what their prognosis is, how long treatment will take, and how much it will cost. Frequently, the directness with which these questions are answered will determine whether or not a patient will remain in treatment. The manner in which these questions are addressed also is important in helping the individual develop a proper perspective on his or her treatment, what can and cannot be done, and what long-term prognosis entails. Although relatively infrequent in comparison to other settings, emergency situations may arise in outpatient settings as well (e.g., suicidal or homicidal ideation) and clinicians should be prepared for such situations.

Medical Settings

Interviewing patients in a general medical setting presents a unique type of challenge. In many cases, medical patients have not requested to see a mental health professional. Rather, referral is frequently the decision of the treating physician, sometimes without consulting with or explaining the need for the interview to the patient. Thus, on occasion, patients in this setting often will be reluctant to communicate and may refuse to be interviewed. A critical factor in such a case is to introduce oneself, explain the nature of the consultation and who requested it, and explain what the relationship with the patient is at this point. An important factor to remember in these situations is that patients see themselves as suffering from a medical disorder, and frequently they do have various medical illnesses. Because they have defined their problems as medical, they do not understand why a mental health professional has been sent to see them. Also, depending on their medical condition, they may be in considerable discomfort, which may influence their ability to respond to questions and the type of response that they give. Thus, the clinician will need to adjust the format and length of questioning based on these factors.

In approaching patients in general medical settings, we have found it advisable to present oneself as an information gatherer, acknowledging the patient's physical condition without suggesting that there is a psychological disturbance, even if one is suspected. These patients may require a period of cultivation before they are willing to discuss their emotional state. Thus, several visits may be warranted before the interviewing task can be completed.

A potential major problem in this setting can arise if clinicians allow themselves to be manipulated into siding with the patient against the physician or other caregiver. Patients in these settings will sometimes complain about physicians and nursing personnel to mental health professionals, and in some cases may seek to prove the physician wrong by getting the interviewer to agree with them or their conceptualization of the presenting problem. It is critical that the clinician assume no specific position in such cases, but rather maintain the stance of investigator with no particular point of view. Consultants must remember that they are invited in by the treating physician to render their expert advice on a particular problem. Statements and judgments about other aspects of the patient's care can have a negative impact on the doctor–patient relationship and can well reduce the interviewer's credibility and effectiveness.

CONFIDENTIALITY

The issue of confidentiality is one of the most critical to be faced in the interview setting. Clinicians are obliged not to disclose information about the patient obtained in the interview without the patient's consent. However, there are some limitations to confidentiality (discussed further below) and patients have a right to know of these limits before the interview begins. Guidelines for psychologists regarding confidentiality are established by the American Psychological

Association in the *Ethical Principles of Psychologists* (American Psychological Association, 2002). Clinicians should be knowledgeable of these ethical principles. In addition to the Ethics Code itself, there are numerous other publications of the American Psychological Association that offer guidance in this area. Finally, state laws regulating the practice of psychologists typically have provisions about confidentiality and guidelines pertaining to the doctor–patient relationship in particular states. It is essential that clinicians are knowledgeable about the laws of the states in which they practice.

The issue of confidentiality will arise in a number of ways. First, patients enter into the interview with the expectation that in divulging information, they do so in confidence. Furthermore, in many cases, whether patients reveal highly personal information will depend on whether or not they feel they can do so in confidence. To some degree, the setting will likely dictate the level of confidence expected. For example, those being interviewed in an emergency room might be seen by more than one clinician, and the interviewer might involve other sources, such as significant others, the police, or employers, in an effort to gather the information necessary to render a diagnosis and make a disposition. On the other hand, in the private consulting room, in many cases, no one else will be involved in the interview.

In recent years, changes in the delivery of health care services have heightened concerns about confidentiality. Specifically, the growth of managed care has increased the role of third-party payers in the health care delivery process. For example, cost containment strategies such as gatekeeping and utilization review have increased the number of individuals with access to mental health care information. Similarly, these procedures typically require clinicians to provide detailed, sensitive mental health care information about the patient to the managed care organization. These procedures may reduce patient's willingness to disclose personal information during psychological assessments and treatment (Kremer & Gesten, 1998). In addition, managed care companies typically store sensitive mental health information in large databases, which are accessible to a growing number of individuals and entities. Given these concerns about the erosion of confidentiality in the patient–doctor relationship due to managed care practices, legislators at both the state and federal levels have proposed and passed laws to protect the rights of patients.

Clinicians should be cognizant of the impact that changes in the health care delivery system may have on the confidentiality of mental health care information and of changes in standards and laws affecting confidentiality. In addition, they should discuss managed care procedures and potential implications for confidentiality with their patients before the interview begins. For a detailed discussion of managed care and confidentiality in mental health, see Gates and Arons (2000).

Next, we turn to a number of other factors that may impinge on confidentiality.

Age

The age of consent or individual responsibility varies among the states. Thus, a 15-year-old adolescent seeking mental health services without parental consent might be able to do so legally in one state but not in another. In a state in which it is legal to provide services to 15-year-olds without parental consent, all confidentiality laws of that state would apply. On the other hand, in some states, persons this age would be considered minors, and no services could be dispensed without parental consent. In this case, the clinician should inform the patient of this requirement before rendering services. The interviewing of minors in most states requires parental consent, and parents have a legal right to know the results of such an interview or assessment. Thus, when working with minors, clinicians should inform them that information they provide may very well be shared with their parents.

Confidentiality of Records

Written records of psychological interviews are confidential documents. Such records may be released to others (including other professionals) only with the patient's written consent. Parameters governing confidentiality are contained in the ethical guidelines developed and promulgated by the American Psychological Association as well as by the state law. It is the responsibility of each professional to provide adequate safeguards for such material. Even though records are normally considered privileged information, they are subject to court subpoena in certain types of criminal cases. This liability may hold even though the communication between doctor and patient may be privileged information under state law. Despite the enormous amount of time and resources required to maintain proper records, this documentation should not be taken lightly for a number of reasons. First, records may be important to a patient for future treatment or third-party reimbursement. Second, the information contained in a record might prove helpful to a clinician reviewing the history of illness and the patient's treatment history. Third, the record conveys the clinician's thoughts about the illness as well as the rationale for treatments used. As such, the record could be extremely important in any disagreement or malpractice claim arising from an interview or treatment. Thus, it behooves the clinician to maintain up-to-date, detailed, and accurate records of each patient contact, including contact via telephone or any other medium.

The security of patient records is the responsibility of everyone in the clinical setting, and in particular, the treating clinician. Records often contain highly personal and intimate information and, as such, should be handled as confidential documents. Written information should not be left lying in open view, but rather should be filed promptly and properly. Records should be kept in locked files with limited access.

Use of electronic media to store mental health care information poses new challenges to protecting confidentiality. On the one hand, storing sensitive information on computers may present a threat to confidentiality because the information may be more easily accessible to many users. On the other hand, computers may offer newer, more secure ways to safeguard against misuse of confidential records and using computers to manage health care information could potentially improve patient care. For a detailed discussion of how new technologies may affect confidentiality and the delivery of mental health services, see Gellman (2000).

Duty to Warn and Protect

During the course of their work, mental health professionals will at times confront the issue of dangerousness. This issue concerns danger that patients represent to themselves (i.e., suicide potential), danger to the clinician, and danger to the society in general or to specific persons. It is the latter that we are concerned with in this section. What are the obligations of a clinician who interviews a patient and learns that the patient harbors aggressive feelings toward others? Also, how does this potential danger relate to the issue of confidentiality and the doctor–patient relationship?

Although clinicians have a legal and ethical obligation to maintain confidentiality of information between themselves and their patients, the straightforward application of the legal and ethical responsibility for confidentiality has been blurred since the landmark *Tarasoff* v. *Regents of University of California* case in 1976. Basically, the decision by the California Supreme Court required clinicians to take steps to protect individuals who are potential victims of their patients. Thus, if an interviewee informs the interviewer of plans to harm an identifiable person, the clinician might incur the responsibility not only to warn but also to take steps to protect the intended victim. For example, it might be sufficient to inform the intended victim and hospitalize the patient.

In recent years, much attention has been given to the complex issues surrounding confidentiality in the area of HIV/AIDS (e.g., Anderson & Barret, 2001; Chenneville, 2000; Melchert & Patterson, 1999). Clinicians who work with individuals with HIV/AIDS may be confronted with difficult decisions about confidentiality and duty to warn and protect. Specifically, patients who knowingly engage in unsafe sexual practices or unsafe needle exchange practices and resist informing their partners of the potential risk of HIV exposure are posing a danger to others. If an HIV/AIDS patient discloses such information to a clinician and identifies his or her partner(s), the clinician may need to make a decision about breaching confidentiality to protect the third party from HIV exposure. However, there is considerable debate about whether Tarasoff principles apply to cases involving HIV/AIDS and the application of Tarasoff principles to date has varied by case and by state. Confidentiality issues in cases of HIV/AIDS are very complex and have both ethical and legal implications. Clinicians should be aware of these issues and of the statutes in their states that address them. For a more detailed discussion, see Chenneville (2000) and Anderson and Barret (2001).

Confidentiality is a serious and complex issue with many ramifications and our intent here is to alert the clinician to it. For more complete coverage of this issue, the reader is referred to Anfang and Appelbaum (1996), Bennett, Bryant, VandenBos, and Greenwood (1990), Stromberg, Schneider, and Joondeph (1993), and *Ethical Principles of Psychologists and Code of Conduct* (American Psychological Association, 1992).

ETHNIC AND RACIAL CONSIDERATIONS

The role of ethnic and racial variables in psychopathological states, diagnosis, the therapeutic relationship, and treatment outcome remain poorly understood. However, there has been a continuous, albeit slow, increment of data over the past several decades that suggests these racial/ethnic variables can be important in the diagnostic and therapeutic process. Unfortunately, most of our clinical training programs do not provide any systematic education on these issues, and few of our textbooks address them in any depth. Thus, not much in the way of understanding the psychology of minority groups has been taught. In short, we still do not have a psychology that addresses the diversity of the American population (Hall, 1997). As a result, clinicians often find themselves thrust into settings that serve primarily ethnic minorities, groups they are ill prepared to serve. Until clinicians are educated and trained to work with an increasingly diverse population, we can only hope that they will learn from their supervisors in the particular settings or that a course of self-education will be pursued.

How important are ethnic and racial variables in the interview process? Although it is difficult to answer this question, there are enough data to suggest that both can be important factors. Next, we discuss the influence of race and ethnicity on the interview and diagnostic processes.

Interview Process

The interviewing process relies on communication between the clinician and patient about the nature and severity of the patient's symptoms and their impact on functioning. The information gathered during the interview process is critical to determining the diagnosis, which in turn is critical to planning treatment. Because of this reliance on communication between the clinician and patient for an accurate diagnosis and subsequent appropriate treatment, it is important to identify and address racial or ethnic factors that might impede or influence communication.

Communication problems may arise due to racial, ethnic, cultural, or socio-economic differences between the clinician and patient. Both verbal and nonverbal communication may be misinterpreted by the clinician, patient, or both during the interviewing process. These problems may be intensified if the patient speaks in a language or dialect different from that of the clinician. Communication problems may be worsened by differences in vocabulary, modes of communication, and expression of distress (Adebimpe, 1981). In addition, the interpretation of certain behaviors may be influenced by racial, ethnic, and cultural variables. For example, one study found that White and Black persons interpreted the same interpersonal behavior during social discourse of persons with schizophrenia in a different manner (Turner, Beidel, Hersen, & Bellack, 1984). Similarly, analog studies have reported that persons of different races who have the same symptom profile or same behaviors are rated differently by clinicians (e.g., Jenkins-Hall & Sacco, 1991; Loring & Powell, 1988; Martin, 1993). Consider, for example, that among certain cultural groups, perceiving visions or voices might be a normal part of religious experience. Clinicians who are unfamiliar with such cultures may misinterpret these experiences as psychotic symptoms (U.S. Department of Health and Human Services [DHHS], 2001). Similarly, clinicians may be biased based on stereotypes of certain racial or ethnic groups. For example, studies suggest that clinicians overpathologize symptoms found in African-Americans and minimize Asian-Americans' reported symptoms due to stereotypes they hold about these groups (DHHS, 2001; Takeuchi & Uehara, 1996).

Another factor that might influence the interviewing process is the clinician's judgment about what "normal" functioning is for a certain person. Clinical judgment is needed to determine if the patient's symptoms interfere with functioning, and what is considered dysfunctional may vary by race, ethnicity, and culture. Thus, clinicians need to be knowledgeable about the patients' culture to accurately assess their psychological difficulties and whether they represent a significant deviation from the norm for that culture.

The attitude of minority patients toward mental health care providers also can affect communication between the patient and the health care provider. Many studies have documented that racial and ethnic minorities are less likely than Whites to seek mental health care (see reviews by DHHS, 2001; Gray-Little & Kaplan, 2000). In addition, minority members often turn to other, more informal forms of help such as clergy, friends, family, and traditional healers (DHHS, 2001). A host of possible reasons for this pattern has been examined including barriers to services such as cost, fragmentation of services, stigma, and mistrust.

Mistrust, in particular, is a factor that may influence the interviewing process. Mistrust of Whites and the health care system is considered to be pervasive among minorities (DHHS, 1999; Whaley, 2001). Given existence of a cultural norm toward seeking help from more informal sources and a skeptical attitude toward psychological services, clinicians will most likely confront many skeptical minorities in the interview setting. Studies of mistrust suggest that African-Americans have varying degrees of mistrust of Whites due to past and current experiences with oppression and racism (Whaley, 2001), and some have referred to this mistrust as a healthy cultural paranoia (Carter, 1974; Ridley, 1984). This mistrust and related paranoid-like behaviors may be misinterpreted by clinicians as clinical paranoia (Adebimpe, 1981; Jones & Gray, 1986; Whaley, 2001). When African-Americans present at a clinic, they may be wary and defensive and also appear apathetic (Block, 1984). Obviously, the ability to interpret such behavior and the ability to address it in a fashion that will allow the needed information to be obtained requires certain knowledge and skill. One indication that patients are aware that he/she needs help is the fact that he/she is in the mental health facility. Therefore, the clinician should not assume that the patient is unwilling to receive or is uninterested in receiving help. Moreover, the interviewer should not be dissuaded by such behavior and should proceed to complete a diagnostic assessment.

Given the problems that may arise when the patient and clinician are not of the same racial, ethnic, or cultural group, researchers have investigated whether patient–clinician matching on these variables improves the therapeutic process and treatment outcome. One might expect that clinician matching would reduce the chances for misunderstandings and facilitate the process of developing rapport and trust between the clinician and patient. However, the available literature has not uniformly supported this view. A recent review of this literature by Gray-Little and Kaplan (2000) found that much of the research on patient–clinician matching has been conducted with analog studies. Overall, such studies have not found improved outcomes for patients who were matched with an ethnically similar clinician compared to those who were not. However, there is some evidence suggesting that minority patients may remain in treatment for a longer period of time when matched to an ethnically similar clinician compared to those who are not. This finding may be viewed as indirect evidence that ethnicity matching may facilitate the therapeutic process and this might be expected to improve outcome assuming that remaining in treatment longer allows their difficulties to be addressed in a better fashion. These issues will need to be addressed in better studies with clinical populations with some focus on types of disorders and types of treatment in order to obtain any degree of clarity.

Some studies suggest that ethnic minorities prefer ethnically similar clinicians but it is unclear to what extent it is this variable per se or inferences made about attitudes, values, and skills that underlie this preference (Coleman, Wampold, & Casali, 1995; Kim & Atkinson, 2002). Gray-Little and Kaplan (2000) concluded that studies on patients' choices appear to depend more on their perception of the clinician as trustworthy and competent than on race per se, but that race may be used to infer these qualities if little other information is available. These studies indicate that race probably is not a major or sole factor with respect to patients' preferences and experience in the therapeutic process, but that when it is an issue, the clinician must be able to identify it.

Diagnosis

An accurate diagnosis is essential to the therapeutic endeavor. The diagnosis dictates the type of treatment and can provide some indication of the likely prognosis and course of the disorder. The diagnosis of a psychiatric disorder requires clinicians to make judgments about the patient's symptom patterns, mental status, and functional impairment, and their observations of the patient's behavior. The final diagnostic decision depends on clinical judgment and interpretation of these variables. These judgments may be influenced by a range of factors including the race and ethnicity of the patient (DHHS, 2001; Gray-Little & Kaplan, 2000).

Over the past two decades, studies have consistently found that race is associated with the differential diagnosis of psychiatric disorders. Specifically, data indicate that minorities are more likely to be misdiagnosed than Whites (see reviews by Adebimpe, 1981, 1994; Gray-Little & Kaplan, 2000; Neighbors, Jackson, Campbell, & Williams, 1989). These patterns exist even though there is no evidence to suggest that there are substantial differences in the prevalence rates of the various major psychiatric disorders among different racial groups (DHHS, 2001; Kessler et al., 1994).

A prime example is the consistent finding of overdiagnosis of schizophrenia and underdiagnosis of affective disorders in African-Americans (Lawson, Hepler,

Holladay, & Cuffel, 1994; Mukherjee, Shukla, Woodle, Rosen, & Olarte, 1983; Pavkov, Lewis, & Lyons, 1989; Simon, Fleiss, Gurland, Stiller, & Sharpe, 1973; Strakowski et al., 1995, 1996a; Strakowski, McElroy, Keck, & West, 1996b; Strakowski, Shelton, & Kolbrener, 1993). Strakowski et al. (1997) found that misdiagnoses in a psychiatric emergency setting were more common among non-Whites than Whites. They then examined whether the misdiagnoses were a result of information variance (i.e., differences in the information patients offer to different clinicians) or criterion variance (i.e., differences in how diagnostic criteria are applied) and if either of these types of variance was related to race. They found that information variance was the cause of diagnostic disagreement in 58% of the cases and criterion variance was the cause in 42% of the cases. However, only the information variance was associated with the race of the patient. Therefore, this study suggests that race influences the information obtained from patients during the clinical assessment process. However, Trierweiler et al. (2000) found that African-Americans and White Americans applied different decision rules to different patients based on race in judging the presence of schizophrenia. Thus, it would appear that both of these factors (criterion and information variance) most likely contribute to the pattern of misdiagnoses among racial and ethnic minorities.

These diagnostic patterns are diminished when diagnoses are made with semistructured or structured interviews rather than unstructured clinical interviews (Adebimpe, 1981; Baker & Bell, 1999; Neighbors et al., 1989). Structured and semistructured interviews ensure that certain questions are asked and that specific criteria are met before a diagnosis is made, and thus seem to control to some degree the influence of race or ethnicity. This likely is due to the fact that information gathered in this fashion decreases the likelihood of information and criterion variance. This means, of course, that when there is nothing to structure the course of the interview, race influences the interviewer as to the assignment of diagnoses, highlighting yet another value to using semistructured interviews rather than the open clinical interview.

We have found that when racial and ethnic issues arise during an interview, it is best to acknowledge them without dwelling on the topic and making them the focus of the interview. If racial or ethnic issues clearly become the paramount focus of attention, it may be that the interview will not prove to be useful. Clinicians must be prepared to acknowledge racial or ethnic biases of their own, as well as those that might be harbored by the patient. In some cases, it might be advisable to bring in an interviewer of the same race or ethnic background as the interviewee either for consultation or to conduct the interview. Decisions in these matters must be made by each individual clinician.

Other factors to consider when interviewing racial and ethnic minorities are that their symptom patterns may differ somewhat from Whites and they may selectively report symptoms in culturally acceptable ways (Kleinman, 1988; Whaley, 1997). Although the core symptoms of many emotional disorders have been found to be similar cross-culturally (Weissman, 1996; Weissman et al., 1994, 1997), secondary symptom patterns can vary markedly. For example, Asians are more likely than other groups to report somatic symptoms such as dizziness, blurred vision, and vertigo (Hsu & Folstein, 1997), but also tend to report more emotional symptoms with more probing (Lin & Cheung, 1999). Similarly, African-Americans are more likely to report somatic symptoms when compared to Whites (Swartz, Landerman, George, Blazer, & Escobar, 1991). In the case of depression, it has been noted that African-Americans, particularly those from the lower socioeconomic strata, often do not present with a depressed mood or the preponderance of cognitive symptoms seen in Caucasians when they are in fact depressed. Rather, multiple somatic and physical complaints predominate (Brown, Schulberg, & Madonia, 1996; Carter, 1974; Myers et al., 2002). For example, Brown et al. (1996) found that African-Americans with major depression reported more severe sleep disturbance than Whites. Myers et al. (2002) found that depressed Latina and African-American women reported significantly more somatic symptoms than Caucasian women. Thus, clinicians must be able to recognize the potential importance of somatic complaints among different patient groups.

Although mental disorders have similar symptom profiles across cultures and are found worldwide (Weissman, 1996; Weissman et al., 1994, 1997), some cultural variations in the presentation of clinical symptoms have led to the discussion of "culture-bound syndromes" (American Psychiatric Association, 1994). Culture-bound syndromes are symptom clusters that appear to be more prevalent in certain cultures. For example, taijin kyofusho is a distinctive phobia in Japan that is characterized by an intense fear that one's body, its parts, or its functions might displease or offend others (e.g., in odor, movements, appearance, or facial expressions). Variations of this condition also have been noted in other Asian groups.

Clinicians should be aware that stress-related disorders occur at an alarmingly high rate among African-Americans. In addition, African-American patients with panic disorder appear to have a higher rate of comorbidity with isolated sleep paralysis (ISP) compared to other groups (Bell & Jenkins, 1994). ISP is a condition characterized by awakening in the night with an acute onset of inability to move. In addition to the comorbidity of ISP with panic disorder, the condition also appears to be present in African-Americans with hypertension. Because hypertension and panic are known to be associated with emotional distress, it has been hypothesized that stress might be the mediator of all these conditions (Neal & Turner, 1991). African-Americans suffering from panic might present with a complaint of any one of these syndromes or other stress-related conditions, and one needs to be more cognizant of the possible interrelationships of the stress-related conditions when interviewing African-Americans.

Issues about race and ethnicity are highly complex and poorly understood, and here we have limited our discussion to some of the issues related to interviewing. It was not our purpose in this chapter to provide the necessary background material for one to adequately assess patients from different cultural or racial groups. Rather, it is to alert the clinician to the importance of these issues. Training programs in psychology, psychiatry, social work, and other mental health professions need to devote the necessary time to these issues in their curricula to ensure that their trainees have some minimal level of knowledge. Currently, minority clinicians are frequently as ignorant as their White colleagues in these matters because they have been trained in the same programs. Most clinical training programs give lip service to the need for training of this type, but few ever implement serious empirically based curriculum and experiential training. Training programs for all the mental health disciplines have the responsibility to ensure that their graduates have some level of knowledge and competence to serve racial and ethnic minorities. If they do not, in our view, this represents programmatic and training malfeasance.

For in-depth coverage, the interested reader is referred to a number of sources that cover this area more comprehensively: Aponte and Wohl (2000); Clark, Anderson, Clark, and Williams (1999); DHHS (2001); Hogue, Hargraves, and Collins (2000); Lee (1997); Lu, Lim, and Mezzich (1995); Neighbors and Jackson (1996); Sue and Sue (1999).

METHODS OF OBTAINING INFORMATION

In recent years, a large number of structured and semistructured schedules have been used to enhance interrater reliability in the interview. The fully structured interview schedules enable the interviewer to follow an established format and sequence. In the semistructured schedules, the interviewer has considerable latitude. Such schedules have improved the diagnostic process by delineating specific targets and types of information that the interviewer must uncover (e.g., Segal, 1997; Sher & Trull, 1996). These interviews ensure that certain questions are asked and that they are asked in a similar fashion by clinicians, while still allowing for the flexibility and rapport needed for a successful interview. Structured and semistructured interview schedules, because of their greater precision than the unstructured interviews, have also enhanced the likelihood of interstudy comparisons for diagnostic research and treatment trials. These schedules have been developed for interviewing both children (e.g., the Kiddie Schedule for Affective Disorders and Schizophrenia for School-Aged Children [K-SADS; Chambers et al., 1985], the Diagnostic Interview Schedule for Children [DISC; Schaffer, 1992], and the Anxiety Disorders Interview Schedule for Children [ADIS-C; Silverman & Nelles, 1988]) and adults (e.g., Structured Clinical Interview for *Diagnostic and Statistical Manual of Mental Disorders*, Fourth Edition [DSM-IV] [SCID-IV; First, Spitzer, Gibbon, & Williams, 1997], and the Anxiety Disorders Interview Schedule [ADIS; Di Nardo, Brown, & Barlow, 1995]).

REFERENCES

Adebimpe, V. R. (1981). Overview: White norms and psychiatric diagnosis of Black patients. *American Journal of Psychiatry, 138*, 279–285.

Adebimpe, V. R. (1994). Race, racism, and epidemiological surveys. *Hospital & Community Psychiatry, 45*, 27–31.

American Psychiatric Association. (1994). *Diagnostic and statistical manual of mental disorders* (4th ed.). Washington, DC: Author.

American Psychological Association (2002). *Ethical principles of psychologists and code of conduct. American Psychologist, 57*, 1060–1073.

Anderson, J. R., & Barret, R. L. (Eds.). (2001). *Ethics in HIV-related psychotherapy: Clinical decision making in complex cases*. Washington, DC: American Psychological Association.

Anfang, S. A., & Appelbaum, P. S. (1996). Twenty years after Tarasoff: Reviewing the duty to protect. *Harvard Review of Psychiatry, 4*, 67–76.

Aponte, J. F., & Wohl, J. (Eds.). (2000). *Psychological intervention and cultural diversity* (2nd ed.). Needham Heights, MA: Allyn & Bacon.

Baker, F. M., & Bell, C. C. (1999). Issues in the psychiatric treatment of African Americans. *Psychiatric Services, 50*, 362–368.

Bell, C. C., & Jenkins, E. J. (1994). Isolated sleep paralysis and anxiety disorders. In S. Friedman (Ed.), *Anxiety disorders in African Americans* (pp. 117–127). New York, NY: Springer.

Bennett, B. E., Bryant, B. K., VandenBos, G. R., & Greenwood, A. (1990). *Professional liability and risk management*. Washington, DC: American Psychological Association.

Block, C. B. (1984). Diagnostic and treatment issues for black patients. *The Clinical Psychologist, 37*, 52–54.

Brown, C., Schulberg, H. C., & Madonia, M. J. (1996). Clinical presentations of major depression by African Americans and whites in primary medical care practice. *Journal of Affective Disorders, 41*, 181–191.

Carter, J. H. (1974). Recognizing psychiatric symptoms in black Americans. *Geriatrics, 29*, 95–99.

Chambers, W. J., Puig-Antich, J., Hirsch, M., Paez, P., Ambrosini, P. J., Tabrizi, M. A., & Davies, M. (1985). The assessment of affective disorders in children and adolescents by semistructured interview. Test–retest reliability of the K-SADS-P. *Archives of General Psychiatry, 42*, 696–702.

Chenneville, T. (2000). HIV, confidentiality, and duty to protect: A decision-making model. *Professional Psychology: Research & Practice, 31*, 661–670.

Clark, R., Anderson, N. B., and Clark, V. R., & Williams, D.R. (1999). Racism as a stressor for African Americans: A biopsychosocial model. *American Psychologist, 54*, 805–816.

Coleman, H. L. K., Wampold, B. E., & Casali, S. L. (1995). Ethnic minorities' ratings of ethnically similar and European American counselors: A meta-analysis. *Journal of Counseling Psychology, 42*, 55–64.

Di Nardo, P. A., Brown, T. A., & Barlow, D. H. (1995). *Anxiety disorders interview schedule for DSM-IV (lifetime version)*. San Antonio, TX: Psychological Corporation.

First, M. B., Spitzer, R. L., Gibbon, M., & Williams, J. B. W. (1997). *Structured clinical interview for DSM-IV axis I disorders*. Washington, DC: American Psychiatric Press.

Gates, J. J., & Arons, B. S. (Eds.). (2000). *Privacy and confidentiality in mental health care*. Baltimore, MD: Paul H. Brookes.

Gellman, R. (2000). Will technology help or hurt in the struggle for health privacy? In J. J. Gates & B. S. Arons (Eds.), *Privacy and confidentiality in mental health care* (pp. 127–156). Baltimore, MD: Paul H. Brookes.

Gray-Little, B., & Kaplan, D. (2000). Race and ethnicity in psychotherapy research. In C. R. Snyder & R. E. Ingram (Eds.), *Handbook of psychological change: Psychotherapy processes & practices for the 21st century* (pp. 591–613). New York, NY: John Wiley & Sons.

Hall, C. C. I. (1997). Cultural malpractice: The growing obsolescence of psychology with the changing U.S. population. *American Psychologist, 52*, 642–651.

Hogue, C. J. R., Hargraves, M. R., & Collins, K. S. (2000). *Minority health in America: Policy implications from the Commonwealth Fund Minority Health Survey*. Baltimore, MD: Johns Hopkins University Press.

Hsu, L. K. G., & Folstein, M. F. (1997). Somatoform disorders in Caucasian and Chinese Americans. *Journal of Nervous and Mental Disease, 185*, 382–387.

Jenkins-Hall, K., & Sacco, W. P. (1991). Effect of client race and depression on evaluations by White therapists. *Journal of Social and Clinical Psychology, 10*, 322–333.

Jones, B. E., & Gray, B. A. (1986). Problems in diagnosing schizophrenia and affective disorders among blacks. *Hospital and Community Psychiatry, 37*, 61–65.

Kessler, R. C., McGonagle, K. A., Zhao, S., Nelson, C. B., Hughes, M., Eshelman, S., Wittchen, H., & Kendler, K. S. (1994). Lifetime and 12-month prevalence of DSM-III-R psychiatric disorders in the United States. *Archives of General Psychiatry, 51*, 8–19.

Kim, B. S., & Atkinson, D. R. (2002). Asian American client adherence to Asian cultural values, counselor expression of cultural values, counselor ethnicity, and career counseling process. *Journal of Counseling Psychology, 49*, 3–13.

Kleespies, P. M. (Ed.). (1998). *Emergencies in mental health practice: Evaluation and management.* New York, NY: The Guilford Press.

Kleinman, A. (1988). *Rethinking psychiatry: From cultural category to personal experience.* New York: Free Press.

Kremer, T. G., & Gesten, E. L. (1998). Confidentiality limits of managed care and clients' willingness to self-disclose. *Professional Psychology: Research & Practice, 29*, 553–558.

Lawson, W. B., Hepler, N., Holladay, J., & Cuffel, B. (1994). Race as a factor in inpatient and outpatient admissions and diagnosis. *Hospital and Community Psychiatry, 45*, 72–74.

Lee, E. (1997). *Working with Asian Americans: A guide for clinicians.* New York, NY: The Guilford Press.

Lin, K., & Cheung, F. (1999). Mental health issues for Asian Americans. *Psychiatric Services, 50*, 774–780.

Loring, M., & Powell, B. (1988). Gender, race, and DSM-III: A study of the objectivity of psychiatric diagnostic behavior. *Journal of Health & Social Behavior, 29*, 1–22.

Lu, F., Lim, R. F., & Mezzich, J. E. (1995). Issues in the assessment and diagnosis of culturally diverse individuals. In J. Oldham & M. Riba (Eds.), *Review of psychiatry* (Vol. 14, pp. 477–510). Washington, DC: American Psychiatric Press.

Martin, T. (1993). White therapists' differing perceptions of Black and White adolescents. *Adolescence, 28*, 281–289.

Melchert, T. P., & Patterson, M. M. (1999). Duty to warn and intervention with HIV-positive clients. *Professional Psychology: Research & Practice, 30*, 180–186.

Mukherjee, S., Shukla, S., Woodle, J., Rosen, A. M., & Olarte, S. (1983). Misdiagnosis of schizophrenia in bipolar patients: A multiethnic comparison. *American Journal of Psychiatry, 140*, 1571–1574.

Myers, H. F., Lesser, I., Rodriguez, N., Mira, C. B., Hwang, W. C., Camp, C., Anderson, D., Erickson, L., & Wohl, M. (2002). Ethnic differences in clinical presentation of depression in adult women. *Cultural Diversity & Ethnic Minority Psychology, 8*, 138–156.

Neal, A., & Turner, S. M. (1991). Anxiety disorders research with African Americans: Current status. *Psychological Bulletin, 190*, 400–410.

Neighbors, H. W., & Jackson, J. S. (Eds.). (1996). *Mental health in Black America.* Thousand Oaks, CA: Sage.

Neighbors, H. W., Jackson, J. S., Campbell, L., & Williams, D. (1989). The influence of racial factors on psychiatric diagnosis: A review and suggestions for research. *Community Mental Health Journal, 25*, 301–311.

Pavkov, T. W., Lewis, D. A., & Lyons, J. S. (1989). Psychiatric diagnoses and racial bias: An empirical investigation. *Professional Psychology: Research & Practice, 20*, 364–368.

Ridley, C. A. (1984). Clinical treatment of the nondisclosing Black client: A therapeutic paradox. *American Psychologist, 39*, 1234–1244.

Schaffer, D. (1992). *Diagnostic interview schedule for children (DISC 3.0) parent version.* New York: Columbia University Press.

Segal, D. (1997). Structured interviewing and DSM classification. In S. M. Turner & M. Hersen (Eds.), *Adult psychopathology and diagnosis* (pp. 24–57). New York, NY: John Wiley & Sons.

Sher, K. J., & Trull, T. J. (1996). Methodological issues in psychotherapy research. *Annual Review of Psychology, 47*, 371–400.

Silverman, W. K., & Nelles, W. B. (1988). The anxiety disorders interview schedule for children. *Journal of the American Academy of Child & Adolescent Psychology, 27*, 772–778.

Simon, R. J., Fleiss, J. L., Gurland, B. J., Stiller, P. R., & Sharpe, L. (1973). Depression and schizophrenia in black and white mental patients. *Archives of General Psychiatry, 28*, 509–512.

Strakowski, S. M., Flaum, M., Amador, X., Bracha, H. S., et al. (1996a). Racial differences in the diagnosis of psychosis. *Schizophrenia Research, 21*, 117–124.

Strakowski, S. M., Hawkins, J. M., Keck Jr., P. E., McElroy, S. L., West, S. A., Bourne, M. L., Sax, K. W., & Tugrul, K. C. (1997). The effects of race and information variance on disagreement between psychiatric emergency service and research diagnoses in first-episode psychosis. *Journal of Clinical Psychiatry, 58*, 457–463.

Strakowski, S. M., Lonczak, H. S., Sax, K. W., West, S. A., Crist, A., Mehta, R., & Thienhaus, O. J. (1995). The effects of race on diagnosis and disposition from a psychiatric emergency service. *Journal of Clinical Psychiatry, 56*, 101–107.

Strakowski, S. M., McElroy, S. L., Keck Jr., P. E., & West, S. A. (1996b). Racial influence on diagnosis in psychotic mania. *Journal of Affective Disorders, 39*, 157–162.

Strakowski, S. M., Shelton, R. C., & Kolbrener, M. L. (1993). The effects of race and comorbidity on clinical diagnosis in patients with psychosis. *Journal of Clinical Psychiatry, 54*, 96–102.

Stromberg, C., Schneider, J., & Joondeph, B. (1993). *The psychologists update number 2 (August)*. Washington, DC: National Register of Health Service Providers in Psychology.

Sue, D. W., & Sue, D. (1999). *Counseling the culturally different: Theory and practice* (3rd ed.). New York, NY: John Wiley & Sons.

Swartz, M., Landerman, R., George, L.K., Blazer, D.G., & Escobar, J. (1991). In L. Robins & D. A. Regier (Eds.), *Psychiatric disorders in America: The Epidemiologic Catchment Area Study* (pp. 220–257). New York, NY: The Free Press.

Takeuchi, D. T., & Uehara, E. S. (1996). Ethnic minority mental health services: Current research and future conceptual directions. In B. L. Levin & J. Petrila (Eds.), *Mental health services: A public health perspective* (pp. 63–80). New York: Oxford University Press.

Trierweiler, S. J., Neighbors, H. W., Munday, C., Thompson, E. E., Binion, V. J., & Gomez, J. P. (2000). Clinician attributions associated with the diagnosis of schizophrenia in African American and non-African American patients. *Journal of Consulting and Clinical Psychology, 68*, 171–175.

Turner, S. M., Beidel, D. C., Hersen, M., & Bellack, A. S. (1984). Effects of race on rating of social skill. *Journal of Consulting and Clinical Psychology, 52*, 474–475.

U.S. Department of Health and Human Services (1999). *Mental health: A report of the Surgeon General*. Rockville, MD: Author.

U.S. Department of Health and Human Services (2001). *Mental health: Culture, race, and ethnicity— A supplement to mental health: A report of the Surgeon General*. Rockville, MD: Author.

Weissman, M. M. (1996). Cross-national epidemiology of major depression and bipolar disorder. *Journal of the American Medical Association, 276*, 293–299.

Weissman, M. M., Bland, R. C., Canino, G. J., Greenwald, S., Hwu, H. G., Lee, C. K., Newman, S. C., Oakley-Browne, M. A., Rubio-Stipec, M., Wickramaratne, P. J., Wittchen, H. U., & Yeh, E. K. (1994). The cross national epidemiology of obsessive compulsive disorder. *Journal of Clinical Psychiatry, 55*(Suppl.), 5–10.

Weissman, M. M., Bland, R. C., Canino, G. J., Faravelli, C., Greenwald, S., Hwu, H. G., Joyce, P. R., Karam, E. G., Lee, C. K., Lellouch, J., Lepine, J. P., Newman, S. C., Rubio-Stipec, M., Wells, J. E., Wickramaratne, P. J., Wittchen, H. U., & Yeh, E. K. (1997). The cross-national epidemiology of panic disorder. *Archives of General Psychiatry, 54*, 305–309.

Whaley, A. L. (1997). Ethnicity/race, paranoia, and psychiatric diagnoses: Clinician bias versus socio-cultural differences. *Journal of Psychopathology and Behavioral Assessment, 19*, 1–20.

Whaley, A. L. (2001). Cultural mistrust: An important psychological construct for diagnosis and treatment of African Americans. *Professional Psychology: Research and Practice, 32*, 555–562.

Wingerson, D., Russo, J., Ries, R., Dagadakis, C., & Roy-Byrne, P. (2001). Use of psychiatric emergency services and enrollment status in a public managed mental health care plan. *Psychiatric Services, 52*, 1494–1501.

Mental Status Examination

Michael S. Daniel and Carrie J. Crider

Introduction

The mental status examination (MSE) is an interview screening evaluation of all the important areas of a patient's emotional and cognitive functioning, often augmented with some simple cognitive tests. The MSE provides the data for formulating a psychiatric diagnosis or developing a working hypothesis regarding psychiatric diagnosis. The MSE is to psychiatric diagnosis what the physical examination is to medical diagnosis (Andreasen & Black, 1987; Hales, Talbott, & Yudofsky, 1994; Trzepacz & Baker, 1993). The MSE also can be used as a basis for developing diagnosis of neurobehavioral disorders due to neurological damage, but this chapter will focus on the psychiatric application of the MSE. Interested readers are referred to Strub and Black's (2000) seminal work on use of the MSE for a neurologically oriented diagnosis.

The MSE is based on observations of the patient's non-verbal and verbal behavior, and includes the patient's descriptions of her/his subjective experiences. Evaluation of a person's emotional and cognitive state by means of interview observations can be subjective. Subjective impressions can lead to an unreliable diagnosis. The purpose of the MSE is to provide an framework for the comprehensive evaluation of mental functioning that increases objectivity and reliability of the data and subsequent diagnosis. There is a high degree of similarity between various MSE formats presented in the literature, suggesting there is a relatively good consensus about what comprises a standard MSE. It is thus important to develop a standardized approach for conducting a MSE that includes assessment of the domains described below. A standardized approach increases reliability of the MSE, that is, the likelihood that the patient would be diagnosed the same way by another professional using an MSE. In addition, with experience, a standardized approach allows a clinician to develop a set of internal norms that

Michael S. Daniel and Carrie J. Crider • School of Professional Psychology, Pacific University, Forest Grove, Oregon 97116.

can provide "a good sense of the range of normal and abnormal responses in a variety of individuals of various ages, educational levels and psychopathological states" (Andreasen & Black, 1987).

Another issue related to reliability of diagnosis is the importance of specifying the behavior on which key interpretations and conclusions are based. If you state the patient is guarded, hostile, anxious, or hallucinating, describe the behavior(s) you observed that led to the conclusion. These behaviors may be statements made by the patient, for example, "I feel like I'm about to come out of my skin," or non-verbal behaviors, for example, "the patient was restless, rapidly bouncing his leg up and down on the ball of his foot and often sitting forward on the edge of his chair." Holding yourself to the standard of citing behavioral data to support your clinical interpretations will make your diagnosis more reliable and clearly communicate to other mental health professionals what data your impressions are based on.

A standardized and comprehensive approach to the MSE must be balanced with the individualization necessary to set the patient at ease and develop rapport. The patient is most likely to feel at ease, and the clinician most likely to obtain valid data, if the MSE flows smoothly and has a conversational quality, especially at the beginning of the interview. Empathy is expressed by a genuine concern for the patient and the circumstances that have brought her/him to the MSE; an earnest attempt to obtain all pertinent information and understand its context, meaning, and implications for the patient will effectively convey the positive regard necessary to develop rapport and is an effective way to collect comprehensive, reliable, and valid data. Developing rapport from the beginning of the MSE will increase the patient's comfort with, and likelihood of good effort on, more structured cognitive tests employed later in the MSE to assess specific cognitive abilities.

Another important element of rapport and obtaining valid MSE results is awareness of the patient's cultural background. Cultural factors will influence the extent of eye contact, how appropriate individuals feel it is to reveal personal and family information, how emotionally expressive they are and their understanding of and response to cognitive tests. Developing a successful working relationship with patients from a different culture will require modification of the MSE in a way that respects their cultural mores. In addition, behaviors and beliefs that often will be interpreted as likely signs of psychopathology in mainstream American culture may be common in sub- and foreign cultures. For instance, it is common in some cultures to believe that certain people possess special powers that enable them to place curses on others or enlist the power of spirits to manipulate others' actions. While these beliefs likely represent delusions in many patients, in some cases they may represent the person's acculturation.

Finally, the MSE is one component of a comprehensive psychiatric evaluation. The information derived from an MSE offers a picture of the patient's functioning at that moment. These data are most meaningful in the context of a thorough psychosocial and psychiatric history. The significance of ambiguous symptoms noted in the MSE often is much clearer when considered in light of the patterns of behavior evident in the patient's history. In addition, many symptoms that may represent psychiatric disturbance also can be caused by medical problems or

Table 1. Domains of the Mental Status Exam

Physical	Emotional	Cognitive
Appearance	Attitude	Orientation
Behavior	Mood and affect	Attention/concentration
Motor activity	Thought and perception	Speech and language
	Insight/judgment	Memory
		Intelligence/abstraction

medications. General knowledge of this overlapping etiology and accurate information about current medical status will prevent misdiagnosis that could have serious consequences.

We divide the MSE into three general domains as shown in Table 1. Certainly, there are various ways of organizing these areas of mental functioning and some mental functions can be included in more than one category (e.g., sometimes speech is as much reflective of a psychiatric process as it is a cognitive ability and behavior is as much a dimension of emotional functioning as physical). We developed this scheme based on the type of data each area is intended to provide for a psychiatrically oriented MSE.

Appearance

Appearance is what the patient looks like. References on MSE encourage the examiner to paint a portrait (e.g., Amchin, 1991; Hales et al., 1994) or take a photograph (Akiskal & Akiskal, 1994) with a description that captures unique features and affords the reader a clear mental image of the patient. Description of the patient's appearance documents an important element of the context in which other MSE data is obtained. Such documentation proves valuable if the patient is evaluated again in the future as it allows comparison and detection of any change in appearance that may be a manifestation of a change in psychiatric status. The person who, appropriately attired and groomed, was diagnosed with a depressive adjustment disorder 9 months ago but now appears disheveled and unshaven may not have availed himself of the recommended psychotherapy and deteriorated into a major depressive disorder or may have an undiagnosed dementia. Often, description of appearance merely will note there is nothing unusual and will not contribute to diagnosis.

Poor *grooming and hygiene* in the form of an unwashed/malodorous body, unwashed/unkempt hair, poor dental hygiene, and dirty fingernails often are signs of a psychiatric disorder such as schizophrenia or severe depression, brain dysfunction such as dementia, or the underprivilege of homelessness. However, body odor also is culturally determined as many non-American cultures bathe less frequently and have what Americans experience as pungent body odor. Unkempt or dirty *attire* or *dress* may be associated with the same conditions just described. Bizarre or outrageous attire may be an indication of mania, psychosis, or dementia.

Seductive or lavish dress, jewelry, or makeup can reflect a histrionic or narcissistic personality style. Sloppy dress and unshaven appearance with adequate hygiene may indicate the patient has no interest in impressing the examiner or is resistant to seeing a clinician for MSE.

Essentially all MSE references instruct the clinician to comment on *whether the patient appears his/her stated age*. Patients who appear younger than their chronological age are either genetically blessed or have had successful cosmetic rehabilitation; this generally does not have clinical significance, with the exception of when the latter is a manifestation of a clinical issue with body image. When patients appear older than their stated age, it may be due to poor physical health, medical problems, alcohol or drug abuse, or a life of severe hardship such as homelessness. Severe or chronic psychiatric disturbance including depression, mania, and schizophrenia may also result in a prematurely aged appearance (Trzepacz & Baker, 1993). *Facial expression* may convey information about mood. Decreased facial expression is common in schizophrenia and can be a side-effect of anti-psychotic medication. An expressionless or mask-like face is typical of Parkinson's and right hemisphere cerebral vascular accident (CVA). *Posture* also can convey information about the patient's emotional state at the moment or mood. Anxiety or resistance to the interview may be manifested in arms tightly crossed across the body. A "kicked back" posture may reflect general comfort with or indifference to the circumstances. Abrupt changes in posture, especially becoming more rigid, crossing arms, or turning away often indicate the patient is having an emotional reaction to or at least is uncomfortable with the topic at hand (Trzepacz & Baker, 1993). *Scars* may represent previous suicide gestures and *tattoos* gang affiliation. If the nature of an unusual physical feature is unclear, it is preferable to inquire about it rather than to ignore it out of concern for social grace (Trzepacz & Baker, 1993).

Eye contact may reflect various features of emotional functioning. Little eye contact with the examiner and downturned gaze may reflect depression, anxiety, awkwardness, or low self-esteem. Glaring may signal hostility. As with many elements of social interaction, eye contact is culturally determined and it is considered rude to make direct eye contact in certain situations in some cultures. Indeed it is important to determine if this is the case especially for patients of non-western cultures.

Any unusual feature should be noted including weight, height, limp, sweating, and signs of intoxication such as conjunctivitis, narrowed eyelids, and dilated pupils.

Akiskal and Akiskal's (1994, p. 28) excellent examples of how appearance may contribute to the MSE diagnostic picture are excerpted below:

> This 20-year-old, self-referred single, Chinese-American student was interviewed in the student counseling center. She is a petite, frail-looking woman appearing much younger than her stated age. She wore no makeup, and was dressed in simple attire consisting of a blue button-down boy's shirt, a pair of cutoff blue jeans, woolen knee stockings, and penny loafers. She carried a knapsack full of books that she held closely on her lap. Throughout the interview, her hands were tightly clasped around her knapsack. Her fingernails were bitten down to the quick.
>
> The description of this patient's appearance gives us clues about a moderate level of anxiety and tension, clues that should be pursued during the remainder of the examination. The next example illustrates a more disturbed patient.

This divorced white woman was brought to the county mental health center by her distraught son and daughter-in-law because she had become increasingly hostile and combative at home and was staying up all night. She was restless during the interview, rising frequently from her chair, looking at every diploma on the walls, making comments about each of them, doing essentially all the talking during the interview. She looked her stated age of 53, but her clothes would have been appropriate only for a much younger person: Although quite obese, she wore orange "hot pants" and a halter top that showed a bare midriff. Her legs had prominent varicose veins. She wore old wooden beach sandals with high spike heels. Her general level of grooming was very poor: Her short gray hair was matted on both sides of an irregular part. Her fingernails were long and yellowed from nicotine; her toenails were also very long, each painted a different color.

The general appearance of this patient suggests a psychotic level of disorder and raises hypotheses of much different nature from those generated by (the) first patient, necessitating further inquiry along the lines of a manic disorder.

The general appearance of (the) third patient suggests entirely different diagnostic possibilities.

A 25-year-old single white engineer was seen in a private office. He was impeccably dressed in a three-piece gray pinstripe suit and matching dress shoes. His hair and mustache were carefully groomed. The secretary noted that when he signed his name on the admission form, his hands were visibly tremulous. He generally appeared uneasy and glanced furtively about the room, paying special attention to electrical outlets, air-conditioning vents, and, most especially, the security camera.

Inquiry along the lines of a delusional disorder is suggested by this patient's general appearance, and differential diagnosis should consider such conditions as amphetamine psychosis and paranoid schizophrenia.

BEHAVIOR

Behavior is how the patient acts. Of course, everything assessed in an MSE is behavior of some type; whether motor, verbal, or affect, it all is behavior. So this section refers to the more general qualities of behavior not subsumed under other sections. Behavior is observed throughout the MSE. As noted above for posture, any abrupt or notable change in demeanor may indicate that the patient is uncomfortable with or threatened by the topic at hand. As with appearance, the MSE description of behavior may merely note there was nothing unusual and will not contribute to diagnosis.

Many MSE references include level of consciousness under behavior. Normal consciousness is in evidence when the patient is alert, normally aware of internal and external stimuli (Strub & Black, 2000), and responds generally appropriately to the interview. Low level of consciousness is manifest in decreased alertness and arousal. The patient may appear lethargic. At more extreme low levels of consciousness, the person is described as obtunded or stuporous (Strub & Black, 2000; Trzepacz & Baker, 1993). Low levels of arousal almost always are due to physiological or other acute medical problems and are referred to as *acute confusional state* or *delirium*. Causes include toxic or idiosyncratic drug reactions, sedative-hypnotic use, infection, metabolic abnormality, or systemic failure (e.g., cardiac, respiratory, renal). Acute confusional state can also occur with the onset of an acute brain event such as CVA. It can occur in the elderly with most any kind of medical challenge. It is common post-operatively, especially in the elderly, who have some pulmonary compromise (e.g., smoke cigarettes, emphysema, asthma). Generally, the most reliable clinical feature distinguishing acute confusional state from other types of brain dysfunction (e.g., dementia) and psychiatric disturbance is general impairment of alertness or "clouding of consciousness"; fluctuations in level of consciousness, variable alertness, and incoherent answers are qualities of an acute confusional state (Strub & Black, 2000).

At the opposite end of the arousal continuum is *hypervigilance*. Hypervigilant patients may restlessly scan the room and attend to every discernible sound and change in visual stimuli; they may be easily startled. *Hyperarousal* is typical of anxiety, mania, and paranoia as well as some medical conditions such as hyperthyroidism; it may be the effect of acute substance abuse (Trzepacz & Baker, 1993).

Trzepacz and Baker (1993) define *mannerisms* as consistent, characteristic, distinctive, apparently purposeful, and highly stylized actions. They are at least unique, and often are atypical actions such as always rubbing the back of your head before speaking. Many people with substantially below average intelligence have stereotyped mannerisms. Alone, mannerisms usually are not specifically diagnostic; the significance of mannerisms is determined by considering them in conjunction with other MSE findings. *Compulsions* are an extreme form of mannerisms; they are stereotyped, often ritualistic, and trivial (Trzepacz & Baker, 1993). Compulsions almost always parallel obsessive thoughts. They can take many forms including repeatedly saying a phrase before responding or doing some repetitive act like washing hands or turning a light switch on and off. The following is Trzepacz and Baker's (1993) most excellent method for MSE evaluation of compulsions. The clinician asks patients if they have any eccentricities or odd habits. If patients respond affirmatively or the clinician observes any unusual or repetitive behavior suggestive of compulsions, the clinician asks patients if they are aware of the behavior, if the behavior occurs in other circumstances, and if the patient would like to stop the behavior but is unable to. If the answer to all these questions is yes, the behavior very likely is a compulsion and further similar inquiry for obsessions is indicated. In addition to Obsessive–Compulsive Disorder, compulsions also occur in Tourette's syndrome. If the patient is not aware of the behavior in question or it is accompanied by an altered level of consciousness (i.e., acute confusional state), it is unlikely a compulsion.

MOTOR ACTIVITY

Motor activity is the type and quality of movements the patient makes. The patient may sit quietly, have no abnormal movements, and move normally. Abnormal movement is broadly divided into the dichotomy of those that are part of a psychiatric disturbance and those that are due to neurological dysfunction.

Decreased level of motor activity is *psychomotor retardation* and often is associated with severe depression. Decreased motor activity due to neurological cause is referred to as *akinesia* (absence of movement), *hypokinesia* (decreased movement), or *bradykinesia* (slowed movement); these terms and psychomotor retardation often are used synonymously. Subcortical disorders such as Parkinson's disease, Huntington's disease, progressive supranuclear palsy, and AIDS-related brain deterioration all result in decreased motor activity. In Parkinson's, the patient frequently also has tremor (described below) as well as rigid posture, problems initiating movements (i.e., getting up from chair and taking the first step when walking) and short-stepped gait. Observations of these other motor qualities will aid in discriminating psychomotor retardation due to psychological versus neurological cause. *Catatonia* is an extreme form of psychomotor retardation (Trzepacz & Baker, 1993) typically seen in schizophrenia. The catatonic patient will remain immobile for prolonged periods of time despite prompts or circumstances that will elicit responses in patients with other psychiatric disorders. *Cataplepsy* or *posturing* is immobility that involves assuming a (often unusual) posture for prolonged periods; sometimes the patient is rigid in this posture. In *waxy flexibility*, the patient's posture can be changed by someone else, but is maintained in whatever position the patient is left, even if it is odd.

Paresis and *plegia* are decreased motor movement due to loss of strength resulting from neurological damage. CVA, traumatic brain injury, and spinal cord injury are the primary causes. Paralysis of a body part also occurs in conversion disorders. Neurological versus psychological etiology of paresis usually is determined by anatomical inconsistencies in the presentation of paralysis and evidence in the history suggesting likely functional basis for the symptom. Muscle weakness (not referred to as paresis or plegia) is a primary symptom of neurological disorders such as multiple sclerosis, Guillian–Barre, and myasthenia gravis.

As the foregoing makes clear, it is important to carefully observe and describe the quality of decreased movement in order to distinguish psychological and neurological causes. In most cases, medical causes of movement disorders are documented by the time MSE is conducted with the patient, although there may be those rare occasions when a neurological problem has been unrecognized prior to MSE.

Obvious active motor signs of emotional states are hand wringing, nail biting, or pacing, all of which may reflect anxiety. Increased overall level of motor activity is referred to as *psychomotor agitation*. It is associated with agitated depression, mania and can occur in acute confusional state (Trzepacz & Baker, 1993); it also can be a byproduct of stimulant drug use.

While psychomotor agitation as defined above is not a common symptom of neurological disease, there are many neurological conditions that produce abnormal involuntary movements. *Tardive dyskinesia* exclusively affects psychiatric patients and results from long-term use of anti-dopaminergic neuroleptic medication. Tardive dyskinesia most commonly affects the muscles of the face, especially the lips and mouth and appears as a writhing or tic-like (see below) movement. *Tremors* are oscillating movements that occur in a relatively consistent rhythm, often occurring in distal body parts such as the hands; tremor can become more pronounced with stress and can be temporarily controlled volitionally (Trzepacz & Baker, 1993). Resting tremors are common in Parkinson's while intention tremors (i.e., with movement) can occur with cerebellum damage. Some elderly people have tremor as a result of nonspecific infirmities of age. *Tics* are involuntary movements or vocalizations that range from simple to complex, including blinking, facial grimacing, neck jerks, shoulder shrugging, and throat clearing; they are associated with obsessive–compulsive disorder and stimulant use (Trzepacz & Baker, 1993). Tourette's syndrome is the most notable psychiatric condition manifesting tics. Tics of three kinds occur in Tourette's: (1) palilalia—patients' repetition of their own words, (2) echolalia—repetition of others' words, and (3) coprolalia—profanity and obscenities (Trzepacz & Baker, 1993). Many people who are mentally and emotionally healthy have tics (Trzepacz & Baker, 1993), so their significance is determined by the overall findings of the MSE. *Choreiform* movements are a wide variety of involuntary movements that have a rapid, highly complex, and jerky quality; they are typical of Huntington's disease. Often people with choreiform movement disorders are skillful at "finishing" the involuntary movement to make it look intentional and functional, and thus disguise its involuntary nature.

ATTITUDE

Attitude is how patients feel and what they think about participating in the MSE. Attitude is inferred from the patient's behavior, including characteristics described above such as facial expression, posture, and eye contact. Other behavioral indicators of attitude are voice tone, how completely or evasively patients answer questions, and their attentiveness and responsiveness to questions (Trzepacz & Baker, 1993). Many patients will participate willingly in the MSE and are usually described as *cooperative, friendly, responsive, open*, etc.

Other patients, however, are not willing participants in the MSE. Attitude is important because if the patient is not sufficiently cooperative, the MSE will not produce valid results. If it appears at the outset that the patients are not willing to engage in the MSE in a productive manner or their attitude changes notably in the course of the MSE, it probably is best to empathically mention your observations, attempt to find out how the persons are feeling (Trzepacz & Baker, 1993) and if anything can be done to enlist their cooperation. "You seem upset by/uneasy with this whole thing/what we're talking about now." Allow patient to confirm or disconfirm. "I was wondering what makes you feel that way?" Allow patient to respond. "What would make you feel better about talking to me/talking about this?" If it is not clear if patients are open and truthful in their responses, you can ask them a question about a potentially delicate topic to which you already know the answer. Comparison of response with collateral information will give some indication of their frankness and may also give you a patients' unique perspective that was not available in other accounts (Trzepacz & Baker, 1993).

Patients may be *guarded or suspicious*: reluctant to answer questions for fear the information they provide will be the basis for bias against them in the hospital, clinic or by the doctor. Other patients may be *hostile* because they are angry about whatever circumstances led to their referral for a MSE; often they feel they have no problems and view their referral for a MSE as part of a malicious plot against them or the failure of others to understand their circumstances. *Passive* patients will not volunteer information; when asked, their answers are incomplete and unelaborated.

The patient's attitude may shed light on psychopathology. The sociopath may be socially skilled and charming but evade giving full or truthful answers to avoid revealing illicit activities. Histrionic patients may be seductive in an effort to manipulate the examiner. Trzepacz and Baker (1993) aptly describe the dynamics of borderline personality disorder. Borderline patients often have difficulty with the ambiguity of simultaneous positive and negative feeling toward a person and so can vacillate between extremes of very positive and very negative feelings for the examiner. This may lead to the patient suddenly and unexpectedly directing anger toward the examiner because the examiner will not grant some request or endorse some point of view favored by the patient. This can be followed by just as abrupt an expression of admiration and affection by the patient for the examiner.

Other attitude characterizations include *childlike, argumentative, resistant, dramatic* (Amchin, 1991) and *flippant, threatening, impatient, preoccupied, sarcastic, arrogant* (Trzepacz & Baker, 1993). It is important to specify the behaviors on which a pejorative attitude attribution is based.

MOOD AND AFFECT

Mood and affect disturbance are the central features of many common psychiatric disorders (Trzepacz & Baker, 1993). While definitions vary somewhat, in general, *mood* is considered the internal emotional state of the patient, and *affect* is the external expression of emotional state. Normally, there is high concordance between mood and affect; however, they may be discordant in patients with psychiatric disorders. Generally, mood is considered more stable, changing over days and weeks, while affect may change moment to moment and is more influenced by context.

Since mood is the subjective experience of the patient, many authors recommend using the patient's self-report to characterize mood (Akiskal & Akiskal, 1994; Kaplan & Sadock, 1995), and quoting patients' statements about their mood is a good way of documenting it. Others suggest that in addition to the patient's self-report, the clinician describe the patient's mood based on clinical impressions; discrepancies between the patient and clinician's formulation may indicate patients have decreased awareness of their mood suggesting the possibility of poor awareness of emotional state or denial (Amchin, 1991). Whether the patient's mood is judged "abnormal" is determined by the degree to which it appears to match present life circumstances (Trzepacz & Baker, 1993). It is important to discuss patients' mood in an empathetic manner, communicating genuine concern if they are experiencing emotional pain.

We use Trzepacz and Baker's (1993) model and characterize mood in one of six categories (see Table 2). *Euthymic* is essentially normal mood without pathology. Unfortunately, many nonmental health professionals who read MSE reports do not

Table 2. Mood Categorizations

Euthymic	Angry
Dysphoric	Apprehensive
Euphoric	Apathetic

Based on material from Trzepacz and Bakers (1993).

know what this word means. *Dysphoric* mood is sad and depressed. It is one of the most common moods in patients referred for an MSE and the hallmark feature of depressive disorders. It also occurs with many other psychiatric disturbances, including bipolar disorders, psychosis, anxiety disorders, personality disorders, and substance-induced states (Trzepacz & Baker, 1993). Many patients with medical problems have dysphoric mood as a direct effect of or reaction to their condition. In addition, sadness and grief are a normal response to substantial loss or trauma. *Euphoria* is at the opposite end of the mood continuum and is typified by extreme and excessive happiness and elation. Most common in manic disorders, it also can occur in schizophrenia and substance-induced states (Trzepacz & Baker, 1993). *Angry* mood often is manifested in antagonism, belligerence, confrontation, and opposition. It is seen in manics who are not euphoric, depressives who are not merely sad and can be the result of substance-induced states. Often it is a consequence of dementia and other brain dysfunction, especially in the prefrontal lobes. Patients with borderline, antisocial, and narcissistic personality disorders express poorly regulated anger when their demands are not met or limits are set on their behavior. Of course, when a patient is angry it is always important to assess the potential for violence and the clinician's safety (Trzepacz & Baker, 1993). *Apprehensive* mood is distinguished by worry, dread, and fear. It is common in anxiety disorders and sometimes is present in depression and paranoid states. *Panic*, an extreme form of apprehension, usually is accompanied by pronounced autonomic nervous system symptoms such as palpitations, hyperventilation, sweating, and sometimes chest pains; as a result, panic frequently is associated with fear of imminent death. Anxiety is a direct symptom of some medical problems such as hyperthyroidism. Patients who suffer respiratory compromise often become very apprehensive because severe symptoms can make persons feel like they are dying (Trzepacz & Baker, 1993). *Apathetic* mood is characterized by disinterest and detachment. Apathy can occur as an acute reaction to severe trauma or emotional shock. It also is associated with severe forms of psychosis such as catatonia and can be a symptom of conversion disorder. Brain dysfunction in the prefrontal–basal ganglia circuit can cause apathy (Trzepacz & Baker, 1993).

Assessment of affect is based on the clinician's observations of the patient's behavior, some of which were discussed above. Obvious characteristics such as crying, laughing, shouting, and startling as well as more subtle qualities such as facial expression, voice tone, and body posture are the behavioral data that define affect. Therefore, it is important to reference the behavioral observations on which the clinical judgment of affect is based. For example, "Affect was anxious as evidenced by rapid sometimes stammering speech, biting the inside of his lip,

TABLE 3. Qualities of Affect: Modified from Trzepacz and Baker (1993)

Quality of affect	Normal	Abnormal
Appropriateness	Congruent with context	Incongruent with context
Range/variability	Full Shows change	Restricted Constricted Labile
Intensity	Strength of emotional response typical for social interactions Animated	Flat Blunted Exaggerated
Responsiveness	Reacts emotionally to changes in context	Nonreactive Unresponsive

near constant shifting in the chair and visible perspiration stains on the under-arms of his shirt."

The primary characterization of affect is type. Trzepacz and Baker (1993) list 51 adjectives describing affect including friendly, pleasant, angry, hostile, elated, euphoric, apathetic, sad, dysphoric, despondent, anxious, apprehensive, worried, and tense. After the type of affect is determined, various qualities of affect typically are assessed. Again, we use a modified version of Trzepacz and Baker's (1993) model and evaluate four qualities of affect (see Table 3).

Appropriateness is the how well the patient's affect matches the circumstances and topic of discussion. Affect is *congruent* if emotional expression matches patients' description of their mood and other verbalizations, for example, acting sad or being tearful when describing recent loss or trauma or acting anxious when discussing a planned potentially painful medical procedure. Affect is *incongruent* when it does not match reported mood or verbalizations, for example, matter of factly discussing recent significant loss, demonstrating great anger about an inconsequential slight, or laughing when nothing humorous occurred or was said; the first is common among histrionic patients, the second among borderline personalities, and the last schizophrenics.

Range or *variability* is the breadth of emotional expression demonstrated. Normally, affective range varies in the course of a social interaction depending upon the topic and idiosyncratic feelings about it. Affective variability can be abnormal in both directions from the normal median. At one extreme, the patient who shows little or no variation in emotional expression despite changes in circumstances has *restricted* or *constricted* affect. Affect may be restricted to any part of the continuum; for example, the patient who is only euphoric has restricted range just as someone who is only sad. Depressed and schizophrenic patients often have restricted affective range, as do some patients with right CVA and many with prefrontal brain injury. At the other end of the continuum is a capricious and often rapid change in emotional expression referred to as *labile*. Labile patients suddenly burst into tears or burst into laughter and regain control with effort, only to repeatedly burst into tears or laughter again. Lability is common among right CVA patients and can occur in schizophrenia.

Intensity is the strength of emotional response. Normal intensity is defined in both normative and contextual terms: that is, how strongly would the average person respond in this situation. In most situations, normal intensity is referred to as *animated*. Intensity can be abnormal in both directions from the normal median. At one extreme, the patient shows little or no animation in emotional expression and has *blunted* or *flat* affect. This is common in severely depressed and schizophrenic patients as well as in patients with prefrontal lobe damage, Parkinson's, and right CVA. *Exaggerated* affect is at the other extreme and is an unusually strong emotional response; histrionic and borderline personalities often have exaggerated affect.

Responsiveness is the degree to which the patient responds emotionally to things people usually respond to. Normally, people will respond to emotionally laden topics. Patients may be *nonreactive* or *unresponsive* in an indifferent manner such as seen in histrionic personalities, or they may be unresponsive in a constricted manner characteristic of schizophrenia.

SPEECH AND LANGUAGE

Language is the use of symbols to communicate. Speech, one of four general modes of language, is what patients say and the quality of how they talk. Before speech can be considered an indication of psychiatric functioning, it must be first established that there is no language impairment due to brain dysfunction. For most patients, it will be clear from the outset that there is no language deficit because their responses to questions reflect comprehension and they are able to express ideas adequately in speech. For these patients, speech and language is normal, no further evaluation of these abilities is necessary and speech can be considered a reliable reflection of thought and perception (discussed below). However, when there is some abnormality of speech or it is not clear the patient reliably comprehends what is said, it is necessary to further assess language in an effort to determine if these problems are due to psychiatric disturbance, brain damage, or both. Although thought disorder and language impairment usually occur independently (Trzepacz & Baker, 1993), there are similarities in the speech anomalies seen in brain damage and psychosis; typically the presence/absence of associated symptoms allows differential diagnosis. If brain damage is suspected, medical concerns are referred for neurological and cognitive issues for neuropsychological or speech pathology consultation.

Only a brief overview of language functioning is possible here; refer to Strub and Black (2000) and Trzepacz and Baker (1993) for a more detailed description of language. From a cognitive perspective, language generally is divided into four domains as illustrated in Table 4. *Aphasia* is impairment of language due to brain damage and is broadly classified into two general syndromes: non-fluent, mostly associated with frontal brain damage, and fluent, mostly associated with temporal–parietal damage. *Non-fluent aphasia* is characterized by slow, labored, halting speech with particular difficulty saying function words: for example, a, the, in, about. Non-fluent aphasics mostly produce content words, primarily nouns, but

TABLE 4. Broad Domains of Language

	Receptive	Expressive
Auditory	Auditory–verbal comprehension	Speech
Visual	Reading	Writing

also verbs, adjectives, and adverbs. Auditory–verbal comprehension is less affected, but often there are comprehension deficits for statements when the grammatical structure is important in conveying the meaning (e.g., distinguishing between "the child called for her mother" and "the mother called for her child" and "the mother was called by her child"). *Fluent aphasia* is characterized by impaired auditory–verbal comprehension and speech that generally is normal in rhythm, intonation, and quantity, but is a meaningless mix of nonsense words (*neologisms* or *jargon*) and real words. For the most part, fluent aphasics are aware of their language deficits while non-fluent aphasics are not. Reading and writing deficits are associated with fluent and non-fluent aphasia. *Dysnomia*, or word retrieval deficits, is a common symptom of most aphasia syndromes. When CVA is the cause of aphasia it often produces symptoms of both syndromes; aphasia also can result from head injury and dementia. Speech deficits will be, for the most part, apparent in conversation. If it appears that the patient is experiencing subtle word finding problems unrelated to psychiatric disturbance referral for neuropsychological or speech pathology evaluation is indicated. If the patient gives unreliable or incoherent answers to questions, comprehension may be at issue and can be tested at a basic level. Place three or four common items in front of the patient (e.g., pen, cup, book, key) and say "I want to make sure you can understand what I'm saying so I'm going to ask you to do some things with these objects on the table. Point to the ——," completing the statement with each item in turn. If the patient is successful at this level then give 3–4 instructions that include two or more objects: for example, "put the pen in the cup … put the key on top of the book … put the cup between the pen and key." You can also use prompts such as "show me the one you use to unlock a door." Anything other than perfect performance indicates the patient is not reliably processing language and it is important to determine if it represents a neurological or psychiatric problem. The patient who passes this simple comprehension screening but still appears to have comprehension deficits that appear unrelated to psychiatric disturbance should be referred for more comprehensive evaluation. *Dysarthria* is distorted pronunciation due to impaired neuromuscular control of oral-facial muscles and results from a number of developmental disorders and acquired brain injury.

From a psychiatric perspective, features of speech such as the *rate, intonation, latency, spontaneity, articulation,* and *volume* may be relevant. Manics often will interrupt or respond without pause with rapid, pressured speech that parallels racing thoughts. Significantly depressed patients will have slow speech of low volume, little variation in intonation, increased response latencies, and no initiation; the speech of some schizophrenics will have the same qualities, but often will have bizarre content (discussed below). Although slurred speech often is the result of intoxication, the possibility of an acute neurological event must be considered. *Mutism* is the complete absence of speech. It can occur after brain injury, but it is relatively rare and is associated with focal lesion of the anterior cingulate. Psychiatrically, mutism may occur in catatonia and should be distinguished from "loss of voice" due to conversion disorder; the latter is distinguished by accurately mouthing words and the ability to communicate adequately in other verbal and non-verbal forms, although it is important to rule out laryngeal pathology in these cases (Akiskal & Akiskal, 1994).

Clinically, the most difficult distinction to make is between fluent aphasia and the bizarre speech of schizophrenia. The disturbed speech of a schizophrenic may contain confused, fragmented utterances with nonsense "made up" words similar to that which occurs in fluent aphasia. However, schizophrenics often will vary between coherent statements, especially in response to structured questions, and confused speech; this type of variation is less common in fluent aphasia where the nonsensical quality of speech is consistent. Syntax usually is preserved in thought disorder but not in fluent aphasia (Trzepacz & Baker, 1993). In addition, a schizophrenic's speech abnormalities are more likely to be accompanied by delusions, hallucinations, and affective disturbance, symptoms uncommon among fluent aphasics. Unless severely psychotic, patients with thought disturbance can read aloud, write to simple dictation, and copy from written material while patients with fluent aphasia will show impairments in these areas that parallel their speech. Even incoherent schizophrenics typically can follow simple instructions, name objects and repeat simple phrases, abilities impaired in fluent aphasia (Trzepacz & Baker, 1993).

THOUGHT AND PERCEPTION

Thought is the internal dialogue that occurs in the patient's mind. *Perception* is the patient's sensory–perceptual experience and interpretation of external events and circumstances. Since thought and perception are internal, they are inferred almost completely from what the patient says (thus the importance of first ruling out neurologically based language impairments). While in some situations, it is to an extent possible to infer thought and perception from the patient's behavior (e.g., if they attend or respond to auditory hallucinations), it is not possible to assess thought and perception if the patient does not express herself through speech, writing, or sign language (Trzepacz & Baker, 1993). Patients who have otherwise significant psychological problems (e.g., mood disturbance), and those who have none, will have logical goal-directed thoughts in adequate quantity, express them in an organized fashion, and will interpret events in a realistic manner; these patients have no thought or perception disorder. Most often, thought and perception disturbance is the hallmark of psychosis, although it can be present in severe mania and depression.

Most references on MSE distinguish two aspects of thought: process and content. *Thought process* is the formulation, flow, and organization of thought

(Trzepacz & Baker, 1993). *Circumstantiality* is the mildest form of thought disorder (and a personal style of many otherwise normal people). Responses are over-elaborative, include much more detail than necessary but eventually get to the point and ultimately are relevant. For example, when asked what resulted in his current admission, the circumstantial patient may begin with a detailed description of a conflict 10 years ago with his mother "where it all began" and give excruciating detail of ensuing events. Circumstantiality may reflect obsessive thinking and is described clinically in temporal lobe epilepsy. *Tangentiality* is a train of thought that strays from the original topic and never returns; the thoughts generally are logical, but digress from the target and at best are minimally relevant. Tangentiality is not diagnostic of psychiatric disturbance in and of itself (Trzepacz & Baker, 1993). *Flight of ideas* is the repeated rapid successive change from one idea to another associated idea. Ideas typically are logical and the association between them clear, however, in severe cases neither may be discernable. In mania, flight of ideas is manifest in pressured speech. *Loose associations* are thoughts without logical basis or based on obscure or bizarre logic (Amchin, 1991). Trzepacz and Baker (1993) note that loosening of associations may be obscured in a completely structured MSE interview, so it is useful to include some open-ended questions and unstructured conversation to allow opportunity for loose associations to emerge. *Word salad* is the most extreme form of thought process disturbance in which even the logical association between words is lost and the patient's speech is a jumble of meaningless words and nonsense words. Most often a sign of schizophrenia, word salad must be distinguished from fluent aphasia (see Speech and Language section).

Other types of thought disturbance include *thought blocking*, which is losing track of a thought before it is completely expressed and is manifest in a pause mid-sentence; if speech resumes, the topic has changed. If asked, patients usually do not remember what they were thinking/talking about prior to speech arrest (Trzepacz & Baker, 1993). *Perseveration* is the repetition of a word, phrase, or idea resulting from failure to properly inhibit and cease a response when it no longer is appropriate. At extreme levels, the patient may repeat the same word or phrase in a mechanical and rote manner, relevant or not, regardless of redirecting prompts; this typically occurs in psychotic and severely brain damaged patients. At a less severe level, the patient may perseverate on a topic or idea that continually intrudes despite change of topic; this may be associated with psychosis or obsessive–compulsive disorder. *Clang associations* are productions of words or phrases based on rhyming sound; for example, the patient may say "My pants are too loose. You must be Toulouse Lautrec. I think I've seen you on Star Trek." *Neologisms* are made up words. The patient may say "They stole my ferckle and I need it to especialate." Neologisms are common in fluent aphasia and need to be distinguished from schizophrenia (see Speech and Language section). Patients who extensively or only repeat what they hear the clinician say have *echoalia*. This also can occur in aphasia and should be distinguished from psychosis. For the most part, the thought disorders in this paragraph are relatively rare (Trzepacz & Baker, 1993).

Thought content is what patients think about, as reflected in what they talk about. *Obsessions* are "undesired, unpleasant, intrusive thoughts that cannot be suppressed through the patient's own volition" (Trzepacz & Baker, 1993) and frequently accompany compulsions. The thought is disturbing to patients and they have insight that it is irrational. In the MSE, *preoccupations* often are an indication of an underlying obsession and are manifest in continually revisiting a topic (Trzepacz & Baker, 1993). The significance of preoccupations can be assessed with Trzepacz and Baker's approach by asking patients if they have any repetitive thoughts that are bothersome and that they cannot stop. If the answer is yes, follow up with inquiry about specifics of content, frequency, accompanying feelings and associated actions. *Phobia* is fear of an object or situation that in fact is not threatening. Phobic patients usually recognize the irrationality of their fears. We will briefly discuss three types of phobias: agoraphobia, social phobia, and simple phobia. *Agoraphobia* is fear of open and/or public places and often results in the patient restricting herself to home. *Panic attacks* frequently accompany agoraphobia; they are characterized by autonomic nervous system symptoms such as sweating, hyperventilation, and rapid heart rate, often giving rise to a feeling of impending death. *Social phobia* is a fear of public humiliation or embarrassment that is so severe it interferes with the patient's social or occupational functioning. *Simple phobia* is inordinate fear of a specific object or situation, for example, spiders, heights, flying. Simple phobias in and of themselves are not indicative of significant psychopathology, but can substantially disrupt the patient's life when the associated avoidance interferes with functioning (Trzepacz & Baker, 1993).

Of course, it is very important to evaluate *suicidal* and *homicidal ideation* since this represents one of the major areas of risk for the patient and others, as well as liability for the clinician. It should be routinely documented in the MSE report whether present or absent. Amchin (1991) recommends using the word "suicide" in at least one question to break possible taboo on using the word. If the patient acknowledges suicidal ideation, distinguish between passive thoughts/desire to die versus intention to actively end life. Ask if the patient has a plan, what the plan is (noting the extent of detail), if the patient has the means to execute the plan (e.g., access to weapons or potentially lethal medication), and has the patient done anything to execute the plan. Other risk factors for suicide that should be assessed are past suicide attempts, attempts by family or friends and alcohol abuse. Chronically depressed and schizophrenic patients are most likely to commit suicide (Trzepacz & Baker, 1993), but any patient with intent is at risk. Homicidal ideation or thoughts of just assaulting someone can be assessed with essentially the same approach. Distinguish between passive thought and active intent. Inquire about plans, means, degree of execution of plan, and past/family history of violence. Psychopathic personalities are the most likely to plan violence.

Perception is the patient's interpretation of external events and circumstances; delusions are impairments in this interpretation. *Delusions* are "firmly held, fixed personal beliefs based on incorrect reasoning and inferences, which are not consistent with widely held religious or cultural beliefs" (Amchin, 1991) and are not dissuaded by evidence to the contrary. Delusions range from plausible (the police are following me) to bizarre (my neighbor's Christmas lights are arranged in code to communicate with aliens). They also vary in their organization. Some delusional systems are stable—change little over time—and systematized—the various features of the delusions are interrelated. Unstable and nonsystematized delusions change frequently with little connection between various features. Cultural factors are pertinent (see Introduction). *Paranoid* delusions, especially *persecutory* ones, are the most common in general psychiatric populations (Trzepacz & Baker, 1993). Persecutory delusions are irrational beliefs that one is the victim or conspiratory target of harm or threat (e.g., my neighbor sends signals through her sewing machine to my mind) and are seen in schizophrenics as well as delirious, dementia, and temporal lobe epilepsy patients (Trzepacz & Baker, 1993). *Grandiose* delusions are of exceptional skills, status, or position. These patients may claim to have great wealth, exclusive knowledge/ability, or to be confidants of prominent people and are most common in mania. *Somatic* delusions are of physical symptoms and medical problems (e.g., there are worms eating my insides). In less severe forms, these delusions are plausible symptoms and it is important to rule out veridical medical pathology. Somatic delusions occur in schizophrenia, brief reactive psychosis, severe depression, mania, dementia, and delirium (Trzepacz & Baker, 1993). *Ideas of reference* are delusions that some unrelated thing has special and specific reference to the patient. Media often is the focus of ideas of reference, for example, "the news reporter was talking about me on television when she did that story about…" or "when they put the flag at half mast that meant I was only going to work for another 2 weeks." Other forms of delusions are: *erotomania*—belief that someone else, usually famous, is in love with me; *delusional jealousy*—unfounded and consuming belief that one's partner is unfaithful; *nihilistic delusions*—belief of some impending or already occurred doom. Some authors refer to *irrational beliefs* that are illogical, but not quite bad enough to be delusional, for instance, believing that cheating on income taxes resulted in physical illness. *Magical thinking* also refers to the belief that there is connection between events when none actually exists.

A *hallucination* is an impairment of sensory experience in which the patient has a perception that is internally generated and not the result of sensory input from the environment, that is, hears, sees, feels, smells something that actually is not there. *Auditory hallucinations* are the most common in psychiatric patients, especially schizophrenia, and usually consist of hearing voices. They may hear a voice calling their name or saying insulting, critical, derogatory things about the patient. If the voices give instructions, they are called *command auditory hallucinations* and it is important to determine if the patient has acted or feels compelled to act on them (Trzepacz & Baker, 1993). Unformed sounds such as ringing and buzzing are more likely to be related to neurological dysfunction. *Visual hallucinations* can occur in psychiatric disturbance, but more likely represent neurological dysfunction. *Olfactory* and *gustatory hallucinations* are most likely related to neurological dysfunction, especially temporal lobe epilepsy. *Tactile hallucinations* such as ants crawling on the skin are common in alcohol withdrawal, drug toxicity, and somatic delusions (Trzepacz & Baker, 1993). *Hypnagogic hallucinations* are part of a sleep disorder in which dreaming occurs with the sleep paralysis that is a normal element of dreaming, but while lying awake; they typically occur when transitioning to sleep or just after awakening and do not represent a psychiatric problem.

INSIGHT AND JUDGMENT

Insight is self-awareness (Trzepacz & Baker, 1993). Insight is the extent to which the patient recognizes he has a problem, recognizes the nature and various elements of the problem, understands that the problem represents a departure from what is considered normal or at least desirable, understands the negative effects of the problem for self and others, and accepts the need for treatment. At the highest levels, insight is the patient's appreciation of how her personality, perceptions, behavior, and past experiences interact with present circumstances to give rise to the problem. Few patients will have insight at all these levels (and a large portion of non-patients will not). Intact cognitive functions are a necessary but not sufficient requisite for good insight. In general, the more severe the patient's psychiatric disturbance or cognitive impairment, the poorer the insight. However, patients with intact cognitive abilities, including some with high intelligence, have impaired insight because of their psychological disorder.

Virtually all psychiatric disorders potentially can impair insight to some degree (Trzepacz & Baker, 1993). Severely psychotic patients will not even recognize they have a problem or that their functioning is impaired. Manic patients often do not know or care they are experiencing or causing problems because of the reinforcing nature of the elation they experience. Histrionic personality and conversion disorders often deny they have a problem or any disruption in functioning/relationships. Borderline personality disorders may acknowledge that a problem exists, but blame others for their own dysfunction. Patients with impaired cognitive abilities often have associated impairment of insight; right hemisphere CVA, dementia, and traumatic brain injury commonly are associated with poor insight.

Ultimately, assessment of insight derives from clinical judgment largely based on what the patient says spontaneously and in response to questions regarding the areas outlined above. Generally, ability to articulate accurately about the areas outlined above, or at least in a reasonable and plausible way not at odds with verified information, is evidence of good insight. By convention, insight is rated as good, fair, or poor. It is most meaningful to reference these ratings with specific examples of the patient's good or poor insight into the specifics of their circumstances.

Judgment is the ability to make and execute good decisions. To make good decisions it is necessary to identify, consider, and weigh important information. Important information includes the advantages and disadvantages of various options, the likely outcomes for self and others, what are morally right and wrong, and long-term consequences. This cognitive process leads to a rational decision. To execute good decisions it is necessary to act in accordance with the decision. Often, good judgment requires cognitive reformulation or restraint of emotional inclinations for behavior. Poor judgment can manifest itself in the most basic inaction, such as not initiating simple hygiene, or in the most complex circumstances, such as when someone repeatedly becomes involved with partners who have addictions. To act emotionally without the guidance of this rational process also can lead to impulsive behavior. Most patients referred for an MSE will show some difficulty with judgment, but the behavioral level at which it occurs will vary depending on the nature and severity of the psychiatric disturbance or cognitive impairment. Similar to insight, virtually all psychiatric disorders potentially can impair judgment to some degree. Schizophrenics may not have the judgment to maintain even basic health. Manics often use bad judgment and engage in outrageous behavior such as spending sprees or audacious social interactions. Borderline personality disorders may assault, vandalize, or make a suicide gesture because of bad judgment.

Insight and adequate cognitive ability are necessary but not sufficient for making good decisions. As with insight, patients with adequate and even superior cognitive abilities have impaired judgment. However, ability to verbalize rational responses to hypothetical scenarios presented in interview is not a reliable predictor of the patient's ability to use good judgment in everyday circumstances. At times, psychiatric and brain damaged patients are able to verbalize accurate knowledge about the appropriate action, but when confronted with the real-life circumstance, this knowledge does not guide their behavior, such as when the brain damaged patient accurately identifies the dangers of using power tools but does it anyway or the codependent patient goes back to an abusive spouse despite being able to articulate the dysfunction and danger of the relationship. Thus, while assessment of judgment is to some degree based on the patient's verbal responses in interview, it is most accurately evaluated based on the patient's past judgment as reflected in behavior. Finally, to some extent, cultural issues determine what is rational good judgment and what is not. For example, presuming to select your child's marriage partner and negotiating the terms of the marriage would be considered bad judgment and irrational in American culture but is expected behavior in others.

ORIENTATION

Orientation is awareness of personal identity, time, location, and circumstances (i.e., what led up to the patients' referral, for MSE and why are they here). Most patients seen for an MSE will be oriented in all these spheres, and it is significant for those who are not. It is not unusual for patients not to accurately know the date, especially if they are hospitalized, but they should at least be able to indicate if it is in the first or last half of the month. Otherwise, perfect performance is expected. Disorientation most often is a sign of brain dysfunction. Delirious patients and those with moderate or worse dementia are disoriented; disorientation is common in the acute phase following CVA and traumatic brain injury. Psychotic patients usually are oriented unless they have severe thought disturbance or hallucinations (Trzepacz & Baker, 1993). Orientation is expected to be accurate in all other forms of psychological disturbance.

Two, and frequently three, aspects of orientation can be surreptitiously assessed in the course of conversation with the patient. Upon first approaching the patient, introduce yourself, and many times the patient, will respond by telling you his or her name; if not, you can say "and what is your name?" After explaining who you are and what you are doing, it is natural to ask the patient "So, tell me what led up to you being here." The patient's response to this question will reveal if they are oriented to location and present circumstances. If the patient's response does not clearly reflect accurate orientation, ask directly. When you begin the cognitive tests (described below), you can ask the patient to write his or her name, date, and address on a sheet of paper. Any dimensions to which the patient is not spontaneously oriented should be assessed with simple multiple choices: for example, are you in a doctor's office, hospital, or clinic? Or for more disoriented patients, are you in a church, hospital, or school? The patient who responds correctly to multiple choices is better oriented than one who does not.

ATTENTION/CONCENTRATION

In more recent neuropsychological models, the cognitive abilities formerly known as attention and concentration are now referred to as *working memory*. However, we will use the terms attention and concentration because they still are used when discussing MSE. Simply put, attention is the ability to focus cognitive processing on the appropriate target and avoid being distracted by irrelevant stimuli. While attention generally is limited to accurately detecting target stimuli, concentration adds the demands of sustaining attention over a longer period of time or manipulating and processing the contents of what is attended to. Attention also is a gateway to other types of cognitive processing. Before language can be comprehended, visual–spatial relationships perceived, information remembered, or problems solved, the stimuli must be attended to. Thus, if attention is impaired, other types of cognitive abilities likely will be impaired as a consequence. Attention and concentration are affected by brain damage of many types and psychological disturbance of many types.

Attention and concentration deficits are common to many types of brain injury including right hemisphere CVA, traumatic brain injury, cortical, and subcortical dementias. Delirium is always accompanied by impaired attention, and many drug-induced states are as well. Impaired attention may reflect an Attention Deficit Disorder (ADD). Anxiety, depression, psychosis, histrionic personality, and somatoform disorder all can affect performance on attention and concentration tests. Usually it is not possible to discriminate between these underlying psychological causes of poor attention based on attention test performance alone; this is determined by findings from other parts of the MSE and the patient's history. For example, patients with ADD, depression, and schizophrenia each may be intermittently inattentive, and it is not possible to distinguish between them based on how many digits each can repeat in order. It is the extra-test behavior that distinguishes them, with the schizophrenic talking back to voices, the depressed patient sitting passively expending little apparent effort, and the patient with ADD losing track of the task when a magazine picture of a motorcycle distracts him. Assessing attention and concentration gives an indication of how reliably the patient processes information and as such serves as a guide for structuring interactions with the patient ranging from simple medicine instructions to psychotherapy approaches.

Attention and concentration are subjectively assessed throughout the MSE by observations of the patient's behavior and verbal responses. More obvious behavioral signs of attention problems are motor restlessness (e.g., frequent shifting in the chair, standing and walking around the room, peering out the window, doors, or at objects in the room), attending to extraneous sounds, being distracted by ambient stimuli, and doing something else while the examiner is attempting to engage in conversation. More subtle signs of attention problems are evident in the quality and cadence of verbal responses. The patient may begin answering a question before it is completed. Tangential answers or irrelevant answers represent problems with attention and concentration. Poorly attentive patients may start answering a question, become tangential and then ask, "What was the question again?" or indicate they do not know what the original question was if a circumstantial answer is interrupted with an inquiry.

The most common test of attention probably is digit span forward and backward. Digit span forward is a measure of attention and digits backward of concentration (using the definitions described above). It is best to have digit sequences written in advance for ready reference and to assure accuracy of scoring the patient's performance (i.e., so you can remember what the digit sequences were!). Different digit sequences should be used for forward and backward to avoid potential confounding of memory for number sequences (which is more likely if the patient uses the superior strategy of "chunking" numbers). Read numbers at the rate of one per second. Average performance is similar for ages 20–64 after which there is a slight decline (see Table 5). In general, individuals with more education will perform at the top of the average range and those with lower education at the lower end.

Other commonly used tests of concentration are to ask the patient to spell a word backward, such as "world" (Folstein, Folstein, & McHugh, 1975). This is an easy task, and failure indicates likely significant problems with concentration; accurately spelling words demonstrates some capacity for concentration but does not rule out concentration problems. Serial calculations also are a favorite MSE test of concentration. An easy version is to start with 1 and count by 3s. Most people can perform 13 trials with no more than one error (usually adding 3 to 19 and getting 21). The more standard format is serial subtraction by 7 starting from 100. Some authors note that chronic patients may perform this test well due to practice effects (Amchin, 1991); in these cases serial subtraction by 6 or 8 can be substituted. Most people can perform serial subtractions with only one or two errors in 14 trials.

TABLE 5. Average Digit Span Performance by Age

| | Age | | |
	20–64	65–69	70–89
Digits forward	6–8	6–8	6–7
Digits backward	5–7	5–6	4–5

Compiled from *Wechsler Memory Scale III* (1997).

MEMORY

Memory is a complex cognitive ability that involves the recall or recognition of previous experience (Kolb & Whishaw, 2001). The formation of new memories involves recognition and registration of the initial sensory input, retention and storage of the information, and recall or retrieval of the stored information (Strub & Black, 2000). Memory impairment is one of the most common sequela of brain damage of all kinds and is the most prominent early deficit of progressive dementias like Alzheimer's. Memory distortion occurs as part of the presentation of many forms of psychopathology, but often the quality of MSE memory performance is different from patients with brain damage. For purposes of MSE, memory can be divided into remote, recent, immediate, and delayed. The first two are recall of events from many years and a few days to months ago, respectively; the latter two are the types of memory evaluated by MSE cognitive tests.

Memory impairment associated with many types of brain injury such as traumatic brain injury, CVA, early- and mid-stage progressive dementia typically is worse for recent information and relatively preserved for past or remote information. In these cases, the patient's memory deficit will be most evident on the memory tests for words and figures given in the MSE and for recall of recent history (i.e., since head injury or CVA, or in the case of dementia, recall of the past few months) with relatively good recall of past personal history (before onset of brain injury or dementia) several years ago. In more advanced stages of dementia and more severe brain injuries, memory is impaired for everything.

Anxiety and mood disturbance also can interfere with memory performance. In these cases, patients likely do not have true memory impairment; rather, psychological processes interfere with their ability to perform to potential. Severe anxiety can greatly interfere with memory test performance but usually is not a factor at low levels. Depression also decreases memory test performance. Often, people who are depressed do poorly on free recall but are accurate on recognition tests. Presence of depressed affect and mood disturbance help confirm that this pattern of memory performance is due to depression. However, this pattern of memory performance and affective change also is seen in many subcortical dementias. Distortions in memory of past events are part and parcel of many types of psychopathology. Patients with histrionic personalities will recall events in exaggerated and dramatic fashion. Borderline personalities will remember relationships in a distorted manner as either idealized or extremely negative. Sociopaths will lie to serve their purposes (Aksikal & Akiskal, 1994). All these circumstances of inaccurately reported memories are the result of personality functioning distorting what is otherwise an intact memory capacity.

Evaluation of remote and recent memory is obtained when taking history of recent events and psychosocial history. Key aspects of this information obtained from the patient are verified (e.g., by family) to determine the reliability of memory in these areas. Impaired attention will interfere with memory of new information and evaluation of attention as described above. When assessing immediate and delayed recall in MSE, the goal is to determine in a screening fashion if the person is capable of recalling new information following delay. Although many references recommend a delay period of 5 min, a 20-min delay is necessary to assure the patient's consolidation and storage is evaluated. While many MSE formats include recall of only verbal information, it is important also to evaluate visual-graphic memory for those rare patients who may have a previously unrecognized cerebral event lateralized to the right hemisphere, and to screen for cognitive deficits among those who have identified cerebral involvement.

Tell patients you are going to say three words that you want them to remember. We use the words *screwdriver, compassion, brown* presented in that order (to minimize the chances of the patient using a visual or verbal mnemonic such as "brown screwdriver"). Say all three words at once, pausing briefly between each. Then have the patient repeat all three. Repeat all three as necessary until the patient can say all three. Then have the patient copy three figures. We use the figures in Figure 1. The patients' accurate copy of the figures indicates that their basic visual–perceptual and construction skills are intact. Difficulty copying the figures may indicate deficits in either of these areas and merits further neuropsychological evaluation. Consistent or exclusive left-sided errors on drawing likely reflect some degree of left inattention or neglect associated with right hemisphere damage. Tell patients you will ask them to draw the figures again from memory later. Continue the MSE for 20 min keeping the patients engaged with other activities to assure they are not rehearsing the words or figures. Then ask them to recall the words. Almost all normal people under the age of 70 will remember the words immediately; people over 70 may spontaneously remember only two and should at least recognize the third in multiple-choice format. For any words not spontaneously recalled, give a cue: for example, "one of the words was a tool/feeling/color." If the word(s) is not recalled with the cue, give multiple-choice recognition: for example, "Was the word: pliers, wrench, or *screwdriver*—frustration, *compassion*, or admiration—*brown*, black, or gray?" Then ask the patient to draw the three figures again. For any figures not spontaneously recalled, horizontally present the target figure with the foils in Figure 2 for multiple-choice recognition; be sure that the target figure appears in a different position (i.e., first, second, or third) for each trial. Most everyone under age 60 will remember all three figures. Ability to recall and draw figures after a delay declines steadily after 60 and many normal people in their 70s and 80s will recall only one or two of the drawings; however, most people older than 60 will recognize the figures in multiple choice format they do not recall spontaneously. Performance below these

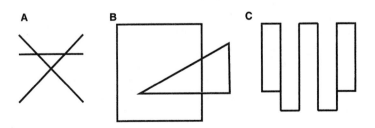

FIGURE 1. Figures for memory test

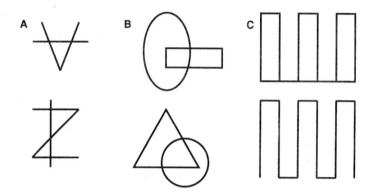

FIGURE 2. Multiple-choice figures for figure recognition

expected levels merits referral for neuropsychological evaluation, especially in the absence of significant findings in other areas of the MSE.

INTELLIGENCE AND ABSTRACTION

Evaluation of *intelligence* and *abstraction* essentially is an attempt to estimate where the patient's abilities fall on a continuum of innate overall cognitive ability. If an accurate measurement of intelligence or abstract thinking ability is needed, the patient should be referred for neuropsychological evaluation. Short of this, these abilities can be only grossly estimated based on the MSE.

The best demographic predictors of an individual's intelligence are education and occupation. In general, people with less than a high school education will have low-average or below intelligence, high school average, college high-average, and graduate education high-average to superior intelligence. There are people for whom education underestimates their cognitive ability, and in these cases, occupational achievement is a better indicator. If someone dropped out of school in the eleventh grade but now owns a large real estate company, is a deacon in his church, and designs web pages as a hobby, the high-average intelligence predicted by these non-academic activities likely is more accurate than the low-average level predicted by education. In general, higher technical and professional occupations require higher levels of intelligence for success than manual labor and clerical jobs. In the MSE, the patient's use of vocabulary, ability to give concise but thorough answers, and ability to independently comprehend the implications of statements are indications of intellectual level.

Abstraction is the capacity to recognize and comprehend relationships that are not immediately or concretely apparent. Most MSE references describe two approaches to assessing abstraction: similarities and proverb interpretation. Similarities involve asking the patient in what way two objects or concepts are alike. Test items range from more obvious and concrete to more abstract in ascending difficulty: for example, celery–carrot, music–sculpture, love–hate, talking–listening. Responses may range from accurate identification of the abstract similarity (they are vegetables), to a correct but concrete similarity (you can eat both of them), to a correct but irrelevant or incorrect response (you buy both in a store). Proverb interpretation is asking the patient to explain the more general meaning of a concrete statement. These also are organized from simple to complex: for example, there's no use crying over spilt milk, a stitch in time saves nine, people who live in glass houses shouldn't throw stones, a rolling stone gathers no moss. Responses are scored along the same lines as described above for similarities. For both similarities and proverb interpretation, patients of low education/occupational status are expected to get only the simplest item of each set correct, high school education/average occupational attainment 2–3 correct, and high education/occupational status all 4 items correct.

Poor performance on these types of items confirms that the patient of limited education and occupational success is of modest innate cognitive ability. However, poor performance by someone of advanced education/high occupational success suggests the possibility of brain dysfunction and should be considered in conjunction with performance on other cognitive screening tests described below. Despite the legacy of considering poor performance on similarities and proverb interpretation tasks as evidence of concrete thinking that is diagnostically significant for schizophrenia, in truth it is not. Akiskal and Akiskal (1994) cite research which shows that poor performance on these types of abstraction tests is unreliable in diagnosing schizophrenia (Andreasen & Black, 1987). Thus, performance on these types of tests is useful for identifying low cognitive ability due to endowment or brain dysfunction but not for identifying psychiatric disturbance.

SUMMARY

The MSE is an interview screening evaluation of all the important areas of a patient's emotional and cognitive functioning, often augmented with some simple cognitive tests. The MSE provides the data for formulating a psychiatric diagnosis or developing a working hypothesis regarding psychiatric diagnosis. A standardized approach increases reliability of the MSE; specifying the behavior on which key interpretations and conclusions are based also is important for MSE reliability. Genuine concern for the patient, awareness of her/his cultural background and some degree of individualization of the MSE is necessary to set the patient at ease, develop rapport, and is an effective way to collect comprehensive, valid, and reliable data. MSE data is most meaningful when considered in the context of a thorough psychosocial and psychiatric history. General knowledge of the overlapping etiology of psychiatric and medical processes is important in preventing misdiagnosis.

A comprehensive MSE includes evaluation of 12 areas. *Appearance* is what the patient looks like. *Behavior* is how the patient acts. *Motor* activity is the type and quality of movements the patient makes. *Attitude* is how patients feel and what they think about participating in the MSE. *Mood* is the internal emotional state of the patient and *affect* is the external expression of emotional state.

Language is the ability to use symbols to communicate and *speech* is what patients say and the quality of how they talk. *Thought* is the internal dialogue that occurs in the patient's mind while *perception* is the patient's sensory–perceptual experience and interpretation of external events and circumstances. *Insight* is the extent to which the patient recognizes the existence, nature, and scope of her/his problems; *judgment* is the ability to make and execute good decisions. *Orientation* is awareness of personal identity, time, location, and circumstances. *Attention* is the ability to focus and sustain cognitive processing on the appropriate target. *Memory* is the ability to recall previous experience as well as store and recall new information. *Intelligence* and *abstraction* are innate cognitive abilities; the former is overall level of cognitive ability, the latter the ability to recognize and comprehend relationships that are not immediately or concretely apparent.

REFERENCES

Akiskal, H. S., & Akiskal, K. (1994). Mental status examination: The art and science of the clinical interview. In M. Hersen & S. D. Turner (Eds.), *Diagnostic interviewing* (2nd ed.). New York, NY: Plenum Press.

Amchin, J. (1991). *Psychiatric diagnosis: A biopsychosocial approach using DSM-III-R.* Washington, DC: American Psychiatric Press.

Andreasen, N. C., & Black, D. W. (1987). *Introductory textbook of psychiatry.* Washington, DC: American Psychiatric Press.

Folstein M. F., Folstein, S. E., & McHugh, P. R. (1975). Mini-mental state: A practical method for grading the cognitive state of patients for the clinician. *Journal of Psychiatry Research, 12,* 189–198.

Hales, R. E., Talbott, J. A., & Yudofsky, S. C. (1994). *The American Psychiatric Press textbook of psychiatry* (pp. 212–217). Washington, DC: American Psychiatric Press.

Kaplan, H. I., & Sadock, B. J. (1995). *Comprehensive textbook of psychiatry/VI* (6th ed.). Baltimore, MD: Williams & Wilkins.

Kolb, B., & Whishaw, I. Q. (2001). *An introduction to brain and behavior.* New York, NY: Worth.

Strub, R. L., & Black, F. W. (2000). *The mental status examination in neurology* (4th ed.). Philadelphia, PA: F. A. Davis Company.

Trzepacz, P. T., & Baker, R. W. (1993). *The psychiatric mental status examination.* New York, NY: Oxford University Press.

Wechsler Memory Scale III: Administration and Scoring Manual. (1997). San Antonio, TX: The Psychological Corporation.

3

Interviewing Strategies

CATHERINE MILLER

INTRODUCTION

Diagnostic interviewing is fundamental to the assessment of clients' presenting problems and overall functioning (Friedman, 1989; Sarwer & Sayers, 1998). Despite an explosion of self-report instruments and questionnaires, interviewing "remains the most basic, most commonly used, and most powerful technique of clinical assessment" (Korchin, 1976, p. 192). Researchers and clinicians may employ direct observation methods, psychological tests, self-report questionnaires, and/or self-monitoring forms in an attempt to assess client issues, but it is the interview that continues to play an instrumental and prominent role in diagnostic evaluations (Rogers, 1995). Historically, clinicians have employed a flexible or unstructured approach to interviewing (Sher & Trull, 1996), relying on client presentation and clinical intuition to focus and guide the interview process. Although clinicians learned basic interviewing skills during graduate training and some informal guidelines on the type of information to collect in an interview, until recently there has been little standardization of interview formats (Friedman, 1989). However, within the past three decades, structured approaches have been developed that have systematized the interview process (Rogers, 2001).

The current chapter will define the main features, advantages, and disadvantages of unstructured and structured approaches. In addition, this chapter will review several specific structured interview formats in an effort to help clinicians make informed choices of assessment instruments.

PSYCHOMETRIC ISSUES

Before discussing specific interviewing strategies, a brief review of psychometric issues is necessary. Just as the psychometric properties of any other diagnostic

CATHERINE MILLER • School of Professional Psychology, Pacific University, Forest Grove, Oregon 97116.

instrument are scrutinized, the reliability and validity of interview formats must be reviewed in order to weigh the merits of various interview strategies (Rogers, 2001).

First, an interview format must demonstrate adequate reliability or replicability. An instrument will be maximally reliable when there is little error variance affecting the scores (Cone, 1998). For interview formats, reliability may be assessed at various levels, such as individual items, symptom clusters, or diagnoses (Rogers, 2001). The majority of studies on interview formats have been focused only at the diagnostic rather than the item or syndrome level.

Regardless of the level of analysis, there are two major ways to assess the reliability of interview formats: interrater reliability and test–retest reliability (Mash & Terdel, 1997; Rogers, 2001; Sattler, 1992). The most commonly employed measure is that of interrater reliability, or agreement between independent interviewers (Rogers, 2001; Summerfeldt & Antony, 2002). To determine interrater reliability, one interview is conducted with a client on one occasion; this interview is observed by two independent clinicians who form diagnostic conclusions based on the respondent's answers. Less commonly assessed is test–retest reliability, which involves administration of interviews by two independent clinicians on two different occasions (typically separated by 1–4 weeks) (Rogers, 2001). Test–retest reliability is generally considered more stringent than interrater reliability for two reasons. First, test–retest assessment includes a time confound that is likely to lower the reliability coefficient (Summerfeldt & Antony, 2002). Second, test–retest reliability is affected by attenuation, which may be defined as the tendency of interviewees to report fewer symptoms on retesting (Shaffer, Fisher, & Lucas, 1999). This common phenomenon has been shown consistently across interviews and other measures (e.g., self-report instruments, ratings by others), and it functions to lower reliability coefficients (Rogers, 2001).

Four different statistical values may be employed to report degree of reliability: percent agreement, Yule's Y, intraclass coefficients (ICCs), and Cohen's kappa (Cone, 1998; Friedman, 1989; Summerfeldt & Antony, 2002). Percent agreement, the percentage of times two interviewers agree on an item, is the least commonly employed measure of reliability, as it can be inflated by chance agreements (Friedman, 1989). Yule's Y also is infrequently reported in the literature, but it is recommended due to its good stability with low base rate phenomena (such as psychiatric diagnoses) (Summerfeldt & Antony, 2002). ICCs are employed in special cases, such as when agreement between more than two interviewers is assessed (Rogers, 2001). The kappa coefficient (Cohen, 1960) is the most commonly used statistic and is considered a conservative measure of reliability, as it corrects for chance agreements (Friedman, 1989). Unfortunately, there are two main problems with the kappa coefficient. First, kappa values tend to drop when there is a low base rate (Robins, 1985). For example, near perfect agreement between interviewers (95% agreement) results in a high kappa of 0.81 with a 50% base rate but drops to a very low kappa of 0.14 with a 1% base rate (Rogers, 2001). Such dramatic differences due to varying base rates make the kappa coefficient difficult to compare across studies. Another problem with the kappa coefficient is that there is no agreement in the literature as to cutoff coefficients (Hodges & Cools, 1990). Kappa coefficients range in value from −1.00 (complete disagreement between observers), through 0 (chance levels of agreement), to +1.00 (complete agreement) (Cone, 1998). Several authors have recommended that a kappa of 0.50 or greater should be considered an acceptable level of reliability (Costello, Edelbrock, Dulcan, Kalas, & Klaric, 1984; Spitzer, Fleiss, & Endicott, 1978). However, others have recommended that 0.40 should be the lower limit of acceptability (Hodges, 1993; Landis & Koch, 1977) Clearly, consensus has not been reached as to cutoffs for kappa coefficients, making interpretation of research findings difficult for clinicians.

Although reliability is necessary, it is also important to establish the validity of interview approaches. There are two major ways to assess the validity of interview formats: criterion-related and construct validity (Rogers, 2001). Criterion-related validity examines how well the interview information corresponds to an independent criterion. The difficulty in establishing criterion-related validity is in finding an adequate, well-validated criterion against which to measure the interview format. In most studies, researchers have utilized diagnostic interviews conducted by highly skilled clinicians as the criterion, a process that is clearly imperfect but widely employed (Rogers, 2001). Criterion-related validity includes both concurrent and predictive validity. Concurrent validity is defined as the extent to which interview information corresponds to information obtained through another method conducted simultaneously. Predictive validity is defined as the extent to which interview information predicts treatment course or outcome (Rogers, 2001; Sattler, 1992). Most studies on interview formats have assessed only concurrent validity and have reported results utilizing the kappa coefficient.

Construct validity is defined as the extent to which the interview measures what it purports to measure (Anastasi, 1988), and it includes both convergent and discriminant validity (Rogers, 2001; Sattler, 1992). Both types of validity assess degree of relationship between information obtained by different methods (e.g., interviews, self-report measures, ratings by others). For example, information about depression obtained in an interview should be maximally similar to information about depression obtained via another method. It is also true, however, that information about depression obtained in an interview should be dissimilar to information about psychosis obtained via another method. In other words, convergent validity assesses the degree of relationship of similar concepts, while discriminant validity assesses the degree of relationship of dissimilar concepts (Rogers, 2001). Most studies assessing construct validity have examined only convergent validity and have reported results via correlation coefficients.

In summary, any assessment of a client should be conducted with psychometrically sound instruments, so that clinicians can rely on the resulting diagnoses. As with any instrument, it is necessary to examine the reliability and validity of interview formats to adequately assess the interview's worth and utility. Specific psychometric results will be discussed in the following review of unstructured and structured interview approaches.

UNSTRUCTURED APPROACHES TO INTERVIEWING

Unstructured approaches to interviewing allow clinicians to formulate their own questions depending on a client's issues and concerns. In addition, unstructured approaches allow clinicians to record client responses in idiosyncratic ways (Rogers, 1995). Utilizing such formats, it is the clinician who is "entirely responsible for determining what questions to ask and how the resulting information is to be used in arriving at a diagnosis" (Summerfeldt & Antony, 2002, p. 3).

The primary advantage of unstructured approaches lies in the flexibility of such a format. The interviewer is free to focus the questioning on concerns evidenced by the particular client. Such flexibility is thought to greatly aid in establishing rapport with the client, as the client's main concerns are the focus of the interview and little time is spent in questioning other areas or symptoms (Mash & Terdel, 1997; Sattler, 1992). However, the flexibility that is the hallmark of unstructured approaches carries with it some disadvantages.

The main difficulty with unstructured approaches is the lack of established reliability and validity (Rogers, 2001). Unstructured interviews are "highly dependent on the specific interviewer, the specific interviewee, the type of interview, and the conditions under which the interview took place" (Sattler, 1992, p. 463). In other words, the flexibility inherent in unstructured formats means that there are an infinite variety of ways an interview may be conducted, depending upon the client's presentation and the clinician's interests. This diversity of styles makes establishing the psychometric properties of unstructured approaches very difficult.

Research has clearly shown that clinicians with similar training in similar working environments are often unable to agree about an individual's diagnosis (Angold & Fisher, 1999). Why this is such a common phenomenon is likely due to the variability inherent in diagnostic interviews. Within an interview, two main sources of variability have been identified: criterion variance and information variance (Ward, Beck, Mendelson, Mock, & Erbaugh, 1962). Criterion variance may be defined as "variations among clinicians in applying standards for what is clinically relevant ... and when the diagnostic criteria are met" (Rogers, 2001, p. 5). Nosological systems such as the current version of the *Diagnostic and Statistical Manual of Mental Disorders*, Fourth Edition (*DSM-IV*; American Psychiatric Association, 1994), which contain explicit diagnostic criteria and a multiaxial system, have substantially reduced criterion variance, but have not eliminated the problem (Lesser, 1997; Rogers, 1995). For example, Blashfield (1992, as cited in Rogers, 1995) found that clinicians employing unstructured interview methods still do not systematically apply diagnostic criteria, resulting in misdiagnosis 60% of the time.

Information variance may be defined as "variations among clinicians in what questions are asked, which observations are made, and how the resulting information is organized" (Rogers, 2001, p. 5). For example, clinicians may ask questions in unique ways that may be understood in different ways by different clients. In addition, clinicians are subject to confirmatory bias. In other words, clinicians tend to form a diagnostic hypothesis before they have collected all the relevant data and then seek information selectively to confirm that hypothesis, ignoring any disconfirming evidence and missing important symptoms (Angold & Fisher, 1999; Rogers, 2001). Finally, clinicians tend to stop the interview process after the first mental disorder is established, so that many diagnoses are missed, particularly disorders that are rare (Rogers, 2001). All of these variations among interviewers lead to different amounts and type of information being collected; this naturally results in different diagnostic formulations (Lesser, 1997).

Ward and colleagues (1962) argued that the majority of diagnostic discrepancies between clinicians arise from criterion and information variance, not from true differences in client symptom presentation. Ward et al. reported that 62.5% of variability in responding results from criterion variance, 32.5% results from information variance, and only 5.0% is the result of true changes in a client's clinical presentation. In other words, how the interview is conducted (information variance) and how the criteria are utilized to score responses (criterion variance) greatly affect the results.

Such findings led to dissatisfaction both with diagnostic classification schemes and with traditional unstructured approaches to interviewing. As previously stated, improvements in the *DSM* over the years have helped to reduce criterion variance. To reduce information variance, researchers discarded the unstructured approach to interviewing, instead developing formats that required interviewers to ask the same questions of all clients. The need to control information variance was the primary impetus behind the development of more structured approaches to interviewing (Lesser, 1997).

STRUCTURED APPROACHES TO INTERVIEWING

Beginning in the late 1970s, researchers concerned about the difficulty of establishing the reliability and validity of unstructured interview formats developed structured approaches to interviewing, in an attempt to improve the psychometric properties of interviews (Rogers, 2001). Use of structured interviews has grown to the point that such a format is standard practice in research settings and many clinical practices currently (Summerfeldt & Antony, 2002). Unlike unstructured formats, structured approaches provide a standardized framework of questions and ratings, allowing for direct comparisons across clinicians, settings, and diagnostic groups (Rogers, 1995).

Currently, structured interview formats exist for both child and adult populations. Although initial studies were conducted with adult interview formats, researchers began developing child structured interview approaches in the late 1970s, with the majority of work being done in the 1980s (Edelbrock & Costello, 1988). The need for psychometrically sound child interviews is clear, as discrepancies are often found between parent and child reports of child symptoms (Hodges, 1993). In particular, researchers have noted that parents and children demonstrate good agreement regarding objective child behavioral symptoms but evidence much less agreement regarding subjective child symptoms, such as depression or anxiety (Edelbrock, Costello, Dulcan, Conover, & Kalas, 1986).

Given this finding that parent and child reports are not interchangeable, clinicians should interview both children and parents for a complete diagnostic picture. The finding that even very young children (i.e., 6 years old) may be reliable reporters of their own symptoms (Herjanic, Herjanic, Brown, & Wheatt, 1975) paved the way for the development of structured interviews for a child population similar to formats developed for adults (Hodges, Gordon, & Lennon, 1990).

There are several advantages of structured approaches over unstructured interview formats, including improvements in the assessment of psychometric properties, coverage of diagnostic categories, ratings of psychopathology, and application of interviews. First and foremost, structured interviews are able to demonstrate adequate psychometric properties, something that was difficult to even assess with unstructured formats (Rogers, 1995). Second, there is more comprehensive coverage of diagnostic categories with structured interviews, including diagnoses that are less prevalent. Such a thorough diagnostic evaluation aids both clients and clinicians. Clients benefit from improved treatment planning, while clinicians benefit from decreased risk of negligence or malpractice allegations (Hodges & Cools, 1990). Third, structured interviews allow clinicians to rate gradations in severity of symptoms and level of impairment, rather than to merely note the presence or absence of symptoms (Rogers, 1995). Fourth, the routine wording and ordering of questions of structured formats greatly eases interview administration and, therefore, expense. Rather than highly trained professionals, lay interviewers or computerized administrations may be utilized for some of the more highly structured interview formats. The improved administration ease and reduced expense may allow thorough diagnostic interviews to be conducted in large settings where few clinicians traditionally are found, such as prisons, residential treatment centers, shelters, etc. (Shaffer et al., 1999).

Although their advantages are convincing, structured interviews have several disadvantages. First, the rigid structure of the interview may interfere with relaxed communication. In other words, without the flexibility to focus on client concerns, rapport may be compromised. If clinicians become too tied to a rigid and inflexible protocol, there is a chance that clients may become disengaged from the diagnostic process (Rogers, 1995). Second, as mentioned earlier, structured interviews specify precise wording of questions and generally do not allow for rephrasing of questions by interviewers. There is a risk that clients may misunderstand questions and then respond inappropriately (Shaffer et al., 1999). Third, interviews cannot cover every diagnosis and symptom presentation; if they did, they would be too long and cumbersome to be helpful. Therefore, they may not do an adequate job assessing atypical symptoms or diagnoses (Shaffer et al., 1999). Finally, these interviews are time consuming to learn and to administer. Training in administration typically takes at least 1 week and often up to 4 weeks. Administration typically takes at least 75 min but may take up to 4 hr with severely disturbed clients.

Most structured interview formats share some common features (Hodges & Cools, 1990; Rogers, 1995). First, these interviews are typically organized by disorder or syndrome, a system called symptom clustering. Although this organization necessarily entails repeated questioning of symptoms contained in several diagnoses, it is advantageous, in that it allows clinicians to quickly rule out specific disorders and to allocate maximum time within the interview to those diagnoses that appear most likely (Summerfeldt & Antony, 2002). Second, structured interviews typically employ unidirectional scoring, meaning that endorsement of an item is a sign of psychopathology. Such a process allows for rapid scoring and diagnostic decision-making. Third, structured interviews typically begin with a series of neutral or less threatening questions and progress to more intrusive questions. This sequencing of topics avoids prematurely intruding on clients, thereby allowing for maximum amounts of information to be obtained. Finally, questions included in many structured interviews directly correspond to diagnostic criteria contained in the *DSM* or some other classification system, such as the Research Diagnostic Criteria (RDC; Spitzer, Endicott, & Robins, 1978). This direct correspondence clearly aids clinicians when attempting to diagnose clients based on interview responses.

Despite common features, structured interviews vary considerably across three main dimensions, including diagnostic coverage, ease of use, and degree of structure (Rogers, 2001). First, structured interviews differ according to breadth and depth of focus, known in the literature as the bandwidth-fidelity issue (Widiger & Frances, 1987, as cited in Rogers, 2001). Due to time constraints, a single interview cannot simultaneously cover all diagnostic categories in considerable depth. Interviews with broad diagnostic coverage sacrifice depth in two ways: by screening out disorders, and by minimizing the number of questions asked. In contrast, interviews with greater depth (i.e., more questions regarding each symptom) restrict coverage to common diagnoses. Second, structured interviews differ according to ease of use. As previously mentioned, interviews that closely follow *DSM* diagnostic criteria and that are organized around symptom clusters simplify administration and scoring (Rogers, 2001). Interviews that require considerable clinical judgment in question formulation and scoring are obviously much more difficult to use.

In addition to diagnostic coverage and ease of use issues, structured interviews also differ according to the level of structure imposed on the clinician. Within the structured interview approach, two main subtypes are recognized: semistructured and highly structured approaches (Rogers, 2001). Highly structured approaches specify the exact wording, order, and coding of each question (Edelbrock & Costello, 1988). Questions must be read verbatim, with no variation or additions. In contrast, semistructured approaches provide only general and flexible guidelines for conducting the interview, allowing clinicians more latitude in pursuing alternative lines of inquiry (Edelbrock & Costello, 1988). Clinicians may even invent their own unstructured questions (Rogers, 1995), allowing semistructured interviews to appear more conversational than highly structured interviews (Edelstein & Berler, 1987). Semistructured formats have been referred to as interviewer-based interviews, as the clinician has some discretion in varying the wording and the ordering of questions (Angold & Fisher, 1999), whereas highly structured formats have been referred to as respondent-based interviews, as the client is required to interpret the meaning of the questions and decide on a reply with minimal or no assistance of the interviewer (Shaffer et al., 1999).

The remaining portion of this chapter will briefly review several semistructured and highly structured interview formats so that clinicians may better evaluate their relative merits. Of the various formats available for both child and adult respondents, five interviews will be reviewed in this chapter, as these five appear to be the most commonly utilized formats in clinical and research settings. It should be noted that structured interviews are works in progress, as they are constantly being revised in order to improve psychometric properties and to reflect changes in diagnostic classification systems (Angold & Fisher, 1999). Due to this constant process of revision, it is difficult to assess the psychometric properties of current versions of interview formats, as the majority of available reliability and validity studies have been conducted with prior versions. Nevertheless, given the similarity in content and format across revisions of various interview formats, information from early studies should remain useful to clinicians and will be reviewed in this chapter.

EXAMPLES OF STRUCTURED INTERVIEWS

Highly Structured Interview Formats

Diagnostic Interview Schedule (DIS)

The DIS for adults (Robins, Helzer, Croughan, & Ratcliff, 1981) was the first highly structured diagnostic interview to be developed. It was designed in 1978 as a research instrument for the Epidemiological Catchment Area project, a large epidemiological study in the United States sponsored by the National Institutes of Mental Health (NIMH). The highly structured format of the DIS can be attributed to budgetary restrictions of the study. In order to minimize the high cost of experienced clinicians, the developers of the DIS utilized a highly structured approach, which minimized clinical inference and judgment, allowing less costly lay persons to administer interviews (Rogers, 2001; Summerfeldt & Antony, 2002). Because it is a highly structured interview, the questions on the DIS must be read verbatim; the interviewer is not given the flexibility to invent his or her own questions (Rogers, 2001).

The DIS is a broad-based measure, designed to assess a wide range of both current and lifetime diagnoses (Summerfeldt & Antony, 2002). Originally, it was based on diagnostic criteria from the third revision of the *DSM* (*DSM-III*; American Psychiatric Association, 1980), and it has been revised several times to reflect updated *DSM* criteria. There have been many versions throughout the years, reflecting advancement not only in diagnostic criteria, but also in psychometric properties and computerized administration/scoring (for a thorough review of DIS versions, see Rogers, 2001).

The current version, DIS-IV (Robins, Cottler, Bucholz, & Compton, 1995), corresponds to *DSM-IV* diagnostic criteria (American Psychiatric Association, 1994). DIS-IV covers more than 30 Axis I diagnoses and 1 Axis II diagnosis (antisocial personality disorder) (Rogers, 2001). Although primarily designed as an adult instrument, DIS-IV covers several disorders that originate in childhood, including Attention Deficit Hyperactivity Disorder (ADHD), Separation Anxiety Disorder, Oppositional Defiant Disorder, and Conduct Disorder (Rogers, 2001). Due to time and length restrictions, several diagnoses are not covered, including most somatoform disorders, dissociative disorders, most sexual disorders, and delusional disorders (Summerfeldt & Antony, 2002). In general, administration time of the DIS-IV is estimated to take approximately $1\frac{1}{2}$–2 hr (Rogers, 2001). However, administration time may be significantly increased for severely ill patients or those with multiple disorders (Summerfeldt & Antony, 2002). It should be noted that hand scoring is not available on the DIS-IV; instead, the interview must be scored via computer.

The interview is organized into 19 diagnostic modules, which are designed to be independent of each other (Rogers, 2001). Within each module, there are optional termination points, which indicate appropriate places to stop questioning if too few required symptoms are endorsed to meet diagnostic criteria. Items in the DIS-IV consist of standard forced choice questions and optional probes. If the respondent answers affirmatively to the standard question, the interviewer may ask optional probes. The purposes of these optional probes are twofold: to assess the clinical significance of a symptom, and to assess potential etiology, including physical conditions or substance use (Summerfeldt & Antony, 2002). The DIS-IV includes detailed instructions on when and how to use these probes (Rogers, 2001).

Based on the respondent's answers to both standard questions and optional probes, each symptom is rated on a 1–5 scale, with a score of 3 required for clinical significance (Summerfeldt & Antony, 2002). What is unique about the scoring on the DIS-IV is that the ratings combine clinical relevance with possible etiology of the symptom, in an attempt to rule out organic disorders due to substance use or medical conditions (Rogers, 2001). For example, based on the respondent's answers, the interviewer may rate clinically relevant symptoms with the following scores: 3, suggesting etiology due to medications, drugs, or alcohol; 4, suggesting etiology due to physical illness or injury; or 5, suggesting etiology due to a psychiatric disorder (Rogers, 2001).

Unfortunately, the psychometric properties of the DIS have not lived up to its promise as a clinical tool. Test–retest studies have reported only modest reliability coefficients for various diagnostic categories. For example, Wells, Burnham, Leake, and Robins (1988) found a median kappa coefficient of 0.57 for current diagnoses over a period of 3 months, while Vandiver and Sher (1991) found median kappa coefficients of 0.46 for current diagnoses and 0.43 for lifetime diagnoses over a period of 9 months. It is important to note that both of these studies limited diagnostic coverage, which may have artificially inflated kappa values. For example, Wells and colleagues (1988) only looked at depression diagnoses, while Vandiver and Sher eliminated disorders believed to be uncommon (Rogers, 2001). In general, higher reliability figures will be found when diagnostic coverage is limited or focused (Rogers, 2001).

Interrater reliability studies examining consistency of diagnoses between lay and professional (i.e., psychiatrist) interviewers also have reported only modest results. For example, Robins and colleagues (1981) reported kappa coefficients of 0.50 or greater for lifetime diagnoses, with the exception of panic disorder (kappa = 0.40). Later studies reported even lower figures. For example, Helzer et al. (1985) reported an average kappa coefficient of 0.43 for lifetime diagnoses, while Helzer, Spitznagel, and McEvoy (1987) reported an average kappa coefficient of only 0.37 for lifetime diagnoses. These authors noted that much of the disagreement between lay and professional interviewers involved borderline cases in which diagnostic criteria were only marginally met. It appears that inter-rater reliability figures may be considerably higher when diagnostic criteria are exceeded.

Concurrent validity studies have compared DIS diagnoses to diagnoses obtained from experienced clinicians. These studies have produced only modest results, with kappa coefficients generally falling well below the 0.50 range. For example, across several diagnostic categories, Helzer et al. (1985) found a median kappa coefficient of 0.40. Overall, more agreement between interviewers is found for substance abuse disorders, with poorer agreement for both mood and anxiety disorders (Rogers, 2001).

Convergent validity studies have produced more promising results, at least for specific diagnostic categories. For example, Whisman et al. (1989) compared diagnoses obtained from the DIS and the interview version of the Hamilton Rating Scale for Depression (Hamilton, 1960); these researchers reported a high median ICC of 0.89. Similarly, Gavin, Ross, and Skinner (1989; as cited in Rogers, 2001) compared diagnoses from the DIS and results from the Michigan Alcoholism Screening Test (Selzer, 1971); these researchers reported a good correlation of 0.65.

Diagnostic Interview Schedule for Children (DISC)

The DISC (Costello et al., 1984) is a highly structured interview modeled after the adult DIS. It was commissioned by NIMH in 1979 for use in epidemiological studies with children ages 6–18 (Edelstein & Berler, 1987). The DISC covers a broad range of symptoms, assessing over 30 of the most common psychiatric diagnoses in children and adolescents. As with the DIS, the highly structured format of this interview requires that all questions be read verbatim.

Although originally designed to reflect *DSM-III* criteria (American Psychiatric Association, 1980), the DISC has been updated several times to correspond to changes in diagnostic criteria (for a review of DISC versions, see Shaffer, Fisher, Lucas, Dulcan, & Schwab-Stone, 2000). The current version, DISC-IV, was developed in 1997 to reflect *DSM-IV* criteria (American Psychiatric Association, 1994) and to provide information regarding lifetime prevalence of mental disorders (Rogers, 2001). There are two parallel versions of the DISC-IV: a child version (DISC-C) and a parent version (DISC-P). Although both formats are designed to elicit similar information, there are some small differences. First, the parent version contains additional questions regarding developmental milestones and certain diagnostic categories (e.g., autism, pervasive developmental disorder). Second, questions on the child version have been simplified to increase child comprehension. For example, complex questions have been divided into several items and question length typically does not exceed 10 words (Rogers, 2001). Parent and child interviews should be administered and scored separately (Hodges & Cools, 1990). Administration of both interviews is necessary and each one takes approximately 1½ hr (Rogers, 2001).

The DISC-IV is organized into six diagnostic modules, which are designed to be independent of each other. The six modules include anxiety disorders, miscellaneous disorders, mood disorders, schizophrenia, disruptive behavior disorders, and substance abuse disorders. Based on the respondent's answers to both standard questions and optional probes, each symptom is rated on a 1–3 scale, with a rating of 2 required for clinical significance (Rogers, 2001). As with the DIS, computer scoring only is available for the DISC.

Overall, the DISC has demonstrated modest to good test–retest reliability figures. However, it should be noted that younger children (i.e., ages 6–9) evidenced less reliability (ICCs of 0.43) than older children (ICCs of 0.71) on the DISC-C (Edelbrock, Costello, Dulcan, Kalas, & Conover, 1985). Not surprisingly, other studies have found that children of all ages evidenced less reliability than parents. For example, retesting after several weeks, Schwab-Stone et al. (1993) reported a kappa coefficient of 0.82 for the DISC-P but only 0.64 for the DISC-C. In light of these findings, it is recommended that with this interview format clinicians give more weight to parent than child reports, particularly in the case of younger children (Rogers, 2001).

Interrater reliability studies have reported modest to good reliability figures. For example, utilizing only professional interviewers, Anderson, Williams, McGee, and Silva (1987) reported a high kappa coefficient of 0.70 for current diagnoses.

Unfortunately, concurrent validity studies of the DISC have produced disappointing results (Rogers, 2001). For example, Schwab-Stone et al. (1995), comparing diagnoses obtained from the DISC and from highly trained clinicians, found that the median kappa coefficient was 0.47 on the DISC-P but only 0.33 on the DISC-C. Clearly, interviewers' and clinicians' diagnoses typically do not agree, particularly when utilizing only child information.

Convergent validity studies have reported more promising results than concurrent studies, at least with the parent version of the DISC. For example, Costello, Edelbrock, and Costello (1985) found a moderate correlation of 0.71 between DISC-P symptoms and those reported by parents on the Child Behavior Checklist (CBCL) (Achenbach & Edelbrock, 1983), a broadband measure of general child impairment. However, the DISC-C did not demonstrate convergent validity with the CBCL, as evidenced by the low correlation of only 0.14 between the two instruments.

Semistructured Interview Formats

Schedule for Affective Disorders and Schizophrenia (SADS)

The SADS for adults (Spitzer & Endicott, 1978) is a semistructured interview that was designed primarily for the diagnosis of mood and psychotic disorders (Rogers, 2001). Rather than *DSM* criteria, the SADS is based on RDC (Spitzer,

Endicott, et al., 1978). In contrast to the broad-based format of the DIS, the SADS covers only 23 RDC diagnoses in great depth (Summerfeldt & Antony, 2002). In addition to this depth of coverage, another advantage of the SADS is its ability to assess the severity and duration of symptoms (Rogers, 2001).

Partly because it is a semistructured interview, there are several different versions of the SADS that have been customized by different researchers (for a review of SADS versions, see Rogers, 2001). By far, the most widely used versions are the original SADS and the SADS-Lifetime (SADS-L) (Summerfeldt & Antony, 2002). The original SADS has two main sections: Part I assesses the current episode, while Part II assesses any prior episodes. The SADS-L is similar to Part II of the original SADS; however, the time period is not restricted and instead covers all current and past symptoms (Summerfeldt & Antony, 2002).

Since it is a semistructured interview, the SADS should be administered by clinicians rather than by lay persons, due to the amount of inference and judgment required during administration. As with highly structured interview formats, the SADS contains standard questions asked of all respondents, as well as optional probes that are used to clarify incomplete or ambiguous responses. In addition to these verbatim questions, however, clinicians are free to construct other unscripted questions if necessary (Rogers, 2001). Clinicians also are allowed to utilize their judgment in skipping questions throughout the interview (Summerfeldt & Antony, 2002). The semistructured format broadens the range of time needed to administer the interview. Typically, Part I takes 45–75 min to administer, while Part II takes an additional 15–60 min (Rogers, 2001). However, administration may take up to 4 hr with severely ill clients (Summerfeldt & Antony, 2002).

Ratings of symptoms on the SADS differ from the highly structured interviews in that they are not based solely on interview responses. Instead, clinicians are encouraged to rate symptoms based on a combination of interview data and information collected from record reviews and/or collateral interviews (Rogers, 2001). Once all ratings have been made, they are summed to produce the following eight scales: depressed mood and ideation, endogenous features, depressive-associated features, suicidal ideation and behavior, anxiety, manic syndrome, delusions/hallucinations, and formal thought disorder (Rogers, 2001; Summerfeldt & Antony, 2002).

Test–retest studies generally have reported high coefficients for both current and lifetime diagnoses. For example, retesting after several days, Spitzer, Endicott, et al. (1978) reported median kappa coefficients of 0.91 for current diagnoses and 0.93 for lifetime diagnoses. Interrater reliability studies have shown promise, as well. For example, Andreasen et al. (1982) reported average ICCs of 0.75. It should be noted that these authors utilized professional interviewers exclusively, as the SADS was not designed to be administered by lay interviewers (Rogers, 2001).

Concurrent and convergent validity studies have demonstrated modest to good findings. For example, Hesselbrock, Stabenau, Hesselbrock, Mirkin, and Meyer (1982), in a concurrent study of the SADS and the DIS, reported a median kappa of 0.76 across four common diagnoses. Endicott and Spitzer (1978), in a convergent validity study, compared the SADS to the Symptom Checklist-90 (Derogatis, 1977), a broad measure of distress. These authors reported a moderate correlation of 0.47, which modestly supports the usefulness of the SADS as a measure of general impairment.

Schedule of Affective Disorders and Schizophrenia for School-Age Children (K-SADS)

The K-SADS (Puig-Antich & Chambers, 1978) is a semistructured interview that corresponds to the adult version of the SADS and was designed for children as young as 6 years of age. Of all of the structured interview formats, the K-SADS appears to have the greatest number of alternative versions that have been studied (for a review of K-SADS versions, see Ambrosini, 2000). The most recent version, K-SADS-IV (Ambrosini & Dixon, 1996) corresponds to *DSM-IV* (American Psychiatric Association, 1994) and RDC (Spitzer, Endicott, et al., 1978). There are parallel child and parent versions of the K-SADS-IV, and both should be administered prior to rating symptoms. It is recommended that parents be interviewed prior to children on all occasions. If discrepancies appear between parent and child reports, then such discrepancies should be pointed out to the child, and reconciliation of the two reports should then be made (Rogers, 2001).

Similar to the SADS, reliability studies have demonstrated adequate to high reliability. An early test–retest study by Chambers et al. (1985) over a short time interval (2–3 days) reported kappa coefficients ranging from 0.24–0.70 across diagnostic categories. Testing over several weeks, Kaufman et al. (1997) reported kappa coefficients between 0.63 and 1.0 for current diagnoses and between 0.55 and 1.0 for lifetime diagnoses. Consistency over time was highest for depression diagnoses and bipolar disorder, with less consistency for ADHD and Post-traumatic Stress Disorder (PTSD) (Kaufman et al., 1997).

Interrater reliability figures also have shown promise. For example, Ambrosini, Metz, Prabucki, and Lee (1989) reported mean kappa coefficients of 0.79 for the child version and 0.86 for the parent version. As with the SADS, professional interviewers were utilized in these studies, as the K-SADS was not designed to be administered by lay interviewers.

Validity studies, overall, have demonstrated only modest results. For example, Carlson, Koshani, Thomas, Vaidya, and Daniel (1987), in a concurrent study comparing diagnoses obtained from the parent version of the K-SADS to clinical diagnoses, found a median kappa coefficient of 0.50. Cashel, Rogers, Sewell, and Holliman (1998), in a convergent validity study, compared results from the K-SADS to the Minnesota Multiphasic Personality Inventory for Adolescents (MMPI-A; Butcher et al., 1992). These authors reported only low to modest correlations (in the 0.30–0.50 range).

Structured Clinical Interview for DSM-IV (SCID)

The SCID for adults (Spitzer, Williams, & Gibbon, 1987) is a semistructured interview that is widely used in research settings (Lesser, 1997; Summerfeldt & Antony, 2002). There are several different versions of the SCID, including both research and clinical versions (for a review of SCID versions, see Rogers, 2001).

All versions provide broad coverage of *DSM-IV* disorders, with the most comprehensive version of the SCID covering 51 Axis I diagnostic categories (Rogers, 2001). For many diagnostic categories, information is obtained regarding both current episode and lifetime prevalence. However, the following conditions are only questioned regarding current episode: dysthymic disorder, generalized anxiety disorder, all somatoform disorders, and adjustment disorder (Summerfeldt & Antony, 2002). Administration time ranges from 1–3 hr, depending upon the version employed and the severity of symptoms (Rogers, 2001).

There are several modules within the SCID, organized by diagnostic categories (Rogers, 2001). Clinicians may customize each interview by administering only those modules of interest (Summerfeldt & Antony, 2002). Within each module, there are standard questions asked of each client, required probe questions, and optional follow-up questions (Summerfeldt & Antony, 2002). In addition, clinicians have the flexibility of developing unstructured questions if desired (Rogers, 2001). Within each module, there are clear decision trees for discontinuation, if required symptoms are not endorsed (Rogers, 2001). Similar to the SADS, final ratings are made based on all sources of data, including client interview as well as record review and/or collateral interviews (Rogers, 2001).

Test–retest and interrater reliability studies have demonstrated modest to good coefficients. For example, Williams et al. (1992), utilizing a test–retest design over a 2-week period, reported a mean kappa coefficient of 0.61 for current diagnoses and 0.68 for lifetime diagnoses. It should be noted that reliability figures were higher for certain diagnostic categories, such as bipolar disorder and alcohol or drug abuse, but were only fair for diagnoses such as major depression and generalized anxiety disorder. Riskland, Beck, Berchick, Brown, and Steer (1987), comparing ratings across interviewers, reported a median kappa coefficient of 0.76 for current diagnoses. As with the SADS, only professional interviewers were utilized for this study, due to the semistructured format of the SCID.

Compared to other structured interview formats, relatively few concurrent or construct validity studies have been conducted with the SCID. The lack of these validity studies may be explained by the close correspondence between the SCID and DSM criteria (Rogers, 2001). Of the studies that have been done, adequate to good validity has been demonstrated. For example, in a concurrent validity study, Maziade and colleagues (1992) compared diagnoses obtained from the SCID diagnoses to diagnoses obtained from expert psychiatrists; these authors reported high levels of agreement (kappa = 0.83).

Summary of Specific Interview Formats

In summary, several different structured interview formats exist for both child and adult populations. These formats differ according to level of structure and breadth of diagnostic coverage. In choosing which structured interview to administer, there is no substitute for actually reviewing each format, in order to directly compare wording and ordering of items. Clinicians should write to developers of structured interviews to request a copy of each format (see Table 1 for contact information).

TABLE 1. Contact Information for Interview Formats

DIS-IV
Lee Robins, PhD, Department of Psychiatry, Washington University School of
  Medicine, 4940 Children's Place, St. Louis, MO 63110-1093
DISC-IV
DISC Development Group, 1051 Riverside Drive, Box 78, NY, NY 10032
SADS
Jean Endicott, Department of Research and Training, New York State
  Psychiatric Institute, Unit 123, 1051 Riverside Drive, NY, NY 10032
K-SADS-IV
Paul Ambrosini, MD, 3200 Henry Avenue, Philadelphia, PA 19129-1137
SCID
Research version: SCID Central, Biometrics Research Department, New York
  State Psychiatric Institute, Unit 60, 1051 Riverside Drive, NY, NY 100032
Clinical version: American Psychiatric Press, Inc., 1400 K Street NW,
  Washington, DC 20005

Once interviews are obtained, clinicians should assess several factors, includ-ing the purposes of the interview, practical matters, and psychometric data (Angold & Fisher, 1999). First, clinicians should review the particular needs the interview should meet. Included in this is an examination of the time frame covered by each interview approach, as some structured formats limit certain diagnostic categories to only current episodes (SCID) while others assess both current and lifetime symptoms (DIS, SADS). Also included is a review of diag-nostic coverage, as some formats assess a broad range of diagnostic categories (DIS), whereas others assess a more narrowly defined range (SADS).

Second, clinicians should review practical issues, such as the time and money involved in training on administration and scoring of each interview. In general, more structured interviews (DIS, DISC) minimize the role of inference, thereby allowing lay persons, or those with minimal clinical training, to conduct these inter-views. Semistructured interviews (SADS, K-SADS), which allow greater interviewer latitude in determining question wording and order as well as in interpreting responses, require clinically sophisticated interviewers (Edelbrock & Costello, 1988).

Finally, clinicians should review the available psychometric properties of each interview format. Although much research has been conducted, overall the evidence for reliability and validity of structured interview formats is modest at best. Out of the interview formats reviewed for this chapter, the SADS and K-SADS appear to demonstrate the best psychometric properties, a surprising finding given the semistructured format of these two interviews.

SUMMARY AND RECOMMENDATIONS

Historically, clinicians have employed unstructured interviews to assess client functioning and diagnostic presentation. The flexibility inherent in unstructured interview approaches allowed clinicians to vary every aspect of the interview process, producing significant information variation among clinicians and contributing to diagnostic confusion. In an effort to combat these problems, researchers over the last 30 years have developed several structured interview formats for both child and adult populations. The primary advantage of structured interview formats is the comprehensive coverage of diagnostic categories. In addition, structured interview formats have adequate psychometric properties, something unstructured approaches have had difficulty establishing. Even if reliability and validity figures for structured approaches generally have been modest, today's managed care environment has forced clinicians to seek out assessment instruments with demonstrated psychometric properties.

Although structured interview formats hold much promise, considerably more research is needed before there will be widespread acceptance of these instruments outside research settings. The resistance of many clinicians to employing structured interview formats may be traced to two factors: (1) a dearth of research on the acceptability of structured formats to clients, and (2) a lack of convincing data on the psychometric properties of these interviews. First, there has been little research on client satisfaction with structured interview formats. Particularly with highly structured interviews, which must be read verbatim, there is a risk that clients may be distanced from the diagnostic process and become bored or frustrated. Even semistructured interview formats may be offensive or insulting to clients if they perceive the repeated questions asked throughout several diagnostic modules to be redundant and evidence that the interviewer is not listening. Finally, most structured interview formats are long. It is possible that over the course of the interview clients may become inattentive or unresponsive. Only one study has even indirectly studied client satisfaction utilizing an alternative administration format for the DISC (Edelbrock, Crnic, & Bohnert, 1999). These authors found that allowing respondents to control the administration order of the diagnostic modules, a large departure from the highly structured format of the DISC, resulted in positive client reactions. Further studies assessing client satisfaction with structured interviews may serve to alleviate clinician concerns and increase the use of these formats.

In addition to client acceptability studies, more research is needed on the psychometric properties of structured interview formats. Clearly, research must be conducted with current versions of interviews, as very few studies have employed updated versions. In addition, reliability studies must expand at the diagnostic level, as research has been conducted with only a handful of diagnostic categories. Therefore, "clinicians should not characterize [an interview] as a reliable interview. Rather, they should discuss the reliability of diagnostic categories (e.g., mood disorders) or specific diagnoses" (Rogers, 2001, p. 66). It is likely that the use of structured interviews would increase greatly if studies could establish the overall reliability of each format. Third, more validity studies should be conducted. For example, valid ways of combining child and adult reports have yet to be studied in depth.

Even though structured approaches appeared on the scene three decades ago, such formats are still in the process of being developed and refined. Clinicians have unanswered questions regarding structured formats and have not yet abandoned unstructured approaches to interviewing. Both structured and unstructured approaches to interviewing may be useful at different times and for different purposes. Just as no one personality instrument or self-report questionnaire serves all assessment purposes, neither will one interview format suffice for all clients. It is incumbent on clinicians to remain informed about the research on various interview formats, so that they can make competent decisions regarding which instrument to employ in each assessment situation.

REFERENCES

Achenbach, T. M., & Edelbrock, C. S. (1983). *Manual for the child behavior checklist and revised child behavior profile*. Burlington, VT: University of Vermont.

Ambrosini, P. J. (2000). Historical development and present status of the Schedule for Affective Disorders and Schizophrenia for School-Age Children (K-SADS). *Journal of the American Academy of Child and Adolescent Psychiatry, 39*(1), 49–58.

Ambrosini, P. J., & Dixon, M. (1996). *Schedule for affective disorders and schizophrenia, childhood version* (4th ed.). Philadelphia, PA: Medical College of Pennsylvania.

Ambrosini, P. J., Metz, C., Prabucki, K., & Lee, J. C. (1989). Videotape reliability of the third revised edition of the K-SADS. *Journal of the American Academy of Child and Adolescent Psychiatry, 28*(5), 723–728.

American Psychiatric Association. (1980). *Diagnostic and statistical manual of mental disorders* (3rd ed.). Washington, DC: Author.

American Psychiatric Association. (1994). *Diagnostic and statistical manual of mental disorders* (4th ed.). Washington, DC: Author.

Anastasi, A. (1988). *Psychological testing* (6th ed.). NY: Macmillan.

Anderson, J. C., Williams, S., McGee, R., & Silva, P. A. (1987). DSM-III disorders in preadolescent children. *Archives of General Psychiatry, 42*, 69–76.

Andreasen, N. C., McDonald-Scott, P., Grove, W. M., Keller, M. B., Shapiro, R. W., & Hirschfeld, R. M. A. (1982). Assessment of reliability in multicenter collaborative research with a videotape approach. *American Journal of Psychiatry, 139*, 876–882.

Angold, A., & Fisher, P. W. (1999). Interviewer-based interviews. In D. Shaffer, C. P. Lucas, & J. E. Richters (Eds.), *Diagnostic assessment in child and adolescent psychopathology* (pp. 34–64). NY: Guilford Press.

Butcher, J. N., Williams, C. L., Graham, J. R., Archer, R., Tellegen, A., Ben-Porath, Y. S., et al. (1992). *MMPI-A manual for administration, scoring, and interpretation*. Minneapolis, MN: University of Minnesota Press.

Carlson, G. A., Koshani, J. H., Thomas, M. D. F., Vaidya, A., & Daniel, A. E. (1987). Comparison of the DISC and the K-SADS-P interviews in an epidemiological sample of children. *Journal of the American Academy of Child and Adolescent Psychiatry, 26*, 645–648.

Cashel, M. L., Rogers, R., Sewell, K. W., & Holliman, N. (1998). Preliminary validation of the MMPI-A for a male delinquent sample: An investigation of clinical correlates and discriminant validity. *Journal of Personality Assessment, 71*, 49–69.

Chambers, W., Puig-Antich, J., Hirsch, M., Paez, P., Ambrosini, P. J., Tabrizi, M. A., et al. (1985). The assessment of affective disorders in children and adolescents by semistructured interview: Test–retest reliability of the K-SADS-P. *Archives of General Psychiatry, 42*, 696–702.

Cohen, J. (1960). A coefficient of agreement for nominal scales. *Educational and Psychological Measurement, 20*, 37–46.

Cone, J. D. (1998). Psychometric considerations: Concepts, contents, and methods. In A. S. Bellack & M. Hersen (Eds.), *Behavioral assessment: A practical handbook* (4th ed., pp. 22–46). Boston, MA: Allyn & Bacon.

Costello, A. J., Edelbrock, C., Dulcan, M. K., Kalas, R., & Klaric, S. H. (1984). *Development and testing of the NIMH Diagnostic Interview Schedule for Children in a clinic population*. (Final report, Contract No. RFP-DB-81–0027). Rockville, MD: Center for Epidemiological Studies, National Institute of Mental Health.

Costello, E. J., Edelbrock, C. S., & Costello, A. J. (1985). Validity of the NIMH Diagnostic Interview Schedule for Children: A comparison between psychiatric and pediatric referrals. *Journal of Abnormal and Child Psychology, 13*(4), 579–595.

Derogatis, L. R. (1977). *The SCL-90 manual: Scoring, administration, and procedures for the SCL-90.* Baltimore, MD: Johns Hopkins University.

Edelbrock, C., & Costello, A. J. (1988). Structured psychiatric interviews for children. In M. Rutter, A. H. Tuma, & I. S. Lann (Eds.), *Assessment and diagnosis in child psychopathology* (pp. 87–112). NY: Guilford Press.

Edelbrock, C., Crnic, K., & Bohnert, A. (1999). Interviewing as communication: An alternative way of administering the Diagnostic Interview Schedule for Children. *Journal of Abnormal Child Psychology, 27*(6), 447–453.

Edelbrock, C., Costello, A. J., Dulcan, M. K., Conover, N. C., & Kalas, R. (1986). Parent–child agreement on child psychiatric symptoms assessed via structured interview. *Journal of Child Psychology and Psychiatry, 27*, 181–190.

Edelbrock, C., Costello, A. J., Dulcan, M. K., Kalas, R., & Conover, N. C. (1985). Age differences in the reliability of the psychiatric interview of the child. *Child Development, 56*, 265–275.

Edelstein, B. A., & Berler, E. S. (1987). Interviewing and report writing. In C. L. Frame & J. L. Matson (Eds.), *Handbook of assessment in childhood psychopathology: Applied issues in differential diagnosis and treatment evaluation* (pp. 163–184). NY: Plenum Press.

Endicott, J., & Spitzer, R. L. (1978). A diagnostic interview: The schedule for affective disorders and schizophrenia. *Archives of General Psychiatry, 35*(7), 837–844.

Friedman, J. M. H. (1989). Structured interviews: The expert's vantage. In S. Wetzler & M. Katz (Eds.), *Contemporary approaches to psychological assessment* (pp. 83–97). NY: Brunner/Mazel.

Hamilton, M. (1960). A rating scale for depression. *Journal of Neurology, Neurosurgery, and Psychiatry, 23*, 56–62.

Helzer, J. E., Robins, L. N., McEvoy, L. T., Spitznagel, E. L., Stolzman, R. K., Farmer, A., et al. (1985). A comparison of clinical and Diagnostic Interview Schedule diagnoses: Physician reexamination of lay-interviewed cases in the general population. *Archives of General Psychiatry, 42*, 657–666.

Helzer, J. E., Spitznagel, E. L., & McEvoy, L. T. (1987). The predictive validity of lay Diagnostic Interview Schedule diagnoses in the general population: A comparison with physician examiners. *Archives of General Psychiatry, 44*, 1069–1077.

Herjanic, B., Herjanic, M., Brown, F., & Wheatt, T. (1975). Are children reliable reporters? *Journal of Abnormal Child Psychology, 3*, 41–48.

Hesselbrock, V., Stabenau, J., Hesselbrock, M., Mirkin, P., & Meyer, R. (1982). A comparison of two interview schedules: The Schedule for Affective Disorders and Schizophrenia-Lifetime and the National Institute of Mental Health Diagnostic Interview Schedule. *Archives of General Psychiatry, 39*(6), 674–677.

Hodges, K. (1993). Structured interviews for assessing children. *Journal of Child Psychology and Psychiatry, 34*(1), 49–68.

Hodges, K. H., & Cools, J. N. (1990). Structured diagnostic interviews. In A. M. La Greca (Ed.), *Through the eyes of the child* (pp. 109–149). Boston, MA: Allyn & Bacon.

Hodges, K. H., Gordon, Y., & Lennon, M. (1990). Parent–child agreement on symptoms assessed via a clinical research interview for children: The Child Assessment Schedule (CAS). *Journal of Child Psychology and Psychiatry, 31*, 427–431.

Kaufman, J., Birmaher, B., Brent, D., Rao, U., Flynn, C., Moreci, P., et al. (1997). Schedule for Affective Disorder and Schizophrenia for School-Age Children—Present and Lifetime Version (K-SADS-PL): Initial reliability and validity data. *Journal of the American Academy of Child and Adolescent Psychiatry, 36*, 980–988.

Korchin, S. J. (1976). *Modern clinical psychology: Principles of intervention in the clinic and community.* NY: Basic Books.

Landis, J. R., & Koch, G. G. (1977). The measurement of observer agreement for categorical data. *Biometrics, 33*, 159–174.

Lesser, I. M. (1997). Cultural considerations using the Structured Clinical Interview for DSM-III for mood and anxiety disorders assessment. *Journal of Psychopathology and Behavioral Assessment, 19*(2), 149–159.

Mash, E. J., & Terdel, L. G. (1997). *Assessment of childhood disorders* (3rd ed.). NY: Guilford Press.

Maziade, M., Roy, A. A., Fournier, J. P., Cliche, D., Merette, C., Caron, C., et al. (1992). Reliability of best-estimate diagnosis in genetic linkage studies of major psychosis. *American Journal of Psychiatry, 149*, 1674–1686.

Puig-Antich, J., & Chambers, W. (1978). *The Schedule for Affective Disorders and Schizoprenia for School-Age Children (Kiddie-SADS)*. NY: New York State Psychiatric Institute.

Riskland, J. H., Beck, A. T., Berchick, R. J., Brown, G., & Steer, R. A. (1987). Reliability of DSM-III diagnoses for major depression and generalized anxiety disorder using the Structured Clinical Interview for DSM-III. *Archives of General Psychiatry, 44*, 817–820.

Robins, L. N. (1985). Epidemiology: Reflections on testing the validity of psychiatric interviews. *Archives of General Psychiatry, 42*, 918–924.

Robins, L. N., Cottler, L., Bucholz, K., & Compton, W. (1995). *The Diagnostic Interview Schedule, Version 4*. St. Louis, MO: Washington University.

Robins, L. N., Helzer, J. E., Croughan, J., & Ratcliff, K. S. (1981). The National Institute of Mental Health Diagnostic Interview Schedule: Its history, characteristics, and validity. *Archives of General Psychiatry, 38*(4), 381–389.

Rogers, R. (1995). *Diagnostic and structured interviewing: A handbook for psychologists*. Odessa, FL: Psychological Assessment Resources.

Rogers, R. (2001). *Handbook of diagnostic and structured interviewing*. New York, NY: The Guilford Press.

Sarwer, D. B., & Sayers, S. L. (1998). Behavioral interviewing. In A. S. Bellack & M. Hersen (Eds.), *Behavioral assessment* (4th ed., pp. 63–78). Boston, MA: Allyn & Bacon.

Sattler, J. M. (1992). *Assessment of children* (revised and updated 3rd ed.). San Diego, CA: Jerome M. Sattler.

Schwab-Stone, M., Fisher, P., Piacentini, J., Shaffer, D., Davies, M., & Briggs, M. (1993). The Diagnostic Interview Schedule for Children—Revised Version (DISC-R): II. Test–retest reliability. *Journal of American Academy of Child and Adolescent Psychiatry, 32*, 651–657.

Schwab-Stone, M., Shaffer, D., Davies, M., Dulcan, M. K., Jensen, P. S., Fisher, P., et al. (1995). The Diagnostic Interview Schedule for Children—Version 2.3 (DISC-2.3). *Journal of American Academy of Child and Adolescent Psychiatry, 35*, 878–888.

Selzer, M. L. (1971). Michigan Alcoholism Screening Test: The quest for a new diagnostic instrument. *American Journal of Psychiatry, 127*, 1653–1658.

Shaffer, D., Fisher, P. W., & Lucas, C. P. (1999). Respondent-based interviews. In D. Shaffer, C. P. Lucas, & J. E. Richters (Eds.), *Diagnostic assessment in child and adolescent psychopathology* (pp. 3–33). NY: Guilford Press.

Shaffer, D., Fisher, P. W., Lucas, C. P., Dulcan, M., & Schwab-Stone, M. E. (2000). NIMH Diagnostic Interview Schedule for Children, Version IV (NIMH DISC-IV): Description, differences from previous versions, and reliability of some common diagnoses. *Journal of the American Academy of Child and Adolescent Psychiatry, 39*(1), 28–38.

Sher, K. J., & Trull, T. J. (1996). Methodological issues in psychopathology research. *Annual Review of Psychology, 47*, 371–400.

Spitzer, R. L., & Endicott, J. (1978). *Schedule for affective disorders and schizophrenia* (3rd ed.). NY: Biometrics Research.

Spitzer, R. L., Endicott, J., & Robins, E. (1978). Research diagnostic criteria for use in psychiatric research. *Archives of General Psychiatry, 35*, 773–782.

Spitzer, R. L., Fleiss, J. L., & Endicott, J. (1978). Problems of classification: Reliability and validity. In M. A. Lipton, A. DiMasco, & K. Killam (Eds.), *Psychopharmacology: A generation of progress* (pp. 857–869). NY: Raven Press.

Spitzer, R. L., Williams, J. B. W., & Gibbon, M. (1987). *Structured clinical interview for DSM-III-R (SCID)*. NY: Biometrics Research.

Summerfeldt, L. J., & Antony, M. M. (2002). Structured and semistructured diagnostic interviews. In A. M. Antony (Ed.), *Handbook of assessment and treatment planning for psychological disorders* (pp. 3–37). New York, NY: Guilford Press.

Vandiver, T., & Sher, K. (1991). Temporal stability of the Diagnostic Interview Schedule. *Psychological Assessment, 3*, 277–281.

Ward, C. H., Beck, A. T., Mendelson, M., Mock, J. E., & Erbaugh, J. K. (1962). The psychiatric nomen-
    clature. *Archives of General Psychiatry, 7*, 198–205.
Wells, K. B., Burnham, A., Leake, B., & Robins, L. N. (1988). Agreement between face-to-face and
    telephone-administered versions of the depression section of the NIMH Diagnostic Interview
    Schedule. *Journal of Psychiatric Research, 22*, 207–220.
Whisman, M. A., Strosahl, K., Fruzetti, A. E., Schmaling, K. B., Jacobson, N. S., & Miller, D. M. (1989).
    A structured interview version of the Hamilton Rating Scale for Depression: Reliability and valid-
    ity. *Psychological Assessment, 1*, 238–241.
Williams, J. B. W., Gibbon, M., First, M. B., Spitzer, R. L., Davies, M., Borus, J., et al. (1992). The
    Structured Clinical Interview for DSM-III-R (SCID): II. Multisite test–retest reliability. *Archives of
    General Psychiatry, 49*, 630–636.

4

Consideration of Neuropsychological Factors in Interviewing

David M. Freed

Introduction

Our world is, first and foremost, a world of other persons. For most individuals, success is based on ability to successfully interact with other individuals, to convey and receive information. The salesman's ability to assess a potential client, an advertiser's sensitivity to consumers, a judge's ability to evaluate an individual's guilt, a suitor's ability to determine receptivity, and a psychologist's ability to infer parental fitness are all examples of the importance of assessment. Assessment is the process by which we acquire information about other individuals.

We learn about or "assess" other individuals by questioning or observing—we either "ask 'em or watch 'em" (Sundberg, 1977). In some cases, we learn about individuals by questioning others who know them or by reviewing historical documents (e.g., medical records, school records, military records), but this occurs only in very specialized contexts. Similarly, assessment through observation (which includes test administration) is performed by a small percentage of highly trained individuals, such as psychologists or psychiatrists. By and large, the vast majority of information that we acquire about individuals is obtained through conversation and by asking questions. Salesmen ask questions of potential clients, advertisers query focus groups of consumers, and family physicians begin their physical examination with "What seems to be the matter today?" The interview process is thus the foundation of all assessment. Put another way, "Clinical interviews compose the essential core of current diagnostic and assessment methods" (Rogers, 1997).

Interviewing is decidedly low-tech and does not have the glamour of magnetic resonance imaging (MRI), quantitative electroencephalography (EEG), or computerized assessment. Most beginning clinicians are more likely to have a

---

David M. Freed • Department of Human Services, Oregon State Hospital, Salem, Oregon 97310.

course in pharmacology than interviewing (despite the critical importance of both topics), just as in a world filled with television, CDs, and the internet, conversation seems to be a lost art. In this author's experience, however, the most highly skilled clinicians are those most skilled in the art of interview. I recall the late Norman Geschwind, who could evoke critical information from a patient in a few short minutes. This efficient use of the clinical interview was the result of vast clinical experience and highly developed observation skills.

The clinical interview can be adapted to a variety of circumstances and diverse patient populations. Such versatility is also the greatest liability of the clinical interview. On scientific grounds, the individuality of interviews and interviewing styles makes standardization impractical and empirical study difficult (Rogers, 1997). This liability can be addressed by crafting structured interviews, but only at the expense of versatility. Experienced clinicians have in their heads a set of questions designed to elicit critical information, perhaps even utilizing structured or semistructured interviews with specific populations. Put simply, seasoned clinicians possess knowledge that efficiently guides the interview. This may sound trivial, but it takes years of practice to know what to ask and how to ask it while avoiding unimportant questions.

THE RELATIONSHIP BETWEEN BRAIN AND BEHAVIOR

Psychology is defined as the study of mental processes or alternatively as the study of human or animal behavior (*Webster's New Universal Unabridged Dictionary*, 1983). Unfortunately, both of these definitions tend to overlook recent trends in neuroscience that emphasize the role of the machinery of the brain as opposed to the theoretical operations of the mind. An understanding of this machinery is vital if a clinician is to recognize neurologic disease or injury. Put another way, there are many individuals who do not understand the operation of the internal combustion engine yet are safe drivers. However, it would be inadvisable to depend on one of these individuals to diagnose a fault with a modern fuel injection system (although they may be perfectly capable of referring you to a qualified mechanic).

The human brain is the most complex system that we are aware of, rivaling the known universe in terms of numbers. For example, it is estimated that there are 10^{12} neurons in the human nervous system (Nauta & Feirtag, 1986). (Neurons come in a great variety of sizes and shapes such that estimates may vary by several orders of magnitude.) Each of these neurons has synaptic connections with an average of perhaps 5,000 other neurons, although again there is enormous variation. This elaborate neuronal network is supported by huge numbers of non-neural glial cells, with estimates suggesting perhaps ten times as many glial cells as neurons (Nauta & Feirtag, 1986). While initially thought of as mere scaffolding, neuroscientists now recognize that glial cells play an important role by transporting, secreting, and sequestering chemical agents important for neuronal communication. More important than sheer numbers, however, is the precise and elaborate arrangement of neurons as well as their inputs and outputs.

The precision of this network is reflected in the consistency of neuronal organization from one individual to another and provides the basis for systematic study that we call neuroanatomy. The overwhelming complexity of cell types as well as their precise and elaborate organization is the basis for the complexity of human behavior.

This elaborate network of neurons is only part of the story, however. Neurons communicate with one another through the use of chemical agents known as neurotransmitters. In addition, there is a variety of chemical compounds that modulate ongoing neuronal activity, and these are known as neuromodulators. Neuromodulators include hormones such as estrogen and testosterone. Taken together, there are dozens of neurotransmitters, neurohormones, and neuromodulators that influence functioning of the central nervous system. Adding to this complexity is the fact that any given neurotransmitter may serve to potentiate neuronal activity in one area and inhibit neuronal activity in another. Similarly, activity of a neurotransmitter may be measured in milliseconds in one area and minutes (or hours) in another. The overwhelming complexity of the physical structure of the nervous system is multiplied many times over by the diversity of neurochemical signaling. The human brain is even capable of monitoring the carbohydrate to protein ratio of our diet in order to modify behavior in terms of food selection (Wurtman et al., 1985.)

Given the tools of modern neuroscience (among them electron microscopes, radioactive tracers, and MRI), how do we study the relationship of brain structure to behavior? Historically, this is an easy question to answer: study abnormal behavior and identify the associated brain regions. This was the approach taken by Paul Broca in the mid-19th century to identify postmortem a brain region essential for fluent speech and which still bears his name. (It should be noted that there are difficulties with this approach, but when the only tool you have is a hammer, problems tend to present themselves as nails.) Neuropsychology was given its greatest impetus by World War I and World War II, when the technology of mass destruction (e.g., high velocity projectiles and shrapnel) met advances in battlefield medicine. The net result was that relatively large numbers of individuals who sustained penetrating brain injuries survived for future study. It has been jokingly said that the greatest advance in neuropsychology was not the computer tomography (CT) scan but the machine gun. Today, clinical neuropsychologists continue to study accidents of nature due to disease or injury. This is still the prevalent approach today, although advances in neuroimaging are starting to provide some other tools. It is like studying a supercomputer by firing bullets at it and later seeing what does not work.

The point of this brief discussion of clinical neuroscience is to illustrate that human behavior is the product of complex neuronal interactions. If this elaborate neuronal network is disrupted in any significant fashion, behavior is also likely to be disrupted. For the neuropsychologist, this means that changes in behavior are often an early indicator of brain dysfunction. Perhaps the clearest demonstration of this fact is revealed in Parkinson's disease. The resting tremor, paucity of voluntary movement, loss of postural reflexes, and hypophonic speech characteristic of this disorder are the result of the loss of a specific neuron type in a circumscribed brain region, the pars compacta of the substantia nigra. The loss of 80% of some half million cells in this brain region results in the clinical disorder that we know as Parkinson's disease (Cote & Crutcher, 1991). Furthermore, administering the building block of the neurotransmitter found in these cells can temporarily reverse the symptoms of Parkinson's disease.

Behavior is often the most sensitive indicator of brain dysfunction. Psychologists have developed an elaborate array of "objective" tests of memory, visuospatial ability, and personality, with new tests being added at a dizzying rate. What is not widely recognized, however, is that these objective tests are simply standardized ways to sample human behavior. We do not measure "memory," only an individual's responses to specific questions. We infer that these responses accurately reflect a mental function such as memory, but it is only the behavioral responses to the questions that are observable, not memory per se. Put another way, objective tests are useful tools, but are frequently misused. Test data can only be interpreted in light of the subject's observed behavior during the testing session and in the context of knowledge of that individual. For example, administering the *Wechsler Memory Scale—Third Edition* to a primarily Spanish-speaking subject tells us nothing about that individual's memory function, only their linguistic and cultural background. Objective tests are not "magic windows" into mental functioning. Furthermore, the relationship between mental processes and brain function in most cases is poorly understood. Unwavering reliance upon objective tests in isolation is a critical mistake. Information obtained during the clinical interview is vital to understanding test performance.

BRAIN DYSFUNCTION AND ITS DIAGNOSIS

It is incumbent upon the practicing psychologist (and particularly, the neuropsychologist) to be sensitive to the possibility that a client's behavioral abnormalities are due to neurologic disease or injury. This is not to say that every problem that is psychological or behavioral in nature is due to obvious brain dysfunction, but simply that many neurobiological issues go unrecognized and undiagnosed. I recently accepted a position in a large, state-run psychiatric hospital after many years in university-affiliated clinics and hospitals. I have been impressed (and disheartened) by the relatively large number of psychiatric patients with unrecognized symptoms related to neurobiologic dysfunction. Two individuals in particular come to mind.

The first individual has spent many years in a maximum-security psychiatric setting due to unpredictable assaultiveness. This individual has spent thousands of hours in ambulatory restraints during the day due to his aggression, and the fact that he reports feeling safer in the restraints. Like many long-term psychiatric inpatients, this individual was abused both physically and sexually as a child. His aggressive episodes are heralded by increasing agitation, hallucinations involving appearance of family members (particularly those who victimized him), and misidentification of individuals around him. While he had a history of behavioral disturbance as a child, the noted psychiatric symptoms presented acutely following a traumatic brain injury involving the right parietal lobe. Neuropsychological testing recently revealed that this individual suffers from prosopagnosia, an inability to recognize familiar faces, likely as a result of the reported traumatic brain injury. It seems apparent that this individual's history of abuse and early behavioral disturbance was compounded by a traumatic brain injury resulting in the current constellation of symptoms.

The second individual is a young man of college age who has been hospitalized for approximately two years. He is in ambulatory restraints due to well-planned attacks on staff that occur on a daily basis. This individual was a good student in high school and displayed no significant psychiatric symptoms. Shortly after enrolling in the university, this young man attended a party where he consumed alcohol and became acutely intoxicated. He left the party on his bicycle and was later discovered disoriented and bloodied. It is unclear whether he fell off the bicycle or was (according to his report) assaulted. Evaluated at the student health center the following morning, his disorientation was assumed to be secondary to acute intoxication and dehydration. His behavior immediately following the accident was clearly disordered, resulting later in his expulsion from the university. Unfortunately, presence of a significant traumatic brain injury was recognized some weeks following the accident, although at that time the observed symptoms appeared to be disproportionate to the extent of injury. The symptoms slowly began to resolve, although agitation and aggression were prominent. The scientific literature is beginning to recognize that traumatic brain injury sustained while acutely intoxicated is associated with slow recovery and poorer prognosis (Tate, Freed, Bombardier, Harter, & Brinkman, 1999).

This individual appeared to be responding to treatment with neuroleptic medications and was later released to the care of his mother. However, following ongoing difficulties with his mother, this young man apparently attempted suicide by "huffing" propane. He was discovered glassy-eyed and unresponsive. Shortly afterward, this individual developed an elaborate delusional system related to a popular television program. Proclaiming his willingness to proceed to the "next level" and his unwillingness to trust anyone, he refused to consume solid food despite repeated and increasingly desperate attempts by staff and physicians. Having lost thirty or more pounds, tube feeding was begun, something this individual actively resisted. More than a year has passed with daily tube-feedings and active resistance necessitating the use of restraints. An enormous array of medications (individually and in combination) has proven ineffective. A compelling argument can be made that this individual's psychiatric presentation is secondary to the interactive effects of a traumatic brain injury, alcohol intoxication, and acute exposure to propane while "huffing."

The point of presenting these cases is 2-fold. First, these two individuals are fairly representative of long-term psychiatric inpatients who typically present with complicated histories of victimization through child abuse, long-term drug abuse, and possible head injuries. The second purpose is to reiterate the long-standing observation that issues once thought to be solely the province of psychiatry are now the province of neurology due to recognized brain pathology. For example, the classic disease of psychiatry, schizophrenia, is now known to respond in many cases to dopaminergic drugs and be associated with dopamine receptor abnormalities as well as well-defined cognitive impairments (Tamminga, 1997). A compelling argument can be made that schizophrenia is a brain-based disease. It is also entirely possible that perinatal factors and early childhood experiences contribute to enduring changes in brain biology that result in certain forms of mental illness. What is most obvious is the extent of our ignorance in regard to the workings of the brain.

While previous conclusions as to psychiatric illness may be controversial, there can be little doubt about the neurologic basis of many other diseases that may be initially encountered by psychologists. It behooves the practicing psychologist to be familiar with the neuropathology and symptoms associated with these relatively common disorders. In school-aged children, Attention Deficit Hyperactivity Disorder (ADHD) and Learning Disabilities are two of the most common disorders encountered by psychologists. As for ADHD, there is accumulating evidence that this is a brain-based disorder, from its increased occurrence in first-degree relatives (*Diagnostic and Statistical Manual of Mental Disorders*, Fourth Edition, Text Revision [DSM-IV-TR], 2000) to the relatively consistent therapeutic response elicited by psychostimulants (DuPaul, Barkley, & Connor, 1998). Learning disabilities are also commonly observed in first-degree relatives, and in the case of reading disorder (or dyslexia), may be associated with subtle abnormalities of neuronal migration in specific left hemisphere brain regions (Galaburda, Sherman, Rosen, Aboitiz, & Geschwind, 1985). Depression has been noted to result in a constellation of cognitive impairments related to attention and memory. Furthermore, symptoms of depression (including the observed cognitive impairments) respond to antidepressant medications, with the most common agents being selective serotonergic reuptake inhibitors (Mayberg, Mahurin, & Brannan, 1997). Symptoms of depression are also commonly encountered following coronary artery bypass surgery, which is also associated with memory dysfunction, but response to antidepressant medications seems to be less favorable than in depression.

Alcohol is the most commonly used psychotropic drug, and long-term abuse can lead to impairments in memory and visuospatial function. Specific thalamic nuclei and regions of the cerebellum are compromised following long-term alcohol abuse (Adams & Victor, 1993). Other more recent recreational drugs, such as ecstasy or methamphetamines, may be even more destructive to brain tissue following long-term abuse. State psychiatric facilities are filled with individuals who committed crimes following an extended period of methamphetamine abuse during which they suffered from hallucinations and paranoia. Certain prescription medications, particularly in the elderly, may also be associated with psychiatric and cognitive changes (McConnell & Duffy, 1994). There can be little doubt that drugs, whether recreational or prescription, can result in psychological symptoms. The careful clinician is wise to explore the use of recreational drugs and prescription medications during the clinical interview.

It is also important to note that chemical exposure in the workplace can result in enduring symptoms, both physical and psychological. Workers involved in electronic manufacturing, the petrochemical industry, agriculture, painting, and welding, to name only a few, may be at risk of occupational exposure to neurotoxins. More than 65,000 chemicals are found in the EPA's inventory of toxic chemicals and over 1,000 notices of intent to manufacture new substances are received annually (Office of Technology Assessment, 1990). The clinical interview should, by necessity, include questions on current and previous jobs. Where occupational exposure is possible, information about specific job duties and chemical use should be obtained. Both duration of exposure and intensity of exposure are of importance. Furthermore, information concerning any industrial accidents or unusual events should be collected.

I was once referred an older adult for evaluation of possible Alzheimer's disease. He was a small business owner who had retired in the past year due to memory impairment. At interview, I noticed that he was completely bald and lacked eyebrows, eyelashes, and even hair on his arms. When questioned whether this was a life-long condition, he reported that the hair loss had occurred in the past year, coinciding in time with onset of memory impairment. Upon further questioning, this gentleman reported that he had owned and operated a dry-cleaning establishment for more than 20 years. As such, he had worked with dry-cleaning solvents such as carbon tetrachloride and later trichlorethylene. With considerable reluctance, he recounted being cited by the state's Environmental Protection Agency for unacceptable levels of solvent vapors just prior to his retirement. Several of his employees suffered from health problems and quit, as did employees of neighboring businesses. With even greater reluctance, this individual described an industrial accident in which a 55-gal drum of dry-cleaning solvent was spilled. Onset of his memory impairment coincided with the aftermath of the accident in which he had to run the business himself due to his employee's illnesses. Laboratory testing conducted at the University of Miami's School of Medicine revealed serum levels of trichlorethylene elevated 50-fold more than a year following the accident. It was concluded that this individual's memory impairment was due to chemical exposure in the workplace. The gentleman's hair started to re-grow and his memory improved slightly over time.

Some of the most common neurologic disorders include traumatic brain injury, Parkinson's disease, cerebrovascular disease, and Alzheimer's disease. It is not unusual for an individual to suffer from these disorders and seek assistance from a psychologist without having been evaluated medically. It is estimated that roughly 410,000 people in the United States suffer head injuries resulting in brain trauma each year (Kraus et al., 1984). Cognitive impairments can also be encountered in individuals with no observable brain pathology, although the impairments tend to be time-limited. More than 1 million Americans suffer from Parkinson's disease, a disorder in which symptoms may evolve slowly over time. Many individuals seek medical attention before the clinical diagnosis can be made with any certainty and may be labeled as hysterical. Cerebrovascular accidents are typically thought of as having a dramatic presentation. Neurologists and neuropathologists point out, however, that subtle evidence of cerebrovascular disease (e.g., lacunar infarcts, mixed dementia, ischemic white matter disease observed on MRI scans) is commonly observed in older adults. These subtle changes may be clinically invisible, that is to say not sufficient for the individual to seek out medical attention acutely but sufficient to produce subtle signs and symptoms (Starkstein and Robinson, 1994). Finally, Alzheimer's disease is estimated to affect 4 million Americans and is associated with an insidious onset. There is no single diagnostic test for this illness that is frequently diagnosed in later stages by its relatively characteristic presentation in the absence of any significant medical findings. Given its insidious onset and characteristically slow progression, psychologists frequently encounter this illness in clinical practice prior to a formal medical diagnosis. In many cases, psychologists may be the first healthcare practitioners to encounter a variety of neurologic disorders. Knowing what questions to ask and when to refer to a medical professional are essential skills in these cases. The clinical interview can be a vital source of information.

THE REFERRAL QUESTION

The clinical interview in neuropsychological settings begins with the referral question. Knowledge of the referring professional (such as their sophistication with neuropsychological issues), the nature of their patients, and referral patterns can help guide the clinical interview before it ever begins. It is sometimes important to clarify the referral question or to read between the lines. For example, a referral for evaluation of possible memory loss may be quite different depending upon the referral source; a neurologist may be asking a very different question from an attorney or a social worker. As a general rule, more sophisticated users provide more useful and focused referral questions. It is also true, however, that healthcare professionals may assume that they have a level of sophistication that is not always in evidence. Diplomacy and good communication skills are then required in order to clarify the referral question (assuming that one cares about future referrals). A good referral question will likely pertain to the central functions of neuropsychological assessment (that is, diagnosis vs. description of the syndrome). In addition, a good referral question will help neuropsychologists develop hypotheses to test during their evaluation of the client.

The next step is to determine what information will be critical in addressing the referral question, with the goal being to develop a plan of action. This plan may include: requesting medical documentation from the referral source prior to the initial appointment, developing a list of needed information (e.g., hospital records, school records, prior psychological evaluations), requesting that a collateral informant accompany the client, sending out a history-taking form to be completed and returned at the initial appointment, mapping out questions that need to be asked during the interview, and deciding upon tests to be administered. Efficiency and clinical effectiveness can be greatly enhanced by careful preparation prior to the evaluation, to the extent that this is possible. Obviously, clinical context will determine to what extent advance preparations are possible—there are great differences between a planned outpatient evaluation and one conducted at bedside in an emergency room. In general, however, the clinical interview in neuropsychological settings is greatly facilitated by a prior review of all available information.

THE VALUE OF CLINICAL OBSERVATIONS

It is the duty of the clinician to collect and integrate information central to the referral question. Utility of the clinical interview is dependent upon the active involvement of the interviewer who must be constantly aware of the type of information that is important to the situation. My own experience suggests that careful history taking and systematic observation are more important than standardized testing. Indeed such history taking provides hypotheses to be evaluated through psychological or neuropsychological testing. For example, an insurance company referred a client for neuropsychological evaluation of a possible traumatic brain injury secondary to a motor vehicle accident. There was no neuroradiologic evidence of injury and the insurance company had doubts about the severity of the reported symptoms, but the possibility of "post-concussive syndrome" needed to be carefully considered. The client arrived for the evaluation wearing dark glasses and I observed him shuffling slowly down the hall, stopping to lean against walls. What was troubling to me was that the client's wife and son walked some distance behind and seemed relatively unconcerned about the displayed disability. When interviewed separately, the client's wife did not express grief or question what was happening with her husband. Not surprisingly, neuropsychological testing in this case was largely uninformative, as the client was quite familiar with the nature of the tests (having been evaluated previously) and may have been "coached." The pattern of test results, but particularly the family's lack of concern, strongly suggested malingering. Tongue-in-cheek, I now refer to the caregiver's emotional responses to the reported symptoms as the "spousal distress test." Good observation skills are critical for the neuropsychologist.

Everything is grist for the skilled clinician's mill. Asking direct questions can be a valuable approach but some clients may be unable or unwilling to provide direct answers. The interview must be augmented by careful observations. Even when working with a compliant client, observations can be invaluable to the clinician. For example, presence of a fine tremor at rest, difficulty arising from a sitting position, shuffling gait, problems with balance, and a soft voice may signal presence of a disorder such as Parkinson's disease. Word-finding difficulty in an older adult (particularly when coupled with objective evidence of memory impairment and a caregiver's report of impairments in activities of daily living) may signal the presence of a dementia such as Alzheimer's disease. Appearance, personal hygiene, mood, sensory and motor function, self-awareness, vocabulary, intonation, speech prosody, the nature of social interactions, fatigue, frustration, awareness of disability, and emotional lability are important to note. Clinical observations will provide information that can guide test selection as well as the need to request ancillary information from an informant or another healthcare provider.

Clinical observations can also have an important impact upon interpretation of test results. I was once asked to evaluate a liver-transplant candidate. As part of the evaluation process, I administered the Controlled Oral Word Association Test (Spreen & Benton, 1969) to this individual. While providing words beginning with the letter "F," an attractive young nurse walked by. The client followed her with his eyes (socially inappropriate), asked about four-letter words (also socially inappropriate), and then provided the following responses: filly, frilly, frolic, flirt, fun, fundamental, fornicate, and so on. The client's quantitative performance on this test fell within the average range but the qualitative nature of his responses suggested mild disinhibition and the possibility of frontal-lobe impairment. Upon further testing, the client's frontal-lobe deficits (likely secondary to alcohol and drug abuse) were readily apparent. Clinical observations (both before and during objective testing) can provide valuable information.

Direct observation of the client, in some cases, can be rendered more useful through the application of well-known rating scales such as the Brief Psychiatric Rating Scale (Overall & Gorham, 1962). However, it should be remembered that the basis of these rating scales is clinical observation.

The Type of Information to Obtain

When neurologic disease or injury is suspected, the history-taking interview should focus on neurobiological factors known to affect behavior including remote historical factors as well as issues proximal to the referral question. Lezak (1995) organizes this information into four domains: medical history, social history, present life circumstances, and circumstances surrounding the evaluation. Consider the example of a young adult referred for evaluation of a traumatic brain injury. It is important to know something about the birth and education of this individual as well as details of the accident itself. In general, every interview should touch upon basic demographics (i.e., age, gender, ethnicity, level of education, occupational history), medical history, family history, legal involvement, special interests or abilities, as well as regionalisms and cultural issues. A good example of regionalisms can be found in the use of the Boston Naming Test (Kaplan, Goodglass, & Weintraub, 1978). The Boston Naming Test contains simple line drawings of 60 objects, ranging from a bed to an abacus. A single response is viewed as correct. However, older adults in West Texas and Oklahoma commonly call a "harmonica" a "mouth organ," call a "helicopter" a "whirlybird," and call a "mushroom" a "toadstool." Strict scoring of the Boston Naming Test in situations such as this would lead to mistakes.

A detailed medical history must begin with events prior to birth and is especially important when working with young children suspected of suffering from neurologic or neurodevelopmental disorders. Maternal illness (including substance abuse) as well as labor and delivery can be important factors for the future development of the nervous system. A neurodevelopmental history is by necessity a mixture of the medical and social information and as such should include the parent's description of the temperament of the infant (mothers typically do this best), handedness, school performance, and any childhood illness or injury. The neurodevelopmental history is particularly important when dealing with children or adolescents as there is less information (relative to adults) that can be used to establish premorbid function. Handedness can be reliably assessed through the use of a specific questionnaire or by inquiring which hand the patient uses to write, throw, and use a toothbrush. The patient's medical history should include major illnesses, surgeries, and injuries (including head injury), prescription medications, as well as alcohol and drug use. A detailed family history is also a mixture of medical and social elements and includes information regarding education, occupation, and medical history of both first- and second-order relatives. Present life circumstances include occupation, hobbies and interests, legal involvement, and interpersonal relationships as well as sleeping, eating, and sexual habits. Finally, circumstances surrounding the evaluation include the nature and onset of symptoms, the individual's emotional reaction and insight, and impact upon daily life. There is no set order in eliciting this information although skilled interviewers typically follow a framework, often chronological or topical (e.g., education, medical, family history), and "standardized" interviews have been published.

No single fact or observation should be considered out of context or viewed as a critical piece of information. The skilled clinician should be assembling a set of facts and observations while also evaluating the consistency of these clinical impressions. Humans are exceedingly complex and the clinician should be cautious about "snap judgments." As human problem solvers, clinicians tend to focus on a relatively small set of information. As sociologists, physicians, and psychologists will tell you, basic demographic data are the most powerful information available, and not surprisingly, these are the data that many clinicians focus on. A note of caution is in order: Basic demographics can occasionally lead you astray by ignoring the complexity of human experience. For example, it is widely understood that years of education, income, certain health factors (such as cigarette and alcohol consumption), and social status are highly correlated. Clinicians may ask about years of education and make certain (usually reliable) assumptions. There are notable exceptions to the reliability of basic demographic data, however.

For example, this author was referred an older gentleman from a rural area for neuropsychological evaluation of possible dementia. He reported 6 years of formal education and his former occupation (he was retired) as machinist. Coupled with his residence in a small town, certain assumptions were entertained. It became apparent during testing, however, that his intellectual abilities greatly exceeded what might be expected from an individual with this background. Upon further questioning, it was revealed that this gentleman dropped out of school during the Depression to help support his family by working as a blacksmith's apprentice. By age 18, he was recognized throughout the county as an accomplished "fix-it," due to his skill in repairing broken clocks, farm equipment, electrical devices, and other machinery. He became a self-taught machinist of considerable skill, manufacturing the parts he needed for his repair orders. During World War II, he went to work on the Manhattan Project, living in the vicinity. This gentleman apparently played a critical role in converting theoretical physics and basic sketches into working machinery. Despite a sixth grade education, this gentleman holds hundreds of patents, including a device still essential for detonating nuclear devices. Machinist, indeed! The take-home message is that the effective clinician must know when to go beyond simple heuristics, however useful those heuristics may be in most cases.

Working with older adults, the clinician is provided with a rich tapestry of life details, provided that s/he is willing to take the time to gather and sift through the information. Young children pose the opposite challenge, and the clinician must generally collect a neurodevelopmental history as well as information about parents and siblings in order to form an accurate picture. For the neuropsychologist, it is impossible to determine the extent of disability without first determining the premorbid level of functioning. Years of education, special interests or hobbies, occupational attainment, friends and associates, dress, speech, and manner of presentation can help the clinician infer premorbid level of functioning.

PARAMETERS OF THE INTERVIEW

Knowing what type of information to obtain is only half the battle. The skilled clinician must also know how to work effectively with clients and their families in order to obtain critical information. Recognizing the clinical context, establishing rapport, communicating information related to informed consent, properly ordering and timing questions, and developing the overall structure of the interview (e.g., recognizing the need for multiple sessions, how to ask follow-up questions, how to end the interview) are important skills that clinicians need to develop.

The clinician must be sensitive to the clinical context and structure the interview accordingly. An interview conducted at bedside in the hospital is likely to be very different from an interview conducted in an office setting. The clinician's manner may also change according to the clinical context. For example, working with young children requires a different approach by the clinician. Similarly, inpatient psychiatric settings or work with forensic patients will require clinicians to modify their approach.

Establishing rapport with the client and family members is vital to the process of obtaining information. It is important to remember that an interview is a dyadic exchange and not simply a list of questions. For example, when working with older adults, a few minutes of small talk followed by information about the clinician's background and skills will generally result in a more effective interview. The clinician may even signal the beginning of the formal interview and apologize for the pace of the questioning. Clients also should receive a description of the evaluation process, not only as part of obtaining informed consent, but also for rapport. When follow-up questions are asked, it is often useful to explain to the client why the information is important.

The clinician must also communicate information about the purpose and nature of the interview as well as the limits of confidentiality in a way that can be readily understood by the client. The purpose of the evaluation, nature of the evaluation process, limits of confidentiality, and who will provide post-evaluation feedback should be described as part of the informed consent process. In addition, it is often useful to ask the clients about how they feel about the evaluation, as this may be important in understanding their responses and evaluating their level of engagement with the evaluation (Lezak, 1995).

Furthermore, the clinician must be sensitive to characteristics of the client in order to adapt the "vocabulary" of the interview, order of the questions, and the overall structure of the interview. A poorly educated or confused client may require fewer and simpler questions, amplifying the need for a collateral informant. An acutely ill client evaluated at bedside may fatigue easily, and the interview will need to be conducted over multiple sessions. These multiple sessions, however, may provide valuable information to the skilled clinician. Does the client recognize the clinician? Does the client's manner reflect the nature of previous encounters? Does the client recall the previous line of questioning? Part of the clinician's sensitivity to the client must naturally include an understanding of the clinician's own biases and experiences. Do they resent having to work with older adults? Are there particular experiences that have colored the clinician's point of view? Unspoken and unrecognized biases can taint the evaluation process.

Finally, the clinician must also know when and how to ask follow-up questions as well as how to end the interview without appearing rude or abrupt. The clinician must know when to use open-ended questions and when to be direct. The overall structure of the interview will differ from client to client and situation to situation.

THE VALUE OF A COLLATERAL INFORMANT

When cognitive or psychiatric impairments are suspected, a collateral informant is generally advisable. As a rule of thumb, the greater the extent of impairment, the greater the need for a reliable informant. "Discovering that a patient is unable to give an adequate account of his or her life and illness should prompt, first, a search for other informants and second, a search for an explanation of the incapacity" (Ovsiew, 1997). Similarly, when an individual presents with significant psychiatric symptoms, a collateral informant is almost a necessity. It must be admitted, however, that the depth of the search may be constrained by clinical context.

There are many other clinical contexts in which a collateral informant can be of great value, however. For example, upon interview many individuals tend to minimize their abuse of alcohol, prescription medications, or recreational drugs. After explaining the importance of the line of questioning, additional information may be forthcoming. Comparing the individual's reported usage with ancillary information from police reports, pharmacy records, or other healthcare providers may provide additional clues. However, a parent or spouse who is affected by the individual's clinical status may provide more accurate information.

In some cases, individuals may be unaware of the nature or extent of their impairments. For example, many individuals with Alzheimer's disease minimize the extent of their memory impairment perhaps due to lack of self-awareness, difficulty in remembering instances of memory failure, fear, or lack of confidence in the provider. Denial of disability is also encountered in other types of neurologic disorders. In Korsakoff's syndrome, the sufferer displays a marked tendency to fill in the gaps through confabulation. Anosagnosia is encountered after circumscribed lesions in which individuals may deny that a useless limb is problematic or that it is their limb at all. In many cases of cognitive impairment, neuropsychological test data and a collateral informant who can report on activities of daily living can be vital to making an accurate diagnosis. In certain cases of psychiatric illness or neurologic disease involving the frontal lobes, paranoia or anergia may severely constrain the information reported by the client. Good observation skills and information from a collateral informant may be essential in these cases. Psychopathy or antisocial personality disorder is also associated with inaccurate reporting. Finally, collateral information may prove essential in cases of malingering.

FORENSIC ISSUES

The practicing clinician must be sensitive to the context of the interview. Information on the legal involvement of the client is often crucial. Individuals referred by an attorney or insurance company for a second opinion are most likely to present challenges for a clinician. Specialty clinics, such as those for ADHD or traumatic brain injury, are also more likely to draw clients with clinicolegal issues.

With regard to traumatic brain injury, there is often a contentious context for the interview and evaluation. An attorney for the plaintiff may be looking for an expert witness who will testify about the permanent and debilitating aftermath of the injury. Vague arguments about "diffuse axonal injury due to shearing effects" may be offered in order to explain why the observed impairments are greater than might be expected from the neuroradiologic evidence of injury. The attorney for the defendant will likely be arguing that the symptoms of depression, irritability, and mood lability are evidence of a preexisting psychiatric condition or a hysterical reaction to the accident itself or mere malingering. Furthermore, the defense attorney will often argue that the individual's premorbid level of functioning was lower than would be expected, making the observed cognitive impairments somewhat suspect. Attorneys may also pointedly question a clinician about previous evaluations of similar clients and whether the plaintiff or defendant retained them. Sorting these clinical issues out, maintaining professional integrity, and defending one's conclusions on the witness stand are not for the ill prepared or the faint of heart.

In an entirely different forensic setting, a client may be referred for evaluation of trial competency or criminal responsibility or both. With regard to trial competency, these are individuals who are facing criminal charges and who are being evaluated for competency to "aid and assist" an attorney in their defense. Criminal responsibility evaluations focus on the state of mind of the defendant at the time of the alleged crime. Frequently, an evaluation performed by a psychologist in the community may be challenged by a district attorney and referred to clinicians at a state hospital or other psychiatric facility for a second opinion. Mandated treatment at a state hospital versus prison time may hang in the balance with the perception (frequently unfounded) that a defendant would spend less time at the state hospital than in prison. Interestingly, many clinicians rely on focused clinical interviews in matters such as these, perhaps augmented by neuropsychological testing where neurologic disease is in question. There is a decided tendency for examiners to be viewed as consistently for the defense or prosecution. In addition, crimes such as murder or pedophilia present particular ethical challenges and dilemmas.

Despite differences in the two forensic settings described above, there are a number of common principles that apply to the interview and evaluation process. First, congruence (or lack thereof) between different data sources is a critical part of the examination. This principle can also be applied directly to the interview itself. By repeating and reframing questions, the interviewer can evaluate the consistency of responses. The interviewee's tendency to endorse rare symptoms or improbable symptoms is another important consideration. Similarly, the interviewee's tendency to indiscriminately endorse symptoms or to endorse obvious or blatant symptoms may be associated with malingering (Rogers, 1997). Congruence of the interviewee's reported symptoms with the observations of emergency medical personnel, law enforcement officers, friends, and acquaintances may also be of value. Furthermore, the careful clinician will be attentive to the possibility and extent of the interviewee's personal gain while conducting forensic interviews. As with all interviews, the clinician's job is to integrate information from as wide a variety of sources as possible.

SUMMARY

This chapter began with a discussion of the value and versatility of the clinical interview. The following section outlined evidence in support of the conclusion that changes in behavior are often an early indicator of brain dysfunction. Several psychiatric and neurologic disorders were then examined including traumatic brain injury, Parkinson's disease, cerebrovascular disease, and Alzheimer's disease. In many cases, psychologists may be the first healthcare practitioners to encounter a variety of neurologic diseases. In order to address the referral question and develop a plan of action, careful preparation for the clinical interview was stressed in the next section. Following this, the value of clinical observations was emphasized due to their importance in test selection, test interpretation, hypothesis testing, and ultimately, diagnosis. The type of information to obtain during a history-taking interview was then reviewed. It was noted that no single fact or observation should be considered out of context or viewed as a critical piece of information. The parameters of the clinical interview were then outlined, including establishing rapport, communicating information about the interview, sensitivity to characteristics of the client, and an understanding of one's own biases. The value of a collateral informant was outlined in the following section of this chapter. Finally, commonly encountered forensic issues were reviewed with a focus on traumatic brain injury, trial competency, and criminal responsibility. It was noted that congruence (or lack thereof) between different data sources is a critical part of the interview process.

REFERENCES

Adams, R., & Victor, M. (1993). Alcohol and alcoholism. In *Principles of neurology* (5th ed.). New York, NY: McGraw-Hill.

Cote, L., & Crutcher, M. (1991). The basal ganglia. In E. R. Kandel, J. H. Schwartz, & T. M. Jessel (Eds.), *Principles of neural science* (3rd ed.). Norwalk, CT: Appleton & Lange.

Diagnostic and statistical manual of mental disorders (4th ed. text rev.). (2000). Washington, DC: American Psychiatric Press.

DuPaul, G., Barkley, R., & Connor, D. (1998). Stimulants. In R. A. Barkley (Ed.), *Attention deficit hyperactivity disorder: A handbook for diagnosis and treatment.* New York, NY: Guilford Press.

Galaburda, A., Sherman, G., Rosen, G., Aboitiz, F., & Geschwind, N. (1985). Developmental dyslexia: Four consecutive patients with cortical anomalies. *Annals of Neurology, 18,* 223.

Kaplan, E., Goodglass, H., & Weintraub, S. (1978). *The Boston Naming Test* (exp. ed.). Boston, MA: Kaplan & Goodglass.

Kraus, J., Black, M., Sullivan, C., Bowers, S., Knowlton, S., & Marshall, L. (1984). The incidence of acute brain injury and serious impairment in a defined population. *American Journal of Epidemiology, 119,* 186–201.

Lezak, M. (1995). *Neuropsychological assessment* (3rd ed.). New York, NY: Oxford University Press.

Mayberg, H., Mahurin, R., & Brannan, S. (1997). Neuropsychiatric aspects of mood and affective disorders. In S. C. Yudofsky & R. E. Hales (Eds.), *American psychiatric press textbook of neuropsychiatry.* Washington, DC: American Psychiatric Press.

McConnell, H., & Duffy, J. (1994). Neuropsychiatric aspects of medical therapies. In C. E. Coffey & J. L. Cummings (Eds.), *American psychiatric press textbook of geriatric neuropsychiatry.* Washington, DC: American Psychiatric Press.

Nauta, W., & Feirtag, M. (1986). *Fundamental neuroanatomy.* New York, NY: W. H. Freeman.

Office of Technology Assessment. (1990). *Neurotoxicity: Identifying and controlling poisons of the nervous system.* Washington, DC: U.S. Government Printing Office.

Overall, J., & Gorham, D. (1962). The brief psychiatric rating scale. *Psychological Reports, 10,* 799–812.

Ovsiew, F. (1997). Bedside neuropsychiatry: Eliciting the clinical phenomena of neuropsychiatric illness. In S. C. Yudofsky & R. E. Hales (Eds.), *American psychiatric press textbook of neuropsychiatry.* Washington, DC: American Psychiatric Press.

Rogers, R. (1997). Structured interviews and dissimulation. In R. Rogers (Ed.), *Clinical assessment of malingering and deception* (2nd ed.). New York, NY: Guilford Press.

Spreen, O., & Benton, A. (1969). *Neurosensory center comprehensive evaluation for aphasia.* Victoria, Canada: University of Victoria Neuropsychology Laboratory.

Starkstein, S., & Robinson, R. (1994). In C. E. Coffey and J. L. Cummings (Eds.), *American psychiatric press textbook of geriatric neuropsychiatry.* Washington, DC: American Psychiatric Press.

Sundberg, N. (1977). *Assessment of persons.* Englewood Cliffs, NJ: Prentice-Hall.

Tamminga, C. (1997). Neuropsychiatric aspects of schizophrenia. In S. C. Yudofsky & R. E. Hales (Eds.), *American psychiatric press textbook of neuropsychiatry.* Washington, DC: American Psychiatric Press.

Tate, P., Freed, D., Bombardier, C., Harter, S., & Brinkman, S. (1999). Traumatic brain injury: Influence of blood alcohol level on post-acute cognitive function. *Brain Injury, 13*(10), 767–784.

Webster's new universal unabridged dictionary (deluxe 2nd ed.). (1983). New York, NY: Simon and Schuster.

Wurtman, J., Wurtman, R., Mark, S., Tsay, R., Gilbert, W., & Growdon, J. (1985). d-fenfluramine selectively suppresses carbohydrate snacking by obese subjects. *International Journal of Eating Disorders, 4,* 89–99.

II

Specific Disorders

5

Anxiety Disorders

Deborah C. Beidel and William T. Nay

Description of the Disorders

Anxiety disorders are the second most common group of psychiatric disorders (after substance abuse), with a 12-month prevalence rate of approximately 17% in the general adult population (Kessler et al., 1994). Complaints of anxiety are common in general practitioners' offices as well as in mental health clinics (e.g., Marsland, Wood, & Mayo, 1976; Weiller, Bisserbe, Maier, & Lecrubier, 1998). In addition, anxiety is often a component of other psychiatric disorders, such as affective disorders (Barlow, DiNardo, Vermilyea, Vermilyea, & Blanchard, 1986; Breier, Charney, & Heninger, 1984; Brown, Campbell, Lehman, Grisham, & Mancill, 2001; Dealy, Ishiki, Avery, Wilson, & Dunner, 1981; Lesser et al., 1988; Uhde et al., 1985; Van Valkenberg, Akiskal, Puzantian, & Rosenthal, 1984) and substance abuse disorders (Kushner, Sher, & Beitman, 1990; Verheul et al., 2000). Furthermore, anxiety is often only one facet of a more pervasive condition, including personality disorders (American Psychiatric Association [APA], 1994). Given anxiety's ubiquitous nature, it is likely that most clinicians will encounter patients seeking treatment for these disorders.

Anxiety patients present with a myriad of symptoms, including physical complaints, intrusive thoughts, dysphoria, and behavioral avoidance. Although most clinicians are familiar with the tripartite model (Lang, 1977), a thorough assessment involves much more than simply an evaluation of the specific anxiety complaints. Factors such as family history, conditioning experiences, medical status, and developmental history are among the areas that must be included in a comprehensive assessment. Although many clinical trials have demonstrated that pharmacological and behavioral treatments are efficacious in reducing anxious symptomatology, certain disorders appear to be more or less amenable to specific interventions. Thus, because treatment implications follow naturally from the overall symptom picture, proper diagnosis is necessary to provide the most

Deborah C. Beidel and William T. Nay • Department of Psychology, University of Maryland, College Park, Maryland 20742.

appropriate intervention. In this chapter, guidelines for interviewing patients with anxiety disorders will be presented.

There are nine anxiety disorders listed in the *Diagnostic and Statistical Manual of Mental Disorders*, Fourth Edition (*DSM-IV*; APA, 1994). Before discussing the unique features of each disorder, a comment about the ubiquitous nature of panic attacks is necessary. Prior to *DSM-IV*, panic attacks were largely thought to be characteristic only of panic disorder. Contemporary research and theory now recognizes, however, that panic attacks may occur within the context of different anxiety disorders and even occur in individuals without psychiatric disorders (Eaton, Kessler, Wittchen, & Magee, 1994; Reed & Wittchen, 1998). Thus, panic attacks should not be automatically equated with panic disorder. Rather, presence of panic attacks should lead the interviewer to look functionally at the relationship between panic attacks and the immediate contexts. Panic attacks are not a necessary diagnostic criteria for any anxiety disorder except panic disorder. However, because panic attacks can occur in all anxiety disorders, differential diagnosis will depend critically upon the interviewer's astute analysis of when, where, and hypothetically why the attacks occur.

In light of this re-conceptualization, the anxiety disorders section of the *DSM-IV* begins with a discussion of panic attacks and their relationship to certain situational triggers. Essentially, panic attacks are conceptualized as one of three types. *Unexpected* (uncued) panic attacks are not associated with an obvious trigger. *Situationally bound* (cued) attacks occur immediately on exposure to, or in anticipation of, a situation (e.g., always panics at the beginning of giving a speech). Finally, there are *situationally predisposed* attacks, which are more likely to be but are not invariably associated with a particular cue (e.g., occasionally panics at the beginning of giving a speech, and at other times is only a bit nervous). It is important to note that the type of panic attack does not have a direct implication for what anxiety disorder is present, except for the greater likelihood of unexpected (uncued) panic attacks to be related to panic disorder. Below, we begin the description of the anxiety disorders with panic disorder.

The primary characteristic of panic *disorder* (with or without agoraphobia) is the occurrence of "spontaneous" panic attacks that appear unexpectedly and are not triggered by situations in which the person was the focus of attention by others. Characterized by a myriad of physical and cognitive symptoms, the individual must experience a minimum of four out of thirteen possible symptoms in order to be considered a panic attack. If fewer than four symptoms are present, the individual is considered to have limited symptom attacks. Unlike previous editions of the *DSM*, frequency of panic attacks is not a crucial indicator of panic disorder (the current criteria require a minimum of only one previous spontaneous/uncued panic attack). Instead, the high degree of interference from "anxious apprehension" (Barlow, 1988) and avoidance due to the possibility of future attacks is now considered critical. Specifically, impairment criteria are defined as "at least one of the attacks has been followed by a month (or more) of: (a) persistent concern about having additional attacks; (b) worry about the implications of the attack or its consequences (e.g., losing control, having a heart attack, ('going crazy'); or (c) a significant change in behavior related to the attacks" (p. 402).

In certain individuals, panic attacks are coupled with *agoraphobia (PDA)*, a fear of situations from which escape is perceived to be difficult or help unavailable. Commonly, feared situations are those in which panic attacks (or subthreshold panic-like physical and cognitive sensations) have previously occurred or are deemed likely to occur in the future. At its core, therefore, agoraphobia is driven not directly by a fear of certain situations, but rather by a fear of possible panic attacks and inability to escape/get help in these particular situations. Situations often avoided or feared include crowded places, such as theaters, shopping malls, restaurants, and churches. In addition, the individual often avoids activities, such as driving on limited access roads, through tunnels, or over bridges; traveling alone; or being "too far" from home. Some patients with panic disorder do not appear to develop extensive patterns of avoidance, although careful assessment often reveals aspects of a restricted lifestyle, even in patients who deny situational avoidance (Turner, Beidel, & Jacob, 1988).

Those who meet criteria for *agoraphobia without history of panic disorder* exhibit a pattern of behavioral avoidance consistent with a diagnosis of agoraphobia but have never had panic attacks that met criteria for panic disorder. Like patients with PDA, these patients fear being trapped in situations in which escape might be difficult or help unavailable. Rather than panic attacks, the fear is of the development of a specific symptom, such as dizziness or falling, depersonalization or derealization, loss of bladder or bowel control, vomiting, or cardiac distress.

The *agoraphobia without history of panic disorder* category presents a conceptual difficulty due to the fact that agoraphobic avoidance is typically (but not unanimously) thought to be a phenomenon that arises secondarily to panic attacks. That is, avoidance is reinforced by staying away from places in which panic attacks may (or did) occur. Although the Epidemiological Catchment Area (ECA) data indicate that agoraphobia without history of panic disorder is present in the general population (2.9%), it is very rarely seen in anxiety disorder specialty clinics (Beidel & Turner, 1991). In an effort to resolve this discrepancy, Jacob and Turner (1988) noted that among those individuals in the ECA study who were diagnosed with agoraphobia without panic, 47% had a history of panic symptoms but of insufficient severity to meet the diagnostic criteria (i.e., they had "limited symptom attacks"). Of the remaining 53%, approximately 40% had another anxiety disorder or depression that was functionally related to the patient's avoidance. When these factors were considered, the prevalence rate for agoraphobia without panic dropped to approximately 1%. Beidel and Bulik (1990) proposed that although a specific behavioral pattern may be consistent with agoraphobia, other aspects of the clinical presentation indicate that consideration should be given to conceptualizing this uncommon disorder as falling within the obsessional spectrum. As is the case with panic attacks, functional assessment of when, where, and why agoraphobic avoidance occurs is critical in appropriate diagnosis (McNally, 1994). For example, fear of crowds may be driven by agoraphobia, but also could be idiographically attributed to social anxiety disorder (described next) if it were determined that the individual was primarily afraid of being observed and evaluated.

Social anxiety disorder (also called social phobia) is a persistent fear of situations in which the individual is open to possible scrutiny by others or fears that he or she may do something that will be embarrassing or humiliating (APA, 1994). Public speaking is the most common situation feared by those with social phobia (Turner, Beidel, Borden, Stanley, & Jacob, 1991). Although many individuals will present for treatment of a circumscribed fear such as public speaking, only rarely is the distress actually limited to one specific situation (Turner et al., 1991). *DSM-IV* provides for a "generalized" social phobia subtype distinction for individuals who present with fears across most social domains. There has been much recent empirical attention given to this issue of subtypes, as well as the association of the generalized subtype with avoidant personality disorder (Brown, Heimberg, & Juster, 1995; Heimberg, Holt, Schneier, Spitzer, & Liebowitz, 1993; Van Velzen, Emmelkamp, & Scholing, 2000; Wittchen, Stein, & Kessler, 1999). However, the exact nature of these relationships remains unclear. Some evidence suggests that the specific (or "non-generalized") subtype of social phobia may be related to stronger physiological reactions to laboratory social tasks than the generalized, and may be more likely the result of direct conditioning events (Stemberger, Turner, Beidel, & Calhoun, 1995). Conversely, the generalized subtype appears to develop earlier in the life span (Herbert, Hope, & Bellack, 1992; Holt, Heimberg, & Hope, 1992; Wittchen, Stein, & Kessler, 1999) and is associated with greater distress and functional impairment (Brown, Heimberg, & Juster, 1995).

The severity of social anxiety disorder appears to have significant treatment implications, and thus careful attention to the specific clinical presentation is necessary. Furthermore, impairment as a result of the fear must be carefully considered because some individuals will focus solely on public speaking concerns and not associate other aspects of social impairment as arising from their social anxiety. Novice interviewers may find use of the Anxiety Disorders Interview Schedule for *DSM-IV* (ADIS-IV; discussed below) particularly helpful in this respect. The ADIS-IV guides the interviewer through symptom severity ratings across most relevant social anxiety domains as well as overall ratings of interference due to social anxiety. As emphasized earlier in this chapter, there is recognition in the *DSM* that the social performance and evaluation distress may take the form of situationally bound or situationally predisposed panic attacks. Therefore, care must be taken when interviewing to discern whether the panic attacks, if they occur, do so only when confronted with a social situation in which the fear is driven by evaluation concerns, and not by the panic attacks in and of themselves (the "fear of fear" common in prototypical panic disorder). Specific descriptions about the manifestation of social anxiety disorder in children also are included in the *DSM*.

Fears that do not concern public scrutiny, being trapped and unable to receive help, or panic attacks are termed *specific phobias*. Although common in the general population, only rarely does an individual present at an anxiety clinic with an isolated specific phobia. Rather, the fear is often accompanied by other psychiatric complaints, or presents as co-occurring with another anxiety disorder (Sanderson, Rapee, & Barlow, 1987). There are four types of specific phobias listed in the *DSM-IV*: animal type, natural environment type (e.g., heights, storms, and water), blood/injection/injury type, situational type (e.g., planes, elevators, or enclosed places). The *DSM-IV* also allows for the diagnosis of atypical specific phobias by providing for the use of an "other" type. In community samples, specific phobias include fears of animals, blood-injury, heights, and enclosed spaces (Agras, Sylvester, & Oliveau, 1969; APA, 1994), although in clinics the most common complaints are situational, followed by natural environment, blood-injury-illness, and animal (APA, 1994; Beidel, Turner, & Alfano, 2003). It is interesting that although there are numerous studies of college students selected on the basis of severe fear of a certain object or situation, studies of anxiety patients seeking treatment for specific phobia are exceedingly rare (Borden, 1992). Like those for social phobia, descriptors of the manifestation of specific phobia in children are included.

Obsessive–compulsive disorder (OCD) consists of (1) recurrent and persistent thoughts, ideas, or impulses (obsessions) that are experienced as intrusive or senseless and (2) repetitive, purposeful, and intentional behaviors (compulsions) that are performed in response to an obsession, according to certain rules, or in a stereotyped fashion (APA, 1994). The diagnostic criteria require presence of obsessions *or* compulsions, but not necessarily both. Also included is a poor-insight type to describe the situation when the person does not recognize that the obsessions and compulsions are excessive or unreasonable. Patients with OCD will attempt (often unsuccessfully) to suppress or ignore the thoughts or impulses. Furthermore, they recognize that these thoughts are products of their own minds. Common content for obsessional thoughts includes dirt and contamination, aggression, inanimate-interpersonal features (e.g., locks, bolts), sex, and religion (Akhtar, Wig, Verna, Pershad, & Verna, 1975; Antony, Downie, & Swinson, 1998). The compulsive behaviors are usually considered to have a neutralizing or preventative function, but the behaviors are clearly excessive. Common compulsive rituals include hand-washing and bathing, cleaning, checking, counting, and ordering (Akhtar et al., 1975; Antony et al., 1998). The astute clinical interviewer must be aware, however, of the potentially unlimited number and type of obsessions and rituals that present idiographically. In certain cases, the repetitive behavior may appear to be totally unconnected to the potential frightening events or obsessions, a fact that most patients clearly acknowledge.

Although the word "stress" is a common part of our vocabulary, *posttraumatic stress disorder* (PTSD) refers to a constellation of symptoms that occurs after an event that is outside the range of usual experience and would be distressing to almost anyone (APA, 1994). Such situations include: (1) serious threats to one's life, bodily integrity, relatives, or friends; (2) sudden destruction of one's home or community; or (3) witnessing another being killed or seriously injured as a result of an accident or physical violence. Many individuals will experience one or more such events in their lifetimes. However, very few develop the chronic and severe symptom profile of PTSD. Thus, diagnosis of this condition requires a second necessary criterion: The person's response involves persistent intense fear, helplessness, or horror. The event is reexperienced through recurrent and intrusive recollections or dreams, acting or feeling as if the event were recurring, and intense psychological distress at exposure to events that symbolize or resemble an aspect of the traumatic event. In addition, there is avoidance of stimuli associated with the trauma or numbing of general responsiveness and persistent symptoms of increased arousal. The disturbance can have an immediate or a delayed onset. Onset is characterized as delayed if the symptoms occur at least 6 months after the trauma. Finally, the disorder is specified as *acute* if symptom duration is 3 months or less or *chronic* if symptom duration is 3 months or more.

DSM-IV (APA, 1994) introduced a new diagnostic category called *acute stress disorder*. Essentially, the diagnostic criteria are the same as those for PTSD. The difference is in symptom duration and onset. In acute stress disorder, the minimum symptom duration is 2 days and maximum duration is 4 weeks. Furthermore, the onset of symptoms occurs within 4 weeks of the traumatic event.

Generalized anxiety disorder (GAD) is characterized by unrealistic or excessive worry about at least two different life circumstances (e.g., one's own physical health or that of a family member, personal finances). The worry must be consistent for a period of at least 6 months and bother the person more days than not. The worry is unrelated to any other Axis I disorder (e.g., the individual is not worrying about public speaking or the occurrence of panic attacks) and does not occur only during the course of a mood disorder. Furthermore, the individual must find it difficult to control the worry. Such worry is accompanied by symptoms of motor tension, autonomic hyperactivity, and vigilance and scanning. In our clinical experience, GAD can be one of the most difficult diagnoses to make reliably. For example, the domains of worry in GAD are not abnormal in and of themselves. Each domain represents what might be considered "typical" concerns (e.g., the health of significant others). Reliable diagnosis depends heavily, therefore, on understanding that, in GAD, it is primarily the uncontrollability, persistence, and extent (i.e., the number of domains) of worry that underlie the presenting symptom constellation. Similarly, as with all anxiety disorders, the interviewer must place appropriate weight on the assessment of functional interference (school, work, and social functioning) as a result of the particular emotional disorder in question. A person may be characterized as a "worrier," for example, yet be able to set aside worries when necessary (e.g., to get work done; to take care of the children) and otherwise not feel overwhelmed by worry. This type of individual would not, based on exclusionary interference criteria, generally be diagnosable with GAD.

Categories introduced in *DSM-IV* for the first time include *anxiety disorder due to a general medical condition* and *substance-induced anxiety disorder*. These disorders refer to the presence of prominent anxiety, panic attacks, obsessions, or compulsions that are secondary to a medical condition or substance abuse. Treatment of these disorders must take into account the treatment of the precipitating condition. Because of these complicating factors, these disorders will not be addressed in this chapter.

As discussed below, there are certain associated features that accompany many of the diagnostic categories previously described, and attention to these factors is necessary for an accurate diagnosis. The next section presents an assessment of the dimensions necessary to ensure diagnostic accuracy.

PROCEDURES FOR GATHERING INFORMATION

As noted, a proper assessment of anxiety requires attention to many different clinical features. Table 1 lists specific domains that should be addressed in the evaluation process. Obviously, this list is not exhaustive, but it confers a sense of the elements to be addressed in order to understand the patient's clinical condition. However, superseding the specifics about what to address in anxiety disorders interviews is the overarching need to effectively incorporate skillful technique and the "non-specific factors" of interviewing (Chapter 1, this volume; Morrison, 1995) and to be aware of the examinee's mental state (Chapter 2, this volume). During the interview, the mental health provider must strike a skillful balance between trying to obtain the requisite information, yet maintain an empathic and understanding position. Ineffective or inappropriate interview tactics may have many undesirable consequences, such as a client's minimization of distress and symptoms, obtaining inaccurate or incomplete information, creating anxiety in the client, and ultimately resulting in a client not returning for treatment.

Returning to the specific considerations listed in Table 1, the first domain addresses characteristics of the presenting complaint, which need to be carefully delineated. Assessment of the individual's typical responses to anxiety provoking events or situations across the three primary response domains (overt behavior, subjective distress, and somatic responses) are essential. Rarely does anxiety occur only within one domain. Therefore, it is inappropriate to assess, for example, only an individual's thoughts in response to an event or situation. Furthermore, it has been consistently observed that the three systems rarely covary (Hugdahl, 1981). Therefore, one cannot infer from one domain (e.g., negative thoughts) that responses in the other systems necessarily follow (e.g., even though one is afraid of crowds, the individual may not avoid crowds for various reasons).

TABLE 1. Domains to be Included in an Anxiety Disorders
Diagnostic Interview

1. Characteristics of the presenting complaint (behavioral, cognitive, and somatic components; situational determinants).
2. Differential diagnosis across anxiety disorders and assessment for the existence of other Axis I disorders that may account for or alter the presentation of the symptomatology or that may affect the treatment outcome.
3. Existence of Axis II disorders that may account more fully for the presenting symptomatology or that may alter or influence the treatment outcome.
4. Existence of medical conditions that may produce, contribute to, or augment the presenting symptomatology.
5. Environmental influences such as conditioning experiences, stressful events, or familial factors that may contribute to or maintain the current clinical picture.
6. Developmental history factors that may have produced, contributed to, or augmented the current symptom picture.
7. Assessment of prior treatment history that may assist in clarifying issues of primary versus secondary symptomatology.

The three response system assessment, as critical as it is, addresses only a small part of the total symptom picture. For example, although most panic patients assume that their panic attacks come "out of the blue," several studies have indicated that these attacks are often related to presence of stressful life events or negative affective states (Turner et al., 1988). Similarly, patients with OCD will often report that panic attacks occur, but usually only when they come into contact with fearful stimuli. Thus, when a patient reveals having experiences that meet criteria for panic attacks, it is important to extend one's investigation broadly (e.g., "typically when do they occur?", "under what circumstances?", "when did they start?", "what was going on at that time?"). Finally, although it is true for patients with any psychiatric disorder, it is likely that the anxiety patient's conceptualization of the presenting complaint may be more circumscribed than the actual clinical presentation. For example, social phobia patients, knowingly or unknowingly, often minimize the extent of their complaints or may not recognize that specific behaviors (e.g., avoidance) serve an anxiety-reducing function (Turner & Beidel, 1989). The same holds true for patients suffering from any of the anxiety disorders.

Second, many individuals suffer from more than one anxiety disorder (Brown et al., 2001; Sanderson et al., 1987). In addition, depression is a common complaint of anxiety disorder sufferers, especially those with PTSD, GAD, panic disorder with and without agoraphobia, and, to a lesser extent, social phobia (Brown et al., 2001), In general, there is a high degree of comorbidity among all these disorders. Boyd et al. (1984) reported an 18.8-fold increased risk of panic disorder and a 15.3-fold increased risk of agoraphobia given a primary diagnosis of major depression. If the individual had a primary diagnosis of agoraphobia, there was an 18-fold increased risk of panic disorder, and there was a 3-fold increased risk of alcohol abuse given panic disorder. Co-occurring substance abuse is fairly common among a variety of anxiety patients (Keyl & Eaton, 1990; Kushner et al., 1990), and although these latter studies used earlier diagnostic criteria, the data probably still apply. Thus, existence of any of these additional disorders obviously serves to complicate both the case conceptualization and the consideration of treatment strategies for those with primary anxiety disorders.

The high degree of comorbidity between anxiety disorders, and between anxiety and other conditions, is undoubtedly reflective of reality. However, the high degree of symptomatic overlap between anxiety disorders (as well as between anxiety and affective disorders) can lead the novice interviewer to arrive at spurious secondary diagnoses and consequent confusion in case conceptualization. This is precisely why familiarity with the topographical features of diagnostic criteria (i.e., isolated symptom lists) cannot replace a clear, holistic understanding of psychopathology. As emphasized throughout this chapter, the interviewer must determine the functional relations between what the patient fears, when the patient fears them, and then conceptualize a possible explanation. For example, a client may fear and avoid dogs. A topographical analysis may end at this point and lead the interviewer to assign a diagnosis of specific phobia: animal type. However, on functional analysis, the client reveals that he perceives dogs to be filthy, germ-infested animals and actually fears contracting disease from them. Further analysis reveals a constellation of object avoidance centered around avoidance of germs, as well as the presence of compensatory ritual behaviors such as constant washing and cleaning (thus, likely OCD). Certainly, in this simplified case, OCD is primary and an additional diagnosis of specific phobia of dogs would be unnecessary and likely inappropriate.

Third, personality disorders are commonly found among those with Axis I anxiety disorders (Mavissakalian & Hammen, 1986, 1988; Reich & Noyes, 1987; Sanderson, Wetzler, Beck, & Betz, 1994; Turner & Beidel, 1989) and, similar to co-occurring Axis I disorders, serve to complicate the diagnostic presentation and the consideration of treatment outcome (Jenike, Baer, Minichiello, Schwartz, & Carey, 1986; Stanley, Turner, & Borden, 1990).

Fourth, many medical conditions have been associated with presence of anxiety disorders. Certain conditions such as thyroid disease can mimic panic disorder (Stein, 1986). Others, such as mitral valve prolapse, vestibular dysfunction, and seizure activity, have been associated with panic disorder, although the exact nature of these relationships and their association with the anxiety disorder have yet to be fully determined (Beidel & Horak, 2001; Crowe, Pauls, Slymen, & Noyes, 1980; Gorman, Fyer, Glicklich, King, & Klein, 1981; Jacob, Moller, Turner, & Wall, 1985; Kathol et al., 1980; Shear, Devereaux, Kranier-Fox, Mann, & Frances, 1984; Stein, 1986). Neurochemical imbalances also have been reported to be associated with several anxiety disorders. For example, results of lactate infusion studies initially suggested that the neurochemical functioning of panic disorder patients might be different from that of normal controls and of patients with other types of anxiety disorders (Gorman et al., 1983; Liebowitz et al., 1984; 1985a; 1985b). However, these results are open to alternative interpretations, including the influence of situational context at the time of the laboratory assessments (Margraf, Ehlers, & Roth, 1986; Turner et al., 1988; Van der Molenen & van den Hout, 1988; Zvolensky, Lejuez, & Eifert, 2000)

Fifth, environmental factors, such as traumatic events, specific conditioning experiences, and familial factors, may play a role in the development or maintenance of the anxiety disorders (Keyl & Eaton, 1990). With respect to etiology, a study by Öst (1987) indicated that specific or traumatic events accounted for the onset of 76.7–84% of panic/agoraphobia, 58% of social phobias, and 45–68.4% of simple phobias. Thus, although a significant proportion of anxiety patients can recall a specific traumatic event associated with the onset of their fears, not all patients can do so. In addition, environmental factors other than direct conditioning experiences may also contribute to the onset of a disorder. In the study cited above, Öst (1987) noted that a substantial proportion of anxiety patients acquired their fear through information or social learning (modeling). Furthermore, for other patients, onset of their disorder was not necessarily associated with a specific incident, but nonetheless occurred during the context of a major life event. For example, Klein (1964) reported that for some women, the onset of panic disorder occurred after the birth of a child. Although he attributed onset of the disorder to the hormonal changes accompanying childbirth, there are alternative nonbiological explanations as well. For example, depression or a major grief episode has been associated with the onset of panic attacks (Keyl & Eaton, 1990).

Similarly Turner and Beidel (1988) reported that onset of OCD is often associated with life-events, such as getting married, purchasing a home, birth of a child, or death of a close relative. Furthermore, these disorders are often exacerbated by ongoing environmental tensions, such as dysfunctional marriages or hostile parent–child relationships (Turner & Beidel, 1988). To summarize, many factors may be associated with the onset of anxiety, and an understanding of the contributory effect of environmental events must be broader than a simple conceptualization of direct conditioning experiences.

Sixth, developmental history is also an important area of diagnostic interviewing. One caveat, however, is that a patient's recall of past events may be colored by the presence of current psychopathology. Nonetheless, family history is an important consideration in making a diagnostic assessment. Although family history data are often interpreted as evidence of biological etiology, other equally important factors must be considered. For example, significantly higher familial rates of a disorder in a family may demonstrate the powerful impact of modeling (as noted above). In addition, Kagan, Reznick, and Snidman (1988) have shown that children considered to be behaviorally inhibited at an early age can become less inhibited if their parents make a concerted effort to expose the children to peer social interactions. Thus, parenting may play a significant role in the remediation or continuation of anxious symptomatology. Furthermore, a study by Messer and Beidel (1994) indicated that parental and familial variables, such as the father's psychopathology and the family environment (anxious children rated their family environments as restricting the children's independence), have significant predictive validity in discriminating anxious and non-anxious children. Even if these factors are reactive rather than causal, it is likely that a restrictive family environment may serve to maintain anxious symptomatology. Thus, although the specific role of these developmental factors is unclear, it is apparent that an assessment of these factors is necessary.

Seventh, prior treatment history may be an important factor, particularly when attempting to determine primacy of depressive or anxious symptoms. For example, for patients whose depression is secondary to their OCD, traditional antidepressants improve their mood but have little or no effect on their obsessions and compulsions (Turner & Beidel, 1988). Thus, prior treatment with antidepressants that results in significantly improved mood and also eliminates obsessional thinking may suggest the primacy of an affective, rather than an anxiety, disorder. Several notes of caution are in order, however. First, diagnosis should never be determined solely on the basis of treatment response. Thus, determining diagnosis by response to antidepressants would be particularly problematic inasmuch as both anxiety and mood disorders respond to the same medications. Second, in the case of this particular example, the assessment of the OCD symptomatology is critical, and the clinician must carefully assess changes in specific frequency and severity of the obsessions and compulsions, rather than just changes in general estimates of mood and OCD symptoms.

This volume is dedicated to diagnostic interviewing and, indeed, the interview is the cornerstone of clinical assessment. In recent years, there has been an increase in the use of structured and semistructured interview schedules designed to assist in the diagnostic process. Among those geared specifically to *DSM-IV* criteria, some, such as the Structured Clinical Interview for *DSM-IV* Axis I Disorders (SCID; First, Spitzer, Gibbon, & Williams, 1994) and the Diagnostic Interview Schedule—Version IV (DIS-IV) (http://epi.wustl.edu/DIS/dishome.htm; 2002), assess psychopathology across a range of diagnostic categories, including the anxiety disorders. The DIS is a structured interview developed for use in epidemiological studies. The interview is administered by lay interviewers, and diagnoses are derived by computer algorithm. This procedure means that although the final diagnostic decision is taken out of the lay interviewer's hands, that interviewer is still responsible for evaluating the clinical significance of the interviewee's responses. Thus, the administrators still need a significant degree of training in order to make judgments of clinical significance. Studies of interrater reliability and validity using earlier versions of the DIS suggest that this scale has only low to moderate reliability and validity coefficients for anxiety disorders categories (Anthony et al., 1985; Helzer et al., 1985; Robins, 1985).

The SCID is a semistructured interview designed to be used by trained clinicians to assist in deriving Axis I diagnoses. In contrast to structured interviews, semistructured interviews provide some basic interviewing questions but allow latitude for clinicians to use their clinical judgment to ask additional follow-up questions and assign a diagnosis. Because of the need to make a clinical judgment, semistructured interviews are not appropriate for use by lay interviewers or those insufficiently trained in psychopathology. Although formal reliability data on the use of the SCID for the diagnosis of anxiety disorders are limited, information from our clinic suggests that with proper training, acceptable interrater reliability ($r = 0.90$) can be achieved.

In addition to interview schedules that cover a broad range of psychopathology the ADIS-IV (Brown, DiNardo, & Barlow, 1994; DiNardo, Brown, & Barlow, 1994) was developed specifically to assess *DSM-IV* anxiety disorders. Since the ADIS-IV is a semistructured interview schedule, it is appropriate for administration only by an individual who has had significant clinical experience. Skilled interviewers achieve good to excellent interrater reliability with the ADIS-IV (Brown, DiNardo, Lehman, & Campbell, 2001). Although there is some attention to non-anxiety disorders, such as depression, this interview schedule is less comprehensive than some others and thus should be augmented by additional assessments.

In addition to clinical interviewing, comprehensive evaluation usually includes assessment via different modalities. Although self-report inventories are among the most common forms of clinical assessment, relatively few instruments have been developed specifically to address the *DSM-IV* anxiety disorders categories. For example, Turner, McCann, Beidel, and Mezzich (1986) demonstrated that instruments such as the State-Trait Anxiety Inventory (Spielberger, Gorsuch, & Lushene, 1970), the Social Avoidance and Distress Scale and the Fear of Negative Evaluation Scale (Watson & Friend, 1969), and the Maudsley Obsessive Compulsive Inventory (Hodgson & Rachman, 1977) did not discriminate among diagnostic groups. In contrast, the Social Phobia and Anxiety Inventory (SPAI) (Turner, Beidel, Dancu, & Stanley, 1989) was developed specifically to assess social phobia and is capable of differentiating patients with this disorder from other diagnostic groups. Nonetheless, although such instruments are useful in clarifying the extent and severity of the clinical presentation, when used to assist in the determination of a diagnosis, they should be used only in conjunction with other sources of information.

Although this chapter is directed toward interviewing, it is important to note that objective observational data often is helpful in clarlifying the diagnostic picture (see Bellack & Hersen, 1998, for a comprehensive introduction to behavioral assessment). Such information gathering can be invaluable to test diagnostic hypotheses and are very useful in pre- to post-treatment outcome assessment. Objective data should be gathered for each response modality (overt behavior, physiological responding, and thought content). The means for gathering such information are potentially unlimited, and thus are not inherently prohibitive in clinical practice.

Idiographically derived Behavioral Assessment (or Avoidance) Tests (BATs; Bernstein, 1973), for example, are often useful when a client presents with complaints of avoidance. Implementation requires the creation or identification of a replicable situation in which approach or avoidance can be objectively measured. For example, an individual with a spider phobia can be asked to approach, from one end of a measured hallway, an uncaged spider at the other end of the hallway. The data of interest, in this case, would be the distance between the spider and individual at the point where the individual no longer can approach the spider. Also, obtaining physiological data during behavior assessment once was considered to be cost-prohibitive. However, inexpensive devices, such as ambulatory heart rate and blood pressure monitors, now exist. Furthermore, physiological data can be a critical factor in case conceptualization and treatment planning.

Daily self-monitoring also can be very helpful in the diagnostic process. Carefully constructed and completed self-monitoring can provide clarification of important elements of the diagnostic picture such as antecedent triggering events, specific negative cognitions, and engagement in maladaptive behaviors (such as substance abuse or caffeine ingestion) that could produce panic attacks. For those with social phobia, self-monitoring may reveal that the distress and avoidance extend to interpersonal interactions, not just public speaking situations. Thus, these paper-and-pencil measures play an important role in the diagnostic process.

Case Illustration

This case illustrates many of the issues involved in the diagnosis of anxiety disorders discussed above. It was selected for its diagnostic complexity and its appropriateness to illustrate many of the issues discussed above. The structure of the interview is based roughly on that found in the ADIS-IV semistructured interview schedule (Brown, DiNardo, & Barlow, 1994).

The patient is a 24-year-old single male, self-referred through a newspaper advertisement offering treatment for patients with social anxiety disorder. He described a severe fear of public speaking that had restricted his occupational choices and resulted in chronic underemployment. Currently, he was unemployed and believed that his fear prevented him from acquiring a position commensurate with his personal abilities. His girlfriend was aware of his social anxiety, but he had not discussed either his fear or his decision to seek treatment with any of his immediate family. He requested that all telephone contact occur through his girlfriend. The following is a transcript of the first three interviews with the patient and begins after the initial introductions and explanation of the interview process:

T: You telephoned the clinic in response to our announcement about treatment for social phobia. Perhaps you could begin by telling me what it was about that announcement that reminded you of yourself.

P: I get very nervous whenever I have to speak in public.

T: The word "nervous" means different things to different people. Can you tell me what it means to you?

P: What I mean is that I get a rush of anxiety whenever I have to give any type of formal presentation. I worry that something is going to go wrong, that I am going to be so anxious that I won't be able to continue.

T: Can you give me an example of a time when this happened?

P: Well, the last time was when I was at an orientation session for my last job. That was two years ago. We all had to get up and say our names. I felt so nervous, like I could not breathe, like I was going to die from the anxiety. I said it, but I felt so foolish, so embarrassed. This was my name, that's all I had to say.

Although this patient responded to an announcement about treatment for social anxiety disorder, the words "going to die" are often used by individuals with panic disorder. Therefore, a decision was made to clarify the circumstances of the first experiences with anxiety to determine whether it might be more consistent with panic disorder than with social anxiety disorder.

T: I understand your feelings of frustration at being unable to do such a simple thing comfortably, and we will discuss it in more detail in a few moments. But first, can you remember the first time that you felt this way?

P: Well, I remember when I was in junior high, around the time of puberty, feeling a little nervous when I would have to speak in class. But the first time that I remember feeling like I could not breathe was when I was a senior in high school.

T: Tell me what happened.

P: I was in current events class and I was called on to read a newspaper clipping. When I started reading, I became really anxious. The anxiety kept building to a crescendo. It came to a point where I could not talk anymore. I just quit speaking. It was very embarrassing.

The situation that the patient described was clearly one of a social nature. However, once again, some of the words used in his description, particularly his physiological state, were more reminiscent of panic disorder. Therefore, it was decided to continue pursuing the existence of panic attacks.

T: Have you ever had a time when you had a very sudden rush of anxiety, when all of a sudden you felt really anxious?

P: Yes.

T: When do these feelings happen?

P: When I am worrying about some event that may have happened that day. I worry that if I did get really anxious, would I pass out? And if I did pass out, could I get help? I worry that I would pass out and look stupid.

T: Do you worry about one of those things more than the other? What I mean is, do you think that you worry more about whether someone would help you or whether you would look stupid?

P: I think that I worry more about looking stupid. I know that if you pass out, nothing bad would really happen. Probably looking stupid is worse.

T: Do the anxiety feelings ever come out of the blue? Do they ever come when you are not in public speaking situations or worrying about public speaking situations?

P: Not just like that [snaps his fingers]. Usually, I have to be thinking about the situation at the time. Initially, I will be nervous about the speaking situation, and then it hits.

T: Does the anxiety come on in every public speaking situation?

P: Not every situation. I usually do very well in job interviews. But the nervousness happens any time I feel that I have to perform. When I feel really pressed to speak. When I feel that there is no escape.

T: When you are thinking about performance situations, how often do you feel the rush of anxiety? Is it as frequently as once a week?

P: No, it is not even as frequent as once per month.

T: What I want you to do now is think about the last time that you were in a speaking situation that made you anxious.

P: That would have been two years ago at the orientation session.

T: Fine. I am going to ask you about different physical symptoms and I want you to tell me if you experience these symptoms when you are anxious, and if so, how severe the symptoms were.

At this point, all physical symptoms typical of panic attacks were reviewed. The patient endorsed severe symptoms of shortness of breath, tachycardia, trembling, moderate dizziness, mild depersonalization, and mild fear of dying.

T: Other than the incidents that we have discussed, were there any other times when you had a fear of dying?

P: Well, when I was in seventh grade, I choked on a hot dog.

T: Tell me about that.

P: I was sitting in the school cafeteria at lunch time. I was with a bunch of my friends. We were talking and laughing. I literally inhaled the hot dog. It was lodged in my windpipe and I could not get any air. I can still remember clearly thinking that I was going to die. I got up and went in search of a teacher. My gym teacher was in the cafeteria and I remember walking toward him. He did not see me and starting walking away from me. I can remember the two of us circling the cafeteria, me following behind him, like some sort of dance. I was chasing him and I finally caught him. He hit me several times on the back and the hot dog popped out. I remember thinking that everyone was looking at me at the time. After that incident, I remember that I was really worried about eating food for the next several days. My mom noticed this and gave me soft foods at first. But she was also very firm about getting me to eat other things again and would encourage me to try. After a couple of weeks, I was eating normally again, but then I started to worry about getting air. Then this led to another worry that I would not be able to hiccup. I carried throat lozenges for a time. I never used them, but they made me feel better.

It is important to note here that even during this traumatic event, the patient was aware of the scrutiny of others and probably felt embarrassed by it.

T: Do you still worry about these things?

P: Well, I still worry about not getting air, but only when I am forced to speak in formal situations. I don't worry about the hiccupping anymore. I don t carry the throat lozenges either.

T: Other than speaking, do you worry about getting air in other situations?

P: Well, if I was in a real small place, like a box, or if I was buried alive, I'd be worried about air. But it's not something that I think about.

T: What about when you are in an elevator?

P: No. I don't really worry about getting air except when I'm forced to speak.

Because the patient kept using the word "worried," it appeared to be a good opportunity to assess for GAD.

T: You know, you have been using the word "worry" a lot. You worry about speaking in formal presentations, you worry about not getting air. Are there other things that you worry about?

P: Well, I worry about getting a good job. I am unemployed because of the layoffs and I keep worrying that my problem, this weakness, is keeping me from getting the job that I think I am capable of.

T: Well, what about nonsocial things? For example, do you worry a lot about your health, your future? Prior to losing your job, did you worry a lot about your financial situation? Do you worry about little things such as being late for appointments?

P: No, I'm not a worrier. [Leans forward.] But I do like to be prompt, and I expect that other people will be prompt too.

T: How about feeling tense, apparently for no reason at all?

P: No, I generally feel very comfortable.

The patient's posture and affect were consistent with his remarks. He was sprawled out quite comfortably in a chair. In addition, his affect was euthymic other than when discussing his public speaking difficulties. Therefore, further assessment of GAD symptoms was not considered necessary.

T: Fine. Let's talk about different situations that might make you uncomfortable. Tell me if any of these situations make you feel nervous or panicky or if you ever worry about feeling trapped and unable to escape if you find yourself in one of them.

Since there was still some uncertainty about whether this individual was suffering from panic disorder or social anxiety disorder, situations commonly feared by individuals with agoraphobia were reviewed. The patient denied fear in any of them, with two exceptions. The transcript surrounding these two situations is presented below.

T: What about riding on buses?

P: Well, it doesn't bother me now, but it did in the past.

T: When was that?

P: When I was in junior high, I would get really nervous riding the bus to school. It was soon after I choked on the hot dog. I think that I was really worried about not getting enough air. I never avoided the bus, but I remember that I would sit near the front.

T: Do you still sit near the front of the bus?

P: No, I don't even think about it any more. It wouldn't even have occurred to me if you hadn't mentioned it.

T: Alright. What about restaurants?

P: You know, that is really weird.

T: What is weird?

P: That you mention restaurants. I get these really strange feelings in restaurants.

T: Are you saying that you feel panicky in restaurants?

P: No, not panicky. Not even nervous. Just a very strange feeling, but definitely not fear.

T: Does it matter where you are sitting in the restaurant?

P: No, not at all.

T: Do you ever avoid restaurants?

P: No, not at all. Like I said, it is not really a fear, just a strange feeling.

The "funny feeling" in restaurants may indicate some degree of generalization related to the incident in the cafeteria. At this point, it was fairly clear that the individual was not suffering from panic disorder. He also denied the presence of any specific phobias. Therefore, a decision was made to further clarify the extent of the social fears.

T: Let's return to the social situations. When you are in a formal speaking situation, are you concerned that you might do or say something humiliating or embarrassing in front of others?

P: Well, if you are considering embarrassing myself by hyperventilating or passing out and others will see that, then the answer is yes.

T: What thoughts come into your head when you are thinking about having to be in one of these situations?

P: What if the panic comes? What will they think of me? I don't want to look stupid in front of these people.

T: Does the panic come every time?

P: Yes.

T: And do you avoid these situations now?

P: Absolutely.

T: I would like to name several different situations where individuals with fears of public speaking can also feel anxious. Just tell me if any of the situations make you feel uncomfortable.

The patient endorsed few other social situations that created distress. He did acknowledge feeling anxious in meetings if he thought that he might have to speak or any time when meeting new people. He also noted some minimal distress when speaking to authority figures and stated that in the past he had felt anxious when writing in front of others.

T: Are there certain types of people that make you feel more uncomfortable when you speak?

P: I am bothered most if the audience consists of males who are my age. My peer group, you might say. I guess I really don't want to embarrass myself in front of them. It is even embarrassing for me to talk about it here. I see it as a weakness and I am not proud that I am weak. I know that I have many abilities and that I am capable of a much better job than I have had so far. But the type of job that I want will require me to speak in meetings and I cannot do that. It is very frustrating.

T: So the fear has really limited your vocational choice and your occupational opportunities. Has it limited you academically or socially?

P: No, not really.

T: We have talked about situations that often elicit anxiety in some people. However, sometimes people have thoughts or images that come into their heads that are quite frightening. Sometimes they are described as silly or nonsensical thoughts that a person cannot stop thinking no matter how hard he or she tries. Not worrying about something, but thoughts that somehow you might have run over someone when you were driving or thoughts that you might have contracted a disease in some unusual way?

P: No, nothing like that.

T: Are there any facts or behaviors that you feel you must do repeatedly or that you must do in a certain way even if it doesn't make sense to you? But, you feel that you must do it because something bad will happen to you if you do not?

P: Well, I do like things to be done in a certain way, but I could change things if I had to.

Although the patient denied the presence of obsessions or rituals, several of his responses suggested the presence of an obsessional thinking style and some compulsive personality traits. A decision was made to delay discussion of that information in order to first finish the assessment of anxious symptomatology.

T: Have you ever had any extremely stressful or life-threatening or traumatic events that have happened to you?

P: Do you mean anything like the hot dog incident?

T: Well, that would be one. Did you ever have any others like that?

P: I do remember one thing that happened when I was young. I don't know if this is exactly what you mean, but when I was three or four years old, my father got into an argument with the neighbor who lived behind our house. I don't remember what started the fight, but I do remember the neighbor coming over to our front door. I opened the door and the man started yelling at me. My father came to the door and the two of them started yelling. Then, they stepped outside. I don't know if they were going to fight it out with their fists or if it was just to get away from me. I remember watching them. They argued for about ten minutes and then the other man left. My father came back into the house, but we never spoke about it. My bedroom window looked directly out at that man's house, and I remember that at night, when I went to bed, I would be worried that the man would come over and try to hurt me.

T: How often did you think of that?

P: Every single night.

T: How long did it last?

P: A year or two.

T: What made you stop worrying about it?

P: We moved to a new house in a different neighborhood. If we had stayed in that house, I think I still would have worried about it.

The patient was assessed for symptoms of PTSD that might have accompanied this incident. He denied the presence of any of these symptoms, other than the aforementioned worry when he would see the man's house through his bedroom window. Another way to interpret this event is in the context of the individual's predominant mode of thinking, which again appeared consistent with an obsessional style.

T: Before we move to other subject matters, are there any other times that you have experienced anxiety that we have not covered?

P: Well, I was really nervous when I began going to kindergarten. For about two weeks, I would cry every time my mother left me. But then I adjusted and did fine.

T: You have mentioned both your mother and your father. Why don't we take a break from talking about anxiety and you can tell me some things about your family.

P: What would you like to know?

T: Are your parents still living? Do you have brothers and sisters?

P: My parents are both living and are still married to each other. My father is retired from a steel mill where he worked as a laborer all of his life. My mother is a housewife. There are four children in our family, but I am the only boy. I have two older sisters and one younger sister. Growing up was pretty much like "Leave It to Beaver." Very traditional. I was always close to my dad. He worried that with all those girls around, I might become a sissy. So he spent a good deal of time with me on weekends fishing, hunting, baseball. He wanted to make sure that I was tough. None of my family knows that I came here. I would be so embarrassed if they knew I had this fear. I did tell my girlfriend and she encouraged me to come here. I did well in school. I had a B average. Math and science were my strongest subjects. I really enjoyed school. I had lots of friends, played varsity football and baseball in high school. I went to trade school after high school and got an associate degree in electronics. There are few jobs in this area. Besides, the electronics degree was a cop-out. I should have gone to college. I wanted to, but I was afraid that I would have to speak in class.

Despite the patient's earlier denial, his social fears had impaired his academic achievement in that he chose to forgo college because of the possibility that he would have to speak in class.

T: Do you know if anyone else in the family has any problems with anxiety?

P: I think that my dad has this same fear. When I think about it, he would always disappear if speaking before a group seemed imminent. But no one else in the family that I am aware of.

His father's "disappearance" when public speaking was imminent suggests that social learning may have been a factor in the etiology of the patient's disorder. The next part of the interview was directed at an assessment of personality disorders that might be associated with social anxiety. In this case, there were several cues that the patient behaved in ways that are characteristic of individuals with obsessive–compulsive personality disorder. Assessment for the diagnosis of the presence of personality disorders is illustrated below.

T: Fine. Now, I want to turn the topic of our conversation away from anxiety to aspects of your behavior that are typical for you, whether or not you feel anxious. The type of behavior that I am talking about is what most people call "personality." In general terms, how would you describe yourself?

P: Well, I think I would say that I am outgoing, honest, stubborn, and impatient.

T: What words would your friends use to describe you?

P: Outgoing, honest, stubborn, impatient.

T: Pretty consistent. Who or what has been the biggest influence in your life?

P: Probably my parents. I get my stubbornness from my dad. My friend Jeff. He and I are a lot alike. I confide in him. My girlfriend. She has been a real source of support.

T: How have you gotten along with these people?

P: I have always been close with my parents. But we are not affectionate. I never have been a very affectionate person. My girlfriend complains about that sometimes. I like people but it is difficult for me to express it.

T: Has the way that you interact with people ever created difficulties for you? For example, have you lost girlfriends because they thought that you did not care or that you did not tell them how you felt?

P: Maybe. I never really thought about that. I do have difficulty when I see inequality. For example, I am not tolerant of people taking advantage of others, of friends not helping each other equally. I have been told that I really set high standards for my friends.

These behaviors suggest the presence of an obsessive–compulsive personality disorder. Therefore, a decision was made to pursue this topic further.

T: Does this sometimes cause you difficulty with your friends? Do they sometimes tell you that you are stubborn?

P: How did you know? Actually, they tell me that often. I hate to give in when I am fighting with my girlfriend, even when I know she is right. They also give me a hard time about my punctuality. I like to be on time and I get irritated if someone keeps me waiting.

T: What about expressing other types of feelings? Is it easy for you to let people know how much you care about them?

P: No, that is difficult for me. I can tell my girlfriend how I feel about her, but she is the only one. I have never told my family how much I care about them. I have tried, but I just can't get the words out.

T: What about expressing your feelings nonverbally? For example, if you see something that you know a friend or family member would really like, would you ever just buy it for that person as a gift? Just because you know that it would make someone happy?

P: Only if I knew that it was a give-and-take situation. That someday, they might do the same for me. I don't mind doing a favor for someone if I know that they will have to return one some day.

T: You mentioned being stubborn. Are you perfectionistic as well?

P: Very much so. I don't like doing things if I cannot do it well. It used to slow me down in school. My instructors would always compliment me on how well I did something, but half the time the job was completed late. I am perfectionistic about my appearance too. My girlfriend teases me that I take as much time with my appearance as a girl. It didn't interfere with my job, though. I mean, there wasn't that much to be perfectionistic about. But I am really stubborn. I've always had trouble letting others do things for me. I worry that they won't do it correctly.

T: Do you every worry about whether you have done something that is morally wrong? Do you ever worry that your friends are behaving immorally?

P: I don't think I worry about it too much, but my friends seem to think so. They will often tell me that the world is not as black and white as I see it. That sometimes people break rules for the greater good. I don't understand thinking like that. For me, a rule is a rule.

T: What about being a workaholic? Do you ever find yourself so involved with work that you forget to have fun?

P: No, I've never had a job where I could do that. I don't know if I would be that way if I had a different type of job—a more professional job, I mean. All of my jobs have required punching a clock. They were never jobs that you could stay late on or take home with you.

T: One last question—are you a pack rat? Do you save things even if you don't need them right now or they don't have some special meaning for you? Do you hold on to things just in case?

P: Only with magazines. I don't know why I keep them, but I cannot throw them away. That's the only thing that I seem to save.

The interview covered aspects of all the various personality disorders, but the patient denied other symptomatology. He also denied any current medical conditions or prior psychological or psychiatric treatment. In summary, the patient's clinical presentation is similar to that of many patients seeking treatment for "fear of public speaking." As with this patient, rarely is the social anxiety limited to one specific fearful situation. Rather, careful questioning revealed a more pervasive form of the disorder. Furthermore, the clinical presentation illustrates the potential overlap between symptoms more commonly associated with panic disorder and those more commonly associated with social phobia. Nonetheless, careful questioning left little doubt that the proper diagnosis was social phobia. This patient also exemplifies the concept of anxiety-proneness. He describes numerous fearful reactions to a variety of life events, suggesting that for him, anxiety is a common response to the occurrence of stressful events. In addition, his father appears to have been an important role model, and the significant social fears that appear to be present in the father suggest the possibility that a biological predisposition coupled with environmental factors such as social learning and traumatic events contributed to the onset and maintenance of the disorder. Finally, this patient met criteria for an Axis II diagnosis of obsessive–compulsive personality disorder, which is quite common among social phobics (Turner, Beidel, & Townsley, 1992). Although the etiological significance of this Axis II disorder is unclear, it is likely that individuals with rigid and perfectionistic standards for behavior would likely be concerned with others' perceptions of their social behaviors.

Critical Information Necessary to Make the Diagnosis

Much of the critical information necessary to diagnose many of the anxiety disorders has been presented above. Specifically, one needs to ascertain the presence of anxiety features and to assure that the complaints cannot be more logically subsumed under a "broader" Axis II disorder. The necessity of making this distinction cannot be overemphasized, as the application of inappropriate treatment strategies could be ineffective or lead to the exacerbation of a condition. For example, it has been observed repeatedly in our clinic that the use of flooding procedures with a patient who has elements of a paranoid personality disorder (or the paranoid "flavor" that is characteristic of some avoidant personality disorder patients) leads to an exacerbation of the paranoia often directed at the therapist. In such cases, the patient might interpret the flooding procedures as a deliberate attempt by the therapist to humiliate the patient. Careful diagnosis would alert the therapist to the fact that this patient is not suffering simply from an anxiety disorder, which realization, in turn, should profoundly affect the selection of a treatment strategy.

Among the anxiety disorders themselves information critical to a differential diagnosis often can be inferred from the presenting symptom pattern. Such information may be useful in making a distinction between agoraphobia and social phobia, for example. First, Amies, Gelder, and Shaw (1983) noted that social phobics were more likely to complain of physical symptoms, such as blushing and muscle twitching, whereas those with agoraphobia were more likely to report dizziness, difficulty in breathing, weakness in limbs, fainting episodes, and buzzing or ringing in the ears. Similarly, agoraphobics fear the occurrence of their physical symptoms, whereas social phobics fear the perception of those symptoms by others. Finally, the core fear of social phobics and agoraphobics is quite different. According to Marks (1970), agoraphobics fear the crowd, whereas social phobics fear the individuals who make up the crowd. Attention to these specific factors will assist in the differentiation of these two disorders.

In summary, when diagnosing anxiety, it is necessary for the clinician to begin with a broad view of the presenting psychopathology, rather than to focus on the patient's initial presentation. In other words, when considering the patient's complaint, the clinician should use a top-down mode of information processing, that is, the clinician should think first in terms of broad diagnostic categories, such as Axis I versus Axis II disorder, medical versus psychological etiology, rather than simply accept the patient's initial complaint at face value (despite any striking similarity to the typical textbook presentation). These possibilities need to be eliminated prior to the consideration of a specific diagnosis.

Dos and Don'ts

There are several caveats that should be observed when assessing anxiety disorders. First, *do not* discount the severity of the patient's emotional distress. For example, a higher than normal incidence of suicide has been associated with the presence of panic attacks and panic disorder (Korn et al., 1992; Weissman, Klerman, Markowitz, & Ouellette, 1989) and social phobia (Schneier, Johnson, Hornig, Liebowitz, & Weissman, 1992). However, careful examination of these data indicate that it is more likely that such attempts and ideation are accounted for by the presence of Axis II disorders rather than by the panic or social phobia per se. For example, the suicidal ideation reported by the panic-disordered patients in the study by Weissman et al. (1989) occurred prior to the onset of the panic attacks. Because the interview format did not assess Axis II disorders, it is likely that the suicidal ideation was related to the presence of a personality disorder. Similarly, the relationship between social phobia and suicidal ideation can be accounted for largely, *but not entirely*, by the presence of a personality disorder (Schneier et al., 1992). However, the presence of suicidal ideation, even if not directly related to the presence of the anxiety disorder, should alert the clinician to conduct a thorough evaluation along both Axis I and II dimensions.

Do assess carefully for the presence of medical conditions that might be etiological or maintaining factors, but do not dismiss anxiety complaints as simply a manifestation of a physical condition. For example, a patient sought treatment at our anxiety disorders clinic for "shaking in public." According to the patient's primary physician, he had a "congenital tremor" of both hands, the etiology of which was unknown, and the condition was not amenable to traditional medical interventions. It was termed congenital because the patient's mother suffered from the same condition. The tremors had a profound influence on his occupational functioning. He had been fired once because his boss suspected the tremors were the result of a problem with alcohol. He feared that the same thing might happen in his current position, should his trembling be noticed by his superiors. In addition, following his job termination, the patient became more concerned over the possibility of trembling in front of others, particularly those who were not aware of his physical condition, and this concern, in turn, increased his tremor. Although the patient was convinced that the etiology of this tremor was biological, nonetheless he admitted that the tremors were exacerbated by social anxiety. Although it was unclear whether the cause of the tremors was biological or emotional, the patient's distress was still in excess of the ramifications of his "physical" disorder. Therefore, a diagnosis of social anxiety disorder would be warranted.

In summary, although patients may present with medical conditions that seem to account for their anxiety, the clinician must carefully consider whether the patient's fears exceed what would be expected for the presence of the physical condition. In such cases, the patient's anxiety would be treated identically to the others.

Summary

The purpose of this chapter has been to discuss interviewing practices for patients who present with anxiety disorders. Due to the ubiquitous nature of anxiety, patients may present with a myriad of complaints. In addition, the anxiety may not be a singular disorder but part of a more complex picture, involving more encompassing Axis I or II disorders or both. Careful diagnostic practices are necessary, because imprecision may result in inaccurate case conceptualizations or inappropriate treatment. Although interviewing remains the primary source of information-gathering, additional strategies, such as self-report or self-monitoring practices, may be used to assist in clarifying the symptom picture. Numerous factors, as outlined in this chapter, need to be considered in order to fully understand the complexity of these disorders.

REFERENCES

Agras, W. S., Sylvester, D., & Oliveau, D. (1969). The epidemiology of common fear and phobia. *Comprehensive Psychiatry, 10,* 151–156.

Akhtar, S., Wig, N. H., Verna, V. K., Pershad, D., & Verna, S. K. (1975). A phenomenological analysis of symptoms in obsessive–compulsive neuroses. *British Journal of Psychiatry, 127,* 342–348.

American Psychiatric Association. (1994). *Diagnostic and statistical manual of mental disorders* (4th ed.). Washington, DC: Author.

Amies, P. L., Gelder, M. G., & Shaw, P. M. (1983). Social phobia: A comparative clinical study. *British Journal of Psychiatry, 142,* 174–179.

Anthony, J. C., Folstein, M., Romanoski, A. J., Von Korff, M. R., Nestadt, G. R., Chahal, R., Merchant, A., Brown, C. H., Shapiro, S., Kramer, M., & Gruenberg, E. M. (1985). Comparison of the lay Diagnostic Interview Schedule and a standardized psychiatric diagnosis. *Archives of General Psychiatry, 42,* 667–675.

Antony, M. M., Downie, F., & Swinson, R. P. (1998). Diagnostic issues and epidemiology in obsessive–compulsive disorder. In R. P. Swinson & M. M. Antony (Eds.), *Obsessive–compulsive disorder: Theory, research, and treatment.* New York: Guilford Press.

Barlow, D. H. (1988). *Anxiety and its disorders.* New York: Guilford Press.

Barlow, D. H., DiNardo, P. A., Vermilyea, B. B., Vermilyea, J. A., & Blanchard, E. B. (1986). Co-morbidity, and depression among the anxiety disorders: Issues in diagnosis and classification. *Journal of Nervous and Mental Disease, 174,* 63–72.

Beidel, D. C., & Bulik, C. M. (1990). Flooding and response prevention as a treatment for bowel obsessions. *Journal of Anxiety Disorders, 4,* 247–256.

Beidel, D. C., & Horak, F. B. (2001). Behavior therapy for vestibular rehabilitation. *Journal of Anxiety Disorders, 15,* 121–130.

Beidel, D. C., & Turner, S. M. (1991). Anxiety disorders. In M. Hersen & S. M. Turner (Eds.), *Adult psychopathology and diagnosis* (2nd ed., pp. 226–278). New York: John Wiley.

Beidel, D. C., Turner, S. M., & Alfano, C. (2003). Anxiety disorders. In M. Hersen & S. M. Turner (Eds.), *Adult psychopathology and diagnosis* (3rd ed. pp. 358–419). New York: John Wiley.

Bellack, A. S., & Hersen, M. (1998). *Behavioral assessment* (4th ed.). Boston: Allyn & Bacon.

Bernstein, D. A. (1973). Situational factors in behavioral fear assessment: A progress report. *Behavior Therapy, 4,* 41–48.

Borden, J. W. (1992). Behavioral treatment of simple phobia. In S. M. Turner, K. S. Calhoun, & H. E. Adams (Eds.), *Handbook of clinical behavior therapy* (2nd ed., pp. 3–12). New York: John Wiley.

Boyd, J. H., Burke, J. D., Gruenberg, E., Holzer, C. E., III, Rae, D. S., George, L. K., Karno, M., Stoltzman, R., McEvoy, L., & Nestadt, G. (1984). Exclusion criteria of DSM-III: A study of co-occurrence of hierarchy-free syndromes. *Archives of General Psychiatry, 41,* 983–989.

Breier, A., Charney, D. S., & Heninger, G. R. (1984). Major depression in patients with agoraphobia and panic disorder. *Archives of General Psychiatry, 41,* 1129–1135.

Brown, T. A., Campbell, L. A., Lehman, C. L., Grisham, J. R., & Mancill, R. B. (2001). Current and lifetime comorbidity of the DSM-IV anxiety and mood disorders in a large clinical sample. *Journal of Abnormal Psychology, 110,* 585–599.

Brown, T. A., DiNardo, P. A., & Barlow, D. H. (1994). Anxiety Disorders Interview Schedule for DSM-IV: Clinician's manual. Albany, NY: Graywind.

Brown, T. A., DiNardo, P. A., Lehman, C. L., & Campbell, L. A. (2001). Reliability of DSM-IV anxiety and mood disorders: Implications for the classification of emotional disorders. *Journal of Abnormal Psychology, 110,* 49–58.

Brown, E. J., Heimberg, R. G., & Juster, H. R. (1995). Social phobia subtype and avoidant personality disorder: Effect on severity of social phobia, impairment, and outcome of cognitive behavioral treatment. *Behavior Therapy, 26,* 467–486.

Crowe, R. R., Pauls, D. L., Slymen, D. J., & Noyes, R. (1980). A family study of anxiety neurosis: Morbidity risk in families of patients with and without mitral valve prolapse. *Archives of General Psychiatry, 37,* 77–79.

Dealy R. R., Ishiki, D. M., Avery, D. H., Wilson, L. G., & Dunner, D. L. (1981). Secondary depression in anxiety disorders. *Comprehensive Psychiatry, 22,* 612–618.

DiNardo, P. A., Barlow, D. H., Cerny, J. A., Vermilya, B. B., Vermilya, J. A., Himaldi, W. G., & Waddell, M. T. (1986). *Anxiety Disorders Interview Schedule-Revised* (ADIS-R). Unpublished manuscript, State University of New Albany.

DiNardo, P. A., Brown, T. A., & Barlow, D. H. (1994). Anxiety Disorders Interview Schedule for DSM-IV: Lifetime version. Albany, NY: Graywind.

Eaton, W. W., Kessler, R. C., Wittchen, H.-U., & Magee, W. J. (1994). Panic and panic disorder in the United States. *American Journal of Psychiatry, 151,* 413–420.

First, M. B., Spitzer, R. L., Gibbon, M., & Williams, J. (1995). Structured clinical interview for Axis I DSM-IV disorders—patient edition (SCID—I/P, Version 2.0). New York: Biometrics Research Department, New York State Psychiatric Institute.

Gorman, J., Fyer, A. F., Glicklich, J., King, D., & Klein, D. F. (1981). Effect of imipramine on prolapsed mitral valves of patients with panic disorder. *American Journal of Psychiatry, 138,* 977–978.

Gorman, J. M., Levy, G. F., Liebowitz, M. R., McGrath, P., Appleby, I. L., Dillon, D. J., Davies, S. O., & Klein, D. F. (1983). Effect of acute β-adrenergic blockade of lactate-induced panic. *Archives of General Psychiatry, 40,* 1079–1082.

Heimberg, R. G., Holt, C. S., Schneier, F. R., Spitzer, R. L., & Liebowitz, M. R. (1993). The issue of subtypes in the diagnosis of social phobia. *Journal of Anxiety Disorders, 7,* 249–269.

Helzer, J. E., Robins, L. N., McEvoy, L. T., Spitznagel, E. L., Stoltzman, R. K., Farmer, A., & Brockington, I. F. (1985). A comparison of clinical and diagnostic interview schedule diagnoses. *Archives of General Psychiatry, 42,* 657–666.

Herbert, J. D., Hope, D. A., & Bellack, A. S. (1992). Validity of the distinction between generalized social phobia and avoidant personality disorder. *Journal of Abnormal Psychology, 101,* 332–338.

Hodgson, R. J., & Rachman, H. (1977). Obsessional–compulsive complaints. *Behaviour Research and Therapy, 15,* 389–395.

Holt, C. S., Heimberg, R. G., & Hope, D. A. (1992). Avoidant personality disorder and the generalized subtype of social phobia. *Journal of Abnormal Psychology, 101,* 318–325.

Hugdahl, K. (1981). The three-systems-model of fear and emotion: A critical examination. *Behaviour Research and Therapy, 19,* 75–85.

Jacob, R. G., Moller, M. B., Turner, S. M., & Wall, C. (1985). Otoneurological examination in panic disorders and agoraphobia with panic attacks: A pilot study. *American Journal of Psychiatry, 142,* 715–720.

Jacob, R. G., & Turner, S. M. (1988). Panic disorder: Diagnosis and assessment. In A. J. Frances & R. E. Hales (Eds.), *Review of psychiatry* (vol. 7, pp. 67–87). Washington, DC: American Psychiatric Press.

Jenike, M. A., Baer, L., Minichiello, W. E., Schwartz, C. E., & Carey, R. J., Jr. (1986). Concomitant obsessive–compulsive disorders and schizotypal personality disorder. *American Journal of Psychiatry, 143,* 530–532.

Kagan, J., Reznick, J. S., & Snidman, N. (1988). Biological bases of childhood shyness. *Science, 240,* 167–171.

Kathol, R. G., Noyes, R., Slymen, D. J., Crowe, R. R., Clancy, J., & Kerber, R. E. (1980). Propranolol in chronic anxiety disorders. *Archives of General Psychiatry, 37,* 1361–1365.

Kessler, R. C., McGonagle, K. A., Zhao, S., Nelson, C. B., Hughes, M., Eshleman, S., Wittchen, H. U., & Kendler, K. S. (1994). Lifetime and 12-month prevalence of DSM-III-R psychiatric disorders in the United States. *Archives of General Psychiatry, 51,* 8–19.

Keyl, P. M., & Eaton, W. W. (1990). Risk factors for the onset of panic disorder and other panic attacks in a prospective, population-based study. *American Journal of Epidemiology, 131,* 301–311.

Klein, D. F. (1964). Delineation of two drug responsive anxiety syndromes. *Psychopharmacologia, 5,* 397–408.

Korn, M. L., Kotler, M., Molcho, A., Botsis, A. J., Grosz, D., Chen, C., Plutchik, R., Brown, S., & van Praag, H. M. (1992). Suicide and violence associated with panic attacks. *Biological Psychiatry, 31,* 607–612.

Kushner, M. G., Sher, K. J., & Beitman, B. D. (1990). The relation between alcohol problems and the anxiety disorders. *American Journal of Psychiatry, 42,* 685–695.

Lang, P. J. (1977). Physiological assessment of anxiety and fear. In J. D. Cone & R. P. Hawkins (Eds.), *Behavioral assessment: New directions in clinical psychology* (pp. 178–195). New York: Brunner/Mazel.

Lesser, I. M., Rubin, R. T., Pecknold, J. C., Rifkin, A., Swinson, R. P., Lydiard, R. B., Burrows, G. D., Noyes, R. Jr., & DuPont, R. L. (1988). Secondary depression in panic disorder and agoraphobia. *Archives of General Psychiatry, 45,* 437–443.

Liebowitz, M. R., Fyer, A. J., Gorman, J. M., Dillon, D., Appleby, I. L., Levy, G., Anderson, S., Levitt, M., Palij, M., Davies, S. O., & Klein, D. E. (1984). Lactate provocation of panic attacks. *Archives of General Psychiatry, 41,* 764–770.

Liebowitz, M. R., Fyer, A. J., Gorman, J. M., Dillon, D., Davies, S., Stein, J. M., Cohen, B. S., & Klein, D. F. (1985a). Specificity of lactate infusions in social phobia versus panic disorders. *American Journal of Psychiatry, 142,* 947–950.

Liebowitz, M. R., Gorman, J. M., Dillon, D., Levy, G., Appleby, I. L., Anderson, S., Palij, M., Davies, S. O., & Klein, D. F. (1985b). Lactate provocation of panic attacks. *Archives of General Psychiatry, 42,* 709–719.

Margraf, J., Ehlers, A., & Roth, W. T. (1986). Sodium lactate infusions and panic attacks: A review and critique. *Psychosomatic Medicine, 48,* 23–51.

Marks, I. M. (1970). The classification of phobic disorders. *British Journal of Psychiatry, 116,* 377–386.

Marsland, D. W., Wood, M., & Mayo, F. (1976). Content of family practice: A data bank for patient care, curriculum, and research in family-practice patient problems. *Journal of Family Practice, 3,* 25–68.

Mavissakalian, M., & Hamann, M. S. (1986). DSM-III personality disorder in agoraphobia. *Comprehensive Psychiatry, 27,* 471–479.

Mavissakalian, M., & Hammer, M. S. (1988). Correlates of DSM-III personality disorder in panic disorder and agoraphobia. *Comprehensive Psychiatry, 29,* 535–544.

McNally, R. J. (1994). *Panic disorder: A critical analysis.* New York: Guilford Press.

Messer, S., & Beidel, D. C. (1994). Psychosocial and familial characteristics of anxious children. *Journal of the American Academy of Child and Adolescent Psychiatry, 33,* 975–983.

Morrison, J. (1995). *The first interview: Revised for DSM-IV.* New York: Guilford Press.

Öst, L. G. (1987). Age of onset in different phobias. *Journal of Abnormal Psychology, 96,* 223–229.

Reed, V., & Wittchen, H.-U. (1998). DSM-IV panic attacks and panic disorder in a community sample of adolescents and young adults: How specific are panic attacks? *Journal of Psychiatric Research, 32,* 335–345.

Reich, J. H., & Noyes, R., Jr. (1987). A comparison of DSM-III personality disorders in acutely ill panic and depressed patients. *Journal of Anxiety Disorders, 1,* 123–131.

Robins, L. N. (1985). Epidemiology: Reflections on testing the validity of psychiatric interviews. *Archives of General Psychiatry, 42,* 918–924.

Sanderson, W. C., Rapee, R. M., & Barlow, D. H. (1987). *The DSM-III-R revised anxiety disorder categories: Descriptors and patterns of comorbidity.* Presented at the annual meeting of Association for Advancement of Behavior Therapy, Boston.

Sanderson, W. C., Wetzler, S., Beck, A. T., & Betz, F. (1994). Prevalence of personality disorders among patients with anxiety disorders. *Psychiatry Research, 51,* 167–174.

Schneier, F. R., Johnson, J., Hornig, C. D., Liebowitz, M. R., & Weissman, M. M. (1992). Social phobia: Comorbidity and morbidity in an epidemiologic sample. *Archives of General Psychiatry, 49,* 284–288.

Shear, M. K., Devereaux, R. B., Kranier-Fox, R., Mann, J. J., & Frances, A. (1984). Low prevalence of mitral valve prolapse in patients with panic disorder. *American Journal of Psychiatry, 141,* 302–303.

Spielberger, C. D., Gorsuch, R. L., & Lushene, R. E. (1970). *The State-Trait Anxiety Inventory: Test manual for form X.* Palo Alto, CA: Consulting Psychologists Press.

Spitzer, R. B., & Williams, J.B, (1986). *Structured clinical interview for DSM-III-R, Axis II.* Unpublished manuscript, Biometrics Research Department, New York State Psychiatric Institute, New York.

Stanley M. A., Turner, S. M., & Borden, J. W. (1990). Schizotypal features in obsessive–compulsive disorder. *Comprehensive Psychiatry, 31,* 511–518.

Stein, M. B. (1986). Panic disorder and medical illness. *Psychosomatics, 27,* 833–840.

Stemberger, R. T., Turner, S. M., Beidel, D. C., & Calhoun, K. S. (1995). Social phobia: An analysis of possible developmental factors. *Journal of Abnormal Psychology, 104,* 526–531.

Turner, S. M., & Beidel, D. C. (1988). *Treating obsessive–compulsive disorder.* New York, Pergamon Press.

Turner, S. M., & Beidel, D. C. (1989). Social phobia: Clinical syndrome, diagnosis and comorbidity. *Clinical Psychology Review, 9,* 3–18.

Turner, S. M., Beidel, D. C., Borden, J. W., Stanley, M. A., & Jacob, R. G. (1991). Social phobia: Axis I and II correlates. *Journal of Abnormal Psychology, 100*, 102–106.

Turner, S. M., Beidel, D. C., Dancu, C. V., & Stanley, M. A. (1989). An empirically derived inventory to measure social fears and anxiety: The Social Phobia and Anxiety Inventory. *Psychological Assessment: A Journal of Consulting and Clinical Psychology, 1*, 35–40.

Turner, S. M., Beidel, D. C., & Jacob, R. G. (1988). Assessment of panic. In S. Rachman & J. D. Maser (Eds.), *Panic: Psychological perspectives* (pp. 37–50). Hillsdale, NJ: Lawrence Erlbaum.

Turner, S. M., Beidel, D. C., & Townsley, R. M. (1992). Social phobia: A comparison of specific and generalized subtypes and avoidant personality disorder. *Journal of Abnormal Psychology, 101*, 326–331.

Turner, S. M., McCann, B. S., Beidel, D. C., & Mezzich, J. B. (1986). DSM-III classification of anxiety, disorders: A psychometric study. *Journal of Abnormal Psychology, 95*, 168–172.

Uhde, T. W., Boulenger, J. P., Roy-Byrne, P. P., Geraci, M. E., Vittone, B. J., & Post, R. M. (1985). Longitudinal course of panic disorder: Clinical and biological considerations. *Progress in Neuro-Psychopharmacology and Biological Psychiatry, 9*, 39–51.

Van der Molen, C. G., & van den Hout, M. A. (1988). Expectancy effects on respiration during lactate infusion. *Psychosomatic Medicine, 50*, 439–443.

Van Valkenberg, C., Akiskal, H. G., Puzantian, V., & Rosenthal, T. (1984). Anxious depressions: Clinical, family history, and naturalistic outcome-comparisons with panic and major depressive disorders. *Journal of Affective Disorders, 6*, 67–82.

Van Velzen, C. J. M., Emmelkamp, P. M. G., & Scholing, A. (2000). Generalized social phobia versus avoidant personality disorder: Differences in psychopathology, personality traits, and social and occupational functioning. *Journal of Anxiety Disorders, 14*, 395–411.

Verheul, R., Kranzler, H. R., Poling, J., Tennen, H., Ball, S., & Rounsaville, B. J. (2000). Axis I and II disorders in alcoholics and drug addicts: Fact or artifact? *Journal of Studies on Alcohol, 61*, 101–110.

Watson, D., & Friend, R. (1969). Measurement of social-evaluative anxiety. *Journal of Consulting and Clinical Psychology, 33*, 448–457.

Weiller, E., Bisserbe, J. C., Maier, W., & Lecrubier, Y. (1998). Prevalence and recognition of anxiety syndromes in five European primary care settings. A report from the WHO study on psychological problems in general health care. *British Journal of Psychiatry, 34*(Suppl.), 18–23.

Weissman, M. M., Klerman, G. L., Markowitz, J. S., & Ouellette, R. (1989). Suicidal ideation and suicide attempts in panic disorder and attacks. *New England Journal of Medicine, 321*, 1209–1214.

Wittchen, H.-U., Stein, M. B., & Kessler, R. C. (1999). Social fears and social phobia in a community sample of adolescents and young adults: Prevalence, risk factors and co-morbidity. *Psychological Medicine, 29*, 309–323.

Zvolensky, M. J., Lejuez, C. W., & Eifert, G. H. (2000). Prediction and control: Operational definitions for the experimental analysis of anxiety. *Behaviour Research and Therapy, 38*, 653–663.

6

Mood Disorders

Paula Truax and Lisa Selthon

Mood disorders are both common and serious. Up to 19.3% of the population may experience either a unipolar or bipolar mood disorder at some point during their lives (Kessler et al., 1994). Unipolar depressive disorders have been estimated to cost the United States $43 billion in death, lost productivity, work absenteeism, and treatment expenses (Greenberg, Stiglin, Finkelstein, & Berndt, 1993) and bipolar conditions have been estimated to cost an additional $45 billion yearly (Wyatt & Henter, 1995). In addition, mood disturbance is the most salient risk factor in attempted and completed suicides (Persson, Runeson, & Wasserman, 1999) and it may increase the chances of death due to accident or cardiovascular event (Wulsin, Vaillant, & Wells, 1999). Timely detection of mood disorders and accurate distinctions between the categories of mood disorders may enhance the probability that effective care will be sought and received. The goals of this chapter are to: (1) describe the mood disorders; (2) review procedures for gathering diagnostic information; (3) provide representative case illustrations of the mood disorders; (4) review the most commonly used standardized interview formats; (5) list the critical information for making diagnoses, and; (6) encapsulate dos and don'ts with mood disorder diagnosis.

Description of the Disorder

Mood disorders are characterized by a disturbance of mood that deviates substantially from a normative mood along with additional physical, behavioral, and cognitive features. Mood may be described as disturbed if it is either too low (depressive state) or too high (manic state). Mood disorders may be either unipolar or bipolar. Unipolar disorders involve primarily depressed mood. The bipolar disorders typically involve cyclic depression and manic symptoms; however,

Paula Truax and Lisa Selthon • Counseling Psychology Program, Pacific University, Portland, Oregon 97205.

technically some of the bipolar disorders can be diagnosed with only manic symptoms. The discussion that follows addresses both unipolar and bipolar disorders.

When assessing mood disorders there are several levels to consider. First, individual *symptoms* need to be assessed. A symptom is a single occurrence or change in functioning that is an indicator of a psychiatric state (e.g., diminished interest or pleasure in activities). Second, if appropriate, the presence of specific *episodes* should be assessed. An episode is a combination of symptoms that are perceived as a whole and make up an element of a psychiatric disorder (e.g., Major Depressive Episode [MDE]). Finally, exclusive *disorders* may be assessed and diagnosed. Disorders are psychiatric syndromes. Diagnoses may be comprised of a combination of episodes (e.g., Major Depressive Disorder [MDD], Bipolar I Disorder) or they may represent a more enduring and non-episodic condition (e.g., Cyclothymic Disorder, Dysthymic Disorder [DD]). Although symptoms, episodes, and disorders each must be carefully assessed, only disorders can be used as diagnoses; symptoms and episodes are non-diagnosable. Careful diagnosis is essential for accurate conceptualization, treatment planning, and prognosis.

Description of Episodes

Many mood disorders are comprised of combinations of episodes (e.g., MDD, Bipolar I Disorder, and Bipolar II Disorder). The ensuing information on specific disorders and symptomatology is based on the fourth edition, text revision of the *Diagnostic and Statistical Manual of Mental Disorders*, Fourth Edition, Text Revision (*DSM-IV-TR*), the most commonly used mental disorders diagnostic manual (American Psychiatric Association, 2000). According to the *DSM-IV-TR* (2000) there are four types of mood episodes: MDE, Manic Episode, Hypomanic Episode, and Mixed Episode.

Major Depressive Episode

An MDE requires *five or more specific symptoms* that have been present *most of the day nearly every day for at least two weeks*. According to the *DSM-IV-TR*, the core symptoms of an MDE are *depressed mood* and/or *a loss of interest or pleasure in activities*. In adults, at least one of these core symptoms must be present for an MDE. In children and adolescents, however, irritability may be substituted for depressed mood. In addition, behavioral, physical, and/or cognitive symptoms are necessary for an MDE. These include the following: a change in *appetite or weight* (either increase or decrease); *sleep disturbance* (either increase or decrease in quantity, or decrease in quality); psychomotor *retardation or agitation* (observable by others); *fatigue* or low energy, feelings of *worthlessness* and/or excessive guilt, *difficulties concentrating* or making decisions, and *suicidal ideation* and/or thoughts of death. Since many of these symptoms are multidimensional and may vary in number from five to nine, clinical profiles may vary widely. This will be discussed further in the following section on information critical to making a diagnosis.

Manic Episode

In stark contrast to an MDE, a Manic Episode is characterized by a *euphoric or irritable mood* that is present for *at least one week and/or results in hospitalization.* Euphoria/mania is a distinct period of abnormally elevated mood in which there is a sense of extreme elation and expansiveness. With primary *euphoric mood, two or more* of the following additional symptoms are needed; if primary mood is *irritable, three or more* symptoms are needed for a Manic Episode. These symptoms include the following: *inflated self-esteem or feelings of grandiosity; decreased need for sleep; pressured speech* or talkativeness; *racing thoughts* and/or flight of ideas; *distractibility;* psychomotor *agitation and/or an increase in goal-directed behavior;* and engagement in *thrill-seeking or pleasurable activities* that can have negative consequences such as gambling or sexual promiscuity.

Hypomanic Episode

The symptoms required for a Hypomanic Episode are identical to a Manic Episode except that they are not as severe (i.e., *cannot result in hospitalization or marked social or occupational impairment*) and have a shorter duration (i.e., *a minimum of four days*). During this time, the mood and behaviors exhibited are observable to others and are clearly atypical of non-symptomatic periods (APA, 2000).

Mixed Episode

A Mixed Episode requires criteria being met for *both a Manic Episode and an MDE* for at least *a one-week period* (APA, 2000). The episodes can either be intermixed or can alternate every few days and either manic or depressive symptoms can predominate. When assessing for one of the other three mood episodes, a Mixed Episode needs to always be ruled out.

As outlined in the *DSM-IV-TR* (APA, 2000), the symptoms for all mood episodes (except Hypomanic Episode) need to cause clinically significant distress that interfere with important areas of functioning such as work, school, family, and/or social activities. Other psychological, medical, or substance-related causal factors must also be ruled out.

Episodic Disorders

The episodic disorders are usually characterized by a sporadic course, comprised of combinations of episodes interspersed with asymptomatic periods. The relationship between the episodes and disorders is presented graphically in Figure 1.

Major Depressive Disorder

MDD is one of the most commonly experienced mood disorders as well as one of the main reasons individuals seek mental health treatment (Kelleher,

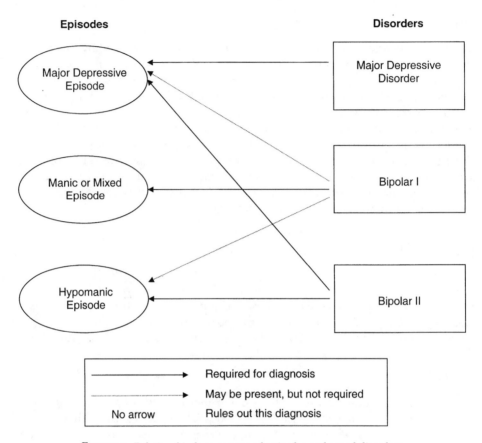

FIGURE 1. Relationship between mood episodes and mood disorders

Talcott, Haddock, & Freeman, 1996). MDD involves no Manic or Hypomanic Episodes and is comprised of one or more MDEs. Although depressed mood typically predominates, a minority of severely depressed individuals (10–15%) may experience a profound loss of interest or pleasure in the absence of depressed mood (Coyne, 1994).

Estimates based on community samples suggest that 10–25% of women and 5–12% of men in the United States will experience MDD in their lifetime (APA, 2000). At any given time, 5–9% of females and 2–3% of males will meet the requirements for MDD (APA, 2000). Early detection and treatment are exceptionally important because, without treatment, MDD may have a chronic impact on those who experience it. Approximately 50–60% of those with one episode of depression will have a second episode; 70% of those with two episodes and 90% of those with three episodes will have another episode (APA, 2000). Additionally, approximately 10% of those initially diagnosed with MDD will eventually develop a Manic or Hypomanic Episode resulting in a diagnostic shift from unipolar to bipolar (Coryell et al., 1995).

Bipolar I Disorder

Bipolar I Disorder is a cyclic disorder comprised of one or more Manic or Mixed Episodes. Paradoxically, although the bipolar title implies the cyclic occurrence of both very high and very low moods, current or past MDEs may exist but are not necessary for a bipolar diagnosis. Thus, any individual who has ever had a Manic Episode, meets criteria for Bipolar I. Those who have had only one Manic Episode and have never before experienced an MDE are likely to be diagnosed with Bipolar I Disorder, Single Manic Episode if the Manic Episode is not better accounted for by any other psychiatric disorder. While Hypomanic Episodes may be present in Bipolar I Disorder, at least one lifetime Manic Episode is necessary. For example, an individual may meet criteria for Bipolar I Disorder, Most Recent Episode Hypomanic with previous Manic Episodes, and a current Hypomanic Episode (APA, 2000). A determination regarding the nature of current and past episodes is central to clarifying the best treatment option and ruling out other possible diagnoses.

Community samples have shown that the lifetime prevalence rate of Bipolar I Disorder ranges from 0.4% to 1.6% (APA, 2000). Results from the Epidemiological Catchment Area (ECA) studies suggest that, on average, 0.8% of individuals will experience Bipolar I Disorder in their lifetime (Weissman et al., 1991). Like MDD, Bipolar I is also characterized by a pattern of increasing risk of future episodes with the occurrence of each new episode. Estimates indicate that more than 90% of individuals who have had one Manic Episode will experience future episodes (APA, 2000). In contrast to MDD, however, women do not appear to be more likely than men to experience Bipolar I Disorder (Winokur, Coryell, Endicott, & Akiskal, 1993).

Bipolar II Disorder

Bipolar II Disorder, like Bipolar I Disorder, is a cyclic disorder. In contrast, however, the elated or irritable mood is milder and significant depression is required, that is, both Major Depressive and Hypomanic Episodes are required for a diagnosis of Bipolar II (APA, 2000). Patients with Bipolar II, who eventually meet criteria for a full Manic or Mixed Episode warrant a diagnostic upgrade to Bipolar I.

Community samples have shown that approximately 0.5% of individuals will experience Bipolar II Disorder in their lifetime (APA, 2000; Weissman et al., 1991). Of more concern is that anywhere from 5–15% of individuals who meet the requirements for Hypomanic Episode will later experience a Manic Episode (APA, 2000).

Non-Episodic Disorders

While the episodic mood disorders have a more intermittent course, the non-episodic disorders tend to have a more chronic and unfluctuating course. The two most prevalent of the non-episodic disorders are DD and Cyclothymic Disorder.

Dysthymic Disorder

The main characteristic of DD is *depressed mood* that does not meet the criteria for an MDE and has been present *more days than not for at least 2 years* (APA, 2000). In addition, at least two of the following cognitive, behavioral, or physical symptoms must be present: *appetite changes* (increase or decrease); *sleep disturbance* (sleeping too much or too little); *low energy or fatigue; low self-esteem; concentration or decision-making difficulties;* and/or feelings of *hopelessness* (APA, 2000). These symptoms need to be present throughout a 2-year period with no symptom-free period greater than 2 months. For children and adolescents, the mood may be primarily irritable and must have lasted only 1 year. Criteria for a Manic, Hypomanic, or Mixed Episode must never have been met for either children or adults.

Approximately 3.2% (Weissman et al., 1991) to 6.4% (Kessler et al., 1994) of individuals will experience Dysthymia in their lifetime while approximately 3% of individuals experience Dysthymia at any particular point in time (APA, 2000; Weissman et al., 1991). In any given year, approximately 10% of individuals with Dysthymia will experience an MDE for the first time (APA, 2000).

Although Bipolar I Disorder, Bipolar II Disorder, and MDD are mutually exclusive disorders, Dysthymia can and often does coexist with other mood disorders, particularly MDD. For a current diagnosis of DD, any MDE must have occurred and fully resolved at least 2 months prior to the development of DD or developed at least 2 years after criteria for DD had been fully met. Low-grade depressive symptoms that begin with an MDE or are interrupted with an MDE during the first 2 years preclude a diagnosis of DD. MDEs that occur after the initial 2 years of DDs suggest the following disorder: MDD superimposed on DD. Colloquially, this is known as "double depression." The ECA program reported that 42% of individuals with DD also met criteria for MDD sometime in their lifetime (Weissman et al., 1991). See the following section regarding Differential Diagnosis for more information about how to make this distinction between DD and MDD, as well as the case conceptualization, treatment planning, and prognosic implications.

Cyclothymic Disorder

Cyclothymic Disorder is a cyclic non-episodic disorder consisting of alternating hypomanic symptoms and depressive symptoms. Although at least one of the hypomanic periods must meet criteria for a Hypomanic Episode, the depressed mood must *not* meet criteria for an MDE (APA, 2000). Cyclothymic Disorder is similar to Bipolar II Disorder, however, the depressed mood is less severe. Like with DD, the symptoms need to be present for at least 2 years (only 1 year in children and adolescents) and individuals must have never met the criteria for a Manic or Mixed Episode. However, after the initial 2-year period of Cyclothymic Disorder, individuals may experience a Manic, Mixed, or MDE superimposed on the Cyclothymia (APA, 2000).

Prevalence rates for Cyclothymia have not been as thoroughly researched as those of other mood disorders. However, the *DSM-IV-TR* indicates that the lifetime prevalence rates of Cyclothymia range from 0.4% to 1% (APA, 2000; Faravelli, Degl'Innocenti, Aiazzi, Incerpi, & Pallanti, 1990).

As with episodic mood disorders, non-episodic mood disorders must also cause clinically significant distress that affects major areas of a person's life. General medical conditions and "direct psychological effects" of a substance must be ruled out as well as other psychiatric complications (APA, 2000). Unlike episodic mood disorders, an individual must presently meet criteria for DD or Cyclothymic Disorder to be diagnosed with the disorder. Past episodes of Dysthymia and Cyclothymia are non-diagnosable.

Other Mood Disorders

Other mood disorders that have not yet been discussed are: Bipolar Disorder Not Otherwise Specified (NOS), Depressive Disorder NOS, Mood Disorder Due to a General Medical Condition, Substance-Induced Mood Disorder, and Mood Disorder NOS. These categories are used for individuals who exhibit some, but not all, of the characteristics necessary for the previously mentioned mood disorders.

Bipolar Disorder NOS

A mood profile that includes manic or hypomanic symptoms but does not meet all of the standard bipolar criteria may be best represented by a Bipolar Disorder NOS diagnosis. For example, the experience of a Hypomanic Episode with no depressed mood may warrant a Bipolar Disorder NOS diagnosis. Similarly, meeting the symptom criteria for Bipolar I or II Disorder, but not the duration criteria may fit into a Bipolar Disorder NOS category.

Depressive Disorder NOS

Unipolar presentations with erratic, atypical, or subthreshold presentations that do not meet criteria for any unipolar diagnosis may be best represented by Depressive Disorder NOS (APA, 2000). Many of the depressive conditions that are currently being researched, but have not yet been accepted as discrete disorders would fit into the Depressive Disorder NOS class. Included in this category are: premenstrual dysphoric disorder; minor depressive disorder; recurrent brief depressive disorder; postpsychotic depressive disorder of Schizophrenia; an MDE superimposed on Delusional Disorder, Psychotic Disorder NOS, or the active phase of Schizophrenia; or situations where a depressive disorder is present, but there is no determination whether it is "primary, due to a general medical condition, or substance induced" (APA, 2000, p. 382).

Mood Disorder NOS

Mood Disorder NOS is a diagnosis that is used when full criteria are not met for any other mood disorder and it is difficult to assess whether a depressive or bipolar course predominates. This diagnosis is reserved for situations in which all other mood disorders are accurately ruled out, yet there appears to be a mood disorder present.

Mood Disorder Due to a General Medical Condition

Mood Disorder Due to a General Medical Condition requires depressed mood or anhedonia and/or an elevated, expansive or irritable mood that is the *"direct physiological consequence of a general medical condition"* (APA, 2000, p. 404). The symptoms must be physiologically related to the medical condition. For example, if an individual has a digestive problem and is depressed because of how the disease affects his or her life, criteria for Mood Disorder Due to a General Medical Condition would not be met because depressive reactions to the sequelae of physical conditions do not warrant this diagnosis. Instead, if an individual's mood presentation is due to the direct physiological consequences of a condition known to have physiologically depressive properties, such as hypothyroidism, then the criteria for MDD due to a General Medical Condition may be met. The medical condition affecting the disorder is listed in the diagnosis (e.g., Mood Disorder Due to Hypothyroidism). A Mood Disorder Due to a General Medical Condition should be determined by laboratory findings, physical examination, and/or a prior history versus merely relying on the client's subjective report (APA, 2000).

General medical disorders can physiologically lead to a variety of symptoms that make up mood disorders. Some common medical disorders that can cause depression are endocrine disorders such as diabetes, hypothyroidism, and hyperthyroidism; infectious disorders such as AIDS and hepatitis; degenerative neurological conditions such as Huntington's chorea, Parkinson's, and multiple sclerosis; cerebrovascular disease such as strokes; autoimmune conditions such as systemic lupus erythematosis; certain cancers; and other medical disorders and complications such as toxic exposure to heavy metals, malnutrition, and vitamin B_{12} deficiency (see Morrison, 1995 for a more comprehensive list). Mania can also be the direct physiological consequence of certain medical disorders such as AIDS, systemic lupus erythematosis, multiple sclerosis, Huntington's chorea, stroke, and influenza (Akiskal & Van Valkenburg, 1994).

Substance-Induced Mood Disorder

As outlined in the *DSM-IV-TR*, a diagnosis of Substance-Induced Mood Disorder requires depressed mood or anhedonia and/or an elevated, expansive, or irritable mood that can be shown to be due to the direct effect of Substance Intoxication or Withdrawal or the known etiological consequence of a medication (APA, 2000). Like with Mood Disorder Due to a General Medical Condition, there needs to be a direct relationship between the mood disorder and the substance use. There are a variety of classes of substances that can lead to substance-induced mood symptoms either through intoxication or withdrawal. Please refer to the *DSM-IV-TR* (APA, 2000) for a comprehensive list of substance classes.

One of the best ways to assess if a mood disorder is primary or secondary is to assess the temporal relationship between the substance use or medical problem and the course of the mood symptoms or episodes (APA, 2000; First, Spitzer, Gibbon, & Williams, 1997). Mood symptoms that occur only while ill or using substances may meet criteria for a Mood Disorder Due to General Medical Condition or Substance-Induced Mood Disorder; whereas, a worsening of pre-existing mood symptoms or mood symptoms that occur both during and after illness or substance use probably would not warrant such diagnoses.

Differential Diagnosis

In order to provide the best possible treatment and prognosis, it is essential that mood disorders be distinguished from one another and from other psychological and physical diagnoses that may mimic them. In addition, a good understanding of the boundaries of mood disorder diagnoses will facilitate accurate diagnosis of comorbid conditions that may affect intervention.

Although the two primary categories of mood disorders (i.e., high mood vs. low mood) may be relatively easy to distinguish from one another, differentiations within each of these categories are somewhat more challenging. Differential diagnosis within the depressed mood diagnoses will be addressed first, followed by diagnoses that involve mania, and finally differentiation between the unipolar and bipolar diagnoses will be presented.

Unipolar Diagnoses

The two diagnostic categories that deal exclusively with depressed mood are MDD and DD. Although both are characterized by primarily depressed mood they differ in length, severity, and onset. MDD is more severe (i.e., *five* symptoms must be present *most of the day nearly everyday*) but usually more acute (i.e., only a *two-week* duration is required) than DD which is less severe (i.e., *two* symptoms must be present *more days than not*) and more chronic (i.e., *two-year* duration is required). These disorders may exist alone or in combination. The tricky differential diagnosis questions will be addressed below.

MDD versus DD. Both quantitative and qualitative differences separate these categories. Quantitatively, MDD requires 2 weeks of at least 5 symptoms (including mood or interest changes); DD requires 2 years of at least 2 symptoms (in addition to low mood). If an individual meets the duration criteria of DD, with the severity level of MDD, then a diagnosis of MDD with a specifier of "chronic" should be given. Qualitatively, some have proposed that MDD is characterized more by somatic symptoms (e.g., sleep disturbance, appetite disturbance, psychomotor changes), whereas DD is characterized more by cognitive and social symptoms (e.g., low self-esteem) (Roberts, Shapiro, & Gamble, 1999; Serretti et al., 1999). Recent data suggest, however, that the difference between chronic and acute depressive disorders may best be described as quantitative rather than qualitative (Klein et al., 1999).

MDD Superimposed on DD versus MDD Without Full Interepisode Recovery. DD and MDD are thought to develop uniquely. DD is defined as a condition that has a gradual onset with a chronic course. MDD has a more acute and sudden onset. As a result, mood episodes that begin abruptly are differentiated from those with a gradual onset. When a chronic course of depression begins with an MDD episode, a diagnosis of DD cannot be given even if there are subsequent 2-year periods with milder depression. Instead, a diagnosis of MDD with a qualifier of "without full interepisode recovery" is given. In contrast, when a chronic course begins with at least a 2-year period of DD (with no episodes of MDD in the initial 2 years) followed by future MDD episodes, the diagnosis is MDD superimposed on DD or "double depression."

The differentiation between these two disorders may have important implications for case conceptualization, prognosis, and treatment. MDD is usually considered an episodic condition characterized by departure from an individual's normal functioning. DD, on the other hand, is often conceptualized as a lifestyle or personality dimension (Akiskal, 1996). McCullough (2000), a prominent researcher and theorist of chronic depression, poses that DD is a developmental disorder in which sufferers never learn to accurately detect the cause and effect relationship between their own behavior and the outcomes of interpersonal interactions. Thus, individuals with chronic DD are purported to have an absence of the skills necessary to reduce their depressed mood, whereas those with MDD may have formerly learned the skills but have difficulty accessing them when in a depressive episode. In addition, in comparison with MDD, those with chronic DD are more likely to have significant global and social impairment (Klein et al., 1996; Klein, Taylor, Dickstein, & Harding, 1988; Klein, Schwartz, Rose, & Leader, 2000), higher rates of personality disorders (Klein et al., 1988), greater substance disorder comorbidity (Klein et al., 1988), more familial psychopathology (Klein et al., 1988), and more severe MDD episodes when they occur (Klein et al., 1988). Further, when DD is coupled with MDD in a double depression (as described above), impairment is even more heightened. In contrast to singular DD and MDD diagnoses, double depressives experience greater social impairment, greater symptom severity, greater work impairment, and poorer financial status (Evan et al., 1996). Consistent with these findings, recovery rates for the unipolar mood disorders can be rank ordered from best to worst as follows: (1) MDD; (2) DD; and (3) double depression (see Wells, Burnam, Rogers, Hays, & Camp, 1992). As noted earlier, however, although recovery rates for MDD may be higher, relapse rates are also high—increasing exponentially with each successive episode (APA, 2000).

These conceptualizations, as well as the existing research, suggest that chronic depression may require treatment approaches different from episodic depression. First, regarding psychotherapy, research on empirically supported treatments indicates that each may require a different focus. Far and away the most frequently supported psychotherapeutic intervention for MDD is cognitive behavioral therapy (see Craighead, Craighead, & Liardi, 1998a for a review). This type of therapy helps clients identify and modify inaccurate or self-defeating thinking while increasing behavioral activity through re-accessing more functional thought and behavior patterns that were used when the individual was not depressed. Those with chronic depression are much less likely to have a favorable response to these interventions (Kavanagh & Wilson, 1989), however. Instead, some recent data suggest that a new psychotherapy entitled Cognitive Behavioral Analysis System of Psychotherapy (CBASP; McCullough, 2000), which focuses on identifying and modifying interpersonal behaviors that are perpetuating the depression, may yield good outcomes with DD (Keller et al., 2000). Second, recommendations regarding psychotropic intervention may differ between these two disorders. Although both MDD and DD share similar patterns of response to psychotherapeutic and psychotropic monotherapies (i.e., good short-term outcome for both medication and psychotherapy; poorer long-term outcome for medication) (Gloaguen, Cottraux, Cucherat, & Blackburn, 1998), the disorders diverge in their response to the combination therapies. For mild to moderate MDD, there appears to be little advantage to combining medication and psychotherapy. Instead, medication, psychotherapy, or the combination of the two appear to yield similar outcomes (Thompson, Coon, Gallagher-Thompson, Sommer, & Koin, 2001). For DD, however, the combination of nefazadone and CBASP may increase the number of responders from approximately 50% to 85% (Keller et al., 2000). In sum, the distinction between chronic unremitting depression and more episodic, acute depression may have important implications for conceptualization, prognosis, and treatment.

Bipolar Diagnoses

The two primary diagnoses that involve both low and high moods—Bipolar I and Bipolar II—also involve some subtle distinctions between categories that may have important implications for conceptualization, prognosis, and treatment. Topographically, the main differences between the two diagnoses are: (1) severity of the manic symptoms (Bipolar I requires a full Manic Episode; Bipolar II requires only a Hypomanic Episode); and (2) necessity of depressive symptoms (Bipolar I allows but does not require depressive symptoms; Bipolar II requires that full criteria for MDE are met at least once).

Although some have argued that Bipolar I and Bipolar II Disorders simply represent quantitative differences in severity (Benazzi, 1999), others have pointed to potentially important qualitative differences. While there are striking similarities between Bipolar I and Bipolar II in successful types of treatment (cf. Tondo, Baldessarini, & Floris, 2001), age of onset (Benazzi, 1999), suicidality (Vieta et al., 1997a), and parental Bipolar I diagnoses (Heun & Maier, 1993), there appear to be some important differences in course and treatment response. For example, amongst untreated bipolar disorders, those with Bipolar II are five times more likely to be rapid cyclers (Baldessarini, Tondo, Floris, & Hennen, 2000) and have more frequent episodes (Vieta, Gasto, Otero, & Nieto, 1997b) than those with Bipolar I. Further, Bipolar II sufferers may be simultaneously less aware of the role of their illness in their symptoms and more distressed about their symptoms (Pallanti et al., 1999). When treated, however, those with Bipolar II are more likely to have a positive response to lithium therapy resulting in a greater reduction in frequency and duration of episodes (Tondo, Baldessarini, Hennen, & Floris, 1998). These findings, coupled with some research pointing to an increased risk of Bipolar II (6.1%) over Bipolar I (1.8%) with parental Bipolar II (Heun & Maier, 1993), suggest that there may be both research and clinical utility in differentiating between Bipolar I and II diagnoses.

Unipolar versus Bipolar

Conceptually, very high and very low moods may be clearly differentiated from one another. In practice, however, these distinctions may be more difficult than they immediately appear. The three issues that make these distinctions especially difficult are differentiating between: (1) normal mood in chronic depression and abnormally high mood; (2) depressive agitation/irritability and manic/hypomanic symptoms; and (3) depressive episodes that are part of bipolar versus unipolar depression. Guidelines for making these diagnostic decisions will be addressed first. Conceptual, treatment, and prognostic rationales will be addressed second.

For clients with chronic depression, a question regarding abnormally elevated mood may be difficult to address. Because any good mood may feel abnormal to clients who are usually depressed, they may respond affirmatively to manic questions. For example, during rare depression remissions, chronic depressives may state that they had periods of increased self-esteem, needed less sleep, talked more quickly than usual, felt their thoughts moving more quickly than usual, and were more involved in pleasurable activities than usual. The key to differentiating between normal good mood and manic symptoms is careful attention to the severity and quality of the manic/hypomanic symptoms. First, each of the symptoms needs to meet duration and pervasiveness requirements. Second, for symptoms to be representative of manic/hypomanic symptoms, the quality should be clearly different from just a good mood. For example, increased self-esteem should be clearly grandiose; need for less sleep should be much less sleep than is needed by most people; pressured speech would be speech that is so fast others noticed and commented; and increased involvement in pleasurable activities would be behaviors with a high potential for negative consequences.

Similarly, depressive symptoms of agitation and irritability can be difficult to differentiate from manic symptoms. According to the *DSM-IV-TR*, agitation is on the symptom list for MDD, and irritability may be a key feature of the bipolar disorders. Yet agitation often appears in mania, and irritation often appears in unipolar depressive episodes. To further complicate the clinical picture, depressive agitation and/or irritability are often combined with other endogenous depression symptoms including difficulty in sleeping and difficulty in concentrating—all possible symptoms of mania. While differentiation between these two disorders may be far from perfect when these symptoms are present, a good rule of thumb is to focus on mood and goal-directedness of the activity. In unipolar depression, the agitation and irritability are typically somewhat diffuse and despite possible intense feelings of restlessness, there is often no press to engage in any particular activity. On the other hand, manic patients often experience agitation or irritability as energizing toward a particular goal. They may feel a strong need to engage in a particular activity as a result of the agitation or irritability. Also the primary mood when the person is feeling less irritable or agitated may provide a clue to the diagnosis. In mania, the mood may shift from irritable to elated; whereas, in depression, the mood may vacillate between irritability and sadness. Finally, as always, ensure that a sufficient number of symptoms are present to make the diagnosis. Three additional symptoms are necessary to make a diagnosis of Manic Episode when irritability is the primary feature. If three symptoms are present along with significant irritability, a bipolar diagnosis may be warranted.

Perhaps the most difficult and imperfect science in diagnosing mood disorders is differentiating between early depressive episodes that are indicative of a recurrent unipolar cycle or a bipolar cycle. Often, the bipolar disorders begin with several depressive episodes prior to the occurrence of Manic or Hypomanic Episodes. Although a bipolar diagnosis cannot be made in the absence of Manic or Hypomanic episodes, some features of depressive episodes may alert clinicians to a possible bipolar course. Compared to those with a unipolar course, those who eventually develop bipolar depression have been shown to be more likely to have atypical depressive episodes characterized by oversleeping, overeating, and interpersonal reactivity (Benazzi, 2001a, 2001b), psychotic depression (Goldberg, Harrow, & Whiteside, 2001), family history of bipolar illness (Goldberg et al., 2001), earlier onset age (Benazzi, 2001b), and nonmelancholic depression (Parker, Roy, Wilhelm, Mitchell, & Hadzi-Pavlovic, 2000).

Although these subtle topographical differences between unipolar and bipolar disorders may seem only academic at first glance, treatment may differ significantly depending upon whether manic symptoms are part of the current or future profile. First, unipolar depression may be successfully treated with psychotherapy, whereas, bipolar disorders often require psychopharmacological interventions (Craighead, Miklowitz, Vajk, & Frank, 1998b). When psychotherapy is used for bipolar patients, the focus would typically be on medication compliance, as well as symptom management (Basco, 2000). In fact, some recent research suggests that the addition of cognitive behavioral therapy to mood stabilizing medication may enhance outcomes over medication alone for bipolar patients (Scott, Garland, & Moorhead, 2001). Second, the type of medication management may vary significantly depending upon the presence of manic symptoms. Not only are bipolar patients less likely to respond to pharmacological interventions targeted at unipolar disorders, they may worsen when treated as if unipolar. A comprehensive literature of review of bipolar treatments by Srisurapanont, Yatham, and Zis (1995) found that all antidepressant treatments not focused on mood stabilization were likely to actually induce a manic/hypomanic switch in bipolar patients. Srisurapanont and colleagues (1995) also concluded in a more recent literature review that antidepressants should never be used as monotherapies for patients with bipolar courses. Instead, mood stabilizers should be used first, followed by the addition of antidepressants, if necessary.

Taken together, these findings suggest that careful assessment and diagnosis are central to successful conceptualization and treatment planning of the mood disorders.

PROCEDURES FOR GATHERING INFORMATION

Accurate diagnosis often requires multimethod, multidimensional assessment. Often clinicians' diagnostic method choices involve balancing practicality with rigor. Below, some methods for gathering diagnostic information will be described along with their relative advantages and disadvantages.

Interview

Perhaps the most common way to obtain diagnostic information from clients is to perform an interview. These diagnostic interviews may be unstructured, semistructured, or structured in format.

Unstructured Clinical Interview

One of the most commonly used, but less reliable interview formats is the unstructured interview (First et al., 1997). An unstructured interview is a highly flexible approach that allows the interviewer to ask general questions. This approach allows the interviewee to answer with more complete information. However, the information gathered may be less accurate and more difficult to categorize. Essential factors in increasing the reliability of the typical clinical interview are the clinician's knowledge and systematic application of that knowledge during the diagnostic portion of the interview. Parts of the following section are adapted from Truax (2002). Minimum knowledge areas include:

1. Diagnostic categories: *DSM-IV-TR symptoms* for the mood disorders; *time frames* necessary for each diagnosis (e.g., at least 2 weeks for MDD); and *severity* (e.g., most of the day, nearly every day for MDD).
2. Differential diagnosis: *DSM-IV-TR* symptoms of other disorders that may overlap or mimic each other.

Application of this knowledge requires:

1. asking specifically about each of the symptoms, time frame, and severity;
2. asking specifically about key symptoms from other diagnoses.

An example of how the diagnostic portion of the clinical interview may begin follows:

T: Now I would like to ask you some fairly specific questions about how you have been feeling recently. I know you said that you have been feeling depressed and that it has been going on for about two months. Has there been a two-week period in the past month in which you felt depressed most of the day, nearly every day?

C: Yes, I have felt depressed most of the day, nearly everyday for the past two months.

T: OK. Can you tell me if the past two weeks have been characteristic of the past two months?

C: If anything, the most recent two weeks have been the worst. That is why I came to see you.

T: OK then, let's focus on the most recent two weeks for the rest of these questions (establishing time-frame). In the past two weeks, have you also lost interest or pleasure in things that you usually enjoyed (checking out specific symptoms)?

C: Yes.

T: Has that been most of the day, nearly every day (severity)?

C: It has been constant. I can't get interested in anything.

T: How about your weight and appetite? You mentioned earlier that you have gained 12 pounds in the past month, because you are eating all the time due to depression. Did I get that right (time-frame, specific symptoms, severity)?

C: Yes, I understand some people lose weight when they feel depressed. I wish that were me.

T: Depression is different for everyone. Weight gain is not uncommon. You also mentioned earlier that you have been having difficulty going to sleep, has that been nearly every day over the past two weeks? (time-frame, specific symptoms, severity)

C: It has been every day over the past two weeks. (interview continues asking about all symptoms for MDD, time-frame, and severity).

T: We've been talking mostly about depressed mood, so far. Now I would like to switch gears a little and ask about other types of moods. Have you ever experienced a time when you felt so happy or elated that others noticed and commented on it (ruling out Bipolar I, Bipolar II, Cyclothymic Disorder)?

C: I wish! No, I have never felt exceptionally happy for more than a minute or two.

T: Now how about the depressed mood, you mentioned that you had been feeling depressed for the past two months. Have you experienced a low-grade depressed mood for the past two years or longer (ruling out DD)?

C: No, not really. The past two months have been really bad, but I was feeling OK before that.

A useful tool for differential diagnosis is drawing a timeline of the mood episodes. This is particularly helpful for differentiating MDD superimposed on DD from MDD in partial remission.

Semistructured Interviews

An alternative to the unstructured clinical interview is a more standardized semistructured interview. These interviews involve a combination of verbatim closed-ended and open-ended questions as well as an option to ask follow-up questions for clarification.

The Structured Clinical Interview for the *DSM-IV* (SCID-IV; First et al., 1997) and the Schedule for Affective Disorders and Schizophrenia (SADS; Endicott & Spitzer, 1978) are examples of semistructured interviews. The SCID is a semi-structured interview that is used to evaluate *DSM* diagnoses. The SCID provides a "breadth of diagnostic coverage and focuses on diagnosis rather than sympto-mology" (Rogers, 2001, p. 104). The SADS is a semistructured interview that is used primarily to assess and diagnose mood and psychotic disorders. The SADS provides in-depth coverage of specific disorders as well as assessing current and prior episodes. One of the major differences between the SADS and the SCID is that the SADS provides more depth, while the SCID provides greater breadth

(Rogers, 2001). This is because the SADS is devoted mostly to Schizophrenia and Affective Disorders while the SCID covers the gamut of *DSM-IV-TR* disorders. Both the SADS and the SCID will be discussed in more depth in the Standardized Interview Format section of this chapter.

Structured Interviews

Structured interviews are standardized interviews that involve asking clients a predetermined set amount of close-ended questions. The purpose of this format is to increase inter-rater reliability and to create a more standardized process in gathering information from clients. All clients are asked the same questions, in the same order. An example of a structured interview format is the Diagnostic Interview Schedule (DIS; Robins, Helzer, Croughan, & Ratcliff, 1981). The DIS is a highly structured interview that is used to assess current and lifetime diagnoses of common mental disorders. Interviewers follow a set of prescribed questions and are informed not to deviate from the structure. One difficulty with structured interviews is that there may be situations where a question is not fully answered or follow-up after an answer is necessary. According to Rogers (2001) "information variance is optimized" with structured interviews while "criterion variance is optimized" with semistructured interviews (p. 27). This means there are fewer variations in the inclusion/exclusion criteria used by clinicians to make diagnoses when semistructured interviews are used. Therefore, there is less disagreement between clinicians about what is clinically relevant. Alternatively, there are fewer variations in the amounts and types of information gathered by clinicians and how this information is organized when structured interviews are used. The DIS will also be discussed in further detail in the Standardized Interview Format section of this chapter.

Self-Report Measures

Self-report paper and pencil questionnaires are economical, efficient methods for diagnostic screening and severity level. Questionnaires should never be used as a substitute for a thorough clinical interview when making diagnostic decisions. Although there is a multitude of self-report measures for the mood disorders, just a few of the most commonly used will be reviewed here. See Nezu, Ronan, Meadows, and McClure (2000) for a comprehensive list of measures for the depressive disorders.

Unipolar Instruments

Two of the most commonly used self-report depression measures are the Beck Depression Inventory—Second Edition (BDI-II; Beck, Steer, & Brown, 1996) and the Center for Epidemiological Studies Depression Scale (CES-D; Radloff, 1977). Both self-report measures are useful in determining the severity level of depression. In addition, a cut-off has been developed for the CES-D to screen for the presence of an MDD diagnosis.

Beck Depression Inventory-II. The BDI-II is a widely accepted and administered 21-item self-rating inventory corresponding to the *DSM-IV-TR* symptoms of depression. It takes 5–10 min to complete and is useful in assessing the severity of depression in individuals 13 and older (Beck et al., 1996). Consistent with the *DSM-IV-TR* criteria for MDD, the answers are based on the preceding 2 weeks, and each item is rated from 0 to 3. For example, one item asks individuals to choose the most accurate statement regarding sadness ("I do not feel sad," "I feel sad much of the time," "I am sad all of the time," or "I am so sad or unhappy that I can't stand it") (Beck et al., 1996). Scoring and interpretation involve totaling the items and comparing the total score to the severity cutoffs in the BDI-II manual (0–13 = minimal; 14–19 = mild; 20–28 = moderate; 29–63 = severe). The BDI-II demonstrates good internal consistency with coefficient alphas of 0.93 and test–retest stability over 1 week ($r = 0.93$, $p < 0.001$). Discriminant and construct validity have been demonstrated with higher correlations between the BDI-II and other depression measures than between the BDI-II and anxiety measures (Steer, Ball, Ranieri, & Beck, 1997). Tests of criterion validity also demonstrate that BDI-II scores are predictive of MDD diagnoses (Arnau, Meagher, Norris, & Bramson, 2001).

Center for Epidemiological Studies—Depression Scale. The CES-D (Radloff, 1977) is a self-report scale of current symptoms of depression that focuses mainly on the affective component of depression. It was initially developed for use in epidemiological studies of depression. The 20 items are scaled by frequency of occurrence during the past week. Scoring requires totaling the scores for each item (taking into account four reverse scored items) yielding scores from 0 to 60. Although, Radloff (1977) originally established a cutoff score of 16 to represent significant risk of current MDD, later research has found that the cutoff may be too lenient. Even though the cutoff of 16 may have exceptional sensitivity, it has low specificity (Santor, Zuroff, Ramsay, Cervantes, & Palacios, 1995). Some authors have suggested cutoffs of 17 and 23 for "possible" and "probable" cases, respectively (Husaini, Neff, Harrington, Hughes, & Stone, 1980); others have proposed different cutoffs based on likelihood ratios (Furukawa, Hirai, Kitamura, & Takahashi, 1997). Overall, however, the CES-D has been demonstrated as internally consistent (0.85 and 0.90 in general and psychiatric patients, respectively) and relatively stable for short periods of time (Radloff, 1977). The CES-D was also shown to have excellent concurrent validity and good known-groups validity as well as being sensitive to change in improvement after treatment (Radloff, 1977).

One study found the CES-D to be more discriminating than the BDI, but found that the CES-D is often less specific (Santor et al., 1995). This finding implies that the CES-D is better at identifying individuals differing in depressive severity whereas the BDI is more precise in identifying if individuals are depressed or not. The BDI has been shown to produce fewer false positives than the CES-D (Santor et al., 1995).

Bipolar Instruments

While self-report measurement is an exceedingly common method of assessment for the unipolar depressions, it is relatively uncommon for the bipolar conditions. Many have been concerned that the manic impairment is so significant that a self-report instrument would be unwieldy. Data from recent studies have suggested, however, that most manic patients can successfully complete brief self-report instruments with adequate internal consistency, test–retest reliability, and predictive and concurrent validity even when psychotic symptoms are present or insight is limited (Altman, 1998). One of the more commonly used assessments of mania will be presented here.

Altman Self-Rating Mania Scale. The Altman Self-Rating Mania Scale (ASRM; Altman, Hedeker, Peterson, & Davis, 1997) was developed to assess the severity of current manic symptoms. The ASRM is composed of five items with each item rated on a 0–4 point scale. A factor analysis of these items suggested that there might be separate subscales including mania, psychotic symptoms, and irritability (Altman et al., 1997). Compared to patients with schizoaffective disorder, schizophrenia, and MDD, bipolar patients scored higher on the mania component and were more likely to have a reduction in total scores after treatment (Altman et al., 1997). The ASRM has also demonstrated very good sensitivity (93%); however, the specificity has been quite low (33%). Together, these findings suggest that the ASRM may be a good screening instrument to determine whether additional assessment of manic symptoms is necessary; however, it may over-identify possible bipolar disorders (Altman, Hedeker, Peterson, & Davis, 2001).

Observation

The methods of gathering information discussed thus far have relied on verbal information; yet there are some fundamental problems with the accuracy of verbal report. First, verbal reports are notoriously flawed. Williams, Lees-Haley, and Price (1998), for example, found that symptom self-reports might be inflated by explicit attention to symptoms. Second, several of the criterion symptoms for the mood disorders require observation of an external observer (e.g., agitation or retardation; speaking more quickly than usual). Third, insight for certain symptoms or constellations may be low, particularly the bipolar disorders (Ghaemi, 1997). Finally, efforts to present socially desirably may affect the accuracy of self-report. Cappeliez (1989) found, for example, that social desirability was negatively related to BDI scores in a sample of older adults. These issues all point to the necessity of alternative methods for collecting diagnostic information.

Direct observation of the client by others may provide important information that cannot be gained through verbal reports. This information may be crucial to diagnostic decisions. Such observations may occur in-session by the therapist or out-of-session by the client him/herself or other third party observers such as a parent, spouse, roommate, friend, or sibling. Although direct observation may address some of the problems inherent in self-report, it has a few problems of its own because most observers are biased in some way. Therapists, for example, tend to rate therapy as more successful than clients do (Weiss, Rabinowitz, & Spiro, 1996) and be poor predictors of therapy outcome based on their observations of the client (Barber et al., 1999). Similarly, external familial observers may be biased by their own mood or other factors (Teri & Truax, 1994). Despite these potential shortcomings, direct observation may provide information that the patient is unaware of or unwilling or unable to report.

The mental status exam (MSE) has traditionally been the mainstay of in-session observation. The goal of the MSE is to observationally assess the client's emotional and cognitive functioning. There are a variety of MSEs; some are structured and more detailed while others are less structured and briefer in format. Rogers (2001) discusses two types of MSEs: comprehensive and cognitive. Comprehensive MSEs are used to assess "cognitive impairment and psychopathology" as well as to assist in diagnosis (p. 36). Cognitive MSEs are utilized to assess memory and other cognitive and intellectual functions. For a thorough history on MSEs and background about specific MSEs, the reader is directed to Rogers (2001).

MSE information can be gained via observation or through the use of specific interviews and activities. Some broad areas that should be observed are: general appearance and behavior (e.g., age, alertness, hygiene, motor activity, eye contact); emotional presentation (e.g., mood, feelings, and affect); orientation to person, time, and place; flow of thought (e.g., distractibility, suicidality, homicidality); speech process (e.g., rate and rhythm of speech); cognitive functioning (e.g., appropriateness of thought content); judgment; insight; and attitude toward the examination and examiner.

An MSE may provide important diagnostic information about depressed mood, psychomotor retardation or agitation, concentration or decision-making, rate of speech, and distractibility. For children or elderly, external observers such as family and caregivers may be able to provide additional observational information regarding sleep, appetite, feelings about self (i.e., guilt, worthlessness, grandiosity), and extent to which activities are engaged in (i.e., interest in few activities or overinterest in hazardous activities). This information may augment the information collected in the interview.

Self-Monitoring

Although direct observation has certain advantages, it is often too intrusive or not feasible for adult clients. In these cases, client self-monitoring may be an alternative. Client self-monitoring may be useful both in and out of session to assess specific symptoms and how they may or may not change. During sessions, self-monitoring can provide a self-analysis of clients' here-and-now affects and perceptions of their symptoms. Out-of-session self-monitoring can assess a client's mood and symptoms over a more prolonged period. Having clients journal their moods and carry out functional analyses may also aid in determining the functional antecedents and consequences of mood shifts. Such analyses may, for example, assist the clinician in making determinations about the role of a substance in mood presentation.

Although descriptions of the representative symptoms and assessments may aid in understanding and identifying the mood disorders, clinical case examples may further clarify the clinical picture.

CLINICAL CASE EXAMPLES

Case examples for MDD, DD, Bipolar I, Bipolar II, Cyclothymic Disorder, and Mood Disorder Due to a General Medical Condition follow. Although these examples are designed to be illustrative, they are in no way intended to mirror all possible clinical presentations of these disorders. With MDD, for example, with all the combinations of symptoms accounted for, there are a myriad of possible symptom combinations.

Major Depressive Disorder

Ms. S is a 24-year-old unmarried nursing student who reports a family history of depression in both her mother and father. She was referred to the college counseling center by her academic advisor, because she said that her failing grades were due to "stress." Ms. S reported that she had been very "stressed," since her break-up with her boyfriend two months ago. Further assessment of her symptoms indicated that she had been feeling "morose" and had been crying daily in response to minor incidents like missing the bus. She said that even her favorite activities could not cheer her up. She also reported that she had been sleeping 12–14 hr a day which interfered with class attendance and studying. She noted that the only good side-effect of being so stressed was that she had lost 15 lbs over the past month with no effort. While she denied being either slowed down or speeded up, she acknowledged that it had been almost impossible to concentrate on anything other than thinking about how worthless she felt because "the love of my life dumped me." She denied feeling suicidal, but said that she chose to walk through the cemetery more frequently now and think about what a relief it would be to be lying peacefully in a coffin. She denied any previous MDEs, Manic Episodes, or Hypomanic Episodes. Although, she admitted that she sometimes coped with feeling stressed by drinking alcohol, she said there had been no change in the quantity of alcohol consumption since she entered college 2 years ago.

Ms. S was diagnosed with 296.22 MDD, Single Episode, Moderate. MDD requires at least one MDE. An MDE requires that at least five of the symptoms on the criteria list be met with at least one symptom being depressed mood or loss of interest. Ms. S met seven of the possible nine symptoms of MDD including both depressed mood and loss of interest. Given that this was her first episode and her symptoms were in excess of the minimum (mild) but below the maximum (severe), qualifiers of Single Episode and Moderate were given. The bipolar disorders were ruled out due to lack of manic/hypomanic symptoms and mood disorders due to medical or substance-induced conditions were ruled out because her depressive symptoms did not correspond to changes in health or substance use.

Dysthymic Disorder

Mrs. W, a 45-year-old divorced female, presented to a community mental health center with the chief complaint of depressed mood. She reported that the depressed mood had been present since she was a teenager and that she could not remember any time in her life since then that her mood had been any different. She denied any periods of extremely low or high mood. She reported feeling hopeless and having a poor self-esteem. She also reported feeling fatigued more times than not in the past 30 years. Client said she had been diagnosed with a chronic pain condition by her primary care physician, but stated that the depression had preceded her medical condition by more than 20 years. She reported having difficulty engaging in social relationships with others, which she stated made her feel even worse about herself and her life. She stated that her marriage made her only briefly happy and ended due to her not being willing to seek out help for her depressed mood. She reported no significant relationships since her divorce and said that she had not had any periods of remission in the past 10 years.

Mrs. W was diagnosed with DD, Early Onset. Minimally, DD requires at least two symptoms in addition to chronic depressed mood lasting at least 2 years with no more than 2 months' remission in the most recent 2-year period. Mrs. W met criteria for three of the possible seven symptoms, in addition to depressed mood for the majority of the past 30 years. MDD was ruled out due to the duration of her symptoms and her less severe symptom profile. MDD due to a General Medical Condition was ruled out due to her symptoms of depression occurring years prior to her chronic pain symptoms. Bipolar I Disorder, Bipolar II Disorder, and Cyclothymic Disorder were ruled out due to no current or prior Manic, Hypomanic, or Mixed Episodes.

Bipolar I

Ms. G, a 32-year-old married accountant, arrived at the mental health clinic to attend a group on sleep hygiene. She expressed significant concern about her bouts of sleeplessness. She tearfully explained that she would go through phases lasting up to a week and a half in which she could not sleep more than an hour or two a night. She said that during these times her thoughts were racing a "million miles an hour" and she talked a "mile a minute." She also reported that she felt a distinct press to get as much done as possible. The last time that she went through one of these phases she stayed home from work and focused on repainting, wallpapering, and refacing all her cabinets. She admitted that she did not feel like herself and did things like hang precariously off the top of the ladder with a circular saw to try to get the project done. She reported being extremely irritable with her family when they would try to interfere with her activities, but mostly felt very elated while engaged in the remodeling project. She said that she felt she could do no wrong and that during this time she felt like an expert cabinetmaker. Both she and her family had confirmed, after this bout passed, that most of her work needed to be redone by a real carpenter. She said that she had felt confused by her unusual behavior, but attributed it to her inability to sleep; thus, she had wanted to learn some sleep hygiene skills. She denied any periods of more than a few days of depression, but reluctantly admitted that her mother was "manic-depressive" and had been institutionalized when Ms. G was a young child. She said she had not been physically sick and was taking no medications or substances.

Ms. G was diagnosed with 296.42 Bipolar Disorder I, Most Recent Episode Manic, Moderate. The diagnosis of Bipolar I requires a least one Manic or Mixed Episode and may include an MDE although depression is not necessary. A Manic Episode requires that, in addition to euphoria, two of the seven symptoms be present for at least 1 week. Ms. G reported at least six of the seven symptoms lasting a week and a half with clinically significant impairment in occupational and familial relationships. The presence of a Manic Episode rules out all other mood disorders.

Bipolar II

Mr. D is a 44-year-old divorced male who is returning to school to get his law degree. Although he has been referred to the clinic under grim circumstances (i.e., having been arrested for assaulting his girlfriend 3 days ago), he appears to be quite jovial. He is talking animatedly with the front desk staff when you greet him. A few minutes into your assessment, he offers to show you the BMW he bought yesterday, and throughout the interview he appears to be entirely unconcerned about the possible consequences of his arrest stating, "They can't catch me, I'm the gingerbread man!" Although, he reports that his sleep has been normal, the interviewer notes that he is talking very quickly and that he says he needs to talk fast to get his thoughts out. When asked how long he had been feeling this euphoric, he indicated about 4 days. He said he normally looked forward to these times of "spinning" because they were a relief from his usual feelings of depression. He said that this was first time he had experienced any real problems as a result of them. He noted that they "never lasted long enough," however (i.e., 5 days or less). Although he was reluctant to talk about his depressed moods because he was afraid that talking about them would bring one on, he acknowledged that he normally felt quite depressed along with eating incessantly, difficulty making decisions, pervasive feelings of guilt, thoughts of suicide, and a significant reduction in his usually pleasurable activities. He said that these depressed times lasted anywhere from 1 to 8 weeks.

Mr. D was diagnosed with 296.89 Bipolar II, Most Recent Episode Hypomanic which requires the presence of at least one lifetime Hypomanic Episode (symptoms identical to Manic Episode except that symptoms may last as little as 4 days and may not result in hospitalization) and one MDE. Mr. D met criteria for a current Hypomanic Episode with euphoria, irritability (assault on girlfriend), feelings of inflated self-esteem, pressured speech, racing thoughts, and excessive or dangerous pleasurable activities. His hypomanic symptoms had never lasted as long as a week and had never resulted in hospitalization. He also met criteria for past MDE with depressed mood lasting as long as 8 weeks with six of the nine symptoms.

Cyclothymic Disorder

Mr. P, a 28-year-old single male, presented to a mental health center with the major complaint of being unable to keep a job. He reported having periods of time at work where he was really productive, which led his supervisors and co-workers to have high expectations of him. This would then be followed by a "slump" in which both quality and quantity of his work declined sharply. With further exploration, Mr. P reported having periods of times in his life where his mood was more elevated than normal. During these 5–7-day periods he reported needing less sleep than usual (4 hr per night), being more talkative than usual, and feeling quite ostentatious. He reported an increase in goal-directed activities, which usually leads to him being more productive at work. He stated that he was a really happy person during these periods. However, he also reported having periods of time after the elevated mood where his mood became depressed and he felt more hopeless and tired than usual. He denied having suicidal ideations and reported no somatic symptoms of depression (e.g., sleep disturbance, eating changes). He stated that these periods of elevated and depressed mood had been occurring since he was around age 21, with no symptom-free period longer than 1 month. Mr. P denied having any periods of time where his elevated mood required him to seek medical treatment. Mr. P denied using alcohol or taking any other substances during these periods or any other times. He also denied any medical problems.

Mr. P was diagnosed with 301.13 Cyclothymic Disorder. He met the requirements for five of the possible eight Hypomanic Episode symptoms including the required symptom of elevated or expansive mood. His symptoms met the duration criteria of at least 2 years, with each Hypomanic Episode lasting at least 4 days. During these periods his mood was uncharacteristic of when he was non-symptomatic and his change in functioning was noticed by others (e.g., co-workers and supervisors at work). Because Mr. P's depressed symptoms did not meet the requirements for an MDE, Bipolar II was ruled out. Similarly, the absence of a full Manic or Mixed Episode ruled out Bipolar I. Mood Disorder Due to a General Medical Condition and Substance-Induced Mood Disorder were ruled out due to Mr. P recently having a physical with no positive findings and due to him denying any use or abuse of alcohol or any other substances.

Mood Disorder Due to a General Medical Condition

Mr. V, a 22-year-old male presented to a mental health clinic with the chief complaint of depressed mood. He reported that for the past 4 weeks he had been experiencing depressive feelings more days than not as well as a decrease in interest in previously desired activities. He also reported feeling very sluggish with a tendency to tire easy and to sleep more than normal as well as a recent weight gain of 15 pounds. He reported that this was the first time he had experienced these symptoms in his lifetime other than "normal" periods of sadness due to life circumstances such as the death of a loved one. Mr. V denied any drug or alcohol use in the past year. He was not aware of a family history of depression.

Mr. V was first diagnosed with MDD, Single Episode, Moderate and was seen in psychotherapy for 2 months with little improvement in his symptoms. At that time, he was referred for a full medical battery where he was diagnosed with Hypothyroidism. His primary care physician prescribed a thyroid replacement medication and his symptoms began to remit after 4 weeks of taking the medication.

After being diagnosed with Hypothyroidism, Mr. V's mental health diagnosis was changed to 293.83 Mood Disorder due to Hypothyroidism, with Major Depressive-Like Episode. Thyroid disorders, especially Hypothyroidism can cause symptoms that appear like an MDE. For example, it is very common for individuals with Hypothyroidism to experience weight gain, weakness, general depressive symptoms, and emotional lability.

There was a distinct temporal relationship between Mr. V's depressive symptoms and his medical condition, which is important when diagnosing a Mood Disorder Due to a General Medical Condition. The specifier *with Major Depressive-Like Episode* was used rather than *with Depressive Features* because all criteria for an MDE were met except for the symptoms not being due to a general medical condition. Bipolar I Disorder, Bipolar II Disorder, DD, and Cyclothymic Disorder were ruled out due to Mr. V never having experienced a Manic, Mixed, or Hypomanic Episode. Substance-Induced Mood Disorder was ruled out due to Mr. V not drinking alcohol or using any other substances or medications at the time of his depressive symptoms.

STANDARDIZED INTERVIEW FORMATS

Although there are a variety of standardized interview formats that address mood disorders in the context of other *DSM-IV-TR* disorders, there are none, to date, exclusively devoted to the mood disorders. The most commonly used semistructured and structured interview formats addressing mood disorder diagnoses will be reviewed below.

The Schedule for Affective Disorders and Schizophrenia

The SADS (Endicott & Spitzer, 1978) is a semistructured interview that was designed to be administered by trained clinicians. While the focus of the SADS is on the differential diagnoses of affective and psychotic disorders, the SADS also covers anxiety disorders as well as alcohol and drug use disorders (Endicott & Spitzer, 1978). The SADS is divided into two parts. Part I evaluates current psychological problems and impairment (for the worst period of the current episode and the current time) while Part II is used to assess past episodes of psychopathology and treatment (Rogers, 2001; Segal, 1997). When used together, Part I and Part II provide information necessary for making both current and lifetime psychiatric diagnoses.

Several other versions of the SADS have been developed. Two of the most prominent are the SADS—Lifetime version (SADS-L) and the version for measuring change (SADS-C; Endicott & Spitzer, 1978). The SADS-L is very similar to Part II of the regular version of the SADS and can be used by itself with clients and non-clients to assess for prior or current episodes of mood disorders. One of the benefits of the SADS-L is that it takes less time to administer than the full SADS. The SADS-C is comprised of 45 symptoms selected from Part I of the regular version of the SADS (Endicott & Spitzer, 1978; Rogers, 2001). The SADS-C is useful in measuring change in symptom level over time. There have also been several specialized versions of the SADS-L, such as the SADS-LB, which was developed to assess bipolar disorders (Rogers, 2001; Segal, 1997).

The SADS was not coordinated with the *DSM* criteria for mental disorders, but rather, it was designed to evaluate the psychiatric disorders as specified by the Research Diagnostic Criteria (RDC; Spitzer, Endicott, & Robins, 1978). The SADS covers 23 RDC disorders and provides subcategories for 3 of the disorders including 11 subtypes of MDD (Rogers, 2001; Segal, 1997; Spitzer et al., 1978). Rogers (2001) states that although there is considerable overlap between the two diagnostic systems (RDC and *DSM*) it is useful for interviewers to be "knowledgeable about the two systems so that they may supplement the SADS with additional questions required to make DSM-IV diagnoses" (p. 85). The full SADS can take from 1 to 2.5 hr to administer depending on the client's history and current presenting issue (Endicott & Spitzer, 1978; Rogers, 2001; Segal, 1997).

The SADS is structured so that questions are organized around specific diagnoses. There are standard questions for specific symptoms to disorders with optional probes. Interviewers are also allowed to ask their own unstructured questions when a situation is ambiguous and the optional probes do not clarify the situation. Most of the questions on Part I are rated using a Likert scale format, which allows for severity and impairment assessment of each symptom (Rogers, 2001; Segal, 1997). Most mood symptoms and behavioral observations are rated on a 6-point scale where a rating of a 3 or higher is considered "clinically significant" (Rogers, 2001). Part II is rated dichotomously due to most individuals being unable to accurately remember the severity of past episodes (Rogers, 2001). There are skip-out options if screening questions reveal that an individual does not meet criteria for a specific disorder.

An initial scoring system was developed for the SADS where items were organized into eight summary scales that were identified through factor analysis: depressive mood and ideation; endogenous features; depressive-associated features; suicidal ideation and behavior; anxiety; manic syndrome; delusions–hallucinations;

and formal thought disorder (Endicott & Spitzer, 1978). These scales were developed to assist in dimensional ratings. For example, the dimension of mood can be differentiated from the dimension of psychotic symptoms.

The SADS has been shown to have excellent interrater reliability for current episodes, which includes individual symptoms, summary scales, and current diagnoses (Rogers, 2001). Endicott and Spitzer (1978) initially evaluated the SADS for reliability using two different samples. The first study looked at 150 inpatients that were jointly evaluated by pairs of raters. This study showed the summary scales to have excellent interrater reliability with interclass correlation coefficients (ICCs) ranging from 0.82 to 0.99. Internal consistency was also shown to be high (0.79–0.97) for all, but two summary scales (formal thought disorder = 0.47 and anxiety = 0.58) in the same study (Endicott & Spitzer, 1978). A second study utilized a test–retest design where 60 inpatients were interviewed twice by independent interviewers. Agreement rates were slightly lower for the second study, but all ICCs were above 0.75 except for anxiety (ICC = 0.67) and formal thought disorder (ICC = 0.49) (Endicott & Spitzer, 1978). The SADS is also comparable to other structured interviews in regard to test–retest reliability on lifetime diagnoses (Rogers, 2001). The reader is referred to Rogers (2001) for a comprehensive summary of reliability and validity studies of the SADS.

Although the SADS may be limited due to its limited breadth of diagnosis (mostly mood and psychotic disorders), the ability of the SADS to provide severity ratings for many current episode symptoms makes it a valuable assessment tool. The SADS can easily be supplemented with other interview formats to obtain important and useful information about other disorders and episodes that are not measured on the SADS. The SADS has been shown to be useful in medical and forensic settings as well as in clinical settings (Rogers, 2001) and is available in several different languages (Rogers, 2001; Segal, 1997). Rogers (2001) also discusses how past research by himself and others has proven the SADS to be sensitive to response styles, which is useful in assessing feigning and response consistency.

The Diagnostic Interview Schedule

The DIS (Robins et al., 1981) is a structured interview that can be used to assess current and lifetime diagnoses of mental disorders including the mood disorders. The DIS was developed to help collect data for the NIMH's ECA Program (Regier et al., 1984). The DIS is a very detailed structured interview that provides information about age of onset, frequency and duration of episodes, and recency of symptoms (Hesselbrock, Stabenau, Hesselbrock, Mirkin, & Meyer, 1982). One reason the DIS is fully structured is because it was specially designed for use by nonprofessional interviewers (Segal, 1997). The DIS was designed to evaluate disorders defined by the *DSM-III* (APA, 1980), the Feighner criteria (Feighner, Robins, Guze, Woodruff, Winokur, & Munoz, 1972), and the RDC (Spitzer et al., 1978).

All questions on the DIS are written to be close-ended and replies are forced choice format and coded as yes or no except for a few open-ended questions at the very beginning of the interview where interviewees are given the opportunity to describe their presenting problem and to provide some background information. Most sections have screening questions that allow the interviewer to skip out if there is no evidence that an interviewee has the symptoms. However, these skip-outs are suggested to be used cautiously due to the structured format of the interview. A set of core questions is asked of all clients, with follow-up questions that are only asked if a preceding core question is answered positively. The DIS also has probes built in to evaluate on a symptom-by-symptom basis the causes of a symptom to assess for organic etiology (attributing to the effects of a general medical condition, substance, or medication) (Robins et al., 1981). The DIS questions and probes are read verbatim. In addition to assessing symptoms, demographic information and psychosocial functioning are also assessed.

The newest version is the DIS-IV that was published in 1995 (Robins, Cottler, Bucholz, & Compton, 1995) and had several minor revisions in 2001 (Rogers, 2001). The DIS-IV was developed to establish compatibility with the *DSM-IV* criteria and was organized into 19 diagnostic modules including the mood disorders. The DIS-IV is estimated to take from 1.5 to 2 hr to administer and is available in both computerized and paper-and-pencil versions. In addition, it has been translated into both Spanish and Chinese (Rogers, 2001).

Initial reliability results of the DIS (Version II) were measured using 216 subjects who were interviewed twice; once by a psychiatrist and once by a lay interviewer (Robins et al., 1981). The concordance rates between lay administration and psychiatrist administration were assessed for the three diagnostic systems: *DSM-III*, Feighner criteria, and RDC. For *DSM-III* criteria exclusively, mania had a kappa of 0.65, and depression had a kappa of 0.63 (Robins et al., 1981). In regard to the interview's ability to accurately detect cases of mood disorders, depression had a sensitivity of 80% and a specificity of 84%; mania had a sensitivity of 65% and a specificity of 97% (Robins et al., 1981). These findings suggest that the DIS appears to be better in establishing the absence rather than the presence of a mood disorder diagnosis.

Compared to the SADS, the DIS covers more *DSM* diagnoses. The DIS also avoids using screening questions and diagnostic hierarchies like the SADS, which decrease the instrument's ability to accurately diagnose individuals who meet criteria for any given disorder (Robins et al., 1981). Finally, the DIS minimizes the use of clinical judgment required and relies on the degree to which questions and probes have been endorsed to make diagnoses (Robins et al., 1981, p. 385). However, the SADS is better for extracting severity ratings of mental disorders than the DIS, especially since the DIS places more emphasis on etiology (Rogers, 2001). The SADS also has clinical guidelines for the assessment of response styles, such as feigning, whereas the DIS can be quite vulnerable to response styles (Rogers, 2001).

The Structured Clinical Interview for DSM-IV Axis I Disorders

The SCID Axis I Disorders (SCID-I; First et al., 1997) is a semistructured interview that was initially developed for both researcher and clinician use. Later, the SCID-I interview was divided into a research version for research settings and a more simplified clinical version (SCID-I-CV) for clinical settings. The research version includes more specific ratings for various subtypes of disorders (e.g., seasonal pattern, melancholic features). The SCID was developed to be administered by clinical interviewers and was originally intended to be used for assessing *DSM-III* criteria for mental disorders (Spitzer, Williams, Gibbon, & First, 1992).

The SCID-I begins with a history overview prior to the structured portion of the interview. This provides relevant background information and allows clients to begin telling their stories in a less structured way (Spitzer et al., 1992). The SCID-I then moves on to diagnosing specific disorders by having the clinician/researcher ask the client questions that are asked verbatim. The SCID-I is not merely a checklist, but rather the interviewer needs to gather enough information to determine if a problem actually exists. If there is not enough information provided by the initial specific questions then verbatim follow-up questions are asked. When verbatim follow-up questions are exhausted, interviewers may ask additional questions of their choosing to clarify, if necessary. Interviewers are encouraged to appropriately challenge a client if they believe the client is not answering a question accurately (Spitzer et al., 1992).

The interview begins with the most current behavior and then moves to lifetime occurrence. For example, if a client was experiencing an MDE at the time of the interview then the clinician would ask the structured questions first about the present episode and then repeat the questions for possible past episodes. However, certain disorders such as Dysthymia and Generalized Anxiety Disorder are only considered in their current state (Segal, 1997). Individual symptoms are based on a 3-point scale where 1 = absent/false, 2 = subthreshold, and 3 = threshold/true. The SCID has skip-out options that allow the interviewer to move on to another section if it is obvious that an individual's symptoms do not meet diagnostic criteria.

The SCID was developed to be less time consuming than other clinical interviews such as the SADS. One way to optimize time usage was to allow for diagnoses to be made as the interview was in progress rather than waiting for all of the information to be gathered and assessed. Diagnoses can be changed as the interview continues and new information is obtained. At the end of each section there is a place to score the severity of the disorder (e.g., mild, moderate, or severe), the course of the disorder if appropriate (e.g., full or partial remission), the onset of symptoms, and the amount of time the symptoms were present in the past 5 years. Like with many other structured interviews, the SCID has probes to assess for organic etiology of disorders as well.

Unlike with the DIS, the interviewer administering the SCID is encouraged to use all available information about the client including previous clinical records and information from family members (Spitzer et al., 1992). When all data are gathered a score sheet is completed that records the presence or absence of each disorder covered by the SCID, a Global Assessment of Functioning rating, and information about the quality of information gathered from the client (Spitzer et al., 1992).

The SCID-CV is divided into modules that can be used independently or together as a comprehensive diagnostic interview. There are six modules: Mood

Episodes, Psychotic Symptoms, Psychotic Disorders, Mood Disorders, Substance Use Disorders, and Anxiety and Other Disorders. To assess for Mood Disorders, the Mood Episodes and Mood Disorders modules should be used together. The administration time for the two mood modules (Mood Episodes and Mood Disorders) is approximately 20 min. Administration time for the entire SCID-CV ranges from 45 to 90 min (First et al., 1997).

Williams et al. (1992) conducted a large test–retest reliability study with the SCID *DSM-III-R* Version. Seven sites participated in the study, six in the United States and one in Germany. A total of 592 individuals participated in the study, 390 clinical and 202 non-clinical subjects. For the 390 clinical participants, the mean kappas for agreement on mood disorders were as follows: bipolar disorder ($\kappa = 0.84$), major depression ($\kappa = 0.64$), Dysthymia ($\kappa = 0.40$) (Williams et al., 1992). According to Rogers' (2001) review of other reliability studies on the SCID, there appears to be "good-to-superb reliability for the diagnoses of current episodes" (p. 108).

The Composite International Diagnostic Interview

The Composite International Diagnostic Interview (CIDI; Robins et al., 1988) is a structured diagnostic interview that combines all items from the DIS and some questions from the Present State Examination (PSE; Wing, Cooper, & Sartorius, 1974). The PSE is used for assessment of symptomatology within the ICD framework. The CIDI was developed at the request of the World Health Organization (WHO)—Alcohol, Drug Abuse, and Mental Health Administration (Robins et al., 1988). According to Robins et al. (1988), the CIDI was developed to "serve cross-cultural epidemiologic and comparative studies of psychopathology" (p. 1069). The CIDI covers 40 *DSM-III* disorders including 7 mood disorders and 63 PSE items (Robins et al., 1988). The administration time ranges from 75 to 105 min, depending on interviewer experience (Rogers, 2001).

The DIS was chosen as a model for the CIDI due to its highly structured format that allows trained interviewers who are not necessarily clinicians to administer it in a timely manner. Another strength of the DIS is that it has been translated into several languages and has been shown to be successful in a variety of international settings (Robins et al., 1988). Like the DIS, the CIDI utilizes computerization of diagnosis.

There were modifications of both the PSE items to fit with the DIS format and the overall CIDI to improve cross-cultural appropriateness. The PSE items had to be altered slightly to transform them into close-ended questions and/or to add recency and severity probes (Robins et al., 1988). Once the PSE items were modified and the CIDI was developed, other modifications were made to make sure all items were applicable to all users, especially individuals in less industrialized countries (Robins et al., 1988).

There have been a handful of reliability and validity studies on the CIDI, but one problem that Rogers (2001) points out is that most reliability studies have compared the CIDI to the DIS even with the revisions of wording and ratings for certain items on the CIDI. For a comprehensive review of validation on the CIDI, the reader is referred to Rogers (2001).

INFORMATION CRITICAL TO MAKING A DIAGNOSIS

Although broad categories of mood disorders are discussed above, the specific symptom presentations may provide important information about treatment and prognosis. The *DSM-IV-TR* uses uniform specifiers to describe the nature, severity, and course of the most recent episodes, as well as the episodic pattern and the time of onset for DD.

Specifiers Regarding the Current Episode

Nature

There are a variety of specifiers that describe the nature of the most recent episode as outlined by the *DSM-IV-TR* (APA, 2000). First, there are specifiers that have to do with symptom features of the mood disorders. There are four specifiers that fall into this category: With Atypical Features; With Melancholic Features; With Catatonic Features; and With Postpartum Features. The specifier of With Atypical Features can be used to characterize the most recent MDE or to characterize the mood presentation during the most recent 2 years of DD (APA, 2001; Morrison, 1995). Individuals with atypical features tend to experience mood reactivity to interpersonal events as well as an increase in appetite or weight, an increase in sleep, a feeling of heaviness in the limbs, and sensitivity to rejection by others (APA, 2001; Morrison, 1995). Atypical features are more common in younger individuals and are 2–3 times more common in women than men (APA, 2000; Morrison, 1995).

Catatonic features can be present with an MDE, a Manic Episode, or a Mixed Episode (APA, 2001; Morrison, 1995). To meet the criteria for this specifier, individuals need to experience at least two of the following symptoms: either motor hyperactivity or inactivity, mutism or extreme negativism, prominent posturing or grimacing, and repeating of other's words or phrases (echolalia) or their gestures (echopraxia) (APA, 2001; Morrison, 1995). According to Morrison (1995), the criteria for this specifier are rarely met and are more likely to be seen in an inpatient psychiatric population.

Melancholic features are "classical" symptoms of depression. When symptoms are the most severe, individuals tend to have a lack of pleasure in most activities and tend not to show improvement to positive experiences or interactions in their life. Some other melancholic features are diurnal mood variation, early waking almost every morning, psychomotor agitation or retardation, decrease in weight and/or appetite, and feelings of inappropriate guilt (APA, 2001; Morrison, 1995). Whereas atypical features appear to be more common in younger individuals, melancholic features appear to be more common in older depressed individuals (APA, 2000; Morrison, 1995).

Women may meet the criteria for With Postpartum Onset if an MDE, Manic Episode, or Mixed Episode begins within 4 weeks after childbirth (APA, 2001; Morrison, 1995). This specifier can be applied to Bipolar I Disorder, Bipolar II Disorder, MDD with Atypical or Melancholic Features, or to Brief Psychotic Disorder (Morrison, 1995).

Severity

A second category of specifiers that describes current or the most recent mood episode has to do with the severity of the symptoms. According to the *DSM-IV-TR* (APA, 2000), the specifiers are: Mild, Moderate, Severe Without Psychotic Features, and Severe With Psychotic Features. These specifiers can be used to describe an MDE, a Manic Episode, or a Mixed Episode. Mild refers to episodes that have the minimum symptoms necessary to meet the diagnostic criteria and only minor impairment is resulting. Moderate refers to episodes where symptoms are neither mild nor severe, but range somewhere in between. According to Morrison (1995), Severe Without Psychotic Features refers to episodes where there are a number of symptoms that are in excess of basic diagnostic requirements, the symptoms are causing marked interference in one's life, and/or almost continual supervision is needed to ensure an individual's safety. Severe With Psychotic Features refers to episodes where an individual is experiencing delusions and/or hallucinations. The psychotic features can either be mood congruent where typical depressive and/or manic themes are present (e.g., inflated self-worth with mania or feelings of guilt with depression) or mood incongruent where the delusions and hallucinations are more similar to what would be seen with someone with a psychotic disorder (e.g., thought insertion, delusions of being controlled) (Morrison, 1995).

Chronicity

A third specifier that describes a current or the most recent mood episode is used only to describe an MDE and is used to indicate if there is a chronic nature to the episode. The specifier of chronic can only be used with MDD or an MDE that is part of the most recent type of mood episode in Bipolar I Disorder or Bipolar II Disorder. To be classified as chronic, the episode must have been continuous for at least 2 years (APA, 2000).

Onset

A final specifier used to describe a current disorder is specific to Dysthymia and has to do with when the symptoms were first apparent. If the age of onset of DD is before 21 years of age, then a specifier of Early Onset is used. If the age of onset of DD is after age 21 years, then the specifier of Late Onset is used (APA, 2000).

Specifiers Regarding the Course of Recurrent Episodes

Interepisodic Recovery

A second set of specifiers describes the course of recurrent episodes. First, there is the specifier that describes the level of interepisode recovery. If there is full remission of symptoms between the two most recent episodes that make up

Recurrent MDD, or Bipolar I, or II Disorders, then the specifier With Full Interepisode Recovery can be used (APA, 2000; Morrison, 1995). If a full interepisode recovery has not occurred, then Without Full Interepisode Recovery is specified.

Cyclic Pattern

A second recurrent episode specifier has to do with the cycling pattern of either Bipolar I Disorder or Bipolar II Disorder. If individuals cycle between high and low episodes four or more times during a year or if they have four separate episodes in one year then they would meet the criteria for With Rapid Cycling (APA, 2000; Morrison, 1995). Separate episodes mean that there is partial or full remission for at least 2 months between two episodes or the episodes are separate due to their polarity in mood. For example, if an individual has an MDE for 2 months and then has a Manic Episode for 2 weeks directly after, the episodes are counted as two individual mood episodes due to their polarity in mood presentation. Also, if an individual has an MDD for 1 month and then has a second MDE 3 months later after a 2-month period of partial remission, then the episodes are counted as two discrete episodes.

Seasonal Pattern

A third recurrent episode specifier characterizes whether the mood disorder has a seasonal pattern or not. If depressive symptoms occur at a specific season for at least a 2-year period with no other non-seasonal MDEs, then an individual meets the requirements for the specifier With Seasonal Pattern. The seasonal pattern cannot be due to other external events in one's life such as being out of school during the spring and summer every year. It is more common to see individuals who are depressed in the fall and winter months rather than in the spring and summer months.

DOS AND DON'TS

While diagnosis can be a valuable tool, inaccurate, incomplete, or improperly used diagnoses can deter helpful treatment and/or cause damaging stigmatization for the client. Some guidelines are presented below for compassionately making, using, and sharing mood disorder diagnoses.

When Making the Diagnosis

First and foremost, clinicians making mood disorder diagnoses should remember that the most important reason for using diagnostic labeling is to enhance client care. In particular, it has been argued that the primary purposes of diagnosing are to: improve communication amongst professionals; hone the process of choosing effective care for the client; increase knowledge about course and prognosis; increase the clinician's ability to use clinical outcome research to make treatment decisions; and to reciprocally contribute to the body of information available regarding treatment and prognosis. Indeed, the refinement of mood disorder diagnoses over the past few decades has allowed for the development, research, and widespread use of highly effective psychotherapeutic and psychopharmacological interventions for those with MDD resulting in 60–70% recovery rates (cf., Craighead et al., 1998a). Likewise, accurate identification of manic or hypomanic symptoms has highlighted the necessity of medication management (Craighead et al., 1998b).

Maximization of the therapeutic goals for diagnosis requires accurate assessment. Although diagnosis may have some limitations, if a diagnostic label is used, it should be reliable across providers and situations. Thus, it is imperative that mood disorder diagnoses be assigned only when full criteria are met and when a full assessment, including a face-to-face interview with the client, is complete. Particular attention should be focused on whether the symptoms are related to clinically significant distress or impairment in social, occupational, or other important areas of functioning. Symptoms that do not cause this level of distress do not meet criteria for a disorder even if all other criteria are met. In addition, issues of diversity, such as culture, ethnicity, race, religion, gender, age, etc. should all be taken into account when making mood disorder diagnoses. An older client, for example, may report having less interest in previously enjoyed activities along with symptoms of insomnia, fatigue, psychomotor slowing, difficulty concentrating, and thoughts of death. Although technically the criteria for MDD would be met, such a symptom profile may be more reflective of the age cohort than depression. Here, careful assessment of clinically significant distress and normative functioning would be essential for evaluating the appropriateness of an MDD diagnosis.

Clinicians should also ensure that the symptoms are not better accounted for by another medical or psychological condition. Assessment should regularly include a full physical examination by a physician who understands that the client is wishing to rule out physical causes for depression. This kind of assessment is exceptionally important with elderly clients who may have dementia symptoms that may be masking or masquerading as depression symptoms. Similarly, a child or adolescent client's irritability, distractibility, and/or impulsiveness may be better accounted for by a diagnosis of Attention Deficit and Hyperactivity Disorder than a mood disorder even if mood symptoms are present.

Since the goal of diagnosis is to enhance care, it is also important that the least severe diagnosis that accurately reflects the client's condition be used. Labels can be damaging for many reasons including: reduced eligibility for healthcare coverage; fewer job opportunities; societal stigmatization affecting employers, family members, and friends as well as the clients themselves; and attribution of symptoms to a disease model that results in passive participation in care. For all these reasons, mood disorder diagnoses should be made with a full understanding of the client's life context. If for example, a diagnosis of Adjustment Disorder with Depressed Mood accurately reflects the client's condition and would appropriately facilitate care, then this diagnosis should be assigned rather than a diagnosis of MDD. Similarly, diagnosis should reflect the client's reasons for seeking care rather than a laundry list of all the diagnoses whose criteria could be met. Even though a client may technically meet criteria for 5 or 6 of the 398 diagnoses currently in the *DSM-IV*, a conservative targeted approach to choosing the primary diagnoses, will be more likely to facilitate care and minimize harm to the client due to the reasons listed above. Finally, mood disorder diagnoses are designed to facilitate and guide care; thus, treatment should be the focus rather than a quest for the perfect label.

When Using the Diagnosis

Once a mood disorder diagnosis is made, the use of the diagnostic label can affect the quality of care and the extent to which the diagnosis becomes stigmatizing for the client. First, it is important that the clinician remember that the diagnosis is a categorization of a constellation of symptoms. The label is a description of symptoms rather than an entity in and of itself. Thus, the label should never be used as a reason for a client's behavior. Instead, a thorough understanding of each symptom's context will be important in helping the client make changes. For example, knowing the important interpersonal interactions before and after increased feelings of hopelessness is probably at least as important in helping a depressed client as knowing that MDD diagnosis criteria are met. Likewise, clinicians should avoid using diagnostic labels in ways that reinforce beliefs—however subtly—that these labels are more than a name for a group of symptoms. In particular, diagnoses should never be used as names for clients (e.g., "My bipolar client is coming in today") or as names for clients' problems. Rather, the unique features of the case and symptom context will provide more helpful and less potentially damaging implications.

When Sharing the Diagnosis with the Client

The American Psychological Association's ethical guidelines emphasize the involvement of clients in their assessment and care (American Psychological Association, 1995). Yet, many clinicians have concerns about the impact of sharing diagnostic assessments with clients. While a thorough debate of the issues involved in determining whether to share the diagnosis is beyond the scope of this chapter, some issues to consider when clinicians choose to share will be discussed. First, clients should be informed about the purpose of diagnosis (i.e., as a label for a group of symptoms to facilitate communication and treatment). Ensure that the diagnosis is not presented as a disease or as some intractable entity. Second, the presentation of diagnosis may be in the context of hope. Such an explanation may include information about prevalence and how knowledge of the diagnosis points to treatment. MDD diagnosis, for example, could be presented to a female client as follows:

> Thank you for your willingness to complete these assessments. This is really going to be helpful in choosing interventions that will be most likely to be helpful to you. One outcome of an assessment like this is identifying a label that describes your group of concerns. In your case, the label that best fits your symptoms is Major Depressive Disorder.

While that may seem like a daunting title, I want to make sure that you understand that this gives us an excellent place to start our work together. Major Depressive Disorder is actually a surprisingly common problem. At least 1 in 5 women will meet full criteria for this diagnosis at some point during their lifetime. So you are actually in good company. What this also means is that we know quite a bit about how to treat depression. The good news here is that although depression may feel very debilitating right now, there is an excellent chance that with the right treatment you will begin to feel better. (Proceed to discuss treatment options.)

SUMMARY

In sum, mood disorders are common, debilitating, and expensive; however, with appropriate treatment, mood disorders can often be well managed. The first step to appropriate treatment is accurate diagnosis. Although the reliability rates on structured and semistructured interviews are far from perfect, they are considerably better than for unstructured clinical interviews. Thus, standardized interviews should be used whenever possible. A close cousin to accurate diagnosis is differential diagnosis. An understanding of how each of the mood disorders are the same and different from one another as well as other mental health and medical disorders will be essential to treatment planning. The bipolar disorders may be treated quite differently, for example, than the unipolar mood disorders. In addition, mood disorder diagnosticians should be acutely aware of the impact of making these diagnoses on the welfare of their clients. Therefore, mood disorder diagnoses should be made carefully and conservatively, the diagnostic label should be used appropriately, and diagnosis should be presented to clients hopefully and gently.

REFERENCES

Akiskal, H. S. (1996). Dysthymia as a temperamental variant of affective disorder. *European Psychiatry,* *11*(Suppl 3), 117s–122s.

Akiskal, H. S., & Van Valkenburg, C. (1994). Mood disorders. In M. Hersen & S. M. Turner (Eds.), *Diagnostic interviewing* (2nd ed., pp. 79–107). New York: Plenum Press.

Altman, E. G. (1998). Rating scales for mania: Is self-rating reliable? *Journal of Affective Disorders, 50,* 283–286.

Altman, E. G., Hedeker, D., Peterson, J. L., & Davis, J. M. (1997). The Altman self-rating mania scale. *Biological Psychiatry, 42*(10), 948–955.

Altman, E. G., Hedeker, D., Peterson, J. L., & Davis, J. M. (2001). A comparative evaluation of three self-rating scales for acute mania. *Biological Psychiatry, 50*(6), 468–471.

American Psychiatric Association. (1980). *Diagnostic and statistical manual of mental disorders* (3rd ed.). Washington, DC: American Psychiatric Association.

American Psychiatric Association. (2000). *Diagnostic and statistical manual of mental disorders* (4th ed., Text Revision). Washington, DC: American Psychiatric Association.

American Psychological Association. (1995). *Ethical principles of psychologists and code of conduct.* Washington, DC: Author.

Arnau, R. C., Meagher, M. W., Norris, M. P., & Bramson, R. (2001). Psychometric evaluation of the Beck Depression Inventory-II with primary care medical patients. *Health Psychology, 20*(2), 112–119.

Baldessarini, R. J., Tondo, L., Floris, G., & Hennen, J. (2000). Effects of rapid cycling on response to lithium maintenance treatment in 360 bipolar I and II disorder patients, *Journal of Affective Disorders, 61,* 13–22.

Barber, J. P., Luborsky, L., Crits-Chirstoph, P., Thase, M. E., Weiss, R., Frank, A., Onken, L., & Gallop, R. (1999). Therapeutic alliance as a predictor of outcome in treatment of cocaine dependence. *Psychotherapy Research, 9*(1), 54–73.

Basco, M. R. (2000). Cognitive-behavior therapy for Bipolar I disorder. *Journal of Cognitive Psychotherapy*, 14(3), 287–304.

Beck, A. T., Steer, R. A., & Brown, G. K. (1996). *Manual for the Beck Depression Inventory* (2nd ed.). San Antonio, TX: The Psychological Corporation.

Benazzi, F. (1999). A comparison of the age of onset of bipolar I and bipolar II outpatients. *Journal of Affective Disorders, 54*(3), 249–253.

Benazzi, F. (2001a). Sensitivity and specificity of clinical markers for the diagnosis of bipolar II disorder. *Comprehensive Psychiatry, 42*(6), 461–465.

Benazzi, F. (2001b). The clinical picture of bipolar II outpatient depression in private practice. *Psychopathology, 34*(2), 81–84.

Cappeliez, P. (1989). Social desirability response set and self-report depression inventories in the elderly. *Clinical Gerontologist, 9*(2), 45–52.

Coryell, W., Endicott, J., Maser, J. D., Keller, M. B., Leon, A. C., & Akiskal, H. S. (1995). Long-term stability of polarity distinctions in the affective disorders. *American Journal of Psychiatry, 152*(3), 385–390.

Coyne, J. C. (1994). Self-reported distress: Analog or ersatz depression? *Psychological Bulletin, 116*, 29–45.

Craighead, W. E., Craighead, L. W., & Liardi, S. S. (1998a). Psychosocial treatments for major depressive disorder. In P. E. Nathan & J. M. Gordon (Eds.), *A guide to treatments that work* (pp. 226–239). New York: Oxford University Press.

Craighead, W. E., Miklowitz, D. J., Vajk, F. C., & Frank, E. (1998b). In P. E. Nathan & J. M. Gordon (Eds.), *A guide to treatments that work* (pp. 240–248). New York: Oxford University Press.

Endicott, J., & Spitzer, R. L. (1978). A diagnostic interview: The Schedule for Affective Disorders and Schizophrenia. *Archives of General Psychiatry, 35*, 837–844.

Evan, S., Cloitre, M., Kocsis, J. H., Keitner, G. I., Holzer, C. P., & Gniwesch, L. (1996). Social-vocational adjustment in unipolar mood disorders: Results of the DSM-IV field trial. *Journal of Affective Disorders, 38*(2–3), 73–80.

Faravelli, C., Degl'Innocenti, B. G., Aiazzi, L., Incerpi, G., & Pallanti, S. (1990). Epidemiology of mood disorders: A community survey in Florence. *Journal of Affective Disorders, 20*(2), 135–141.

Feighner, J. P., Robins, E., Guze, S. B., Woodruff, R. A., Winokur, G., & Munoz, R. (1972). Diagnostic criteria for use in psychiatric research. *Archives of General Psychiatry, 26*, 57–63.

First, M. B., Spitzer, R. L., Gibbon, M., & Williams, J. B. W. (1997). *Users guide for the Structured Interview for DSM-IV Axis I Disorders—Clinical Version*. Washington, DC: American Psychiatric Press.

Furukawa, R., Hirai, T., Kitamura, T., & Takahashi, K. (1997). Application of the Center for Epidemiologic Studies Depression Scale among first-visit psychiatric patients: A new approach to improve its performance. *Journal of Affective Disorders, 46*(1), 1–13.

Ghaemi, S. N. (1997). Insight and psychiatric disorders: A review of the literature, with a focus on its clinical relevance for bipolar disorder. *Psychiatric Annals, 27*(12), 782–790.

Gloaguen, V., Cottraux, J., Cucherat, M., & Blackburn, I. (1998). A meta-analysis of the effects of cognitive therapy in depressed patients. *Journal of Affective Disorders, 49*(1), 49–72.

Goldberg, J. F., Harrow, M., & Whiteside, J. E. (2001). Risk for bipolar illness in patients initially hospitalized for unipolar depression. *American Journal of Psychiatry, 158*(8), 1265–1270.

Greenberg, P. E., Stiglin, L. E., Finkelstein, S. N., & Berndt, E. R. (1993). The economic burden of depression in 1990. *Journal of Clinical Psychiatry, 54*, 405–419.

Hesselbrock, V., Stabenau, J., Hesselbrock, M., Mirkin, P., & Meyer, R. (1982). A comparison of two interview schedules: The Schedule for Affective Disorders and Schizophrenia—Lifetime and the National Institute for Mental Health Diagnostic Interview Schedule. *Archives of General Psychiatry, 39*, 674–677.

Heun, R., & Maier, W. (1993). The distinction of bipolar II disorder from bipolar I and recurrent unipolar depression: Results of a controlled family study. *Acta Psychiatrica Scandinavica, 87*(4), 279–284.

Husaini, B. A., Neff, J. A., Harrington, J. B., Hughes, M. D., & Stone, R. H. (1980). Depression in rural communities: Validating the CESD-D scale. *Journal of Community Psychology, 8*, 20–27.

Kavanagh, D. J., & Wilson, P. H. (1989). Prediction of outcome with group cognitive therapy for depression. *Behavior Research and Therapy, 27*(4), 333–343.

Kelleher, W. J., Talcott, G. W., Haddock, C. K., & Freeman, R. K. (1996). Military psychology in the age of managed care: The Wilford Hall model. *Applied & Preventive Psychology, 5*(2), 101–110.

Keller, M. B., McCullough, J. P., Klein, D. N., Arnow, B., Dunner, D. L., Gelenberg, A. J., Markowitz, J. C., Nemeroff, C. B., Russell, J. M., Thase, M. E., Trivedi, M. H., & Zajecka, J. (2000). A comparison of nefazodone, the cognitive behavioral-analysis system of psychotherapy, and their combination for the treatment of chronic depression. *New England Journal of Medicine, 342*(20), 1462–1470.

Kessler, R. C., McGonagle, K. A., Zhao, S., Nelson, C. B., Hughes, M., Eshleman, S., Wittchen, H. U., & Kendler, K. S. (1994). Lifetime and 12-month prevalence of DSM-III-R psychiatric disorders in the United States: Results from the National Comorbidity Survey. *Archives of General Psychiatry, 51*, 8–19.

Klein, D. N., Kocsis, J. H., McCullough, J. P., Holzer, C. E. 3rd, Hirschfeld, R. M., & Keller, M. B. (1996). Symptomatology in dysthymic and major depressive disorder. *Psychiatric Clinics of North America, 19*(1), 41–53.

Klein, D. N., Schatzberg, A. F., McCullough, J. P., Dowling, F., Goodman, D., Howland, R. H., Markowitz, J. C., Smith, C., Thase, M. E., Rush, A. J., LaVange, L., Harrison, W. M., & Keller, M. B. (1999). Age of onset in chronic major depression: Relation to demographic and clinical variables, family history, and treatment response. *Journal of Affective Disorders, 55*(2–3), 149–157.

Klein, D. H., Schwartz, J. E., Rose, S., & Leader, J. B. (2000). Five-year course and outcome of dysthymic disorder: A prospective, naturalistic follow-up study. *American Journal of Psychiatry, 157*(6), 931–939.

Klein, D. N., Taylor, E. B., Dickstein, S., & Harding, K. (1988). Primary early-onset dysthymia: Comparison with primary nonbipolar nonchronic major depression on demographic, clinical, familial, personality, and socioenvironmental characteristics and short-term outcome. *Journal of Abnormal Psychology, 97*(4), 387–398.

McCullough, J. P. Jr. (2000). Treatment for chronic depression: *Cognitive behavioral analysis system of psychotherapy (CBASP)*. New York: The Guilford Press.

Morrison, J. (1995). *DSM-IV made easy: The clinician's guide to diagnosis*. New York: The Guilford Press.

Nezu, A. M., Ronan, G. F., Meadows, E. A., & McClure, K. S. (Eds.). (2000). *Practitioner's guide to empirically based measures of depression*. New York: Kluwer Academic/Plenum.

Pallanti, S., Quercioli, L., Pazzagli, A., Rossi, A., Dell'Osso, L., Pini, S., & Cassano, G. B. (1999). Awareness of illness and subjective experience of cognitive complaints in patients with bipolar I and bipolar II disorders. *American Journal of Psychiatry, 156*(7), 1094–1096.

Parker, G., Roy, K., Wilhelm, K., Mitchell, P., & Hadzi-Pavlovic, D. (2000). The nature of bipolar depression: Implications for the definition of melancholia. *Journal of Affective Disorders, 59*(3), 217–224.

Persson, M. I. I., Runeson, B. S., & Wasserman, D. (1999). Diagnoses, psychosocial stressors and adaptive functioning in attempted suicide. *Annals of Clinical Psychiatry, 11*(3), 119–128.

Radloff, L. S. (1977). The CES-D Scale: A self-report depression scale for research in the general population. *Applied Psychological Measurement, 1*, 385–401.

Regier, D. A., Myers, J. K., Kramer, M., Robins, L. N., Blazer, D. G., Hough, R. L., Eaton, W. W., & Locke, B. Z. (1984). The NIMH Epidemiologic Catchment Area Program: Historical context, major objectives and study population characteristics. *Archives of General Psychiatry, 41*, 934–941.

Roberts, J. E., Shapiro, A. M., & Gamble, S. A. (1999). Level and perceived stability of self-esteem prospectively predict depressive symptoms during psychoeducational group treatment. *British Journal of Clinical Psychology, 38*(4), 425–429.

Robins, L. N., Cottler, L., Bucholz, K., & Compton, W. (1995). *Diagnostic interview schedule, version IV*. St. Louis: Washington School of Medicine.

Robins, L. N., Helzer, J. E., Croughan, J., & Ratcliff, K. S. (1981). National Institute of Mental Health Diagnostic Interview Schedule: Its history, characteristics, and validity. *Archives of General Psychiatry, 38*, 381–389.

Robins, L. N., Wing, J., Wittchen, H. U., Helzer, J. E., Babor, T. F., Burke, J., Farmer, A., Jablenski, A., Pickens, R., Regier, D. A., Sartorius, N., & Towle, L. H. (1988). The Composite International Diagnostic Interview: An epidemiologic instrument suitable for use in conjunction with different diagnostic systems and in different cultures. *Archives of General Psychiatry, 45*, 1069–1077.

Rogers, R. (2001). *Handbook of diagnostic and structured interviewing*. New York: The Guilford Press.

Santor, D. A., Zuroff, D. C., Ramsay, J. O., Cervantes, P., & Palacios, J. (1995). Examining scale discrim-inability in the BDI and CES-D as a function of depressive severity. *Psychological Assessment, 7,* 131–139.

Scott, J., Garland, A., & Moorhead, S. (2001). A pilot study of cognitive therapy in bipolar disorders. *Psychological Medicine, 31*(3), 459–467.

Segal, D. L. (1997). Structured interviewing and DSM Classification. In S. M. Turner & M. Hersen (Eds.), *Adult psychopathology and diagnosis* (3rd ed., pp. 24–57). New York: John Wiley & Sons.

Serretti, A., Jori, M. C., Casadei, G., Ravizza, L., Smeraldi, E., & Akiskal, H. (1999). Delineating psy-chopathologic clusters within dysthymia: A study of 512 out-patients without major depression. *Journal of Affective Disorders, 56*(1), 17–25.

Spitzer, R. L., Endicott, J., & Robins, E. (1978). Research diagnostic criteria for use in psychiatric research. *Archives of General Psychiatry, 35,* 773–782.

Spitzer, R. L., Williams, J. B. W., Gibbon, M., & First, M. B. (1992). The Structured Clinical Interview for DSM-III-R (SCID): History, rationale, and description. *Archives of General Psychiatry, 49,* 624–629.

Srisurapanont, M., Yatham, L. N., & Zis, A. P. (1995). Treatment of acute bipolar depression: A review of the literature. *Canadian Journal of Psychiatry, 40*(9), 533–544.

Steer, R. A., Ball, R., Ranieri, W. F., & Beck, A. T. (1997). Further evidence for the construct validity of the Beck Depression Inventory-II with psychiatric outpatients. *Psychological Reports, 80*(2), 443–446.

Teri, L., & Truax, P. (1994). Assessment of depression in dementia patients: Association of caregiver mood with depression ratings. *Gerontologist, 34*(2), 231–234.

Thompson, L. W., Coon, D. W., Gallagher-Thompson, D., Sommer, B. R., & Koin, D. (2001). Comparison of desipramine and cognitive/behavioral therapy in the treatment of elderly outpa-tients with mild-to-moderate depression. *American Journal of Geriatric Psychiatry, 9*(3), 225–240.

Tondo, L., Baldessarini, R. J., & Floris, G. (2001). Long-term clinical effectiveness of lithium maintenance treatment in types I and II bipolar disorders. *British Journal of Psychiatry, 178*(Suppl 41), s184–s190.

Tondo, L., Baldessarini, R. J., Hennen, J., & Floris, G. (1998). Lithium maintenance treatment of depres-sion and mania in bipolar I and bipolar II disorders. *American Journal of Psychiatry, 155*(5), 638–645.

Truax, P. (2002). Major depressive disorder. In M. Hersen & L. Krug Porzelius (Eds.), *Diagnosis, concep-tualization and treatment planning for adults: A step-by-step guide.* Mahwah, NJ: Lawrence Erlbaum Associates.

Vieta, E., Benabarre, A., Colom, F., Gasto, C., Nieto, E., Otero, A., & Vallejo, J. (1997a). Suicidal behav-ior in bipolar I and bipolar II disorder. *Journal of Nervous & Mental Disease, 185*(6), 407–409.

Vieta, E., Gasto, C., Otero, A., & Nieto, E. (1997b). Differential features between bipolar I and bipolar II disorder. *Comprehensive Psychiatry, 38*(2), 98–101.

Weiss, I., Rabinowitz, J., & Spiro, S. (1996). Agreement between therapists and clients in evaluating therapy and its outcomes: Literature review. *Administration and Policy in Mental Health, 23,* 493–511.

Weissman, M. M., Bruce, M. L., Leaf, P. J., Florio, L. P., & Holzer, C. III. (1991). Affective disorders. In L. N. Robins & D. A. Regier (Eds.), *Psychiatric disorders in America: The Epidemiologic Catchment Area Study* (pp. 53–80). New York: The Free Press.

Wells, K. B., Burnam, M. A., Rogers, W., Hays, R., & Camp, P. (1992). The course of depression in adult outpatients: Results from the Medical Outcomes Study. *Archives of General Psychiatry, 49*(10), 788–794.

Williams, C. W., Lees-Haley, P. R., & Price, J. R. (1998). Self-attention and reported symptoms: Implications for forensic assessment. *Professional Psychology: Research & Practice, 29*(2), 125–129.

Williams, J. B., Gibbon, M., First, M. B., Spitzer, R. L., Davies, M., Borus, J., Howes, M. J., Kane, J., Pope, H. G., Jr. Rounsaville, B., & Wittchen, H. U. (1992). The Structured Clinical Interview for DSM-III-R (SCID): Multisite test–retest reliability. *Archives of General Psychiatry, 49,* 630–636.

Wing, J. K., Cooper, J. E., & Sartorius, N. (1974). *The measurement and classification of psychiatric symptoms.* Cambridge, UK: Cambridge University Press.

Winokur, G., Coryell, W., Endicott, J., & Akiskal, H. (1993). Further distinctions between manic–depressive illness (Bipolar Disorder) and primary depressive disorder (unipolar). *American Journal of Psychiatry, 150*(8), 1176–1181.

Wulsin, L. R., Vaillant, G. E., & Wells, V. E. (1999). A systematic review of the mortality of depression. *Psychosomatic Medicine, 61*(1), 6–17.

Wyatt, R. J., & Henter, I. (1995). An economic evaluation of manic–depressive illness. *Social Psychiatry and Psychiatric Epidemiology, 30,* 213–219.

7

Schizophrenia

STEVEN L. SAYERS, KIMBERLY CARSIA, AND
KIM T. MUESER

DESCRIPTION OF THE DISORDER

Schizophrenia is a complex and confusing illness that can baffle family members, friends, the patient, and mental health professionals alike. Schizophrenia can be contrasted to psychiatric illnesses such as major depression, manic-depression, and anxiety disorders that were described long ago by Hippocrates as common behavioral disturbances. Schizophrenia has been recognized only over the past 100 years as a separate illness with its own unique pattern of onset, symptomatology, course, and treatment. The diagnosis of schizophrenia can be complicated by two important factors. First, the symptoms of the illness overlap with many other disorders (e.g., affective disorders, substance abuse), requiring careful attention to issues of differential diagnosis. Second, patient self-report is critical in establishing the diagnosis of schizophrenia, yet many patients deny the characteristic symptoms or are inconsistent in their report of these internal experiences. While there are difficulties inherent in the assessment of schizophrenia, accurate diagnosis has important implications for pharmacological and psychosocial intervention for the disorder. Indeed, misdiagnosis can result in ineffective treatment and a poor outcome. In order to diagnose schizophrenia accurately, the interviewer must possess an adequate fund of knowledge about the psychopathology of the illness, the relative merits of available assessment instruments, interviewing techniques, and methods for obtaining information necessary for the assessment. We begin this chapter with an overview of the nature of schizophrenia, including its prevalence, course, and outcome, followed by a review of its symptomatology and the criteria for its diagnosis.

STEVEN L. SAYERS AND KIMBERLY CARSIA • Department of Psychiatry and Philadelphia Veterans Affairs Medical Center, University of Pennsylvania Health System, Philadelphia, Pennsylvania 19104. KIM T. MUESER • NH-Dartmouth Psychiatric Research Center, Concord, New Hampshire 03301.

Basic Facts about Schizophrenia

Schizophrenia is a severe adult psychiatric illness that has pervasive effects on patients' interpersonal relationships, ability to work, and self-care skills. Evidence suggests that schizophrenia is a biological illness that can be precipitated or made worse by environmental stress. Family studies indicate that the vulnerability to developing the illness is determined partly by genetic factors, with concordance ratios of schizophrenia in monozygotic twins ranging from 15% to 75% (Walker, Downey, & Caspi, 1991). The causes of schizophrenia are not known at this time, but the major theories hypothesize that symptoms are the result of an imbalance in brain neurotransmitters, structural brain anomalies, or altered blood flow and activation of specific brain regions, and are believed to be the result of an underlying neurodevelopmental disorder (Buchsbaum, 1990; Crow, 1990; Davies, Russell, Jones, & Murray, 1998).

The lifetime risk for developing schizophrenia is approximately 1%, which is consistent across gender, different cultures, and countries. Persons from lower socioeconomic classes appear to be at increased vulnerability to develop schizophrenia and other psychiatric disorders (Bruce, Takeuchi, & Leaf, 1991), a phenomenon that appears to reflect the effects of stress on precipitating onset of the illness (Fox, 1990). Schizophrenia usually develops gradually over a period of months, and in some cases years, between the ages of 16 and 30. Childhood onset of schizophrenia before the age of 12 is rare, as is an onset after 35 years of age. Most people who develop schizophrenia do not show an obvious pattern of maladaptive behavior in childhood or adolescence before the onset of the illness. However, retrospective and prospective research indicates that subtle impairments in the following areas that are indicative of deviant development (Davies et al., 1998): attentional processes (Cornblatt, Lenzenweger, Dworkin, & Erlenmeyer-Kimling, 1992), motor and interpersonal behavior (Walker & Lewine, 1990), and social and sexual adjustment (Done, Crow, Johnstone, & Sacker, 1994; Zigler & Glick, 1986).

Once schizophrenia has developed, its longitudinal course is usually a chronic but episodic one, with the intensity of symptoms fluctuating over time. Patients with schizophrenia can usually be managed effectively in the community, with occasional inpatient hospitalizations required for the treatment of acute symptom exacerbations. Most schizophrenia patients are substantially disabled throughout their lives, even between symptom exacerbations, and require assistance in daily living, such as self-care, handling financial matters, and the like. Over the individual's lifetime, the symptoms of schizophrenia gradually improve, and many patients experience total or partial remission in later life (Harding, Brooks, Ashikaga, Strauss, & Breier, 1987). Women with schizophrenia tend to have a more benign course of illness, characterized by a later age of onset, fewer hospitalizations, a higher rate of marriage, better social adjustment, and better social skills (Goldstein, 1988; Mueser, Bellack, Morrison, & Wade, 1990). Similarly, persons living in underdeveloped countries tend to have a less severe course of schizophrenia (Jablensky & Sartorius, 1975).

Antipsychotic medications are the pharmacological treatment of choice for schizophrenia and are useful for both the treatment of acute symptoms and the prevention of symptom relapses. Despite the undisputed efficacy of antipsychotics, the vast majority of patients continue to experience residual symptoms between episodes. The severity of impairment and course of schizophrenia has been shown to be improved by several psychosocial interventions, including psychoeducational and behavioral family therapy (Bustillo, Lauriello, Horan, & Keith, 2001; Mueser & Glynn, 1999), social skills training (Bellack, Mueser, Gingerich, & Agresta, 1997; Liberman, DeRisi, & Mueser, 1989), cognitive-behavior therapy for psychosis (Gould, Mueser, Bolton, Mays, & Goff, 2001), and supported employment (Bond et al., 2001; Bond, Drake, Becker, & Mueser, 1999).

Psychopathology

The historical roots of the classification of schizophrenia are relatively modern, dating back primarily to the contributions of Kraepelin and Bleuler. Kraepelin (1919), more than any of his predecessors, is credited with distinguishing schizophrenia (which he termed *dementia praecox*) from manic-depressive illness and organic psychoses. According to Kraepelin, schizophrenia is characterized not only by the presence of specific psychotic symptoms in the absence of affective symptoms, but also by its chronic, deteriorating course, compared to the relatively stable episodic course of manic-depressive illness. Current diagnostic criteria for schizophrenia reflect Kraepelin's focus on descriptive psychopathology. Although the course of schizophrenia is no longer assumed to be a deteriorating one, symptoms must be present for a minimum of 6 months to make the diagnosis according to *Diagnostic and Statistical Manual of Mental Disorders, Fourth Edition (DSM-IV)* criteria (American Psychiatric Association, 1994).

Bleuler (1950) theorized that delusions and hallucinations were secondary features of schizophrenia that were the result of primary disturbances in *affect* (flat or inappropriate), *associations* (loose or blocked), *autism* (preoccupation with fantasy), and *ambivalence* (rapid shifting from one idea or action to another). The focus on these more interpretative symptoms of schizophrenia influenced diagnostic practices particularly in the United States, where schizophrenia was for many years diagnosed less on the basis of specific symptoms than on the basis of the clinical interviewer's intuition. Bleuler's observations regarding impairments in affect and associations (i.e., disorganized speech) are included in current *DSM-IV* criteria, although their presence is not required for the diagnosis of schizophrenia.

The diagnostic criteria for schizophrenia according to *DSM-IV* criteria are summarized in Table 1. If the characteristic symptoms have been present for more than 1 week but less than 6 months, then the person meets the criteria for schizophreniform disorder, which most often evolves into schizophrenia.

For descriptive purposes, the symptoms of schizophrenia can be divided into three broad categories: negative symptoms, positive symptoms, and affective disturbances (Kay & Sevy, 1990). *Negative symptoms* are defined by the *absence* or relative paucity of behaviors, cognitions (or cognitive abilities), or emotions that are ordinarily *present* in healthy individuals. Common negative symptoms include: *blunted/flattened affect* (diminished vocal and facial expressiveness), *anhedonia*

TABLE 1. *DSM-IV* Criteria for the Diagnosis of Schizophrenia

---

A. *Characteristic symptoms*
   Two (or more) of the following, each present for a significant portion of time during a 1-month period (or less if successfully treated):

   1. delusions
   2. hallucinations
   3. disorganized speech (e.g., frequent derailment or incoherence)
   4. grossly disorganized or catatonic behavior
   5. negative symptoms, that is, affect flattening, alogia, or avolition

   Note: Only one Criterion A symptom is required if delusions are bizarre or hallucinations consist of a voice keeping up a running commentary on the person's behavior or thoughts, or two or more voices conversing with each other.

B. *Social/occupational dysfunction*
   For a significant proportion of the time from the onset of the disturbance, one or more major areas of functioning such as work, interpersonal relations, or self-care are markedly below the level achieved prior to the onset (or when the onset is in childhood or adolescence, failure to achieve expected level of interpersonal, academic, or occupational achievement).

C. *Duration*
   Continuous signs of the disturbance persist for at least 6 months. This 6-month period must include at least 1 month of symptoms (or less if successfully treated) that meet Criterion A (i.e., active-phase symptoms), and may include periods of prodromal or residual symptoms. During these prodromal or residual periods, the signs of the disturbance may be manifested by only negative symptoms or two or more symptoms listed in Criterion A present in an attenuated form (e.g., odd beliefs, unusual perceptual experiences).

D. *Schizoaffective and mood disorders exclusion*
   Schizoaffective Disorder and Mood Disorder With Psychotic Features have been ruled out because either (1) no Major Depressive, Manic, or Mixed Episodes have occurred concurrently with the active-phase symptoms; or (2) if mood episodes have occurred during active-phase symptoms, their total duration has been brief relative to the duration of the active and residual periods.

E. *Substance/general medical condition exclusion*
   The disturbance is not due to the direct physiological effects of a substance (e.g., a drug of abuse, a medication) or general medical condition.

F. *Relationship to a pervasive developmental disorder*
   If there is a history of Autistic Disorder or another Pervasive Developmental Disorder, the additional diagnosis of schizophrenia is made only if prominent delusions or hallucinations are also present for at least a month (or less if successfully treated).

Adapted from *Diagnostic and statistical manual of mental disorders-IV*, American Psychiatric Association, 1994.

(diminished ability to feel pleasure), *asociality* (lack of social drive and libido), *apathy, alogia* (poverty of speech or content of speech), *attentional impairment*, and *motor and psychomotor retardation*.

Positive symptoms are the opposite of negative symptoms, in that they are defined as the *presence* or excess of behaviors, cognitions, or perceptions ordinarily *absent* in healthy persons. The most common positive symptoms are *hallucinations* and *delusions*. Auditory hallucinations occur most frequently, followed by visual hallucinations, with tactile, olfactory, and gustatory hallucinations occurring less often. Common delusions include *persecutory delusions, delusions of control* (i.e., thought insertion and withdrawal), *delusions of reference* (e.g., the television is talking to the patient), and *delusions of grandeur*. Less common positive symptoms include *loose associations, stereotypic behaviors, mannerisms and posturing*, and *word salad* (disordered syntax). Note that in the *DSM-IV*, symptoms reflective of thought disorder are captured in disorganized speech, which illustrates the emphasis on observable phenomena in the diagnostic criteria (see Table 1).

Common mood disturbances in schizophrenia include *depression, anxiety, anger*, and *hostility*. These disturbances often occur secondary to positive symptoms. For example, paranoid delusions may be accompanied by anger and hostility, whereas delusions of reference can provoke severe anxiety. Most schizophrenia patients experience depression, which often presages relapses of psychotic symptoms. Approximately 50% of schizophrenia patients attempt suicide at some time during their lives, and 10% successfully commit suicide (Roy, 1986).

Schizoaffective Disorder

Schizoaffective disorder is a hybrid psychiatric diagnosis that includes symptoms of both schizophrenia and major affective disorder. The *DSM-IV* criteria for schizoaffective disorder are presented in Table 2. Inspection of Table 2 reveals that in order to meet criteria for schizoaffective disorder, the patient must have a history of schizophrenia symptoms for at least 2 weeks *in the absence of* any affective symptoms and at some other time must have experienced an affective syndrome (either manic or depressive) accompanied by schizophrenia symptoms. That schizoaffective disorder is closely related to schizophrenia is indicated by an accumulating body of evidence, including studies of genetic vulnerability, course of illness, and response to pharmacological treatments (Kramer et al., 1989; Levinson & Levitt, 1987; Mattes & Nayak, 1984). Hence, we include schizoaffective disorder here in our discussion of clinical interviewing for the diagnosis of schizophrenia.

TABLE 2. *DSM-IV* Criteria for the Diagnosis of Schizoaffective Disorder

---

A. An uninterrupted period of illness during which, at some time, there is either a Major Depressive Episode, a Manic Episode, or a Mixed Episode concurrent with symptoms that meet Criterion A of Schizophrenia.
   Note: The Major Depressive Episode must include the symptom, depressed mood.

B. During the same period of illness, there have been delusions or hallucinations for at least 2 weeks in the absence of prominent mood symptoms.

C. Symptoms meeting the criteria for a mood disorder are present for a substantial portion of the total duration of the active and residual periods of the illness.

D. The disturbance is not due to the direct physiological effects of a substance (e.g., a drug of abuse, a medication) or a general medical condition.

Specify type
Bipolar type: If the disturbance includes a Manic or a Mixed Episode (or a Manic or a Mixed Episode and Major Depressive Episodes)
Depressive type: If the disturbance only includes Major Depressive Episodes

---

Adapted from *Diagnostic and statistical manual of mental disorders-IV*, American Psychiatric Association, 1994.

PROCEDURES FOR GATHERING INFORMATION

The diagnosis of schizophrenia depends most heavily on the assessment of the patient's subjective experiences (e.g., delusions and hallucinations), with less emphasis placed on behavioral observation of symptoms, such as flattened affect or looseness of associations (see Table 1). Positive symptoms tend to be less stable over time than negative symptoms, in part due to their subjective quality (Lewine, 1990; Mueser, Douglas, Bellack, & Morrison, 1991). Furthermore, patients may be reluctant to admit experiencing positive symptoms for reasons such as paranoia, an awareness that these symptoms are out of the range of ordinary experience, or negative experiences with prior discussions about these symptoms (e.g., ridicule or denial by family members, attempts to hospitalize the patient). Therefore, whereas the interview is at the heart of diagnostic assessment, the diagnostician must utilize all available resources to determine whether the patient meets the criteria for schizophrenia.

The most useful sources of collateral information about patients' symptomatology include their medical records, the observations of family members, and reports of mental health professionals involved in the patients' long-term treatment. How these sources of information are utilized in conjunction with the patient interview depends on the availability of the resources and the setting of the interview. When possible, it is desirable for the interviewer to examine the patient's medical records prior to the interview in order to identify past symptoms and diagnoses. Sometimes this chart review is impossible (e.g., when the patient has no previous psychiatric hospitalizations) or impractical (e.g., when the patient is being evaluated for hospitalization in a psychiatric emergency room). In such cases, meeting with a relative or friend to briefly discuss the patient's behavior over the past several weeks and the circumstances leading up to the psychiatric evaluation can help guide the diagnostic interview.

Some diagnosticians prefer to limit the amount of information they learn about the patient before the first meeting in order to maximize their objectivity in the interview. Following the interview, the diagnostician may seek additional information from family members and professionals and, when necessary, meet again with the patient to clarify specific points. We have found that this approach provides a balance between objective assessment and the utilization of all relevant sources of information.

Case Example

A 27-year-old Catholic woman was involuntarily admitted to the hospital by her mother because of severe social withdrawal, poor personal hygiene, and increased religious preoccupation. Her chart indicated that she had had two previous psychiatric admissions and had been given diagnoses of paranoid schizophrenia and manic-depression, although the specific content of her delusions was not described. During the interview, the woman denied auditory hallucinations and, while she admitted to being religious, insisted that her beliefs were not delusional compared to those of others in the Charismatic Catholic church to which she belonged. The mother reported that her daughter had recently arranged for a priest to exorcise her and cleanse her apartment with holy water, but the patient refused to explain her actions.

The evidence from the interviews with the patient and her mother was strongly suggestive of schizophrenia, but not sufficient to establish the diagnosis. However, interviews with inpatient staff members indicated that the patient had been observed stuffing tissues into her mouth and talking downward toward the ground to "the Devil." A subsequent meeting with the patient indicated that she used the tissues to prevent the Devil from talking through her mouth, which she had experienced and found very distressing. Thus, observation of the patient's behavior provided valuable additional information that allowed the interviewer to confirm the presence of delusions and auditory hallucinations, thereby confirming a diagnosis of schizophrenia, paranoid subtype.

The diagnosis of schizophrenia requires obtaining a wide range of information from the patient during the interview, including the onset of the illness, a description of events leading up to the current episode, and past and present symptomatology. As with any assessment procedure, the validity of the diagnostic interview can be threatened if it is not conducted in a relatively standardized fashion across different patients. One method for standardizing the diagnostic assessment across both patients and interviewers is the use of structured interview schedules.

Structured Diagnostic Interview Instruments

Prior to the development of objectively based criteria for the diagnosis of schizophrenia in *DSM-III* (American Psychiatric Association, 1980), the reliability of this diagnosis was notoriously low (Matarazzo, 1983) and schizophrenia was widely overdiagnosed in the United States (Kuriansky, Deming, & Gurland, 1974). In addition to the establishment of explicit criteria for the diagnosis of schizophrenia, the use of structured clinical interviews to assess patients' history of illness and symptomatology has also improved the reliability of diagnosis. A variety of semi-structured interview schedules have been developed over the past 20 years, with the most common instruments for the diagnosis of schizophrenia including the Structured Clinical Interview for *DSM-IV* (SCID) (First, Spitzer, Williams, & Gibbon, 1996), the Schedule for Affective Disorders and Schizophrenia (SADS) (Endicott & Spitzer, 1978), the Present State Examination (PSE) (Wing, 1970), and the Diagnostic Interview Schedule (DIS) (Robins, Cottler, Bucholz, & Compton, 1995). Reliability studies of these instruments have demonstrated high sensitivity and specificity across interviewers (for a review, see Morrison, 1988). The SCID is at present the most widely used structured interview in the United States and the PSE is most widely used in England. The DIS was developed for use in epidemiological studies and designed so that it could be administered by a lay person. In general, the DIS is considered to be less precise than the other instruments.

The primary advantage of using structured interviews to diagnose schizophrenia is that they provide a standardized approach for eliciting symptoms, thereby reducing the variability of the assessment across different patients. A related advantage is that structured interview instruments provide guidelines for determining whether a specific symptom exists and for making decisions about ruling out other related disorders (e.g., manic-depressive illness). A final consideration is the availability of training in structured diagnostic interviews. Extensive training opportunities are available for all the instruments described above, including seminars, videotaped interviews, and detailed training books, and training is critical to achieving accurate diagnoses. The major pitfalls of structured interview instruments are the time required to administer them (usually about 90 min) and the training needed to conduct the interview reliably.

CASE ILLUSTRATIONS

Introducing the Interview

During the first meeting, it is important for the interviewer to present himself or herself in an objective, nonjudgmental, empathic manner in order to ease the patient as much as possible and convey the feeling of concern. Patients with delusions or hallucinations frequently experience severe anxiety, depression, and anger because of these psychotic symptoms.

The diagnostic interview should be introduced to the patient clearly in order to gain the greatest cooperation. The clinician may start by saying, "I am going to ask you some questions about problems and difficulties you may have. I will also ask you about difficulties you may have had in the past. As we talk, I will make some notes. Do you have any questions before we begin?" (First et al., 1996). It is important to give the patient an opportunity to express any misgivings about the context of the interview, such as conflicts that might have occurred immediately prior to the interview about which the clinician should be aware. Concerns about the interview should be clarified and other problems acknowledged before proceeding with the interview.

Obtaining the Overview and the History

The first stages of the diagnostic interview cover general information about the patient's age, where and with whom the patient is living, and the patient's source of income (including disability status or occupation). This gives that interviewee a warm-up phase by focusing on easy-to-answer factual questions. These items can be asked directly using questions such as: "What is your source of income?" "How do you support yourself?" "You mentioned that you receive a check—is that a disability check?" "How far did you go in school?" If the patient did not finish high school, the interviewer should ask what happened that prevented him or her from finishing.

In many inpatient settings, the interviewer will have access to demographic and background information. Rather than omit questions about these data, it is preferable to confirm the details with the patient in order to help establish rapport and the flow of the interview. Information can be obtained by saying: "I want to confirm a couple of details about your living situation. Prior to coming to the hospital, you lived at your mother's house at 110 South Greene Street. Do we have that correct?" "Now, who else stays with you and your mother?"

The interviewer then obtains an overview of the present episode by asking, "How did you come to be in the hospital?" or "I understand that you have been experiencing more problems with [major psychotic symptom]. Tell me what difficulties you have been having recently." Often, it is necessary to pursue a denial of problems. For example, if the patient states only that he or she has become more nervous lately, the interviewer might say, "Can you tell me a little more about that?" If the patient denies serious difficulties again, one might say, "Isn't there something else? People aren't usually admitted to psychiatric hospitals just for being nervous." It is also important to assess whether there are stressors associated with the current symptomatology. This information can be gathered by asking: "How were things going when you started having these problems?" "Were you having difficulty with your family?" "How about where you were living?" The last part of the overview of the present episode should include an assessment of medical problems, medications, and alcohol and drug use. Questions similar to the following will suffice: "How has your health been?" "What medications do you take?" "How much alcohol do you drink per week?" "What drugs have you taken—what about street drugs such as marijuana and cocaine?"

A brief historical overview of the patient's illness is also necessary. The interviewer can ask: "How many times before have you had the difficulties you are having now?" or "How many times have you been hospitalized for emotional or psychiatric problems?" The clinician should get a brief outline of the hospitalizations, or discrete episodes, by asking: "Let's review the first time you were hospitalized [or had difficulty]. When was that?" "What problems or symptoms were you having?" "Was it different from what you are experiencing currently?" "Where were you hospitalized?" or "Where did you go for treatment?" Each episode identified by the patient should be explored with these questions. Often, the patient is a poor reporter of the chronology of his or her disorder, so that the interviewer may wish to ask about episodes reported by friends, family, and other mental health professionals. For example, the clinician could ask, "I understand that you were in Temple Hospital for four weeks in January of 2001. Could you tell me about how you came to be in the hospital? What were some of the problems you were experiencing before being admitted?"

In all, the overview need not require more than 10–25 min. It is important that the clinician have this background so that he or she can explore the course of the disorder, the patient's important life events, and the patient's previous and current level of functioning. For many patients this information must come from sources other than the clinical interview. However, these details must be obtained before a diagnosis can be made, and often the interview can be enhanced when the clinician has the information in advance.

Eliciting Symptoms of the Current Episode

There are two major sources of information during the interview: First, the clinician evaluates the content and the logical flow of the patient's verbalizations. The content of the patient's speech may indicate the presence of symptoms such as delusions and hallucinations, whereas the logical flow may indicate the presence of loose associations, circumstantiality, and thought blocking. Second, during the interview, the clinician uses observation of the patient's behavior and affective expressivity to detect symptoms such as blunted or inappropriate affect.

One of the most common symptoms that the interviewer should explore is hallucinations. The clinician may start by asking an open-ended question about a more general complaint. The example below illustrates this tactic with a 38-year-old patient with a 15-year history of psychiatric hospitalizations.

INTERVIEWER: You mentioned that you were suicidal when you came to the hospital this time. What was going on that led you to be suicidal?

PATIENT: I had started to hear people talk outside of my door. I'd go outside and nobody would be there and I heard them laughing about it. Making fun of me, making me feel stupid. I started to drink because I was trying to get them to stop.

I: Where did the voices come from?

P: I don't know. I guess inside my head. I thought outside, but they weren't there. Every time I hear them I end up going to the hospital.

Delusions are also assessed by evaluating the content of the patient's verbalizations. With some patients, delusions are readily assessed because the patient is preoccupied with the theme or idea. Other patients must be engaged into a lengthier discussion before they begin to reveal much about their delusional ideas. When the interviewer successfully scratches the surface of the delusion by discussing related material, the patient may readily expound on his or her beliefs. Thus, it is helpful to find out from other sources of information (i.e., admitting records) what the possible content of the delusion may be before beginning the interview. The interviewer can start with broader questions about delusions.

I: Did it ever seem that people were talking about you or taking special notice of you?

P: I was walking down the street and a white van came up and I could hear them saying, "Let's wait 'til the next light and then jump out and grab her."

I: What did you do?

P: I stopped and stood still so they would have to continue in the traffic. I stood there about 8 or 9 hours so they couldn't get me.

I: How did that work to keep them from grabbing you?

P: I was protected while I was standing still. They couldn't get me. A trolley went by 4 times and the driver asked if I wanted a ride, but I said no. Where would I go, anyway?

In this excerpt, the interviewer's questions were derived largely from the patient's responses. By showing interest and concern, the clinician is able to draw out more details of the delusional system than by using rote, predetermined questions. Other types of general questions that can start this type of dialogue include the following: "Does it seem that something or someone is controlling your thoughts or your behavior?" "What about putting thoughts into your head?" "Do you have ideas or beliefs that others find difficult to believe or understand?"

While asking questions about the patient's beliefs and experiences, the clinician should take note of the logical flow of the patient's verbalizations for evidence of formal thought disorder. The severity of thought disorder can range from very mild to very severe. Mild thought disorder can be difficult to detect, but is often manifested by occasional idiosyncratic word use, neologisms, and non sequiturs in the flow of the interview. The interviewer may find that he or she has lost track of the point the patient was trying to make. This is a cue to consider whether the patient is exhibiting digressive, vague, or circumstantial speech (prodromal or residual symptoms); additionally, the patient may be exhibiting loose associations, as illustrated below. Close examination of this transcript of an actual diagnostic interview reveals a thread of loosely connected ideas that are difficult to follow in conversation.

I: Have you received special messages from the way things are arranged around the room, or have you received special messages from the radio or TV?

P: I like football and sports. When I was home the next door neighbors—well they were married in '70 and they have four kids—they have a pool about the size of this room and I was the lifeguard. I did that last summer.

I: But did you receive special messages from the TV?

P: Nah. I relate to war movies, I guess. The plane is hit by the enemy—Korea and Viet Nam—and has to bail out over water and 50 states of rescue planes, PBY's, throw a life raft. Well, I did it with 50 states of ships. The face of—and 50 states of PT boats. And you build them with the San Diego Naval Base, the Brooklyn Navy Yard and you open up navy yards all—I tried to open up a navy yard where I live—and go to work there. I had a job application in at the Frankford Hospital but I couldn't go to work because my arms—I tell you, I have been trying to get strength in this arm and it won't form. I eat and eat. I'm anemic. It's blood diserialosis and I'm anemic.

CRITICAL INFORMATION FOR MAKING THE DIAGNOSIS

The essence of the diagnostic process is to decide when the threshold for a diagnostic criterion has been met. It is easy to regard diagnostic criteria as a checklist and to make these decisions superficially. However, skilled clinicians recognize the need to clarify any ambiguity in a diagnostic situation by gathering sufficient information. In the past, some of the ambiguity in the diagnostic process stemmed from the lack of *operationalized criteria* of the dominant nosological systems in use. Prior to *DSM-III* (American Psychiatric Association, 1980), DSM diagnostic criteria were written to reflect hypothesized underlying psychological etiological mechanisms (e.g., rather than observable behavior). The introduction of the *DSM-III* operationalized the criteria, vastly improving the clinician's ability to tie his or her observations to a set of criteria.

Despite these improvements in the major diagnostic systems, the clinician is asked to make a number of difficult judgments. We will discuss the critical information needed to fulfill the diagnostic criteria for several areas. First, specific symptomatic criteria, such as hallucinations and delusions, will be discussed. Second, we will discuss the information needed to establish whether the threshold of the *decrease in functioning* criterion has been met. Last, we will examine the criteria with respect to the other clinical syndromes, including affective disorders, drug abuse, or organic factors that need to be considered and ruled out before the diagnosis is made.

Symptomatic Criteria

Some symptoms are assessed by evaluating the content of a patient's verbalizations, such as the case of delusional beliefs. What yardstick is the clinician to use in evaluating the beliefs? To a great extent, the interviewer must rely on his or her own norms of human behavior and experience. This approach may be flawed, however, because the patient may have been raised in a subculture that supports beliefs that seem delusional in the dominant culture. Obviously, making an appropriate judgment depends on the extent of the interviewer's knowledge of beliefs in that subculture. However, more than a superficial knowledge is necessary. It is best for the interviewer to seek the consultation of a colleague who is familiar with that culture for assistance in understanding what beliefs are common and accepted.

In assessing delusions in which the person's subculture is not an issue, an interviewer may simply invite the patient to say as much as possible about the specific topic at hand. Usually, suspected delusional material will become increasingly apparent as the patient is given time to respond to questions, if the interviewer demonstrates genuine concern and interest. It is often instructive to ask a patient whether others share his or her beliefs. In addition, relatives are often available to confirm or disconfirm important aspects of the patient's beliefs. The interviewer may evaluate the internal consistency of the patient's story. Contradictions may point the interviewer to delusional material.

Changes in how bizarre delusions are handled in the *DSM-III-R* (American Psychiatric Association, 1987) and current *DSM-IV* criteria (American Psychiatric Association, 1994) for schizophrenia have caused an increase in the diagnostic importance of this symptom. As noted by Flaum, Arndt, and Andreasen (1991), it is possible to diagnose schizophrenia (in the active phase) on the basis of the presence of a bizarre delusion as sole Criterion A symptom; in the *DSM-III* (American Psychiatric Association, 1980), an earlier edition of the *DSM*, the bizarre delusion was only one of several classes of symptoms that could be used to diagnose schizophrenia in the active phase. Unfortunately, Flaum et al., (1991) reported that the overall reliability of judgments for bizarre delusions is poor, regardless of the rater's level of training or the definition used. The best reliability can be obtained for the bizarre delusions that illustrate the classic Schneiderian first-rank symptoms of thought broadcasting (i.e., the belief that one's thoughts can be heard by others), thought insertion (i.e., the belief that others can put thoughts into one's mind), and "made" (or imposed) volitional acts (i.e., delusion of being controlled by an external force) (see Mellor, 1970). Other types of bizarre delusions, such as somatic or grandiose delusions, led to the lowest reliability. However, as noted below, Schneiderian first-rank symptoms should not be considered pathognomonic of schizophrenia, given the evidence that patients with substance abuse without schizophrenia can also exhibit these symptoms.

These considerations suggest that the diagnostician should take great care in cases in which a patient meets criteria for schizophrenia in the active phase based solely on the presence of a bizarre delusion. Maximum effort should be made to evaluate the presence of other symptoms that might alleviate the diagnostician of the burden of depending on a symptom that cannot be reliably diagnosed. We suggest that interviewers considering the diagnosis of schizophrenia based on a sole bizarre delusion restrict the diagnosis to cases in which the delusion is one of the types found to be most reliably rated by Flaum and colleagues. Perhaps future revisions of the *DSM* will provide greater guidance in the evaluation of bizarre delusions.

Evaluating the presence or absence of hallucinations often requires as much detective work as the assessment of delusions. In some cases, hallucination-like experiences may occur transiently while the patient is in a semisleeping state before deep sleep. When this is the only time "hallucinations" occur, the phenomenon is considered a *hypnagogic experience*, rather than a true hallucination. When a patient is inconsistent about the report of hallucinations, it is useful to observe the patient for signs that he or she is responding either verbally or physically to internal stimuli that may be hallucinations. Patients are often distracted or upset by hallucinations; asking about hallucinations when the patient seems preoccupied can lead to the patient's acknowledgment that he or she is indeed hearing voices.

Criterion of Decrease in Functioning

One important criterion for the diagnosis of schizophrenia is a decrease in social functioning, occupational functioning, and self-care. How does one assess whether the patient has experienced a decline in functioning? Family and friends, and sometimes the patient, can indicate how he or she was functioning in these areas. Sometimes the patient's physical appearance indicates that his or her self-care is so poor that there is likely to have been a decrease from previous levels. A diagnostic interview that includes an overview, as discussed above, will give the interviewer some initial clues as to how the patient was functioning before the current episode. The interviewer must then ask specific questions about activities the patient is not able to manage at this time. For example, "What activities were you able to do before your current difficulties?" "When did you last work?" "When did you last go to your day program?" For patients who have never worked outside their homes, the questions could center around household responsibilities that have been neglected recently: "Were you able to clean the house and care for your children better before your present difficulties?" "Did you begin to have problems taking care of yourself—like eating and showering?" "Did your family notice a change?" Many of the judgments must inevitably rest on subjective accounts by the patient and family members. However, greater accuracy is gained by gathering as much specific information about the patient's actual activities as possible.

Diagnosis of Schizophrenia and the Importance of Longitudinal Information

As mentioned above, 6 months of disturbance in relation to the current episode is necessary to establish a diagnosis of schizophrenia. In general, schizophrenia is seen as a chronic disorder, often with impaired social and psychiatric functioning in between episodes. Recent prospective research focused on the prediction of schizophrenia symptoms from prodromal symptoms supports that the absence of these symptoms likely means that the patient does not have the disorder, although the presence of these symptoms predicts a subsequent diagnosis of schizophrenia in 49.4% of cases (Klosterkötter, Hellmich, Steinmeyer, & Schutze-Lutter, 2001). Patients with longer histories of illness yield more reliable diagnoses because of the greater availability of collective information relevant to establishing a valid diagnosis (Kirby, Hay, Daniels, Jones, & Mowry, 1998). It is clear that the consistency of the diagnosis is less than 100% from initial episodes, although in hospital settings, it is one of the most stable diagnoses (about 90% continue to meet criteria at a subsequent hospitalization; Schwartz et al., 2000). In general, one might expect to be able to achieve greater confidence in inpatient settings compared to outpatient settings, because of the level of functioning of the patient and the range of information that becomes available during a hospitalization.

Patients with schizophrenia exhibit great heterogeneity in their premorbid functioning and current symptomatology, so that *relatively* better premorbid functioning should not be construed as evidence against a diagnosis of schizophrenia. In one large study of diagnosis stability up to 2 years after a first-admission diagnosis of schizophrenia, Schwartz et al. (2000) identified several clinical characteristics that predict changes in the diagnosis patients received. These factors included relatively higher global functioning and lower levels of positive and negative symptoms, compared to stably diagnosed schizophrenia patients. Patients in this study who received a stable diagnosis of schizophrenia after their initial hospitalization had poorer premorbid adjustment in adolescence, lack of lifetime substance abuse, and more negative symptoms at 6 months after the initial hospitalization, compared to psychotic patients as a whole. But diagnosticians must be cautioned not to avoid using the schizophrenia diagnosis simply because the patient has relatively better premorbid functioning or a lower level of symptomatology than other psychotic patients (e.g., depression with psychosis or psychotic symptoms associated with bipolar disorder). Indeed, the hypotheses that patients who meet criteria for schizophreniform disorder (i.e., symptom duration less than 6 months) have a different course than patients with diagnoses of schizophrenia has received inconsistent support (Zarate, Tohen, & Land, 2000; cf. Zhang-Wong, Beiser, Bean, & Iacono, 1995).

Other Relevant Syndromes

The novice interviewer may consider a diagnosis of schizophrenia likely when confronted with a patient with psychotic symptoms. However, there is a myriad of psychiatric and medical conditions that are commonly characterized by psychotic symptoms. Thus, the presence of many other syndromes must be assessed and ruled out before assigning the diagnosis of schizophrenia.

Every patient receiving a psychiatric evaluation should be given a screening physical examination to rule out medical illnesses. The physical examination should include assessment of five areas: (1) vital signs, (2) autonomic system dysfunction, (3) heart and lung dysfunction, (4) neurological dysfunction and head trauma, and (5) abnormalities of the eyes (Shea, 1998). It is not necessary that the physical examination occur before the interview, but in most hospitals and psychiatric institutions the patient will be given an examination on admission.

It is important that medical and nonmedical professionals alike be familiar with many of the conditions that can commonly result in a presentation of psychotic symptoms. Examples include temporal lobe epilepsy, thyroid disorder, and meningitis. For a comprehensive list of organic causes of psychosis, consult Shea (1998).

Schizoaffective disorder and mood disorders are the disorders most commonly confused with schizophrenia by novice interviewers. It is a common misconception that the apparent predominance of psychotic symptoms versus affective symptoms is the only consideration for differentiating between schizophrenia, schizoaffective disorder, and affective disorders. Careful consideration of the *DSM-IV* criteria for these disorders requires the clinician to uncover several crucial pieces of information, including the onset, course, and duration of each of the types of symptoms (psychotic and affective symptoms). The relative timing of psychotic and affective symptoms is crucial to establishing the correct diagnosis. For example, one patient may present as extremely paranoid and somewhat loose and rambling. He may also exhibit pressured speech, grandiosity, and irritability. If the patient had not been paranoid or loose in the absence of the affective symptoms in the course of the disorder, he could not have schizophrenia or schizoaffective disorder, but would more likely have bipolar disorder. It may take several discussions with the patient or family members or both in order to obtain reliable information about the timing of psychotic and affective symptoms.

Post-traumatic stress disorder (PTSD) has emerged as a highly relevant disorder when assessing patients for schizophrenia, in particular because of the high rates of exposure to trauma of these patients, high rates of PTSD comorbidity with schizophrenia, and the overlap in symptom presentation between the disorders. Estimates for exposure to interpersonal violence within the past year for persons with serious mental illnesses (SMIs) range as high as 98% (Mueser et al., 1998), and 29–43% of SMIs meet criteria for PTSD (Mueser, Rosenberg, Goodman, & Trumbetta, 2002).

The presence of psychotic symptoms in PTSD may complicate the evaluation of the patient for schizophrenia. Psychotic symptoms occur in as many as 35% of people with PTSD (Sautter et al., 1999), and there are higher rates of psychotic symptoms in patients who have experienced combat-related traumas (Deering, Glover, Ready, Eddleman, & Alarcon, 1996). Patients with PTSD and psychotic symptoms may exhibit greater severity of paranoia, aggression, and general psychopathology than patients who are either psychotic or manifest PTSD alone; this is true whether or not the psychotic patient with PTSD actually meets criteria for schizophrenia (Sautter et al., 1999). Symptoms that may be interpreted as psychotic, may in fact be dissociative or re-experiencing symptoms such as trauma-related auditory and olfactory phenomena and flashbacks (Deering et al., 1996). As noted above, however, the rates of comorbidity of schizophrenia and PTSD suggest that one should not dismiss potential symptoms of schizophrenia when it is apparent that the patient has experienced a trauma.

Concurrent or recent drug abuse constitutes another important aspect of the clinical presentation that complicates the diagnosis of schizophrenia. This judgment is often difficult because a person with schizophrenia is much more likely to have a substance abuse or dependence disorder than a person without schizophrenia (see Mueser, Bellack, & Blanchard, 1992; Reiger et al., 1990). Indeed, the lifetime prevalence of rate of substance abuse among people with schizophrenia is close to 50% (Mueser, Bennett, & Kushner, 1995). Furthermore, there is evidence that stimulant abuse can lead to an earlier onset of schizophrenia in biologically vulnerable individuals as well as precipitate relapses in patients who already have the illness. Alcohol, cannabis, and hallucinogen abuse have also been linked to increased risk of relapse in schizophrenia (Pristach & Smith, 1996). Thus, the fact that substance use may exacerbate symptoms may mislead novice diagnosticians to attribute the symptomatology to illicit substance use, without considering that the pattern of psychotic symptoms may predate the current episode of substance use.

One "truism" that has often been repeated is that the presence of visual or tactile hallucinations or both is pathognomonic of substance abuse or withdrawal. The opposite has been purported to be true of auditory hallucinations, namely, that it is indicative of schizophrenia rather than drug abuse. However, surveys indicate that a wide range of different types of hallucinations are present in schizophrenia, with auditory hallucinations most common (72%), followed by visual (16%), and tactile (17%), and olfactory/gustatory hallucinations (Mueser, Bellack, & Brady, 1990). Visual hallucinations are even more prevalent in samples of chronic schizophrenia patients, with some estimates exceeding 50% (Bracha, Wolkowitz, Lohr, Karson, & Bigelow, 1989). Thus, the diagnostician must use other evidence for ruling drug abuse in or out as an etiological factor in the presenting psychotic symptoms.

The differential diagnosis of schizophrenia or drug-induced psychosis is made primarily by examining the history and pattern of the drug abuse relative to the psychotic symptoms. In addition to the symptoms necessary for the diagnosis of schizophrenia, a deterioration in social and occupational functioning must be found to have occurred prior to the beginning of the suspected drug or alcohol abuse. Recent research suggests that two specific psychotic symptoms, formal thought disorder and bizarre delusions, may increase the odds that psychotic patients with recent substance abuse meet criteria for schizophrenia, when compared with patients with substance-induced psychosis (i.e., not meeting criteria for schizophrenia) (Rosenthal & Miner, 1997). However, it should be noted that patients with bizarre delusions are only required to have one "Criterion A" symptom (see Table 1), which may represent a virtual tautology when predicting the diagnosis of schizophrenia from such a key definitional symptom. It must be clearly established that the patient experienced psychotic symptoms in the absence of current drug abuse.

We have found that patients often readily admit their drug use when the interviewer carefully examines all classes of drugs. The interviewer places a list of drugs in front of the patient and asks him or her to identify the drugs that have been used (see Table 3). The SCID utilizes this method, and it can be quite effective even when the patient denies drug use in initial questioning.

TABLE 3. Commonly Abused Drugs by Patients with Schizophrenia

---

Sedatives-hypnotics-anxiolytics ("downers")
Quaalude ("ludes"), Seconal ("reds"), Valium, Xanax, Librium, barbiturates, Miltown, Ativan, Dalmane, Halcion

Cannabis
Marijuana, hashish ("hash"), THC, "pot", "grass", "weed", "reefer"

Stimulants ("uppers")
Amphetamine, "speed", "glass", crystal, meth, dexadrine, ritalin, diet pills, "crank", "black beauties"

Opioids
Heroin ("smack", "skag"), morphine, opium, Methadone, Darvon, codeine, Percodan, Demerol, Dilaudid, Oxy Contin, Percocet

Cocaine
Snorting, IV, freebase, "crack", "speedball", "coke"

Hallucinogens ("psychedelics")
LSD ("acid"), purple haze, mescaline, peyote, psilocybin, STP, mushrooms

Dissociative anesthetics
PCP, "angel dust", "peace pill", "wack", "rocket fuel", Ketamine, "Special K"

Other
Steroids, "glue", ethyl chloride, nitrous oxide ("laughing gas"), whippets, amyl or butyl nitrate ("poppers"), Ecstasy ("X", "Adam"), MDA, MDM, GHB, nonprescription sleep or diet pills

---

Adapted from First et al. (1996). A complete list can be found on the website of the National Institute of Drug Abuse (www.nida.nih.gov).

Dos and Don'ts

A well-conducted diagnostic interview has many essential components that have been discussed at length elsewhere. Instead of repeating information already available, we will discuss guidelines for interviewing schizophrenic patients in light of the special challenges they present. Psychotic patients are often interviewed at the height of an exacerbation after an involuntary admission to a psychiatric facility. The patient in this situation may be frightened due to hallucinations and delusions he or she is experiencing. Alternatively, he or she may be angry about the admission. Thus, it is possible that the interviewer would get little more than superficial cooperation from the patient. It is particularly important to develop empathy and rapport in order to maximize the usefulness of the interview. We will present a number of specific ways to achieve this. Interview procedures to avoid also will be presented.

Dos

Outline the information to be covered. It is important to help to the patient be at ease by describing exactly what will happen in the interview. Even if the patient knows that there is information that he or she is not willing to reveal, it makes the interview more predictable and thus more comfortable for the patient (see the section entitled "Introducing the Interview" above).

Use both general and specific questions for difficult topics. When addressing an area about which the patient is upset, such as conflict with family members, it is useful to start with general questions and then gradually become more specific. This technique will help reduce the defensiveness that the patient may have about the topic. This is illustrated below.

I: I understand that things were not going well between you and some of your family members before you came to the hospital. Could you tell me a little about that?

P: There ain't nothing to tell. It's all my sister's fault. If she wasn't so mean, I wouldn't be here.

I: It sounds like you think she may not be on your side.

P: She just is sneaky and doesn't want me at home anymore. I didn't do anything to her. I don't know why she wants me gone.

I: Are there some things that you believe she does to you when you aren't watching.

P: I'm not sure, but I think it's with the food.

I: What do you think she is doing to your food?

P: Rat poison, what else? I really got her for it too. Zapped her right on the forehead. She won't forget that lesson for a while.

Use follow-up questions. The dialogue above also illustrates the importance of follow-up questions. By remaining on the topic and asking follow-up questions, the interviewer gradually acquires more information about a particular area. Follow-up is especially crucial for the assessment of delusions. If the patient is somewhat disorganized or exhibiting loosened associations, follow-up questions may be necessary to redirect the patient back to the topic. The clinician can say, for example, "You mentioned a moment ago that you felt your sister was doing something to hurt you, perhaps even poisoning you. Can you say more about why she would do this?" At other times, the interviewer can simply follow-up by asking: "Could you tell me a little more about that?"

Adjust language to the individual patient. To help the patient feel as comfortable as possible and understand the questions put to him or her, the interviewer should use the patient's language for describing symptoms or events. For example, if the patient describes the initial psychotic break or subsequent exacerbation of schizophrenia as "having a nervous breakdown," the clinician can ask: "You mentioned that you had a 'nervous breakdown' last year. Did you hear voices at that time?" The clinician should also recognize the difference in education that often exists between him or her and the patient and accordingly limit technical jargon and use plain language instead.

Gently pressure the patient only when necessary. Novice diagnostic interviewers often use pressure when faced with inconsistencies or with apparent attempts to conceal important information. It can be frustrating to interview a patient who is uncooperative or evasive when this information is sought. The interviewer needs to bear in mind that most people with schizophrenia have experienced negative social consequences when discussing their symptoms with others, such as being told they are "crazy" when talking about delusions or that auditory hallucinations are "just in their imagination." These unpleasant social reactions have the understandable effect of making many patients reticent to discuss their private perceptions and thoughts. Pressure or confrontation should not be a routine interviewing technique, because it usually increases the patient's defensiveness. When inconsistencies appear in the patient's account of his difficulties, the interviewer can request more information about the topic without pointing out the contradiction. This may be done, for example, by asking a patient who had denied hallucinations prior to admission: "We were talking a minute ago about hearing voices. I noticed that you seemed distracted or bothered by something a moment ago. Can you tell me what you were seeing or hearing?"

Don'ts

Don't apologize for questions. It is unnecessary for a clinician to apologize for the questions asked in a diagnostic interview, even if the interviewee reacts incredulously to queries about delusions or hallucinations. Some patients might initially deny these symptoms, and to apologize for asking may legitimize the denial.

Don't use leading questions. Leading questions imply to the patient what the correct answer is. An example of this type of question is: "*Weren't* you hearing voices when you first came to the hospital?" The preferable way of asking this question is: "*Were* you hearing voices when you first came to the hospital?" Likewise, the interviewer should be cautioned against asking leading questions that suggest that a particular symptom was *not* present, for example, "*You weren't* feeling sad or blue when you first started hearing the voices, *were you?*"

Don't repeat questions. When an interviewer believes that a symptom is present, despite the patient's denial of the symptom, do not simply keep repeating the same question in the hope that the patient will relent and say "Yes." For example, some clinicians might ask: "Did you feel that your family was trying to hurt you?" followed by "So you didn't feel your family was trying to hurt you?" As an alternative, the interviewer might ask for more detailed information about the situation by saying: "I'd like you to describe a little bit about how you have been getting along with your family. Every family has disagreements, so I'd like you to tell me about some things that have bothered you about them or that they have complained about to you over the last month."

Don't try to correct the patient's delusional ideas. If the patient becomes upset when discussing symptoms, the interviewer should empathize with his or her feelings without colluding with the patient by implying that the psychotic beliefs are true [e.g., "It must be very upsetting for you to hear these voices putting you down all the time" (Shea, 1998)]. Attempts to confront and convince patients with schizophrenia that their delusions are false invariably fail, and often paradoxically increase the patient's degree of conviction about the belief (Milton, Patwa, & Hafner, 1978). In rare instances, the patient may directly inquire whether the interviewer believes his or her delusion. In such cases, the interviewer may either refocus the patient back to discussing his or her experiences (e.g., "I would like to concentrate here on what *you* believe, rather than what *I* believe") or state frankly that they have a difference of opinion (e.g., "I don't think that you are being pursued by the FBI and the Mafia, but it's okay for you and I to have different opinions about this").

Don't redirect the interview unless necessary.   Patients should be given as much time as possible to talk about their difficulties so that they feel free to give their version of events. Even in structured interviews, the patient should be given time to describe incidents, problems, or interpretations without frequent interruption so that he or she feels comfortable. Of course, patients who are more disorganized, tangential, or circumstantial will need more redirection and structure. Redirection can be accomplished in some such fashion as this: "Let's back up to where we were talking about when you left your residential home because I want to understand more about what that was like for you. Were you getting the feeling that the people there were going out of their way to give you a hard time or trying to hurt you?"

Summary

Schizophrenia is one of the most difficult psychiatric disorders to diagnose, both because its characteristic symptoms overlap with those of many other disorders and because patients are often reticent to discuss their symptoms. Until recently, the diagnosis of schizophrenia was considered by many to be a wastebasket diagnosis for patients with severe, psychotic symptoms that were not easily classified into other diagnostic categories. The development of operationalized diagnostic criteria and standardized interview instruments over the past 20 years has enabled schizophrenia to be diagnosed reliably.

Special care is required to conduct a diagnostic interview with a patient suspected of having schizophrenia. Efforts must be made to ensure that the patient is as comfortable as possible with the interview situation, to provide the patient with an opportunity to tell his or her story without excessive interruptions or challenges, and to follow up hints of delusions or hallucinations that may be critical to establishing the correct diagnosis. Additionally, other sources of information about the patient usually need to be tapped, such as medical records and reports of significant others. Despite the prominence of thought disorder in many patients with schizophrenia, the vast majority of patients are cooperative during the diagnostic interview and are responsive to a warm, empathic, frank interpersonal style. Strong interviewing skills are necessary to confirm or rule out the diagnosis of schizophrenia, which subsequently has important pharmacological and psychotherapeutic treatment implications. Advances in pharmacological interventions (Jibson & Tandon, 1998; Kane, 1997) and psychosocial treatments for schizophrenia (Mueser, Bond, & Drake, 2001) underscore the importance of establishing an accurate diagnosis in order to link these patients with the treatment services most likely to improve the prognosis of this chronic psychiatric illness.

References

American Psychiatric Association. (1980). *Diagnostic and statistical manual of mental disorders* (3rd ed.). Washington, DC: Author.

American Psychiatric Association. (1987). *Diagnostic and statistical manual of mental disorders* (3rd ed., revised). Washington, DC: Author.

American Psychiatric Association. (1994). *Diagnostic and statistical manual of mental disorders* (4th ed.). Washington, DC: Author.

Bellack, A. S., Mueser, K. T., Gingerich, S., & Agresta, J. (1997). *Social skills training for schizophrenia: A step-by-step guide.* New York: Guilford.

Bleuler, E. (1950). *Dementia praecox or the group of schizophrenias* (J. Zinken, Trans. [1911]). New York: International Universities Press.

Bond, G. R., Becker, D. R., Drake, R. E., Rapp, C. A., Meisler, N., Lehman, A. F., Bell, M. D., & Blyler, C. R. (2001). Implementing supported employment as an evidence-based practice. *Psychiatric Services, 52,* 313–322.

Bond, G. R., Drake, R. E., Becker, D. R., & Mueser, K. T. (1999). Effectiveness of psychiatric rehabilitation approaches for employment of people with severe mental illness. *Journal of Disability Policy Studies, 10,* 18–52.

Bracha, H. S., Wolkowitz, O. M., Lohr, J. B., Karson, C. N., & Bigelow, L. B. (1989). High prevalence of visual hallucinations in research subjects with chronic schizophrenia. *American Journal of Psychiatry, 146,* 526–528.

Bruce, M. L., Takeuchi, D. T., & Leaf, P. J. (1991). Poverty and psychiatric status. *Archives of General Psychiatry, 48,* 470–474.

Buchsbaum, M. S. (1990). The frontal lobes, basal ganglia, and temporal lobes as sites for schizophrenia. *Schizophrenia Bulletin, 16,* 379–389.

Bustillo, J., Lauriello, J., Horan, W., & Keith, S. (2001). The psychosocial treatment of schizophrenia: An update. *American Journal of Psychiatry, 158,* 163–175.

Cornblatt, B. A., Lenzenweger, M. F., Dworkin, R. H., & Erlenmeyer-Kimling, L. (1992). Childhood attentional dysfunctions predict social deficits in unaffected adults at risk for schizophrenia. *British Journal of Psychiatry, 161*(Suppl. 18), 59–64.

Crow, T. J. (1990). Meaning of structural changes in the brain in schizophrenia. In A. Kales, C. N. Stefanis, & J. Talbott (Eds.), *Recent advances in schizophrenia* (pp. 81–94). New York: Springer-Verlag.

Davies, N., Russell, A., Jones, P., & Murray, R. M. (1998). Which characteristics of schizophrenia predate psychosis. *Journal of Psychiatric Research, 32,* 121–131.

Deering, C. G., Glover, S. G., Ready, D., Eddleman, H. C., & Alarcon, R. D. (1996). Unique patterns of comorbidity in posttraumatic stress disorder from different source of trauma. *Comprehensive Psychiatry, 37,* 336–346.

Done, D. J., Crow, T. J., Johnstone, E. C., & Sacker, A. (1994). Childhood antecedents of schizophrenia and affective illnesses: Social adjustment at ages 7 and 11. *British Medical Journal, 309,* 699–703.

Endicott, J., & Spitzer, R. L. (1978). A diagnostic interview: The Schedule for Affective Disorders and Schizophrenia. *Archives of General Psychiatry, 35,* 837–844.

First, M. B., Spitzer, R. L., Williams, J. B. W., & Gibbon, M. (1996). *Structured Clinical Interview for DSM-IV—Patient Edition (SCID-P, Version 2.0).* New York: Biometrics Research Department, New York State Psychiatric Institute.

Flaum, M., Arndt, & Andreasen, N. (1991). The reliability of "bizarre" delusions. *Comprehensive Psychiatry, 32,* 59–65.

Fox, J. W. (1990). Social class, mental illness, and social mobility: The social selection-drift hypothesis for serious mental illness. *Journal of Health and Social Behavior, 31,* 344–353.

Goldstein, J. M. (1988). Gender differences in the course of schizophrenia. *Journal of Psychiatry, 145,* 684–689.

Gould, R. A., Mueser, K. T., Bolton, E., Mays, V., & Goff, D. (2001). Cognitive therapy for psychosis in schizophrenia: A preliminary meta-analysis. *Schizophrenia Research, 48,* 335–342.

Harding, C. M., Brooks, G. W., Ashikaga, T., Strauss, J. S., & Breier, A. (1987). The Vermont longitudinal study of persons with severe mental illness, I. Methodology, study sample, and overall status 32 years later. *American Journal of Psychiatry, 144,* 718–726.

Jablensky, A., & Sartorius, N. (1975). Culture and schizophrenia. In H. M. Van Praag (Ed.), *On the origin of schizophrenia psychoses* (pp. 99–124). Amsterdam: De Erven Bohn.

Jibson, M. D., & Tandon, R. (1998). New atypical antipsychotic medications. *Journal of Psychiatric Research, 32,* 215–228.

Kane, J. M. (1997). The new antipsychotics. *Journal of Practical Psychiatry and Behavioral Health, 3,* 343–355.

Kay, S. R., & Sevy, S. (1990). Pyramidical model of schizophrenia. *Schizophrenia Bulletin, 16*, 537–545.

Kirby, K. C., Hay, D. A., Daniels, B. A., Jones, I. H., & Mowry, B. J. (1998). Comparison between register and structured interview diagnoses of schizophrenia: A case for longitudinal diagnostic profiles. *Australian and New Zealand Journal of Psychiatry, 32*, 410–414.

Klosterkötter, J., Hellmich, M., Steinmeyer, E. M., & Schutze-Lutter, F. (2001). Diagnosing schizophrenia in the initial prodromal stage. *Archives of General Psychiatry, 58*, 158–164.

Kraepelin, E. (1919). *Dementia praecox and paraphrenia*. Edinburgh: Livingston.

Kramer, M. S., Vogel, W. H., DiJohnson, C., Dewey, D. A., Sheves, P., Cavicchia, S., Litle, P., Schmidt, R., & Kimes, I. (1989). Antidepressants in "depressed" schizophrenic inpatients. *Archives of General Psychiatry, 46*, 922–928.

Kuriansky, J. B., Deming, W. E., & Gurland, B. J. (1974). On trends in the diagnosis of schizophrenia. *American Journal of Psychiatry, 131*, 402–408.

Levinson, D. F., & Levitt, M. M. (1987). Schizoaffective mania reconsidered. *American Journal of Psychiatry, 144*, 415–425.

Lewine, R. R. J. (1990). A discriminant validity study of negative symptoms with a special focus on depression and antipsychotic medication. *American Journal of Psychiatry, 147*, 1463–1466.

Liberman, R. P., DeRisi, W. J., & Mueser, K. T. (1989). *Social skills training for psychiatric patients*. New York: Pergamon Press.

Matarazzo, J. D. (1983). The reliability of psychiatric and psychological diagnosis. *Clinical Psychology Review, 3*, 103–145.

Mattes, J. A., & Nayak, D. (1984). Lithium versus fluphenazine for prophylaxis in mainly schizophrenic schizo-affectives. *Biological Psychiatry, 19*, 445–449.

Mellor, C. S. (1970). First rank symptoms of schizophrenia. *British Journal of Psychiatry, 117*, 15–23.

Milton, F., Patwa, V. K., & Hafner, R. J. (1978). Confrontation vs. belief modification in persistently deluded patients. *British Journal of Medical Psychology, 51*, 127–130.

Morrison, R. L. (1988). Structured interviews and rating scales. In A. S. Bellack, & M. Hersen (Eds.), *Behavioral assessment: A practical handbook* (3rd ed., pp. 252–278). New York: Pergamon Press.

Mueser, K. T., Bellack, A. S., & Blanchard, J. J. (1992). Comorbidity of schizophrenia and substance abuse: Implications for treatment. *Journal Consulting and Clinical Psychology, 60*, 845–856.

Mueser, K. T., Bellack, A. S., & Brady, E. U. (1990). Hallucinations in schizophrenia. *Acta Psychiatrica Scandinavia, 82*, 26–29.

Mueser, K. T., Bellack, A. S., Morrison, R. L., & Wade, J. H. (1990). Gender, social competence, and symptomatology in schizophrenia: A longitudinal analysis. *Journal of Abnormal Psychology, 99*, 138–147.

Mueser, K. T., Bennett, M., & Kushner, M. G. (1995). Epidemiology of substance use disorders among persons with chronic mental illnesses. In A. F. Lehman & L. B. Dixon (Eds.), *Double jeopardy: Chronic mental illness and substance use disorders* (Vol. 3, pp. 9–25). Langhorne, PA: Harwood Academic.

Mueser, K. T., Bond, G. R., & Drake, R. E. (2001). Community-based treatment of schizophrenia and other severe mental disorders: Treatment outcomes. *Medscape Mental Health (online journal), 6*, http://psychiatry.medscape.com.

Mueser, K. T., Douglas, M. S., Bellack, A. S., & Morrison, R. L. (1991). Assessment of enduring deficit and negative symptom subtypes in schizophrenia. *Schizophrenia Bulletin, 17*, 565–582.

Mueser, K. T., & Glynn, S. M. (1999). *Behavioral family therapy for psychiatric disorders* (2nd ed.). Oakland, CA: New Harbinger.

Mueser, K. T., Goodman, L. B., Trumbetta, S. L., Rosenberg, S. D., Osher, F. C., Vidaver, R., Auciello, P., & Foy, D. W. (1998). Trauma and posttraumatic stress disorder in severe mental illness. *Journal of Consulting and Clinical Psychology, 66*, 493–499.

Mueser, K. T., Rosenberg, S. D., Goodman, L. A., & Trumbetta, S. L. (2002). Trauma, PTSD, and the course of severe mental illness: An interactive model. *Schizophrenia Research, 553*, 123–143.

Pristach, C. A., & Smith, C. M. (1996). Self-reported effects of alcohol use on symptoms of schizophrenia. *Psychiatric Services, 47*, 421–423.

Reiger, D. A., Farmer, M. E., Rae, D. S., Locke, B. Z., Keith, S. J., & Judd, L. L. (1990) Co-morbidity of mental disorders with alcohol and other drug abuse: Results from the Epidemiological Catchment Area (ECA) Study. *Journal of the American Medical Association, 264*, 2511–2518.

Robins, L. N., Helzer, J. E., Ratcliff, K. S., & Seyfried, W. (1982). Validity of the Diagnostic Interview Schedule, version II: DSM-III diagnoses. *Psychological Medicine, 12*, 855–870.

Robins, L. N., Helzer, J. E., Croughan, J., & Ratcliff, K. S. (1981). National Institute of Mental Health Diagnostic Interview Schedule: Its history, characteristics, and validity. *Archives of General Psychiatry, 38*, 381–389.

Robins, L. N., Cottler, L., Bucholz, K., & Compton, W. (1995). *Diagnostic Interview Schedule for DSM-IV*. St Louis: Washington University.

Rosenthal, R. N., & Miner, C. R. (1997). Differential diagnosis of substance-induced psychosis and schizophrenia in patients with substance use disorders. *Schizophrenia Bulletin, 23*, 187–193.

Roy, A. (1986). Suicide in schizophrenia. In A. Roy (Ed.), *Suicide* (pp. 97–112). Baltimore: Williams & Wilkins.

Sautter, F. J., Brailey, K., Uddo, M. M., Hamilton, M. E., Beard, M. G., & Borges, A. H. (1999). PTSD and comorbid psychotic disorder: Comparison with veterans diagnosed with PTSD or psychotic disorder. *Journal of Traumatic Stress, 12*, 73–88.

Schwartz, J. E., Fenning, S., Tanenberg-Karant, M., Carlson, G., Craig, T., Galambos, N., Lavelle, J., & Bromet, E. J. (2000). Congruence of diagnoses 2 years after a first-admission diagnosis of psychosis. *Archives of General Psychiatry, 57*, 593–600.

Shea, S. C. (1998). *Psychiatric interviewing: The art of understanding* (2nd ed.). Philadelphia: W.B. Saunders Company.

Walker, E., Downey, G., & Caspi, A. (1991). Twin studies of psychopathology: Why do the concordance rates vary? *Schizophrenia Research, 5*, 211–221.

Walker, E., & Lewine, R. J. (1990). Prediction of adult-onset schizophrenia from childhood home movies of the patients. *American Journal of Psychiatry, 147*, 1052–1056.

Wing, J. K. (1970). A standard form of psychiatric Present-State Examination and a method for standardizing the classification of symptoms. In E. H. Hare & J. K. Wing (Eds.), *Psychiatric epidemiology: An international symposium* (pp. 93–108). London: Oxford University Press.

Zarate, C. A., Jr., Tohn, M., & Land, M. (2000). First-episode schizophreniform disorder: Comparisons with first-episode schizophrenia. *Schizophrenia Research, 46*, 31–34.

Zhang-Wong, J., Beiser, M., Bean, G., & Iacono, W. G. (1995). Five-year course of schizophreniform disorder. *Psychiatry Research, 59*, 109–117.

Zigler, E., & Glick, M. (1986). *A developmental approach to adult psychopathology*. New York: John Wiley & Sons.

8

Personality Disorders

JILLAYNE Z. MCCLANAHAN, SOONIE A. KIM, AND MICHELLE BOBOWICK

INTRODUCTION

Assessment of personality disorders, AXIS II conditions in the 5-axes diagnostic system of the *Diagnostic and Statistical Manual of Mental Disorders* (*DSM-IV*) (American Psychiatric Association, 1994) is an often neglected but important area of concern. Comorbidity of Axis I and Axis II disorders is extremely common (Dolan-Sewell, Krueger, & Shea, 2001). The presence of a personality disorder can greatly complicate treatment of co-occurring Axis I disorders, simply by adding to the complexity of the presenting problem, but also through interfering with or otherwise disrupting the therapeutic alliance. In addition, when Axis II pathology is unrecognized or mistaken as an AXIS I condition, the therapist can be misled in attempts to develop an appropriate treatment plan. Until recently, prognosis for treatment of personality disorders has been quite poor. However, with publication of empirical studies showing effectiveness of some manualized, cognitive behavioral approaches, such as Linehan's (1993) Dialectical Behavior Therapy for the treatment of Borderline Personality Disorder (BPD), perceptions of what is clinically feasible in treating Axis II conditions is rapidly changing.

Individuals with personality disorders often come to treatment because of one or more Axis I conditions. Although the therapist may accurately assess these conditions and implement the appropriate treatment, as time goes on, individuals with coexisting personality disorders may not respond as anticipated. At this point, the therapist usually does one of two things: labels the condition as atypical or the client as unmotivated or resistant to change. In either case, the end result

JILLAYNE Z. MCCLANAHAN, SOONIE A. KIM, AND MICHELLE BOBOWICK • Portland Dialectical Behavioral Therapy Program, Portland, Oregon 97237.

is often the same. Whether on the part of the therapist or the client, a potentially helpful treatment is changed, discarded, or otherwise terminated.

Linehan (1993) has described the presence of interpersonal and other problems associated with personality disorders that undermine effectiveness of treatment protocols for certain Axis I conditions as "therapy interfering behaviors" (p. 131). She describes three specific kinds of behavior in this category: (1) behaviors that interfere with the client receiving the therapy (missing or arriving late to sessions, not talking in session, not completing homework assignments); (2) behaviors that interfere with other clients' receiving or benefiting from the therapy (aggressive or intrusive comments that are disruptive to other group members' progress); and (3) behaviors that result in therapist burnout (phoning the therapist too frequently, demands that the therapist solve problems outside of her control, threatening the therapist).

Concerning the latter, one of the most challenging aspects of working with individuals with personality disorders can be the impact on the therapeutic alliance. Clearly, in order for any treatment to be effective, the client needs to be sufficiently and productively engaged in the therapeutic relationship. Because personality disorders are so linked to interpersonal functioning and impact the ability to form trusting relationships, development and maintenance of the therapeutic relationship may be more difficult, taking a longer period of time to foster, coupled with a greater likelihood of reoccurring ruptures. The therapist must be sensitive to the kinds of interpersonal triggers likely to create problems for the client and may need to proactively employ strategies for relationship enhancement and repair.

A primary goal of assessment is to arrive at an accurate diagnosis and plan for treatment. This process becomes more complicated in the case of personality disorders, where the symptomatology frequently results in confusion as to what the diagnosis is and what aspects of the presentation should be the initial focus of attention. Having a clear understanding of AXIS II conditions as well as some idea about how to organize and implement treatment is essential. An example of this approach is found in Linehan's (1993) treatment for BPD. Her manualized approach outlines specific protocols for treating the many facets of the disorder, as well as providing a treatment hierarchy, which is essential in prioritizing therapy goals. Implementation of this blending of principle or theory-driven conceptualization (dialectics, the biosocial model) with protocol-driven strategies (manualized, step-by-step approaches to specific symptoms or maladaptive behaviors) is not limited to the diagnosis and treatment of Axis II disorders. However, Linehan's (1993) approach highlights the importance of accurate assessment and diagnosis in developing adequate protocols to treat more complex, multidiagnostic, difficult-to-manage cases.

Personality

Efforts to describe personality date back as far as Hippocrates in the 5th century BC, who proposed that particular humors or elemental fluids dictate the balance of personality characteristics. Other theories have posited that phrenology (the shape of one's skull), or one's morphology (physiological type), is indicative of personality. The dominant view for most of the 20th century was the psychodynamic perspective, which proposed that intrapersonal dynamics and unresolved early conflicts form the basis of personality in adulthood (Millon & Everly, 1985).

A current perspective gaining prominence is that personality is the product of biosocial processes. These processes involve the interaction over time of an individual's biological predisposition, hypothesized to be influenced by a variety of factors, such as genetics, pre- and peri-natal conditions, early childhood events that may permanently affect the brain in some way, and learning experiences: the complex of family, school, societal, and cultural interactions that make up the infant/child's world (Linehan, 1993; Millon & Everly, 1985). Examples might include daily interpersonal interactions among family members or friends, the degree of stability and predictability in the environment, and acute or pervasive trauma such as separation from significant caregivers or the experience of childhood neglect or abuse. In addition, the developmental stage at which the child is exposed to any of the above can significantly affect the impact of these factors (Millon & Everly, 1985).

Thus, these interactions result in cognitive, emotional, and overt expressions of behavior that begin in earliest childhood and are the product of the repeated interaction of both biological and environmental factors. As certain behaviors are repeated over time, they become, as Millon and Everly (1985) describe, more predictable and emerge as "preferred patterns of behaving" (p. 4). Personality then, according to the biosocial model, refers to the set of co-occurring, well-established ways of perceiving and responding to oneself and the world that are (1) consistent across many kinds of situations, (2) persist over time, and (3) are relatively resistant to change. The biosocial perspective is an inclusive one that acknowledges the complexity and variability of biological, cognitive, and environmental factors and their interactions in the development of personality.

Personality Disorders

The purpose of categorization of mental illness, including personality disorders, is primarily one of clinical efficacy. As Millon and Everly (1985) point out, categories are merely symbols used by therapists to describe groups of behavior in ways that are meaningful to aid in diagnosis and treatment. Disadvantages of classifying or labeling individuals with personality disorders include the potential for stigmatization, overgeneralization of characteristics associated with the diagnosis, thereby obscuring important individual characteristics, and the danger of the label becoming a de facto explanation of behavior resulting in a kind of "circular logic" (p. 23). An example of the latter would be the case of a person with antisocial personality disorder who is thought to behave destructively because he has antisocial personality disorder. In addition to its being fundamentally flawed in terms of logic, this type of tautology does not provide any useful information to understand or treat the problematic behaviors in question. Despite the potential pitfalls described above, the usefulness of categorization of personality disorders, when conscientiously applied, is clear. It allows therapists to communicate accurately, to develop and refine theoretical conceptualizations based on objectively identifiable behavior, and to develop and validate effective treatments.

Debate about the most accurate method of categorizing personality disorders centers around the question of whether to adopt a categorical or dimensional approach. A categorical approach suggests that personality disorders are separate, distinct pathologies, essentially unrelated to other types of mental disorders. Discrete categories based on number and type of symptoms are the result of this approach. A dimensional model, on the other hand, places personality disorders on a continuum and assumes that they are simply more severe versions of other, Axis I disorders (Livesley, 2001). From the latter perspective, some personality disorders (Paranoid and Schizotypal) would be seen as more closely linked with the thought disorders, whereas others (Dependent and Avoidant) would be described as more attenuated versions of an anxiety disorder or alternatively, of a mood disorder (Borderline and Histrionic) (Millon & Everly, 1985).

Regardless of whether one adopts a categorical or dimensional approach, identifying and classifying behaviors as maladaptive is to some extent dependent on context and cultural/societal norms. Those aspects of personality deemed to be pathological have changed over time, and those changes cannot be understood in isolation from the social context in which they occurred. Likewise, the determination of how to classify personality disorders is to a degree an artifact of the times in which those determinations are made. The history of diagnosis and treatment of the range of mental disorders illustrates the fact that what is seen as maladaptive changes over time according to context and the evolution and imposition of social authority within the institutions of medical and mental health care.

METHODS OF ASSESSMENT

It is unlikely that in most clinical settings a therapist would narrow the focus of an initial interview solely to personality. It is understood, therefore, that attention to diagnosis of personality disorders occurs within a broader context of a general clinical interview in which the therapist is screening for a wide range of possible conditions. A number of structured and semistructured interview formats have been developed in recent years with the aim of improving the validity and reliability of the diagnosis of personality disorders. (See Rogers, 2002 for a comprehensive review.) We recommend a less structured approach, using a clinical interview that incorporates certain questions from structured interviews and emphasizes a detailed relationship history, direct observation of the client in session, and gathering collateral information as the primary bases for diagnostic decision-making.

Structured and Semistructured Interviews

Examples of structured interviews for personality disorders currently available include the Structured Interview for *DSM* Personality Disorders (SIDP-IV) (Pfohl, Blum, & Zimmerman, 1995) and the Personality Disorders Examination

(PDE) (Loranger, 1988; Loranger, Susman, Oldham, & Russakoff, 1987). Rogers (2002) notes that the International Personality Disorder Examination *DSM-IV* module (IPDE) (Loranger, 1999a, 1999b), which includes the minor criteria changes in the *DSM-IV* (1994) "corresponds closely to the PDE in its clinical inquiries, organization of items, and ratings" (p. 219) and that therapists have the option of using either the PDE or IPDE *DSM-IV* module. These instruments are well supported by empirical data as to their validity and reliability (Rogers), with the SIDP-IV particularly useful in terms of its "natural flow" (p. 383) and use of questions phrased in a way that makes inference by the client about psychopathology unlikely. Another attractive feature of this instrument is its ability to distinguish between Axis II disorders, with few questions that overlap within clusters (Rogers). In assisting the therapist to tease out Axis I and Axis II conditions, Rogers states that "The SIDP is the obvious interview of choice when considering how Axis I–Axis II interactions may affect treatment outcome" (p. 383). He points out that the PDE has been validated with Axis II disorders in outpatient settings and is contraindicated for use where severe Axis I (psychotic or extreme depression) disorders are in evidence (Rogers). Advantages specific to the PDE are: (1) its particular suitability for multicultural settings, (2) dimensional ratings that can be helpful in noting clinical changes across time, and (3) the ability for therapists to indicate early versus late onset of the disorder (Rogers).

In addition to these instruments is the more familiar Structured Clinical Interview for *DSM-IV*-Axis II (SCID-II) (First, Gibbon, Spitzer, Williams, & Benjamin; 1997). The SCID-II consists of approximately 120 questions and is organized around specific diagnostic criteria found in the *DSM-IV* (1994). One advantage of this instrument is that it can help to streamline the assessment process in situations in which time is particularly limited. Rogers (2002), on the basis of recent studies, notes that reliability and validity remain adequate for its use in clinical settings.

The Personality Disorders Interview-IV (PDI-IV) (Widiger, Mangine, Corbitt, Ellis, & Thomas, 1995) is a 317-question, semistructured interview (specified interview questions with follow-up inquiry) designed to assess each of the *DSM-IV* criteria for the 10 established personality disorders as well the 2 personality disorders presented in the appendices. Given its length, the required time for administration may make this instrument less appealing in settings in which time considerations predominate. Rogers'(2002) review of the PDI-IV highlights a number of issues that need to be addressed in order to firmly establish the validity and reliability of this instrument. However, he notes that a strength of the PDI-IV is its efficacy as a "valuable template for evaluation of personality disorders and the provision of standard questions that closely reflect the diagnostic criteria" (p. 250).

The Interpersonal Interview

Whether the therapist employs a structured or semistructured approach to the clinical interview, the task in the initial assessment is to garner sufficient breadth and depth of information about the client's history and current functioning to make an accurate evaluation and diagnosis. This requires the therapist to take on the role of, as Soloff (1994) describes it, " a detective uncovering his client's modus operandi" (p. 131). The task is accomplished by attending to both the content of the client's responses and the process in the immediate interpersonal interplay between therapist and client in the assessment session. Sullivan (1954) emphasized that data obtained in any interview between therapist and client are entirely the result of a process of "participant observation" (p. 3). He states that:

> [the therapist's] principle instrument of observation is his self—his personality, *him* as a person. The processes and changes in processes that make up the data which can be subjected to scientific study occur, not in the subject person nor in the observer, but in the situation that is created between the observer and his subject (p. 3).

The assessment interview represents a powerful interpersonal microcosm in which the client's responses will likely reflect interpersonal dynamics in evidence elsewhere in his or her life. Likewise, the therapist's own responses to the client's interpersonal process are an important source of information in this regard. The interpersonal assessment provides an opportunity to generate hypotheses about the client's interpersonal skills, ability to tolerate ambiguity, relationship to authority, and interpersonal openness or guardedness. Likewise, the relationship between or consistency of content of responses and observed process provides an additional lens through which to view the client's functioning and degree of insight. Achieving a meaningful integration and interpretation of these sources of information is to a significant degree, the art of the effective assessment interview.

Central to assessment of any mental disorder is the task of obtaining a thorough developmental, relationship, work, and academic history. In the assessment of personality disorders, however, special attention to the client's relational experiences will provide critical information in identifying those pervasive patterns of maladaptive interpersonal functioning that are central to the definition of personality disorders. Here again, the therapist will note the interplay between the content of client responses and the process observations made in the client's initial relational interactions with the therapist.

It is important to spend sufficient time exploring the relationship history of the client, and to approach this topic from a variety of directions. For example, the therapist might inquire about important past and present relationships; how relationships typically begin and end and what kinds of individuals the client seems to gravitate toward in their friendships and partners. In addition, the therapist might ask the client to describe him or herself and then ask how someone who knows the client well would describe him or her. Would that differ from how a brief acquaintance might respond? How does the client experience him or herself differently in different contexts or situations? Does the client notice any common themes in relationships or behaviors that seem to trigger particular responses? By allowing sufficient inquiry in this area the therapist will gain critical information about patterns of interpersonal functioning and, just as important, the client's internal experience and interpretations about him or herself and others.

Collateral Information

Obtaining collateral information, standard practice in the diagnosis of any mental disorder, is particularly important with personality disorders. Under these conditions, in which subjective states may substantially influence the reliability or validity of the client's report, it is important to include perspectives from a wide range of other sources. For example, clients with BPD may typically characterize the behavior of others toward them as quite extreme, moving between idealization and devaluation. This type of characterization is often described as "black or white" thinking. It is helpful, therefore, to obtain accounts of events from others whose perceptions may differ to provide a wider perspective and counter the extreme subjectivity of the client's report. On the other hand, subjective and extreme, but accurate, reports may be discounted by the therapist suspecting a personality disorder. Therefore, it is helpful to corroborate client accounts as much as possible.

Description of Personality Disorders

DSM Description of Personality Disorder

The most widely accepted classification system in use today is the *DSM* (American Psychiatric Association, 1994). This text has undergone a series of revisions and significant expansion since its initial publication in 1952. The most recent version, *DSM-IV*, was published in 1994. In it, personality disorders are defined as:

> An enduring pattern of inner experience and behavior that deviates markedly from the expectations of the individual's culture and is manifested in a least two of the following areas: cognition, affectivity, interpersonal functioning, or impulse control. This enduring pattern is inflexible and leads to clinically significant distress or impairment in social, occupational, or other important areas of functioning. The pattern is stable and of long duration, and its onset can be traced back at least to adolescence or early adulthood. The pattern is not better accounted for as a manifestation or consequence of another mental disorder and is not due to the direct physiological effects of a substance or a general medical condition (p. 630).

The *DSM-IV* (1994) uses three subcategories, called "clusters," to categorize the various personality disorders. Cluster A diagnoses include Paranoid, Schizotypal, and Schizoid Personality Disorders; Histrionic, Antisocial, Borderline, and Narcissistic Personality Disorders comprise Cluster B; and Obsessive–Compulsive, Dependent, and Avoidant Personality Disorders are included in Cluster C.

The *DSM-IV* presents criteria sets for each of the personality disorders and specifies the minimum number of criteria (e.g., four of the following seven criteria must be present) necessary to make a diagnosis. As indicated in the general description of personality disorders, these criteria must represent an enduring pattern that has been relatively rigid or inflexible over time and has been present since adolescence or by early adulthood. These longitudinal factors are often important in distinguishing Axis I and Axis II conditions; however, they are not absolute and a continuing point of disagreement is how to interpret the gray area between long-standing Axis I symptoms versus Axis II's "pervasive patterns" criteria. Dolan-Sewell et al. (2001) note that: "The distinction between persistent patterns of emotional, cognitive, and interpersonal functioning (i.e., personality traits) and problematic functioning during more circumscribed periods of time (i.e., episodic, state, or syndrome disorders) is more blurry than implied by assigning these domains to separate axes" (p. 85). Likewise, Widiger and Shea (1991) note that despite practical and conceptual rationales for placing these disorders on separate axes, the functional distinctions between them are sometimes "illusory" (p. 400).

CLUSTER A PERSONALITY DISORDERS

The Cluster A personality disorders include Paranoid, Schizoid, and Schizotypal Personality Disorders. All three are characterized by impoverishment in emotional expression and absence of long-standing and meaningful interpersonal relationships. The *DSM-IV* (1994) labels this cluster as "odd and eccentric" (p. 634).

Comorbid and Differential Diagnosis

When under stress, people with Cluster A personality disorders may experience "transient psychotic episodes which last from a few minutes to a few hours" (*DSM-IV*, 1994, p. 642). Therefore, careful attention must be paid to distinguish these transient episodes from the enduring symptoms of an Axis I disorder. Psychotic Disorders, Personality Change due to General Medical Condition, and Mood Disorder With Psychotic Features are all examples of Axis I disorders that may be confused with Cluster A personality disorders. Differentiation between Axis I and Axis II disorders is also complicated by the fact that what appear to be Axis II symptoms may in fact be characteristics of a prodromal phase of Schizophrenia or another Axis I disorder (Widiger, Mangine, Corbitt, Ellis, & Thomas, 1995b).

Paranoid Personality Disorder

Paranoid Personality Disorder is characterized by "a pervasive distrust and suspiciousness of others such that their motives are interpreted as malevolent" (*DSM-IV*, 1994, pp. 637–638). Four of the following seven criteria must be in evidence to diagnose the disorder: (1) anticipates exploitation and deception to himself by others, (2) questions the loyalty and honesty of friends even without substantial evidence, (3) avoids sharing information with others for fear it will be used against him, (4) interprets words and events as threatening and devaluing, (5) maintains grudges, (6) assumes others are attacking him although not obvious to others, and responds with anger; (7) questions the fidelity of his sexual partner without evidence (*DSM-IV*). Individuals with Paranoid Personality Disorder are predisposed to interpret innocuous or innocent statements by others as direct attacks, and their hypersensitivity to perceived danger often results in accusations against the perceived attacker (Millon & Everly, 1985). This frequently results in a "self-fulfilling prophecy" of actual mistreatment by others. The paranoid personality has a tendency to enlarge injustices or oversights on the part of others (Maxmen & Ward, 1995), and to perceive them as the result of careful planning or scheming (Widiger et al., 1995). These individuals pay particular attention to power distribution and hierarchies in groups or organizations, aspiring to reach the highest levels of influence themselves. While they may describe themselves as highly rational individuals, in practice they are often quick to assume an aggressive or attacking stance when they feel threatened (Kaplan & Sadock, 1998). Paranoid clients rarely self-refer for treatment and more commonly arrive at the request of an employer or family member (Maxmen & Ward, 1995).

Structured/Semistructured Interview

The following is a representative sample of questions from the PDI-IV (Widiger, Mangine, Corbitt, Ellis, & Thomas, 1995a) under the section on Paranoid Personality Disorder.

> Are you concerned that you might be exploited, harmed or deceived by somebody?
> Is it better not to confide in people?
> Do your neighbors or people at work ever do subtle things that seem to be intentionally hostile, demeaning, or even threatening to you?

Administration of the PDI-IV may be particularly challenging with individuals suffering with Paranoid Personality Disorder due to their suspiciousness of others. Direct questions related to misinterpretations and false suspicions may be particularly problematic. Widiger et al. (1995b) note that it may therefore be necessary to abandon this direct line of questioning, change the order of questions or temporarily change the subject, ask less challenging questions, and/or deliver a paper-and-pencil questionnaire to augment the interview.

Interpersonal Assessment and Relationship History

The initial interview may pose special problems if the client's presentation is particularly provocative, quarrelsome, or hostile (Millon & Everly, 1985). At the very least, these individuals present as very guarded and uncooperative. They may seem to scan the environment for evidence of malevolent intent on the part of the therapist or clinic staff. Emotional expression is usually quite restricted, with the exception of feelings of anger about perceived current or past maltreatment. If a mistake or misunderstanding occurs on the part of the therapist, an apologetic and honest response is recommended, as any sign of defensiveness is likely to result in increased mistrust (Kaplan & Sadock, 1998). Given the fact that these clients may be particularly prone to turn to litigation to address their grievances, it is essential that therapists follow strict protocol, especially with regards to informed consent, and appropriate and complete documentation (Maxmen & Ward, 1995).

Clients with Paranoid Personality Disorder are likely to report having few lasting friendships or romantic relationships. Problems typically occur related to their mistrust of others' motives and actions, which they perceive as threatening or malevolent (Maxmen & Ward, 1995). Themes of trickery, deceit, unfairness, and illegal actions taken against the client predominate in accounts of relational experiences. There may be a history of multiple lawsuits or threatened litigation (Kaplan & Sadock, 1998; Maxmen & Ward, 1995). These individuals may express pride in their independence and autonomy, as reliance on others is perceived as a personal weakness (Millon & Everly, 1985). When they recount instances in which they have placed their trust in others, themes of jealousy and betrayal are common (Kaplan & Sadock, 1998).

Schizoid Personality Disorder

Schizoid Personality Disorder is characterized by "a pervasive pattern of detachment from social relationships and a restricted range of expression of emotions in interpersonal settings..." (DSM-IV, 1994, p. 641). Schizoid Personality Disorder may be diagnosed when four out of the following seven criteria are met: (1) lacks desire or pleasure from close relationships, (2) prefers activities which are done alone, (3) expresses minimal to no interest in sexual relationships, (4) finds little to no pleasure in most activities, (5) identifies few to no close friends outside of immediate family members, (6) displays an emotional separation from both praise and criticism, (7) displays restricted range of affective expression (DSM-IV).

Individuals with Schizoid Personality Disorder demonstrate a significant degree of discomfort in social interactions. They are often perceived by others as loners who are somewhat cold, distant, and aloof (Millon & Everly, 1985). Because the kinds of social deficits described above are not likely to be experienced as problematic for the individual with Schizoid Personality Disorder, it is rare for such an individual to seek psychotherapy services on his or her own behalf (Millon & Everly, 1985). These individuals may seek services to address symptoms related to the presence of an Axis I disorder, such as mood or substance abuse disorder, but typically will not offer concerns related to interpersonal functioning as the basis for the visit.

Structured/Semistructured Interview

Specific questions designed to assess for Schizoid Personality Disorder in the SCID-II (First et al., 1997) include:

> Is it not important to you whether you have any close relationships?
> Would you almost always rather do things alone than with other people?
> Do you find that nothing makes you very happy or very sad? (pp. 5–6)

Interpersonal Assessment and Relationship History

Diagnostic assessment of individuals with Schizoid Personality Disorder can be particularly difficult due to the client's reserved and restrained style of interpersonal relating. The client will assume a serious and task-oriented stance toward the interview, answering questions succinctly, with minimal details (Kaplan & Sadock, 1998). The therapist may note little to no change in the client's body posture or facial expression during the session (Widiger et al., 1995b) and it may feel as if one is sitting in the room with the Tin Man or Mr. Spoc. The client's vagueness and superficiality in responding to questions (Millon & Everly, 1985) can substantially impede the therapist's ability to accurately understand his experience. The therapist will want to be cautious about making any effort to use body language or eye contact to put the client at ease as these individuals may feel increasingly uncomfortable with such attempts to develop a therapeutic alliance. Similarly, light-hearted or spontaneous conversation is unlikely to provide the client with relief (Kaplan & Sadock, 1998). The therapist may feel somewhat uneasy as usually successful strategies for establishing the therapeutic alliance fall short. It is recommended that the therapist respect the client's discomfort with social contact by not overwhelming him with attention or the expression of empathy (McWilliams, 1994), and to recognize that in these cases, the quality of the interpersonal process, as opposed to the content of responses, may ultimately be the most productive source of information.

Questions related to the client's history of relationships will be helpful in distinguishing between the kind of long-standing history of social isolation associated with this disorder and the more acute social isolation that might follow a significant loss. What is distinct about individuals with Schizoid Personality Disorder is their comfort with the absence of interpersonal relationships. The therapist should not discount the client's desire for a solitary life or assume he is troubled by it. The lack of interest in social relationships extends into all spheres of life including employment, personal activities, and long-term goals. Descriptions of those relationships that do exist are likely to be vague and lacking in emotional depth. The client's employment is likely to involve minimal contact with others and it is not uncommon for these clients to work a night shift or to be employed at a job in which they work alone (Kaplan & Sadock, 1998). Likewise, their interests or hobbies are usually of a solitary nature (Millon & Everly, 1985).

Schizotypal Personality Disorder

DSM-IV (1994) defines Schizotypal Personality Disorder as "a pervasive pattern of social and interpersonal deficits marked by acute discomfort with, and reduced capacity for, close relationships as well as by cognitive or perceptual distortions and eccentricities of behavior" (p. 645). Five of the following nine items are required to meet criteria for diagnosis of Schizotypal Personality Disorder: (1) ideas of reference, (2) odd beliefs and magical thinking, (3) unusual perceptual experiences, (4) odd thinking and speech, (5) paranoid ideation, (6) inappropriate affect, (7) unusual or eccentric behavior or appearance, (8) identifies few to no close friends outside of immediate family members, (9) extreme anxiety related to social situations regardless of familiarity (DSM-IV).

Individuals with Schizotypal Personality Disorder often present as slightly odd, with bizarre or mismatched clothing and unusual mannerisms or speech patterns. They may be especially interested in telepathy or fortune-telling and may participate in groups that are considered on the margins of conventional society (Widiger et al., 1995b). Expressions of affect are sometimes inappropriate or unexpected given the context, and they may interpret events or posit explanations for their problems that involve unusual perceptions or abilities. Communication with individuals diagnosed with Schizotypal Personality Disorder can be challenging, as their speech may include peculiar phrases, odd associations, and unusual combinations of words that slightly miss conventional usage (Maxmen & Ward, 1995).

With regard to the client's physical presentation, it is important that the therapist take pains to distinguish the type of presentation associated with this disorder from what may be appropriate attire within a particular subculture. Likewise, the therapist should attend to the potential impact of socioeconomic factors on dress and hygiene and to language differences that might better be accounted for by cultural factors, nationality, or lack of facility with English (Widiger et al., 1995b).

Structured/Semistructured Interview

Some questions from the PDI-IV (Widiger et al., 1995a) used to assess for the presence of Schizotypal Personality Disorder are:

> Have you ever experienced any odd coincidences or occurrences that might have had some special significance for you?
> Do you have any unusual superstitions?
> Did you ever sense the presence of a force or a person that wasn't there? (pp. 52–53)

While these questions are suggestive of the types of odd experiences associated with the disorder, it should be noted that they are somewhat general and open to a rather broad interpretation. The therapist needs to be mindful of the potential for confusion here and should ask for specific examples to be certain he or she is not assuming a level of pathology that is not in fact present.

Interpersonal Assessment and Relationship History

The therapist interviewing an individual with Schizotypal Personality Disorder for the first time may be struck by the client's unusual or bizarre attire. Clothing may be wrinkled, mismatched, or over or undersized (Widiger et al., 1995b). Accounts of very unusual perceptual experiences or information obtained via heightened senses or intuition are not uncommon. The therapist may note affective responses that seem strange or inappropriate given the content of the client's narrative, with unusual expressions or combinations of words used to describe experiences. Though somewhat difficult to follow, the general meaning conveyed by the client is typically discernable and does not share the types of derailment, or loose associations associated with Axis I psychotic disorders (Maxmen & Ward, 1995). Like the Schizoid personality, these clients have a marked tendency to maintain interpersonal distance and may be uncomfortable in directly discussing their internal experiences. Like the Paranoid personality, they may appear suspicious and reluctant to reveal information about themselves. Expressions of empathy and overt interest by the therapist should be kept to a minimum, as they may increase the client's feeling of uneasiness. Throughout the interview, it may be necessary for the therapist to assuage the client's mistrust by reviewing the purpose of the interview in the context of the client's stated presenting problem. Though obtaining information can be challenging, the therapist is advised not to demand more information than the client is willing to provide.

Clients with Schizotypal Personality Disorder typically describe having had few long-standing or significant relationships, suggesting deficits in the ability to form and maintain stable attachments with others (Millon & Everly, 1985). Descriptions of the client's interactions in social situations will suggest a high degree of social anxiety present even in low-pressure situations (Widiger et al., 1995b). The client may profess an interest in having relationships with others, but the persistent avoidance of social contact, along with the generally odd presentation and manner, decrease the likelihood of establishing satisfying interpersonal connections, whether in personal, academic, or employment contexts. Not surprisingly, others may respond negatively to these individuals and their histories may include examples of social embarrassment, isolation, and rejection.

Case Illustration: Paranoid Personality Disorder[1]

Ms. A is a 46-year-old woman who is currently separated from her husband of 5 years. She begins the interview by asking a number of questions about the therapist's credentials and competence in a manner that is challenging to the point of intimidation. The therapist is aware of what appears to be veiled hostility and vigilance in the voice and manner of the client. The therapist answers Ms. A's questions directly and specifically, and then begins making non-invasive, open-ended inquiries about the client's concerns. She states she seeks therapy at the request of her husband, who is considering a reconciliation of the marriage. Ms. A reports that her husband left her explaining that she is unjustifiably suspicious and jealous all of the time. Ms. A reports having an unusual intuitive capacity that she has relied on in forming her belief that her husband has had extramarital affairs. Despite her certainty, Ms. A admits she has never been able to provide any concrete evidence that her husband has been unfaithful. In addition to her concerns about her marriage, Ms. A notes that she is no stranger to relationships in which she has been deceived. She describes situations with past employers, family members, and friends, all of whom engaged in some kind of deceit that resulted in negative consequences for her. At the end of the initial interview, Ms. A agrees to return, but makes the comment she is still not sure that therapy will make a difference.

CLUSTER B PERSONALITY DISORDERS

Cluster B Personality Disorders are characterized as "dramatic, emotional, or erratic" (*DSM-IV*, 1994; p. 630). This cluster is comprised of the Antisocial, Borderline, Histrionic, and Narcissistic Personality Disorders. All four of these disorders share poor impulse control and a strong desire for immediate gratification, often without regard for the needs of other people. Although all these individuals may be experienced by others as being manipulative and self-serving, the dynamics underlying these maladaptive relational behaviors are likely to be quite different depending on the disorder.

---

[1]Case illustrations are fictional and do not represent any actual person.

Comorbid and Differential Diagnosis

Commonly co-occurring Axis I disorders include mood and anxiety disorders, eating disorders, impulse control disorders, and substance-related disorders (Dolan-Sewell et al., 2001).

In Kim and Goff's (2000) experience, differential diagnosis between Axis I and Cluster B disorders can be especially challenging. For example, in the case of the client with BPD presenting with symptoms of Bulimia the question arises: Is the disordered eating behavior better viewed as a primary Axis I eating disorder or as one of the impulsive, mood-regulating behaviors associated with BPD? Without attending to a possible relationship between behaviors that initially present as Axis I conditions and personality disordered behavior, the focus of treatment may be misplaced.

Another example would be the confusion that sometimes arises in making distinctions between the rapid mood fluctuation associated with BPD versus a rapid cycling Axis I Bipolar disorder. Dolan-Sewell et al. (2001) note that this difficulty arises partly because the criteria for BPD include "criteria considered to be hallmarks of bipolar disorder" (p. 92). They go on to make the helpful distinction that whereas the mood shifts associated with bipolar disorder are largely independent of responses to environmental conditions, in BPD those mood changes are often reactive in nature. This distinction may not be entirely clear from the client's report in session, however, which emphasizes the importance of therapist awareness of these areas of potential confusion and preparedness to make inquiries that will make that distinction evident.

In terms of differential diagnosis within the Cluster B category, emotional lability, dramatic presentation, and deficits in empathic response to others typical of Histrionic Personality Disorder may overlap considerably with the other Cluster B personality disorders, making differential diagnosis particularly challenging. Millon and Everly (1985) note that co-diagnoses among the Cluster B disorders are not uncommon.

Antisocial Personality Disorder

Antisocial Personality Disorder is described as "a pervasive pattern of disregard for and violation of the rights of others occurring since age 15 ..." (DSM-IV, 1994; p. 649). Unlike the other personality disorders, Antisocial Personality Disorder requires a pre-existing diagnosis, in this case Conduct Disorder or evidence that criteria for Conduct Disorder would have been met prior to age 15. In addition, diagnosis of Antisocial Personality Disorder requires three of the following criteria: (1) repeated failure to conform to laws often resulting in numerous arrests, (2) history of dishonesty for personal gain, (3) impulsivity without thought of future consequences, (4) frequent aggression directed toward others (5) disregard for the safety of self and others, (6) irresponsibility with regard to employment and finances, and (7) absence of remorse or guilt (DSM-IV).

It is common for these individuals to experience considerable difficulty in work and social settings resulting from consistent failure to act responsibly.

Their disregard for accepted social conventions and rules often alienates them from others. Impulsivity may be expressed in thrill-seeking behaviors, anger, or overtly aggressive or violent acts with little concern for the consequences of their actions either for themselves or others (Sperry, 1995; Widiger et al., 1995b). These individuals have the capacity to present as charming and easy-going initially, but a veneer typically wears thin rapidly in situations in which they encounter opposition from others or are otherwise frustrated in attempts to gratify their immediate desires (Kaplan & Sadock, 1998). They may have particular difficulty deferring gratification and frequently use deceit and/or manipulation to attain their goals (*DSM-IV*, 1994). These individuals do not appear to experience empathic understanding or concern for the feelings of others, though they may be quite proficient at behaviors that mimic or suggest these feelings when they serve as a means to desired ends (Millon & Everly, 1985). These persons may present for treatment as a consequence of legal action or for symptoms related to an associated Axis I disorder.

Structured/Semistructured Interview

The PDI-IV (Widiger et al., 1995a) includes questions focused on establishing the existence of Conduct Disorder prior to age 15. However, Widiger et al. (1995b) recommend first ruling out Antisocial Personality Disorder as a possible diagnosis, as this will eliminate unnecessary questioning. The following sample questions reflect the type of information associated with criteria for Antisocial Personality Disorder:

> Have you ever destroyed someone's property or threatened someone?
> Have you ever made sudden or impulsive decisions regarding your job or a criminal act?
> Have you felt guilty or remorseful for [*insert act*]? (if "*yes*":) What have you done about it? (pp. 3–9).

Widiger et al. (1995b) note that one issue of concern may be the veracity of responses to questions of this nature, as they are transparent in meaning and persons with Antisocial Personality Disorder may give less than candid responses. They emphasize the importance of obtaining collateral information whenever possible to provide the therapist with additional perspective.

Interpersonal Assessment and Relationship History

Sperry (1995) describes the interpersonal, cognitive, and emotional style of the individual with Antisocial Personality Disorder as being marked by impulsivity, aggressiveness, and general irritability. This is not to say, however, that these persons may not appear very likeable in an initial meeting, particularly if the client has an agenda or potential for personal gain by presenting well in the interaction. The therapist may note a pattern of externalizing blame for problems and lack of concern about the impact of behavior on others. While the therapist may have a number of emotional responses to the client as more detailed information emerges, it is important to maintain as neutral an approach as possible. As Soloff (1994) notes, these individuals are aware of the unacceptability of their actions in the eyes of general society and may be disinclined to be forthcoming about current problems, but may be less defensive about past behaviors and more willing to provide an account of those experiences if the therapist adopts an interested yet non-judgmental stance.

The relationship histories of the Antisocial Personality are notable for their volatility and instability. Romantic relationships are often portrayed in terms of sexual conquest (Maxmen & Ward, 1995) and there may be a history of domestic or partner abuse (Kaplan & Sadock, 1998) or failure to care for dependents (*DSM-IV*, 1994). In all cases, concern for the distress caused to others is minimal and situations will tend to be presented in ways that justify the client's behavior or suggest the other person deserved the treatment received. As might be expected, these persons respond negatively to any interference with their autonomy and their histories will usually reflect considerable conflict in relationship to authority figures (Sperry, 1995). Consequently, employment histories are typically erratic, with frequent abrupt moves, job changes, or dismissals. Collateral information will prove extremely helpful in cases where Antisocial Personality Disorder is suspected.

Borderline Personality Disorder

The central feature of BPD as described in the *DSM-IV* (1994) is "a pervasive pattern of instability of interpersonal relationships, self-image, and affects, and marked impulsivity" (p. 654). At least five of the following nine criteria must be met to diagnose BPD: (1) frantic efforts to avoid abandonment, either real or perceived, (2) alternating between extremes of idealization and devaluation of others, (3) unstable self-image, (4) impulsive behaviors that do not include self-mutilation, (5) recurrent self-harm behaviors including suicidal behaviors, gestures, threats, or self-mutilation, (6) intense instability of affect, (7) chronic feelings of emptiness, (8) intense inappropriate anger, (9) dissociative or paranoid symptoms that are transient and related to stress (*DSM-IV*).

Individuals with BPD typically exhibit a low tolerance for frustration (Sperry, 1995) along with intense and rapid shifts in mood that may be expressed openly, or may be masked by a more impassive exterior. They are highly sensitive individuals who are frequently adept at reading the environment for cues they may interpret as evidence of rejection or impending abandonment. Their behavior is characterized by extreme and impulsive responses to intense emotional distress, and these oscillations in mood are often associated with destructive and self-harming behavior (e.g. gambling, over-spending, substance abuse, sexual promiscuity). The client's narrative will frequently include a history of overt self-harm behaviors, suicidal ideation, suicidal gestures, and/or actual suicide attempts. These persons tend to vacillate between idealization and devaluation of others. They are typically very sensitive to any potential interpersonal abandonment and may over-interpret any interpersonal distance, responding impulsively in any of the ways described above. As noted previously, individuals with BPD may experience brief, psychotic-like symptoms when under stress. Sperry (1995) describes these episodes as characterized by: "ill-defined, strange thought processes, especially noted in response to unstructured rather than structured situations, and may take the form of derealization, depersonalization, intense rage reactions, unusual reactions to drugs, and intense, brief paranoid episodes" (p. 56).

Structured/Semistructured Interview

The following selection from the SCID-II (First et al. 1997) provides an example of the types of questions that are useful in the assessment of this disorder:

> Have you often become frantic when you thought that someone you really cared about was going to leave you?
> Are you different with different people or in different situations so that you sometimes don't know who you really are?
> Have you ever cut, burned, or scratched yourself on purpose? (pp. 29–31)

Interpersonal Assessment and Relationship History

Individuals with BPD vary considerably in terms of their presentation at any given time. Depending upon the current level of distress, the client may appear quite capable, socially adept, and appropriate in the session, or at the other extreme, may engage in intense affective displays that appear quite inappropriate given the circumstances or setting. The array of symptoms and problems described by these clients in the initial interview can be overwhelming for therapists, who may have a sense of not knowing where to begin. The client may describe emotions as unbearable or urges to impulsive behavior as uncontrollable and the therapist may note a marked lability of affect within the session. They frequently express feelings of emptiness or uncertainty about their identity (Sperry, 1995). Emotional distress may be expressed in hostile, sarcastic, or aggressive language directed at the therapist or others, or, alternatively, the client may appear extremely passive, refusing to communicate at all. These individuals may initially present as quite compliant and may express idealized notions about the therapist's ability to help them. However, the client's initial idealization of the therapist may give way rapidly to the opposite extreme, particularly if efforts to encourage more adaptive functioning are perceived as being a criticism by the therapist or a withdrawal of the therapist's support.

The relationship histories of these individuals provide critical information for assessment. Typically the client will describe relational patterns characterized by what Sperry (1995) calls "paradoxical instability"(p. 55) in which the individual moves between extremes in perception from idealization to intense devaluation, with little ability to experience others as both valued and fallible. Themes of actual or feared abandonment by others are common, as are descriptions of frantic attempts to prevent separation. Relationships often begin and end impulsively and are marked by intense and turbulent emotion that has an "all or nothing" quality to the estimation of self and other. Response to feared rejection or affective distress frequently takes the form of high risk, impulsive behavior that is often interpreted by others as overtly manipulative, with predictably negative consequences on relationships. Family members and friends may feel helpless, fearful, and frustrated in the face of the client's heightened sensitivity and response style. Unfortunately, all too often, the client's extreme attempts to avoid abandonment by others result in just that consequence, with both personal and professional relationships suffering accordingly as the client's life circumstances become increasingly unstable.

Histrionic Personality Disorder

The current version of the *DSM-IV* (1994) describes the primary features of Histrionic Personality Disorder as "pervasive and excessive emotionality and attention-seeking behavior" (p. 657). Five of the following criteria must be met to be identified to diagnose an individual with Histrionic Personality Disorder: (1) experiences discomfort when she is not the center of attention, (2) interacts with others in a sexually provocative manner, (3) rapid changes in emotions which are shallow in presentation, (4) draws attention to self, (5) uses impressionistic and nonspecific language, (6) displays dramatic mannerisms and over exaggerates her emotional experience, (7) follows others without question, (8) perceives relationships to be more intense than they are (*DSM-IV*).

Individuals with Histrionic Personality Disorder are characterized by an especially dramatic presentation. Sperry (1995) describes these clients as tending to be "exhibitionistic and flirtatious in their manner" (p. 97). The key feature of the disorder is a persistent need to be the center of attention. They may experience dysphoric mood when they are not the focus of attention and are willing to engage in provocative or dramatic behaviors that will ensure they become so (*DSM-IV*, 1994). This attention-seeking behavior is often expressed in exaggerated appearance or dress. Their manner of speaking may be intense or forceful, but typically is overly general and lacks specificity of content. Interpersonally they tend to be superficial with rapidly changing emotional displays. While others often respond quite positively to these persons initially, their lack of real empathy or tolerance for being outside the center of attention typically results in short-lived or superficial relationships (Widiger et al., 1995b). The *DSM-IV* (1994) notes the importance of attending to possible cultural, gender, and age-group differences in assessing the extremity of presentation and the fact that symptoms must cause significant distress for the behavioral pattern to be considered pathological.

Structured/Semistructured Interview

The PDI-IV (Widiger et al., 1995a) includes the following questions under the section on Histrionic Personality Disorder:

> Do people tend to notice you a lot; do you easily catch people's attention?
> Does your mood tend to have a life of its own, shifting from one time to another?
> Do people ever notice you because of the way you appear or dress? (pp. 25–28)

Interpersonal Assessment and Relationship History

In the initial interview, these individuals may appear quite charming, socially at ease, and engaging. Soloff (1994) notes the tendency for these clients to exert control over the interview, noting that "the client creates an illusion of instant rapport and emotional contact, sets a highly emotional tone to each session...and controls the flow of the interview...conveying an impression of great distress with little substantive detail" (p. 133). The task of the therapist can be a challenging one given this presentation and will necessarily include strategies to maintain the focus on discussing issues of concern in sufficient detail to contribute effectively to the assessment, while providing enough validation of the client's experience to keep her engaged in the process. It may be necessary to take a more directive and active approach with this population, as these clients tend to shift from topic to topic rapidly with little sustained focus on the line of questioning pursued by the therapist. In addition, given their rather vague or superficial language, it may be necessary for the therapist to verify the accuracy of interpretation of the client's responses. The fact that the therapy interview makes the client the primary object of attention is very reinforcing for these clients (Kaplan & Sadock, 1998) and may be used to advantage by the therapist as a relational contingency.

Individuals with Histrionic Personality Disorder tend to enter into relationships quickly (Maxmen & Ward, 1995) and may assume an intensity or reciprocity of intimacy that is not shared by others (*DSM-IV*, 1994). Relationships will tend to be short-lived (Kaplan & Sadock, 1998) and are often characterized by intense and dramatic displays of emotion. Others may be drawn to these individuals in social situations but this initial attraction often gives way to frustration and annoyance as the attention-seeking behavior and lack of consideration for others' feelings becomes more apparent (Widiger et al., 1995b). Sperry (1995) describes the cognitive style of these persons as "impulsive, thematic...and field dependent" (p. 97), suggesting an external locus of control consistent with the high degree of suggestibility described in the *DSM-IV* criteria. When difficulties or conflicts arise in work and personal relationships, it is common for these individuals to simply leave the situation rather than attempting to work through issues of concern (Millon & Everly, 1985).

Narcissistic Personality Disorder

The *DSM-IV* (1994) describes the prominent features of Narcissistic Personality Disorder as "a pervasive pattern of grandiosity, need for admiration, and lack of empathy..." (p. 658). Five of the nine following criteria must be met prior to assigning a diagnosis of Narcissistic Personality Disorder: (1) has a sense of grandiosity or exaggerated self-importance, (2) has a preoccupation with success and power, (3) perceives self as unique and surrounds self with those with high stature, (4) insists upon adoration by others, (5) believes that he should receive special treatment and have all needs met, (6) uses other people to achieve own goals, (7) lacks empathy, (8) experiences jealousy and believes others are envious of him, (9) displays arrogance both in thoughts and actions (*DSM-IV*).

Sperry (1995) describes the interpersonal, cognitive, and behavioral characteristics of Narcissistic Personality Disorder as typified by a presentation of self-confidence, assurance, and the appearance of ease in social situations, all of which belies a fundamental lack of self-esteem and emotional resilience

(Widiger et al., 1995b). While these individuals often initially appear extremely charming and easy-going, this façade is easily disrupted if their sense of grandiose self-importance is shaken, which typically results in feelings of intense rage and/or humiliation that may or may not be openly expressed (Sperry, 1995). Like individuals with Histrionic Personality Disorder, the Narcissistic personality tends to use impressionistic language and, as Sperry (1995) notes: "They take liberties with the facts, distort them, and even engage in prevarication and self-deception to preserve their own illusions about themselves and the projects in which they are involved" (p. 114). Because these individuals lack empathy or compassion for the experience of others, they may engage in emotional exploitation as a means of satisfying their own immediate wishes. They typically seek validation by others via overt signs of admiration and respect. Their sense of uniqueness or entitlement can lead to displays of impatience, arrogance, and disdain for others who are less valued or seen to be lower in status (Widiger et al., 1995b).

Structured/Semistructured Interview

Some examples of questions designed to assess for Narcissistic Personality Disorder from the SCID-II (First et al., 1997) include:

> Have people told you that you have too high an opinion of yourself?
> Do you think that it's not necessary to follow certain rules or social conventions when they get in your way?
> Are you not really interested in other people's problems or feelings? (pp. 25–27)

Interpersonal Assessment and Relationship History

The interview experience with the client with Narcissistic Personality Disorder differs in significant ways from other clients with Axis II disorders (Sperry, 1995). Othmer and Othmer (1994) describe a sense in the therapist that he or she is there to "endorse [the client's] self-promoted importance" (p. 403) and that as long as she does not challenge the client's self-construct, she is likely to be viewed in glowing terms. The client may adopt a collegial stance with the therapist, emphasizing his own areas of expertise or the reliance others place on him to support them in dealing with their troubles. Like the individual with BPD, persons with Narcissistic Personality Disorder often swing between extremes of idealization and devaluation of others, depending on circumstances and affect. The therapist may find him or herself responding to the client with feelings of frustration, boredom or anger, as the client persists in monopolizing the interview with lengthy accounts of achievements, of the admiration and respect he has garnered, and of his frustration with the short-comings of others (Sperry, 1995).

Accounts of relationships will tend to reflect the client's need to be seen as superior by others. The client may highlight those relationships with persons thought to be of great importance or standing and emphasize the close connection they share. Themes of entitlement, frustration at the failure of others to recognize the client's merit, lack of empathy, and envy for others' achievements are common

(*DSM-IV*, 1994). It may be especially helpful for the therapist to obtain permission to speak with collateral sources in these cases, as others' accounts of relational experiences with the client may differ considerably from those obtained in the interview.

Case Illustration: Borderline Personality Disorder

Ms. B is a 26-year-old divorced female who presents with multiple stressors in her life, including difficulties with her current boyfriend, employer, and ex-husband. She reports living in a state of panic for the last couple of weeks, but notes, "This isn't anything abnormal, my life is one big roller-coaster ride." She explains she is surprised that she made it to the initial appointment as she has not left the house in 5 days. When asked what has been going on at home, Ms. B explains that since her recent breakup with her boyfriend, she has been trying to contact him by calling him and emailing him repeatedly. She reports that her family members have expressed concern because 2 years ago when she broke up with her husband she was hospitalized for a suicide attempt involving alcohol and an overdose of her psychotropic medication. Ms. B's affect in session is depressed and anxious. When asked about previous treatment, she shares an extensive mental health history going back to high school, including treatment for eating disorders, alcohol and drug dependence, and sexual assault. When the therapist informs Ms. B that the session is almost over, Ms. B becomes noticeably more emotional and expresses urgent concerns about what to do for the rest of the day. After the therapist suggests scheduling another appointment, Ms. B calms down and apologizes for her "out-of-control behavior."

Cluster C

Cluster C includes those diagnoses that share characteristics described as "anxious or fearful" (*DSM-IV*, 1994, p. 630). The specific diagnoses in Cluster C are the Avoidant, Dependent, and Obsessive Compulsive Personality Disorders.

The disorders in this cluster all demonstrate anxiety as a fundamental feature and each expresses a different means of attempting to reduce the associated emotional distress. As the name implies, the Avoidant Personality copes with fears of negative evaluation and social rejection by reducing or eliminating exposure to circumstances that could conceivably result in those experiences. The Dependent Personality manages fears related to inadequate support or personal resources by clinging to significant others, while the Obsessive Compulsive Personality attempts to decrease anxiety via strict adherence to rule-based behavior or standards.

Comorbidity and Differential Diagnosis

The highest comorbidity of Axis I disorders with the Cluster C personality disorders is among the anxiety, mood, eating, and somatoform disorders, with co-occurrence of anxiety disorders and Cluster C disorders especially significant (Dolan-Sewell et al., 2001).

Distinctions between Avoidant Personality Disorder and Generalized Social Phobia, have been particularly difficult to make in the past, as there was significant overlap in the definitions of the disorders in previous versions of the *DSM* (Dolan-Sewell et al., 2001). The *DSM-IV* (1994) seeks to clarify the differences in these conditions, with the criteria for Avoidant Personality Disorder suggestive of a more "general self-conscious introversion rather than simply a social discomfort" (Widiger et al., 1995, p. 73). In practical terms, however, fears associated with initiating interpersonal relationships, and potentially negative evaluation by others, characteristic of Avoidant Personality Disorder, also closely resemble features of generalized Social Phobia or the avoidance associated with Agoraphobia. The therapist should be aware of specific differences in presentation that might suggest comorbid as opposed to differential diagnosis (Widiger et al., 1995b).

Obsessive Compulsive Personality Disorder can be distinguished from the Axis I Obsessive Compulsive Disorder by the relative lack of intrusive obsessive thoughts and/or compensatory, ritualistic behaviors, which characterize the Axis I syndrome. However, persons with Obsessive Compulsive Personality Disorder may engage in ritualistic behavior such as following a prescribed set of behaviors in certain situations, but these behaviors are experienced as being ego-syntonic as opposed to the symptoms associated with the Axis I disorder, which the individual experiences as ego-dystonic (Sperry, 1995).

Avoidant Personality Disorder

The *DSM-IV* (1994) defines Avoidant Personality Disorder as: "A pervasive pattern of social inhibition, feelings of inadequacy, and hypersensitivity to negative evaluation, beginning in early adulthood and present in a variety of contexts" (p. 664). The diagnosis requires at least four of the following specific criteria: (1) avoidance of occupational activities because of feared rejection/judgment by others, (2) avoidance of relationships unless certain of being liked, (3) interpersonal restraint in relationships due to fears of negative evaluation, (4) preoccupation with fears of criticism or rejection in social situations, (5) feelings of inadequacy and inhibition in new relationships, (6) self-concept as socially inept or unappealing to others, (7) avoidance of new activities or personal risks because of potential embarrassment (*DSM-IV*).

One of the primary characteristics common to individuals with Avoidant personality is the intense desire for intimacy and relational connection, countered by an equally strong conviction that they will be rejected, embarrassed, or otherwise negatively evaluated by others. The inherent tension produced by the opposing desires for connection and avoidance of interactions that could facilitate connection, results in very real and pervasive psychological distress.

Structured/Semistructured Interviews

Some questions from the SCID-II (First et al., 1997) specifically targeting Avoidant Personality Disorder are:

> Have you ever avoided jobs or tasks that involved having to deal with a lot of people?
> Do you avoid getting involved with people unless you are certain they will like you?
> Do you often worry about being criticized or rejected in social situations? (pp. 3–4)

Interpersonal Assessment and Relationship History

In the assessment interview, the individual with Avoidant Personality Disorder will exhibit an interpersonal stance that is typically quite guarded initially, and the individual may appear nervous, tense, or apprehensive. Responses to interview questions are likely to be short, non-detailed, and somewhat circumstantial. It may be difficult to elicit answers with sufficient detail and the therapist may find himself or herself working quite hard in the interview. The therapist will find the most effective stance is one that emphasizes empathy and validation of the client's feelings. As the client is likely to pay close attention to the therapist's responses, seeking cues of either acceptance or rejection, the therapist has the opportunity to use these more contextual cues to communicate empathy, acceptance, and reassurance. Sperry (1995) points out that once the client feels assured of the therapist's acceptance, he or she may begin to present quite differently, with a much more relaxed give-and-take exchange in the conversation.

Information related to the relationship history of the avoidant individual will be notable for the difficulty in initiating relationships and the significant level of emotional distress associated with the early phases of establishing relationships. This distress is related to the expectation that others will negatively judge the client, which will lead to embarrassment and rejection. These clients may express general satisfaction with their employment, for example, but will avoid work-related social activities. They typically avoid novel social interactions unless evidence of approval, acceptance, or shared interest is offered in advance. Once sufficient assurance is given, however, the client will describe the ability to establish satisfying connections with others. Past positive experiences do not seem to generalize to current functioning, as the fear of rejection remains the most salient cognitive feature for these individuals and often results in them having few close relationships outside of family members.

Dependent Personality Disorder

The *DSM-IV* (1994) defines the fundamental feature of Dependent Personality Disorder as a "pervasive and excessive need to be taken care of, that leads to submissive and clinging behavior and fears of separation..." (p. 668). The diagnosis requires that at least five of the following criteria are present: (1) problems with everyday decision-making and need for excessive advice from others, (2) need for others to take responsibility for important areas of the client's life, (3) problems with voicing disagreement with others' opinion due to fear of disapproval or loss of support, (4) problems taking the initiative in projects and lacks confidence in going her own way, (5) excessive lengths to gain nurturance from others, (6) difficulty tolerating being alone with exaggerated separation anxiety and fear of abandonment, (7) urgent efforts to replace lost relationships immediately, (8) pervasive and unrealistic preoccupation with fears of being left alone to care for oneself (*DSM-IV*).

While such dependency has been described in different ways in the various versions of the *DSM*, the current emphasis is on the perceived need for care by others, anxiety and preoccupation with being left alone, and resultant clinging behavior. Sperry (1995) describes the interpersonal/behavioral style of persons with Dependent Personality Disorder as typified by a non-assertive, passive, reassurance-seeking stance. These persons may present as particularly naïve or suggestible and may be easily influenced by the opinions of others. Benjamin (1993) notes dichotomous thinking typical of the Dependent Personality in which the relational continuum consists of either a position of control over, or submission to, the other, with the dependent person taking the submissive position. They may also lack critical thinking skills, which can subject them to undue persuasion (Sperry 1995). The affective stance of these individuals tends to be insecure and anxious. They may ruminate about the possibility of being left alone to cope without the assistance of others and may experience any separation as evidence of abandonment (Sperry; Widiger et al., 1995b).

Structured/Semistructured Interviews

Some of the specific questions featured in the PDI–IV (Widiger et al., 1995a) for Dependent Personality Disorder are as follows:

> Do you like to get advice and suggestions of others, even for everyday decisions?
> Is it difficult for you to openly disagree with others?
> Are you often afraid that you will be alone, without someone to love or care for you? (pp. 20–21, 24).

In the discussion of these items, authors Widiger et al. (1995b) stress that while asking advice about everyday decisions may be quite commonplace in the general population, it is the excessive nature of the assurance seeking and the subjective distress experienced by the individual that suggests a clinically significant level of dependency. Again, care must be taken to avoid confusing the normative cultural or gender standards of some groups with pathological behavior. When working with individuals from non-dominant cultural backgrounds, additional attention should be given to fully understand the cultural and social factors influencing the development of any pervasive behavioral pattern.

Interpersonal Assessment and Relationship History

Individuals with Dependent Personality Disorder often present as very agreeable persons who make a concerted effort to defer to the therapist in initiating conversation. While they will typically answer direct questions with well-elaborated responses, they may fall silent if not prompted by the therapist to continue. As Sperry (1995) notes, it is not uncommon for these individuals to express this discomfort with statements such as: "I don't know what to say," or "Ask me questions so I'll know what's important to talk about" (p. 85). In general, the therapist will not have difficulty establishing a therapeutic alliance with these clients. This process can be facilitated by the therapist communicating an empathetic and supportive stance. The dependent individual will often seek to discern and meet perceived expectations of the therapist and, as Sperry notes, will likely be able to tolerate exploration of their own affective states within an overtly empathetic, supportive context. However, as the therapist moves to a more confrontational stance, questioning the effectiveness of the client's behaviors, it will be much more difficult for the client to stay engaged in the process and may result in early termination of therapy. It is important for the therapist to be aware of the potential for her own behavior to be shaped by the differential reinforcement of more supportive or advice-giving interventions, as compared with more confrontational ones, and not to avoid challenging the client to examine the function of certain maladaptive behaviors.

The relationship history of individuals with Dependent Personality Disorder is typically marked by a pattern of heavy reliance on significant others in a number of important areas of daily life. There may be a tendency to idealize important persons, and these clients often make excessive efforts at being agreeable, taking unusual pains not to disagree with, offend, or alienate others at any cost (Widiger et al., 1995b). When a relationship ends, these persons often experience prolonged impairment or may engage in urgent efforts to establish another such connection as soon as possible. As Sperry (1995) points out, in some cases reinforcement of dependent behaviors in these persons may result in developing a pattern of somatic complaints, which not uncommonly co-occur in persons with this disorder (Dolan-Sewell et al., 2001).

Obsessive Compulsive Personality Disorder

Obsessive Compulsive Personality Disorder is characterized by a long-standing "pattern of preoccupation with orderliness, perfectionism, and mental and interpersonal control, at the expense of flexibility, openness, and efficiency" (DSM-IV, 1994, p. 672). The DSM-IV diagnosis requires that the individual exhibit four of the following eight specific criteria: (1) preoccupation with details, rules, order, or schedules at the expense of the primary focus of the activity; (2) perfectionism that results in an inability to complete tasks for fear of not meeting strict standards; (3) excessive focus on work and productivity to the extent that other important life activities are forsaken; (4) inflexibility or being over-scrupulous about morals, ethics, or values (not associated with cultural or religious beliefs); (5) inability to discard old or worthless objects; (6) problems in delegating tasks without maintaining strict control over the outcome and process; (7) greedy attitude about money and spending both in regard to self and others; (8) pattern of rigidity and stubbornness.

Individuals with Obsessive Compulsive Personality Disorder typically emphasize rule-based behaviors and show a marked lack of cognitive and behavioral flexibility. The resulting response patterns include a tendency to become lost in the details of projects, excessive focus on work, insistence that others comply with standards or methods perceived as being correct, and procrastination that derives from an inability to make decisions as a result of over-thinking and deliberation to ascertain the "right" course of action (Sperry, 1995). These individuals may also exhibit a keen awareness of status and hierarchy and may present themselves quite differently when dealing with superiors as opposed to peers. Sperry (1995) notes a tendency for these persons to behave in an approval-seeking or even obsequious manner with persons they perceive to be in authority, while taking a more condescending stance with peers or persons with less status.

Structured/Semistructured Interview

The SCID-II (First et al., 1997) includes the following questions among those included for the assessment of this disorder:

> Do you sometimes get so caught up with [EXAMPLES] that you lose sight of what you are trying to accomplish ?
> Do you have trouble finishing jobs because you spend so much time trying to get things exactly right?
> Do you have trouble throwing things out because they might come in handy one day?
> (pp. 8–9)

Interpersonal Assessment and Relationship History

Establishing rapport during the interpersonal assessment process is typically quite difficult with persons with Obsessive Compulsive Personality Disorder. Sperry (1995) notes that whereas clients with Avoidant or Dependent Personality Disorder will seek out expressions of empathy from the therapist and find such expressions reassuring, the individual with Obsessive Compulsive Personality Disorder is likely to discount such communications as irrelevant. Some progress toward building rapport may be gained by establishing client confidence in the therapist's competence and expertise in problem-solving as opposed to providing a supportive context for the exploration of feelings. The client may present with speech that is somewhat circumstantial or rambling, and this can be particularly frustrating for the interviewing therapist who is attempting to gain as compre-hensive a picture as possible of the client's overall functioning. The therapist may note a particular emphasis on details and a sense that the client is avoiding answering questions about affective experience by attempting to control the inter-view process. These clients may be especially uncomfortable with ambivalence as reflected by their attempts to limit the scope of questioning or a tendency to be confused by, or to answer very concretely, less structured questions (Sperry). Sperry (1999) describes these individuals as exhibiting a great deal of ambivalence about the therapy relationship, as they do not believe their problems can be suc-cessfully addressed, particularly if that might mean relaxing the degree of control they exert in their lives. While establishing a robust therapeutic alliance is espe-cially challenging in these cases, he notes that a kind of "pseudo-collaboration" often occurs in early sessions, in which the client attempts to present as a "model client" (p. 168). However, when the therapist begins to examine the client's feel-ings or fears, such initial enthusiasm dissipates quickly, replaced by discomfort and reluctance to discuss the present-moment process of emotions and relational experience in the session. Attempts on the part of the therapist to build an emo-tional bond in the therapy alliance may backfire, resulting in early termination. Confining the conversation to more intellectual or conceptual material will often result in the client experiencing an increased sense of control over the exchange, which will tend to lessen anxiety in the session (Sperry, 1999). Therefore, a more productive stance and emphasis in the initial session will be one that stresses the theoretical bases and conceptualization of treatment, concrete goal-setting, contracting for change, structured homework, and problem-solving strategies (Sperry, 1999).

The characteristics described above significantly influence the establishment and maintenance of relationships for these individuals. Avoidance of affect results in deficits in expression of empathy for others, and spontaneity in relationships is experienced as extremely aversive and is typically avoided (Sperry, 1999). Likewise, the need for control can interfere with relational functioning. Interpersonal skills are typically underdeveloped as is the flexibility to tolerate relational ambivalence. Therefore, persons with Obsessive Compulsive Personality Disorder may tend to engage in relationships that are quite circumscribed, and they often exhibit rather restrictive or inhibited social behaviors.

Case Illustration: Obsessive Compulsive Personality Disorder

Mr. C is a 46-year-old single businessman who describes himself as an extremely dedicated and loyal employee. His supervisor at work referred Mr. C to the EAP program. Mr. C. explains that his supervisor frequently compliments him on his final work product, along with his qualities of timeliness and orderliness. In spite of these strengths, Mr. C has not been promoted into a managerial level position. He has been told that before he can be promoted, he needs to develop skills to manage his stress, and also to increase his ability to work collaboratively. Mr. C explains that he finds it difficult to work with his peers because they do not strive for the highest possible performance. He also describes being frustrated with others, because they typically work only their required 40-hour week. Mr. C prefers to work extra hours on the weekend to improve the product, often laboring for extended periods of time over very small details. Additionally, Mr. C experiences social discomfort with other employees who often tease him for his frugality, insistence on routine, and stockpiling of office supplies.

PERSONALITY DISORDER NOT OTHERWISE SPECIFIED

Inclusion of the Personality Disorder Not Otherwise Specified (PD NOS) category is a practical and useful one acknowledging that the current *DSM-IV* (1994) diagnoses do not represent the full range of possible Axis II conditions. A diagnosis of PD NOS may be used in the following situations: (1) in instances in which an individual has features of one or more specific personality disorders but does not meet criteria for any single personality disorder and (2) in cases in which the client meets criteria for one of the personality disorders recognized as research diagnoses in the *DSM-IV* appendices. In all cases, the individual must meet the stated general criteria for personality disorder in order to receive the NOS diagnosis.

There are two examples of proposed personality disorder diagnoses in the current *DSM-IV* (1994) edition. They are Depressive Personality Disorder and Passive Aggressive Personality Disorder. One of the issues of concern with the diagnosis of Depressive Personality Disorder is the overlap in criteria between it and the existing Axis I diagnosis of Dysthymia (Widiger et al., 1995b). This point aptly illustrates some of the problems inherent in making categorical distinctions between similar Axis I and Axis II conditions. In the case of Passive Aggressive Personality Disorder, a number of concerns remain as to specificity of criteria and difficulty distinguishing situational passive-aggressive features from a more pervasive personality pattern (Widiger et al., 1995a).

Dos and Don'ts

A primary task of the diagnostic interview is to identify and understand current symptom presentation in context. Specific symptoms may appear as dominant threads in the fabric of the client's experience, but it is the background against which those symptoms lie that makes the diagnostic picture intelligible. By taking a biosocial perspective, we suggest that assessment of behavior cannot be separated from assessment of environmental factors that influence behavior. The immediate and larger social environments are both significant in the development and maintenance of client behaviors and experience. These immediate and larger environmental factors include, but are not limited to, interactions with family and friends, culture, and societal influences in general.

It is important to be clear about the purpose of the diagnostic interview. For therapists, it is sometimes difficult to remain focused on information gathering and critical assessment when sitting with a client in emotional distress. This can be particularly true in the case of clients with an Axis II disorder, where the affective presentation may be extreme and insistence is on obtaining immediate relief. It is essential to keep in mind that effective treatment to ameliorate client symptoms in the long term depends largely on accurate diagnosis. If the therapist moves prematurely toward treating symptoms and problem-solving, critical diagnostic information may be overlooked.

The task of diagnostic assessment is complex and made more challenging by the time constraints imposed on therapists, especially in the current managed-care environment. Typically, therapists must reach a diagnosis in one or, at most, two hour-long sessions. This means the therapist must be able to maintain enough flexibility to adjust to the client's interpersonal style and presentation, while providing the structure and direction necessary to cover the territory sufficiently. It is important that therapists not fall prey to the temptation of attending more to content than to process, or to draw premature diagnostic conclusions.

Given past biases as to prognosis for treatment of personality disorders and the stigma sometimes attached to these conditions, therapists may be hesitant to diagnose on Axis II after only an initial session or two. However, it is important to attend to and document features consistent with an Axis II disorder, even if a firm diagnosis cannot be made in the initial interview. While diagnostic impressions may change over time with additional information, it is essential that initial observations be made available as part of the record. This information can significantly impact treatment planning decisions and the approach taken by the treating therapist. The Provisional designation is useful in this regard as is the option to record features of the various personality disorders or to give an NOS diagnosis if full criteria are not met.

SUMMARY

This chapter discusses the current *DSM-IV* (1994) personality disorders from a biosocial perspective that emphasizes the complex interaction of individual and environmental factors in the development and maintenance of those longstanding patterns of behavior we define as personality. In addition, the chapter provides a method of assessment using a clinical interview that incorporates certain questions from structured interviews and emphasizes a detailed relationship history, direct observation of the client in session, and gathering collateral information as the primary bases for diagnostic decision-making.

The accurate diagnosis of Axis II disorders is important for a number of reasons. First, recent development of empirically validated treatment approaches for these conditions has resulted in a shift in perspective about the prognosis for individuals diagnosed with personality disorders. Second, presentation and treatment of Axis I conditions can be complicated significantly by co-occurring personality disorders. Therefore, correct diagnosis is essential for effective treatment planning. Finally, presence of a personality disorder can greatly impact the quality of the therapeutic alliance. Understanding implications of Axis II pathology for the development and maintenance of therapy relationship can greatly facilitate the effectiveness of treatment and prevent therapist burn-out.

REFERENCES

American Psychiatric Association. (1994). *Diagnostic and statistical manual of mental disorders* (4th ed.). Washington, DC: Author.

Benjamin, L. S. (1996). *Interpersonal diagnosis and treatment of personality disorders.* New York: Guilford Press.

Dolan-Sewell, R. T., Krueger, R. F., & Shea, M. T. (2001). Co-occurrence with Syndrome Disorders. In W. J. Lively (Ed.), *Handbook of personality disorders* (pp. 84–104). New York: Guilford Press.

First, M. B., Gibbon, M., Spitzer, R. L., Williams, J. B. W., & Benjamin, L. S. (1997) *Structured clinical interview for DSM-IV axis II personality disorders (SCID-II).* Washington, DC: American Psychiatric Press. [Copyright 1997 Michael B. First, Miriam Gibbon, Robert L. Spitzer, Janet B.W. Williams, Lorna Smith Benjamin.]

Kaplan, H. I., & Sadock, B. J. (1998). *Synopsis of psychiatry: Behavioral sciences/clinical psychiatry.* (8th ed.). New York: Lippincott Williams & Wilkins.

Kim, Soonie A., & Goff, Brian C. (2000). In M. Hersen (Ed.), *Effective brief therapies: A clinician's guide* (pp. 335–354). San Diego, CA: Academic Press.

Linehan, M. M. (1993). *Cognitive–behavioral treatment of borderline personality disorder.* New York: Guilford Press.

Livesley, J. W. (2001). Conceptual and taxonomic issues. In W.J. Livesley (Ed.), *Handbook of personality disorders* (pp. 3–38). New York: Guilford Press.

Loranger, A. W., Susman, V. L., Oldham, J. M., & Russakoff, L. M. (1985). *The Personality Disorder Examination (PDE): A structured interview for DSM-III-R personality disorders.* Unpublished manuscript, New York Hospital—Cornell Medical Center, White Plains, NY.

Loranger, A. W. (1988). *Personality disorder examination (PDE) manual*. Yonkers, NY: DV Communications.

Loranger, A. W. (1999a). *International personality disorder examination (IPDE) manual*. Odessa, FL: Psychological Assessment Resources.

Loranger, A. W. (1999b). *International personality disorder examination (IPDE) screening questionnaire*. Odessa, FL: Psychological Assessment Resources.

Maxmen, J. S., & Ward, N. G. (1995). *Essential psychopathology and its treatment* (Rev. 2nd ed.). New York: W.W. Norton.

McWilliams, N. (1994). *Psychoanalytic diagnosis: Understanding personality structure in the clinical process*. New York: Guilford Press.

Millon, T., & Everly, G. S., Jr. (1985). *Personality and its disorders*. New York: John Wiley & Sons.

Othmer, E., & Othmer, S. C. (1994). *The clinical interview using DSM IV. Volume 1: Fundamentals*. Washington, DC: American Psychiatric Press.

Pfohl, B., Blum, N., & Zimmerman, M. (1995). *The structured interview for DSM-IV Personality: SIDP-IV*. Iowa City: University of Iowa.

Rogers, R. (2001). *Handbook of diagnostic and structured interviewing*. New York: Guilford Press.

Soloff, P. H. (1994). Personality disorders. In M. H. Hersen & S. M. Turner (Eds.), *Diagnostic Interviewing* (2nd ed., pp. 129–154). New York: Plenum Press.

Sperry, L. (1995). *Handbook of diagnosis and treatment of the DSM-IV personality disorders*. New York: Brunner/Mazel.

Sperry, L. (1999). *Cognitive behavioral therapy of DSM-IV personality disorders*. Philadelphia: Brunner/Mazel.

Sullivan, H. S. (1954). *The psychiatric interview*. New York: W.W. Norton.

Widiger, T. A., Mangine, S., Corbitt, E. M., Ellis, C. G., & Thomas, G. V. (1995a). *Personality disorder interview*. Odessa, FL: Psychological Assessment Resources.

Widiger, T. A., Mangine, S., Corbitt, E. M., Ellis, C. G., & Thomas, G. V. (1995b). *Personality disorder interview: A semi-structured interview for the assessment of personality disorders*. Odessa, FL: Psychological Assessment Resources.

Widiger, T. A., & Shea, T. (1991). Differentiation of Axis I and Axis II disorders. *Journal of Abnormal Psychology, 100*(3), 399–406.

9

Alcohol Problems

David C. Hodgins and Katherine M. Diskin

Description of the Disorder

Alcohol problems can be broadly defined as negative consequences that people experience as a result of their use of alcohol. People may drink alcohol for a number of reasons: to promote feelings of relaxation, to increase feelings of sociability, to elevate mood, to conform to social expectations, or to reduce feelings of stress (Anonymous, 2000). Information from the US National Household Survey on Drug Abuse (NHSDA) for 2000 indicates that approximately 86% of adults surveyed reported alcohol use sometime during their lifetime, 65% reported they had used alcohol during the year preceding the survey, and 50% reported using alcohol in the 30 days preceding the survey.

As well as measuring frequency of alcohol use, the 2000 NHSDA survey also included measures related to drinking quantity. The report stated that approximately 21% of the adults sampled engaged in binge drinking (consuming 5 or more drinks on a single occasion) in the 30 days preceding the survey and 5.5% engaged in heavy drinking (5 or more binges during the preceding 30 days). These findings suggest that over 39.5 million adults were engaging in drinking at a level that is potentially problematic (Dawson, 1994; NIAAA, 1995), and almost 10.5 million were engaging in even heavier and potentially more hazardous alcohol use. Essentially, then, there is at minimum a one in five chance that an adult encountered in clinical practice in the United States has engaged in at least one binge-drinking episode in the past 30 days. Alcohol problems are highly influenced by environmental exposure and cultural norms, thus there is considerable cross-cultural variation in the prevalence of alcohol problems. Nonetheless, despite the difference in prevalence rates, the expression of alcohol problems is similar across cultures (Helzer et al., 1990).

According to the 2000 NHSDA survey, 21-year-olds reported the highest levels of alcohol use, with current alcohol use reported by 65% of the sample,

David C. Hodgins and Katherine M. Diskin • University of Calgary Addiction Center, Foothills Hospital, Calgary, Alberta, Canada T2N 1N4.

binge drinking reported by 45%, and heavy drinking by 17%. Rates of current alcohol use in individuals aged 21–25 were slightly lower (62%) and were further reduced in older age groups (58% in adults aged 26–34; 43.2% in adults aged 60–64; and 32% in individuals 65 and over). These findings are similar to reports from previous prevalence studies (Grant & Dawson, 1999). Although rates of heavy alcohol use are known to decrease with age, heavy alcohol use at an early age may have long lasting consequences, influencing the level of education attained, subsequent employment, and involvement with the legal system.

Just as alcohol use occurs along a continuum from no use to heavy use, alcohol problems may also range in intensity from mild to severe, and, over time, from acute to chronic. Longitudinal studies (as supported by the NHSDA data) indicate that the highest incidence of problem drinking occurs in young adulthood, however only 20–30% of individuals with early alcohol problems continue to have problems in later adulthood (Larimer & Kilmer, 2000). For some individuals alcohol problems follow a progressive course, for others problematic alcohol use either remains constant or resolves over time. Those diagnosed with alcohol problems in middle age are more likely to continue to have problems over time (Larimer & Kilmer, 2000).

Any attempt to describe alcohol problems is complicated not only by questions of intensity and duration, but also by the different ways alcohol problems may be manifested in different individuals. Problem alcohol use can affect physical functioning and may result in neurological consequences, increased susceptibility to infectious diseases, cardiovascular illnesses, or liver disease. It may affect mental functioning, resulting in impaired cognition, depression, or anxiety. Problem drinking can also affect marital and family relationships and work performance, and may precipitate legal problems. Some of the social consequences of alcohol problems include fetal alcohol syndrome, accidents resulting from driving while under the influence of alcohol, and increased levels of aggression and violence. Individuals may experience one or a combination of these negative consequences of problem drinking. Heather and Robertson (1997) noted that "many problem drinkers show some or all of the following problems: they develop serious physical illnesses, they commit suicide, they experience severe depression and anxiety, they suffer prosecutions, evictions, and multiple legal suits, their marriages split up, they become isolated and friendless, they develop low self esteem, and they die younger than they should" (pp. 124–125). Contextual issues must also be considered, with societal expectations influencing the perception of alcohol problems. For example, getting drunk on the weekend may be considered acceptable (or at least tolerable) behavior for college students of both genders, but not for middle-aged women, who may resort to secrecy to avoid being shunned for such behavior.

It is essential to be alert regarding the possibility of alcohol-related problems when dealing with clients. Most people with severe alcohol problems (four out of five) do not seek formal treatment (Institute of Medicine, 1990, p. 213). People who do seek treatment tend to wait an average of 10 years after symptoms appear (Schuckit et al., 1995, as cited in Larimer & Kilmer, 2000). Often individuals do not develop a full range of alcohol related problems, but are affected in one or two areas. They may present with family problems, difficulties at work, emotional issues, or physical problems. Such an individual may appear in the clinical setting "sober, well groomed and with no telltale aura of alcohol. He or she will complain of any of a variety of medical and emotional problems" (Schuckit, 2000, p. 70). For purposes of diagnosis and assessment, an understanding of alcohol problems that incorporates consideration of biological, social, and psychological elements is likely to prove most useful (Institute of Medicine, 1990). When engaging in the assessment process it is necessary to focus on the symptoms and consequences experienced by the particular individual. Due to the widespread use of alcohol, and to the variable nature of the problems that excessive alcohol use can cause or exacerbate, it is important to include questions about alcohol use in any clinical encounter.

PROCEDURES FOR GATHERING INFORMATION

Clinicians need to be able to screen all clients for alcohol problems, make a formal diagnosis of alcohol abuse and dependence, and conduct a comprehensive assessment for the purposes of treatment planning and evaluation. A variety of procedures are available to help the clinician accomplish these three tasks. Semistructured and unstructured interviews are the most readily available and practical method. In some settings, self-completion questionnaires administered in paper-and-pencil format or via computer are feasible. Medical settings may have laboratory and medical support for biochemical adjuncts to assessment such as liver functioning and blood alcohol levels.

ROUTINE SCREENING FOR ALCOHOL PROBLEMS

Regardless of the client's presenting complaint or problem, screening for alcohol use and related problems is advisable. Alcohol is often considered the "great mimicker" of mental health disorders. It is important to rule out alcohol as the underlying cause or contributor to a person's difficulties. For example, depressive symptoms frequently occur with heavy alcohol consumption and typically endure for a number of weeks following abstinence (Brown, Inabe, Gillin, Schuckit, & Stewart, 1995). Alcohol withdrawal, which is experienced beginning at the time that the blood alcohol level begins to drop and which lasts for 48–72 hr, is typically characterized by feelings of anxiety as well as dysphoria. In rare instances, intermediate and major withdrawal symptoms are experienced. In intermediate withdrawal, individuals can experience auditory or visual hallucinations, although the individuals typically recognize that the experience is unreal. The term *alcoholic hallucinosis* has been used to describe this rapid onset presentation that is frequently misdiagnosed as schizophrenia (Surawicz, 1980). Major alcohol withdrawal, often referred to as *delirium tremens* (DTs), involves severe agitation, global confusion, disorientation, and auditory, visual, or tactile hallucinations. DTs occur after 4 or 5 days of severe withdrawal (Kahan & Wilson, 2000).

Alcohol is also associated with a variety of stress-related symptoms and disorders, including gastrointestinal problems, chronic pain syndromes, headaches, insomnia, fatigue, and sexual dysfunctions such as impotence. Cognitive functioning difficulties are also associated with heavy drinking. If screening is not part of a routine evaluation, then it should be initiated in response to any of these client concerns or clinical observations.

APPROACHES TO SCREENING

Interview Methods

Screening involves asking clients specific questions about alcohol consumption. Integrating these questions into a review of health status is often the least threatening approach. The following questions generally provide a reliable indication of consumption:

In the last week, how many days did you have a drink of alcohol, including wine, beer, or liquor? On each of these days, how many drinks did you have? Was the last week typical?

The use of specific questions helps avoid vague responses such as "social" or "light drinking." Providing a list of common drinks containing alcohol is also prudent to ensure that beer or wine coolers are included in the client's report. It is also important to provide the client with a definition of a standard drink and to ask about the size of a typical serving or to obtain descriptions of quantity in terms of bottle size. Table 1 provides pertinent conversion information.

How much is too much? What level of consumption constitutes a positive screen and indicates that the clinician should ask further questions? One standard for evaluation of quantity involves comparing weekly consumption with empirically

TABLE 1. Standard Drink Conversions

Beverage (% alcohol)	Usual bottle size, ml (oz)	Standard drinks	Usual serving, oz (ml)	Standard drinks
Beer (5)	340 (12)	1.0	12 (340)	1.0
Wine (12)	750 (26.4)	5.3	5 (140)	1.0
	1000 (35.2)	7.0		
	1500 (52.8)	10.6		
Fortified wine (18)	750 (26.4)	7.5	3 (85)	1.0
Spirits (40)	340 (12)	8.0	1.5 (43)	1.0
	710 (25)	16.6		
	1135 (40)	26.6		
Wine coolers (5–7)	340 (12) variable sizes from 750 ml to 2 L	1.0–1.4	12 (340)	1.0–1.4
Pre-mixed liquor beverages (5–7)	340 ml (12)	1.0–1.4	12 (340)	1.0–1.4

derived guidelines for low risk drinking versus hazardous drinking. For example, guidelines produced by the Addiction Research Foundation in Toronto recommend drinking no more than two standard drinks per day with a weekly limit of 14 for men and 9 for women (Kahan, 2000). Higher levels of consumption are associated with increased likelihood of psychosocial or physical problems. The US National Institute on Alcohol Abuse and Alcoholism (NIAAA, 1995) guidelines recommend the same weekly limit but include, in addition, a maximum daily limit of four drinks for men and three drinks for women. Another commonly used indicator of potential problems, regardless of typical weekly quantity, is the consumption of five or more drinks on one occasion (Dawson, 1994; NIAAA, 1995).

The CAGE is a widely used screening interview for alcohol problems (Ewing, 1984; Mayfield, McLeod, & Hall, 1974). The CAGE assesses lifetime problems and has been validated for use in both general and clinical populations. The CAGE is comprised of four questions:

C: Have you ever felt the need to *cut* down on your drinking?

A: Have you ever felt *annoyed* by someone criticizing your drinking?

G: Have you ever felt bad or *guilty* about your drinking?

E: Have you ever had a drink first thing in the morning to steady your nerves or get rid of a hangover (*eye-opener*)?

A positive response to two CAGE questions suggests that further assessment is advisable, although there is evidence that one positive response for women is the optimal cut-off (Bradley, Boyd-Wickizer, Powell, & Burman, 1998).

An alternative interview questionnaire, the TWEAK, was developed for use with women, particularly inner city African American women (Russell et al., 1994). The TWEAK has also been used to screen for harmful drinking in male and female samples of the general population, outpatient samples, and hospital inpatients (Chan, Pristach, Welte, & Russell, 1993). The five questions of the TWEAK are:

T: How many drinks can you hold? (3+ suggests *tolerance* and is scored 2 points)

W: Have your close friends or relatives *worried* or complained about your drinking in the past year? (2 points)

E: Do you sometimes take a drink in the morning when you first get up? (*Eye-opener*, 1 point)

A: Has a friend or family member ever told you about things you said or did while you were drinking that you could not remember? (*Amnesia* or blackout, 1 point)

K: Do you sometimes feel the need to cut down on your drinking? (*K(c)ut down*, 1 point)

A score of three or more points is the recommended cut-off.

Self-Completion Questionnaires

The CAGE and the TWEAK can be administered in a self-completion format or can be integrated into a clinical interview. Another well-validated screening scale is the Alcohol Use Disorders Identification Test (AUDIT; Babor, de la Fuente, Saunders, & Grant, 1992), which is a 10-item multiple-choice scale (Table 2).

TABLE 2. Alcohol Use Disorders Identification Test (AUDIT)

Circle the number that comes closest to your actions during the past year.

1. How often do you have a drink containing alcohol?
   Never   (0)
   Monthly or less   (1)
   2 to 4 times a month   (2)
   2 to 3 times a week   (3)
   4 or more times a week   (4)

2. How many drinks containing alcohol do you have on a typical day when you are drinking?
   1 or 2   (0)
   3 or 4   (1)
   5 or 6   (2)
   7 to 9   (3)
   10 or more   (4)

3. How often do you have six or more drinks on one occasion?
   Never   (0)
   Less than monthly   (1)
   Monthly   (2)
   Weekly   (3)
   Daily or almost daily   (4)

4. How often during the past year have you found that you were not able to stop drinking once you had started?
   Never   (0)
   Less than monthly   (1)
   Monthly   (2)
   Weekly   (3)
   Daily or almost daily   (4)

5. How often during the last year have you failed to do what was normally expected from you because of drinking?
   Never   (0)
   Less than monthly   (1)
   Monthly   (2)
   Weekly   (3)
   Daily or almost daily   (4)

6. How often during the last year have you needed a first drink in the morning to get yourself going after a heavy drinking session?
   Never   (0)
   Less than monthly   (1)
   Monthly   (2)
   Weekly   (3)
   Daily or almost daily   (4)

7. How often during the last year have you had a feeling of guilt or remorse after drinking?
   Never   (0)
   Less than monthly   (1)
   Monthly   (2)
   Weekly   (3)
   Daily or almost daily   (4)

8. How often during the last year have you been unable to remember what happened the night before because you had been drinking?
   Never   (0)
   Less than monthly   (1)

TABLE 2. (Continued)

Monthly	(2)
Weekly	(3)
Daily or almost daily	(4)

9. Have you or someone else been injured as a result of your drinking?

No	(0)
Yes, but not in last year	(2)
Yes, during the last year	(4)

10. Has a relative or friend or a doctor or other health worker been concerned about your drinking or suggested you cut down?

No	(0)
Yes, but not in last year	(2)
Yes, during the last year	(4)

Record sum of item scores: _____

Scoring: Each answer is weighted from 0 to 4 as indicated in the brackets. Please note that questions 9 and 10 are scored, 0, 2 or 4. A score of 8 or more indicates that a harmful level of alcohol consumption is likely.

The AUDIT is most easily administered in a paper-and-pencil version, but it can also be administered orally or via computer. The AUDIT covers three domains: alcohol consumption, alcohol dependence, and alcohol-related problems. It was developed for a six-nation World Health Organization study on brief interventions conducted by primary care physicians and was designed to be appropriate for use in a number of cultures and languages. Norms for specific populations (e.g., primary care, students, emergency room patients) are increasingly available (see Allen, Litten, Fertig, & Babor, 1997, for a review). A cut-off of eight is recommended for general use.

Before the development of the AUDIT, the Michigan Alcoholism Screening Test (MAST; Selzer, 1971) was the most extensively used screening tool for many years. The MAST has 25 true or false questions although a variety of short versions exist (e.g., Hedlund & Vieweg, 1984; Selzer, Vinoker, & van Rooijen, 1975). In comparison to the AUDIT, which was designed to identify individuals along a continuum of alcohol problems and focuses on current problems, the MAST items focus on extreme consequences of alcohol problems and, therefore, screen for lifetime alcoholism (i.e., severe dependence).

Laboratory Markers

Current alcohol consumption (i.e., blood alcohol levels) can be validly assessed with breath, blood, saliva, and urine samples. Of these, breath samples measured with a hand-held breathalyzer are the easiest to obtain, and they provide immediate results. Despite this, even alcohol specialists are unlikely to use breathalyzers routinely.

Laboratory markers can be useful adjuncts for screening for recent but longer term heavy alcohol consumption. These markers commonly include a number of liver enzymes, mean red blood cell volume (MCV) and carbohydrate-deficient transferrine (CDT), a glycoprotein involved in transporting iron to body tissues. The liver enzymes commonly include GGT (gamma glutamyl transferase), AST (aspartate aminotransferase), and ALT (alanine aminotransferase). These markers vary considerably in their sensitivity and specificity but are generally less accurate than are self-report measures. Efforts are being made to validate algorithms that use combinations of these markers with or without self-report scales (Allen & Litten, 2001).

Diagnosis

Diagnosis involves the determination of whether an individual meets the specific criteria or symptoms required for a disorder either currently (i.e., in the last month) or over his or her lifetime. Two alcohol use disorders are contained in the *Diagnostic and Statistical Manual of Mental Disorders*, Fourth Edition (*DSM-IV*), Alcohol Abuse and Alcohol Dependence. Both Alcohol Abuse and Dependence require that an individual's alcohol use and its consequences lead to clinically significant impairment or distress, with the symptoms clustering in a 12-month period.

The diagnosis of Alcohol Abuse requires one or more of four criteria:

1. Recurrent drinking resulting in a failure to fulfill major role obligations at work, school, or home.
2. Recurrent drinking in situations in which it is physically hazardous (e.g., driving a car, operating machinery).
3. Recurrent alcohol-related legal problems (e.g., arrests for disorderly conduct).
4. Continued drinking despite having persistent or recurrent social or interpersonal problems caused or exacerbated by drinking (e.g., fights with spouse about alcohol).

In addition, the individual cannot have ever met the criteria for alcohol dependence, which are outlined below. To determine whether the abuse criteria are met requires specific questions in each of these areas, focusing on a specific time period. The time period is most often the past year (currently) or the time in the past when the person had been drinking the most frequently or heavily. For example, "During your early twenties when you were first working at the law firm, did drinking ever cause problems for you with your family? Your wife? Your boss or people at work? Your friends? What about acquaintances? Did you continue to drink despite these problems?" Clinical judgment determines whether difficulties are "recurrent or persistent".

The diagnosis of Alcohol Dependence requires three of seven criteria to be met in a 12-month period:

1. *Tolerance* (either a need for markedly increased amounts to achieve the desired effect or markedly diminished effect with the same amount). Most social drinkers experience some increase in tolerance as they become regular drinkers. This criterion refers to a marked increase in tolerance.

> *Does it take more drinks for you to get drunk than it used to? Can you drink more than you used to drink? Do you find that drinking the same amount has less of an effect than before?*

2. *Withdrawal* (either experiencing two or more withdrawal symptoms including hand tremor, increased heart rate, insomnia, nausea or vomiting, anxiety, transient hallucinations, psychomotor agitation, grand mal seizures or drinking to avoid experiencing withdrawal symptoms)

> *Do you have a drink in the morning to calm your nerves? How often do you experience sweating or shakiness the morning after drinking?*

3. *Drinking more or longer than intended*

> *How often do you end up drinking more than you intend to drink or stay longer in the bar than you planned?*

4. *Persistent desire or unsuccessful efforts to cut down*

> *Have you ever tried to cut back or quit? Were you successful? Have you thought about this a lot? Have you made rules for yourself about drinking, in order to limit your drinking?*

5. *Preoccupation with drinking.* This criterion refers to a narrowing of behavioral repertoire so that the person is spending a great deal of time drinking, planning to drink, or being hung-over.

> *Do you spend a lot of time planning when or how you will be able to drink?*

6. *Important social, occupational, or recreational activities are reduced or given up*

> *Does your drinking cause you to miss work or spend less time with friends or family? Have you given up activities (e.g., sports, playing music) because of drinking?*

7. *Continued use despite a recurrent physical or psychological problem caused or exacerbated by drinking.* This criterion involves two aspects: The individual must experience both an alcohol-related problem and continue to drink despite knowing that it is harmful. For example, an individual has a gastric ulcer but does not stop drinking.

> *Has drinking caused psychological problems or made problems worse (e.g., depression, moodiness, sleep problems, anxiety, blackouts)? What about physical problems? Did you continue to drink anyway?*

The formal criteria for the alcohol use disorders have evolved with each revision of the *DSM*. In the first edition (1952), alcohol problems were classified as personality disorders. In the last three editions, the general conceptualization has been stable although the boundaries between the abuse and dependence categories have been adjusted. In the *DSM-III-R*, alcohol dependence required evidence of tolerance or withdrawal and alcohol abuse was a residual category. These criteria resulted in a more restricted definition of dependence than the current one. According to the *DSM-IV*, dependence does not require tolerance or withdrawal.

In the *DSM-IV* a diagnosis of alcohol dependence at any time in a person's life preempts a diagnosis of alcohol abuse. In other words, if individuals are assessed as being alcohol dependent at one time they no longer qualify for an alcohol abuse diagnosis at a later time period. Instead, course specifiers are used to indicate the current status of the dependence diagnosis. Having some symptoms but meeting fewer than the three required criteria is referred to as partial remission. Finally, the diagnostic criteria for other drugs of abuse (abuse and dependence) are identical to those of the alcohol use disorders.

Assessment

Assessment complements diagnosis by providing a more complete picture of the individuals' context and situation, allowing for more effective treatment planning. Assessment establishes a baseline for functioning that can be used by the clinician to evaluate progress during treatment. Table 3 outlines the important domains that should be included in a comprehensive assessment. In some of these areas standardized instruments are available that can serve to decrease interviewer time. Table 3 includes some of the more commonly used instruments, although a more comprehensive list is available through the NIAAA website (www.niaaa.nih.gov/publications/assinstr.htm). For the majority of the listed instruments, interpretation guidelines are available based upon normative data.

In introducing instruments to clients, it is important to elicit full cooperation by explaining that they will receive feedback on their results and that this information will assist in developing a realistic treatment plan. The tenor for the assessment interview should be collaborative, with the assessor and client jointly committed to discovering those client features that will contribute to important decisions about future clinical management (NIAAA, 1995). The client should also be assured of confidentiality, and limitations to confidentiality should be clearly articulated.

Alcohol dependence syndrome, the first dimension listed in Table 3, is a construct that underlies the current *DSM* and International Classification of Diseases diagnostic systems. The syndrome, first articulated by Edwards and Gross (1976) consists of a constellation of psychological and physical features, including a narrowing of drinking repertoire, salience of drink-seeking behavior, increased tolerance, withdrawal, relief or avoidance of withdrawal symptoms with drinking, a subjective awareness of compulsion to drink, and reinstatement of the syndrome after abstinence. Not all of these features need to be present at one time to indicate alcohol dependence, and the syndrome is conceptualized on a continuum of severity that is related to, but independent from, alcohol quantity and consequences. Severity of dependence is a modest predictor of outcome generally and of appropriateness of treatment goals in particular. More severe alcohol dependence is associated with less chance of successful moderation of drinking (Rosenberg, 1993). There are a variety of assessment instruments available to measure this construct. The Alcohol Dependence Scale (Skinner & Allen, 1982) and the Short Alcohol Dependence Data (Raistrick, Dunbar, & Davidson, 1983) are brief, easy to use and have interpretation guidelines that are useful in providing feedback to clients.

Assessment of *alcohol quantity* was discussed in the alcohol screening section above. A common feature of the recommended instruments for assessing quantity (Table 3) is that each provides a structure that enhances memory cues in order to

TABLE 3. Important Domains in the Assessment of Alcohol Problems

General dimension	Specific construct	Standardized tools
Alcohol dependence syndrome	Tolerance Withdrawal (including seizures) Impaired control	Alcohol Dependence Scale (Skinner & Allen, 1982) Short Alcohol Dependence Data Questionnaire (Raistrick et al., 1983)
Alcohol quantity	Lifetime history Recent daily use (past month)	Lifetime Drinking History (Skinner & Sheu, 1982) Timeline follow-back method (Sobell & Sobell, 1992) Form 90 (Miller, 1996)
Consequences	Health (liver, hypertension, nutritional, gastrointestinal, insomnia) Family Social relationships Employment and financial Emotional (self-esteem) Spiritual Legal	DrInC (Miller et al., 1995)
Association/circumstances of drinking	Functional analysis	Inventory of Drinking Situations (Annis, Graham, & Davis, 1987)
Comorbid psychiatric disorders	DSM Axis 1 and 2	SCID, DIS, CIDI, PRIME-MD (see below)
Other drug use	Prescription and illicit drugs Nicotine, caffeine	
Family History	Biological and family exposure to alcohol	
Treatment history	Programs started and completed 12-step involvement Periods of abstinence or nonproblematic drinking	
Treatment goal	Goal (abstinence or moderation) Self-efficacy	Brief Situational Confidence Questionnaire (Breslin, Sobell, Sobell, & Agrawal, 2000)
Motivation	Readiness to change Reasons to change Family and social support	SOCRATES (Miller & Tonigan, 1996) Readiness to Change Questionnaire (Rollnick et al., 1992) Readiness to Change—Clinician Version (Hodgins, 2001)

help the individual reconstruct drinking patterns. For each of these instruments reliability and validity is good.

The *consequences of heavy alcohol* use are potentially wide ranging and include health, family, social, legal, employment, financial, emotional, and spiritual consequences. Individuals are typically forthcoming about these effects when they are well engaged with the interviewer, although a less direct way to inquire about consequences is to ask whether others have been concerned about the potential for consequences for the drinker. For example, "Has your wife ever worried about the effect of your drinking on the family?" The Drinker Inventory of Consequences (DrInC; Miller, Tonigan, & Longabaugh, 1995) is a self-report instrument that inquires about 50 common consequences occurring over the past 3 months or over the individual's lifetime. A briefer, 15-item version is also available.

Many treatment approaches include relapse prevention training, which involves preparing an individual to cope with a variety of precipitants to drinking. *Functional analysis* is used to identify the circumstances surrounding an individual's use, in particular, conditioned cues or "triggers." Specific instances of drinking are identified and examined in detail including the internal (e.g., emotional) and external (e.g., situational) triggers. For example, negative affective states, which are internal triggers, are a prime precipitant to alcohol relapse (Hodgins, el-Guebaly, & Armstrong, 1995).

Alcohol use frequently co-occurs with other drug use and other psychiatric disorders. These disorders often complicate the course and outcome of alcohol problems and as a consequence have major implications for treatment planning. *Comorbid disorders* can also serve to enhance the motivation of individuals to address their drinking problem and may, therefore, hasten recovery. Diagnosing comorbid psychiatric disorders is challenging for a variety of reasons, including the fact that heavy alcohol use can mimic other disorders (e.g., depression, anxiety). As well, heavy alcohol use can be symptomatic of a primary psychiatric disorder. For example, heavy use may be associated with the acute phase of bipolar disorder or with the impulsivity associated with borderline personality disorders. Structured diagnostic interviews (see below) can be helpful in identifying comorbid disorders, but a longitudinal approach to assessment using all the available sources of information is often required for a valid diagnosis.

Table 3 outlines a number of additional important assessment domains, including *family history* and *treatment history*. These domains are typically assessed through a clinical interview. An understanding of an individual's exposure and reaction to twelve-step programs such as Alcoholics Anonymous (AA) is included because this variant of the disease model of alcohol problems is predominant in formal treatment programs in North America. AA is also a readily accessible resource for those clients who affiliate successfully with the program.

The clients' *personal consumption goal* of abstinence or reduction in drinking is another relevant assessment domain. Consistent with the disease model orientation, most North American treatment programs require that the client's treatment goal be abstinence from drinking. Elsewhere in the world, greater flexibility is allowed, in particular, with clients with less severe alcohol dependence. Research indicates that clients prefer to choose their own goal and that clients who begin with the goal of moderating their drinking may also modify their goals over time, typically through a trial and error process (Hodgins, Leigh, Milne, & Gerrish, 1997).

Self-efficacy, the client's belief in their ability to resist heavy drinking, is an important related construct that changes with treatment involvement and is predictive of outcome. One approach to measurement of self-efficacy involves having the client rate their degree of confidence for a large number of potential drinking triggers. Low self-efficacy in a particular area provides an individualized direction for treatment intervention.

The final general assessment domain listed in Table 3 is *motivation*. This domain includes the client's readiness to change, reasons for change, and family and social support. Readiness to change is typically conceptualized using Prochaska and DiClemente's model of the stages of behavior change (Prochaska, DiClemente, & Norcross, 1992). Readiness to change is viewed as a fluid construct that is influenced by the therapist and other life context factors. According to the model, interventions are more likely to be effective if they are stage appropriate. For example, individuals in the pre-contemplation stage are more likely to respond to general information about alcohol problems than to benefit from action-oriented therapy (e.g., drink refusal skills training). Table 3 includes three measures of readiness to change. SOCRATES (Miller & Tonigan, 1996) and the Readiness to Change Questionnaire (Rollnick, Heather, Gold, & Hall, 1992) are brief inventories that clients complete. The third measure is a clinician version of the Readiness to Change Questionnaire that the clinician completes after a face-to-face assessment has been conducted so as to reduce the burden on the client of a lengthy assessment. The clinician version shows good agreement with the client version (Hodgins, 2001).

Assessing reasons for change not only provides helpful information for treatment planning, but can also serve to enhance the client's readiness. When queried, clients typically identify a number of different reasons for change, some of which have been less in their awareness than others. The assessment process underscores these concerns for the client.

Finally, family and social support for change cannot be assumed and are therefore important to assess. Problem drinkers typically have family and friends who are also heavy drinkers who, as a result, may be ambivalent toward changes in the client's behavior.

STANDARDIZED INTERVIEW FORMATS

Diagnostic Interviews

A number of standardized and structured interview formats are available for both diagnosis and assessment of alcohol problems. For *DSM* diagnosis, the most widely used instrument is the *Structured Clinical Interview for DSM—Patient Edition* (SCID; First, Spitzer, Gibbon, & Williams, 1997). The SCID includes an alcohol use module as well as modules for most other Axis 1 disorders. Questions are provided for each diagnostic criterion and the clinician is expected to probe responses to determine whether or not a specific threshold is reached. The SCID is designed to be administered by clinicians trained in its use, and good reliability and validity have been demonstrated for alcohol use disorders (Kranzler, Kadden, Babor, Tennen, & Rounsaville, 1996). The SCID is available commercially.

Two alternative diagnostic interviews are the Diagnostic Interview Schedule (DIS; Robins, Helzer, Cottler, & Goldring, 1998) and the Composite International Diagnostic Interview (CIDI; World Health Organization, 1997). The DIS and CIDI are very similar instruments that were developed for use by lay interviewers in epidemiological studies. In contrast to the SCID, they are fully structured interviews that do not require clinical judgment. The inter-rater reliability has been demonstrated to be excellent and the test–retest reliability and validity are good (Andrews & Peters, 1998; Robins et al., 1998). The DIS instrument and training are available commercially and the CIDI and information about training are available on the World Health Organization website (www.who.int/msa/cidi/index.htm).

The PRIME-MD (Spitzer et al., 1994) is a briefer alternative to the more lengthy diagnostic interviews described above. It was developed for use by primary care physicians and provides *DSM* diagnoses of mood, anxiety, somatoform, and alcohol use disorders, the disorders most commonly seen in primary care. A one-page screening questionnaire is completed by patients in a self-report format (which includes questions similar to the CAGE described above) that is followed with a structured interview in the areas of potential problems. The PRIME-MD showed good agreement with clinical diagnoses including alcohol abuse and dependence (Spitzer et al., 1994). Moreover, the instrument has also been used to identify comorbid psychiatric disorders in patients with alcohol disorders (Johnson et al., 1995).

Assessment Interviews

Structured and semistructured assessment interviews cover many of the major domains outlined in Table 2. One of the most widely used in both clinical and research settings is the Addiction Severity Index (ASI; McLellan, Luborsky, O'Brien, & Woody, 1980; McLellan et al., 1992). The ASI is a semistructured interview designed to address seven potential problem areas: medical status, employment, drug use, alcohol use, legal status, family/social status, and psychiatric status. In about one hour, an interviewer can gather information on recent (past 30 days) and lifetime problems in all of the problem areas. The ASI provides an overview of problems related to substance use, rather than focusing on any single area. It has been used with mental health, homeless, pregnant, and prisoner populations, but its major use has been with adults seeking treatment for substance abuse problems (Hodgins & el-Guebaly, 1992; McLellan, Luborsky, Cacciola, & Griffith, 1985). The ASI provides two scores: interviewer severity ratings, which are subjective ratings of the clients' need for treatment, and composite scores, which are measures of problem severity during the prior 30 days that are calculated by a computerized scoring program. The composite scores are sensitive to change and are typically used to evaluate outcome. The ASI can be obtained from the National Institute of Drug Abuse (http://www.nida.nih.gov/).

The Comprehensive Drinker Profile (CDP; Miller & Marlatt, 1984) is a longer commercially available structured interview covering consumption, related problems, medical history, other drug use, and motivations for drinking and change. Card sorts are used to help the client provide information about drinking settings and preferences and other drug use. The CDP incorporates the MAST questions as well as a grid to determine typical drinking patterns. The interview takes about 2 hr to complete, although a briefer version is available. The CDP was used as the model in developing Form 90, which was the major assessment instrument used in Project Match, a large multisite outcome study. Reliability and validity of Form 90 has been extensively investigated and is generally good in the research context (Tonigan, Miller, & Brown, 1997).

CASE ILLUSTRATION

Ted is a 31-year-old man with one year of a vocational college program. He has been divorced for 8 years after 3 years of marriage. His 10-year-old daughter lives with his ex-wife although he sees her regularly and has a good relationship with her. He lives in the basement of his mother's house in a self-contained apartment. Ted works as a long distance truck driver but is currently on disability for depression. He has been on disability for 2 weeks since he made a suicide attempt following the end of a relationship with a girlfriend. His family physician noted elevated MCV and GGT values following routine blood work and, as a result, briefly screened for alcohol problems. Ted scored 4/4 on the CAGE questions and acknowledged that he often drinks more than 5 drinks per occasion. A referral was made to a specialized substance abuse treatment center.

The treatment center routinely administers the ASI as part of its intake procedure. The ASI identified that Ted has concerns and treatment needs in the social, employment, psychological, and alcohol areas. He began drinking socially at age 16 and by age 18 was consuming 26 oz of rye on Fridays and Saturdays (17 standard drinks each day) plus 2–3 beers each weekday night (totaling 45 drinks per week). This pattern continued until 5 years ago when he attempted to control his drinking, with periods of abstinence interspersed with 3–4-day binges every 3 months or so. During these binges he consumed about three 40-oz bottles of liquor (80 standard drinks). He smokes cigarettes but uses no street or prescription drugs. Ted was drinking when he made the recent suicide attempt but has been abstinent since.

Ted had attended a number of AA meetings over the past few years but had never successfully affiliated with the program. He has no other treatment involvement.

Ted was diagnosed with current alcohol dependence, meeting all of the seven *DSM-IV* criteria. Ted also reported that he continued to feel very distressed about the loss of his relationship, although he no longer felt suicidal. He was somewhat hopeful about his future.

The therapist completed the Readiness to Change Questionnaire (Hodgins, 2001) that indicated that Ted had a strong willingness to take action. He identified a goal of abstinence, recognizing that his previous attempts to cut down on drinking had been unsuccessful. The Brief Situational Confidence Questionnaire (Breslin, Sobell, Sobell, & Agrawal, 2000) revealed that he was confident in his ability to abstain when pressured socially to drink and when having pleasant times with others but, in particular, lacked confidence in resisting drinking when in conflict with others.

Ted agreed to attend a day treatment program at the center. The goals were to help him develop the coping skills needed to abstain from alcohol and prevent relapse.

Anger management was identified as a particular area of need. He was also encouraged to attend AA as a potential longer term support and as a vehicle to make non-drinking friends. Further assessment of his vocational skills was undertaken, and Ted formulated a plan to return to school in about 2 years. Finally, his mood was monitored and further assessed during a period of abstinence, and no mood or personality disorder was identified. Ted elected to continue to see an individual therapist after discharge from the treatment center to work on interpersonal relationship issues.

Information Critical to Making an Assessment

Alcoholics continue to have the reputation of having a predisposition toward denial and minimization and, as a result, are often believed to be less than honest in their self-reports of drinking and its consequences. At a recent medical school lecture, one professor recommended that clinicians assume that their patients are drinking double the amount that they report. Research evidence, on the other hand, suggests that self-reports are generally accurate (Institute of Medicine, 1990), although individual variability exists. Validity of self-report can be maximized when: the client is alcohol-free and not experiencing acute withdrawal symptoms; rapport has been established and the client understands the limits to confidentiality, the client does not have an obvious reason to distort the information, the interviewer is non-judgmental; questions are specific and structured; and finally, the client believes that self-reports will be checked against other sources of data (Institute of Medicine, 1990). Use of multiple sources of data is highly recommended and can include collateral reports, official records, and laboratory markers. Collateral reports can be obtained from spouses, parents, adult children, and friends and are more accurate when the collateral has greater opportunity to observe the client's drinking. Several studies have shown that when reports between clients and collaterals are discrepant, the clients have typically presented themselves more negatively than the collaterals (Sobell, Sobell, & Nirenberg, 1988).

Finally, a longitudinal approach to assessment can be helpful in increasing validity. It is important not to regard assessment as a single activity performed at a single point in time. Inaccuracies in information provided are often revealed over time and the assessment and treatment plan is modified or fine-tuned.

A final critical aspect of any alcohol assessment is suicide risk. Completed suicides and suicide attempts are very common among alcohol dependent individuals, with the depressed alcoholic group at highest risk (Winokur & Black, 1987). Suicidal risk has implications for treatment planning since many treatment venues are not equipped to monitor and support suicidal clients.

Dos and Don'ts: General Guidelines for Assessment

1. Do become familiar with a variety of treatment options. In most communities, a variety of treatment options exist for people with alcohol problems,

ranging from mutual support groups such as AA, outpatient therapy or counseling to more intensive day and residential programs. Although the majority of treatment providers in North America adhere to the twelve-step disease orientation, alternative models also exist (e.g., cognitive behavioral orientation). We do not have validated guidelines for matching clients to treatment settings; however, client preference as well as cost and availability are important considerations.

2. Do become familiar with the basic concepts and language associated with the recovery movement. Given the dominance of the twelve-step disease model, therapists may be able to better engage clients if they understand the organization and major tenets of the AA program. Literature is readily available that describes the "big book," open and closed meetings, the twelve steps and twelve traditions, and so forth. It is also helpful to be able to understand and use the colloquialisms associated with the "program." For example, popular terms include "walking the walk" (being in personal recovery), "stinking thinking" (distorted negative cognitions), and "going back out" (relapsing).

3. Do recognize the potential secondary impact of conducting screening and assessment. Simply asking about alcohol consumption and related difficulties and providing normative feedback can enhance clients' motivation for change and help them formulate personal goals for improvement. Research on such "brief interventions" reveals that these small interactions with clients can lead to lasting change in drinking behavior (Bien, Miller, & Tonigan, 1993).

4. Don't assume that you and the client are speaking the same language. Ensure that you are both using the same definitions of terms such as standard drinks, blackouts, flashbacks, intoxication, and sobriety. Ted, in the case example above, described experiencing the "DTs" many times when he was, in fact, describing moderate withdrawal symptoms.

5. Don't assume reliability of client report without client abstinence. As discussed, alcohol use may be associated with invalid self-reporting. A related guideline is that the therapist is not able to judge accurately whether or not a client has consumed alcohol. The routine use of a breathalyzer is recommended.

6. Don't assume that a face-to-face clinical interview is superior to self-report questionnaires administered in paper or computer format. As well as increasing time efficiency, self-completion questions can engender less defensiveness on the part of the client. This may be particularly true when the client understands that some normative feedback will be available based upon his or her personal responses.

7. Do watch your use of labels. Use of emotionally loaded terms such as "alcoholics" and "alcoholism," or "drug addict" by the therapist is unnecessary in conducting an assessment and will often encourage denial or minimization of problems.

8. Do point out discrepancies gently. Discrepant information will often surface during the course of an assessment. The clinician can point these discrepancies out in a low key and respectful way to help the client provide an accurate answer. Discrepancies will often reflect the client's ambivalence about his or her problems and not necessarily represent dishonesty (Miller & Rollnick, 1991). In the case example above, Ted was asked during the ASI interview about his relationship with his boss, which he described as good. Later in the interview

he described frequently missing work because of drinking. The interviewer noted the discrepancy by saying "earlier you said you had a good relationship with your boss but you also recognize that you often missed work." Ted clarified that his boss had, in fact, been very concerned about Ted's drinking.

9. Do get specific in your questions. It is good clinical practice to begin your interview and each new area of inquiry during the interview with open-ended questions to enhance engagement, but the clinician must move to specific questions in order to obtain reliable information.

SUMMARY

Many clinicians consider alcohol problems to be a specialty area of practice. Indeed, many specialized treatment options exist for this population. However, the existence of specialized treatments does not excuse generalists and specialists in other areas from the need to screen for, diagnose, and assess alcohol problems. A variety of effective methods are available, which allow clinicians to tailor approaches that fit well with their typical population and practices.

REFERENCES

Allen, J. P., & Litten, R. Z. (2001). The role of laboratory tests in alcoholism treatment. *Journal of Substance Abuse Treatment, 20*, 81–85.

Allen, J. P., Litten, R. Z., Fertig, J. B., & Babor, T. (1997). A review of the Alcohol Use Disorders Identification Test (AUDIT). *Alcoholism: Clinical and Experimental Research, 21*, 613–619.

Andrews, G., & Peters, L. (1998). The psychometric properties of the Composite International Diagnostic Interview. *Social Psychiatry and Psychiatric Epidemiology, 33*(2), 80–88.

Annis, H. M., Graham, J. M., & Davis, C. S. (1987). *Inventory of drinking situations. Users' guide*. Toronto: Addiction Research Foundation.

Anonymous. (2000). Health risks and benefits of alcohol consumption. Alcohol Research & Health. *The Journal of the National Institute on Alcohol Abuse & Alcoholism, 24*(1), 5–11.

Babor, T., de la Fuente, J. R., Saunders, J., & Grant, M. (1992). *The Alcohol Use Disorders Identification Test: Guidelines for use in primary health care*. Geneva: World Health Organization.

Bien, T. H., Miller, W. R., & Tonigan, J. S. (1993). Brief interventions for alcohol problems: A review. *Addiction, 88*, 315–336.

Bradley, K. A., Boyd-Wickizer, J., Powell, S. H., & Burman, M. L. (1998). Alcohol screening questionnaires for women: A critical review. *Journal of the American Medical Association, 280*, 166–171.

Breslin, F. C., Sobell, L. C., Sobell, M. B., & Agrawal, S. (2000). A comparison of a brief and long version of the Situational Confidence Questionnaire. *Behaviour Research and Therapy, 38*, 1211–1220.

Brown, S. A., Inabe, R. K., Gillin, J. C., Schuckit, M. A., & Stewart, M. A. (1995). Alcoholism and affective disorder: Clinical course of depressive symptoms. *American Journal of Psychiatry, 152*, 45–52.

Chan, A. W. K., Pristach, E. A., Welte, J. W., & Russell, M. (1993). Use of the TWEAK test in screening for alcoholism/heavy drinking in three populations. *Alcoholism Clinical and Experimental Research, 17*(6), 1188–1192.

Dawson, D. A. (1994). Consumption indicators of alcohol dependence. *Addiction, 89*, 345–350.

Edwards, G., & Gross, M. M. (1976). Alcohol dependence: Provisional description of a clinical syndrome. *British Medical Journal, 1*, 1058–1061.

Ewing, J. (1984). Detecting alcoholism: The CAGE questionnaire. *Journal of the American Medical Association, 252*, 1905–1907.

First, M. B., Spitzer, R. L., Gibbon, M., & Williams, J. B. W. (1997). *Structured Clinical Interview for DSM-IV Axis I Disorders—Clinician Version (SCID-CV)*. Washington, DC: American Psychiatric Press.

Grant, B. F., & Dawson, D. A. (1999). Alcohol and drug use, abuse, and dependence: Classification, prevalence, and comorbidity. In B. S. McCrady & E. E. Epstein (Eds.), *Addictions: A comprehensive guidebook* (pp. 9–29). New York: Oxford.

Heather, N., & Robertson, I. (1997). *Problem drinking* (3rd ed.). New York: Oxford University Press.

Hedlund, J. L., & Vieweg, B. W. (1984). The Michigan Alcoholism Screening Test (MAST): A comprehensive review. *Journal of Operational Psychiatry, 15*, 55–64.

Helzer, J. E., Canino, G. J., Eng-Kung, Y., Bland, R. C., Lee, C. K., Hwu, H., & Newman, S. (1990). Alcoholism—North America and Asia: A comparison of population surveys with the diagnostic interview schedule. *Archives of General Psychiatry, 47*, 313–319.

Hodgins, D. C. (2001). Stages of change assessments in alcohol problems: Agreement across self and clinician reports. *Substance Abuse, 22*, 87–96.

Hodgins, D. C., & el-Guebaly, N. (1992). More data on the Addiction Severity Index; Reliability and validity with the mentally ill substance abuser. *Journal of Nervous and Mental Disease, 180*, 197–201.

Hodgins, D. C., el-Guebaly, N., & Armstrong, S. (1995). Retrospective and prospective reports of mood states prior to relapse to substance use. *Journal of Consulting and Clinical Psychology, 63*, 400–407.

Hodgins, D. C., Leigh, G., Milne, R., & Gerrish, R. (1997). Drinking goal selection in behavioral self-management treatment of chronic alcoholics. *Addictive Behaviors, 22*, 247–255.

Institute of Medicine. (1990). *Broadening the base of treatment for alcohol problems*. Washington, DC: National Academy Press.

Johnson, J. G., Spitzer, R. L., Kroenke, K., Linzer, M., Brody, D., deGruy, F., & Hahn, S. (1995). Psychiatric comorbidity, health status, and functional impairment associated with alcohol abuse and dependence in primary care patients: Findings of the PRIME MD-1000 study. *Journal of Consulting and Clinical Psychology, 63*, 133–140.

Kahan, M. (2000). Metabolism and acute effects. In E. Brands (Ed.), *Management of alcohol, tobacco, and other drug problems* (pp. 71–75). Toronto: Centre for Addiction and Mental Health.

Kahan, M., & Wilson, L. (2000). Alcohol withdrawal. In E. Brands (Ed.), *Management of alcohol, tobacco, and other drug problems* (pp. 76–86). Toronto: Centre for Addiction and Mental Health.

Kranzler, H. R., Kadden, R. M., Babor, T. F., Tennen, H., & Rounsaville, B. J. (1996). Validity of the SCID in substance abuse patients. *Addiction, 91*, 859–868.

Larimer, M. E., & Kilmer, J. R. (2000). Natural history. In G. Zernig, A. Saria, M. Kurz, & S. O'Malley (Eds.) *Handbook of alcoholism* (pp. 13–28). Boca Raton, FL: CRC Press.

Mayfield, D., McLeod, G., & Hall, P. (1974). The CAGE questionnaire: Validation of a new alcoholism screening instrument. *American Journal of Psychiatry, 131*, 1121–1123.

McLellan, A. T., Luborsky, L., O'Brien, C. P., & Woody, G. E. (1980). An improved diagnostic instrument for substance abuse patients: The Addiction Severity Index. *Journal of Nervous and Mental Disorders, 168*, 26–33.

McLellan, A. T., Kushner, H., Metzger, D., Peters, R., Smith, I., Grissom, G., et al. (1992). The fifth edition of the Addiction Severity Index. *Journal of Substance Abuse Treatment, 9*, 199–213.

McLellan, A. T., Luborsky, L., Cacciola, J., & Griffith, J. (1985). New data from the Addiction Severity Index: Reliability and validity in three centers. *Journal of Nervous and Mental Disease, 173*, 412–423.

Miller, W. R. (1996). *Manual for Form 90: A structured interview for drinking and related behaviors. Project Match Monograph Series, Volume 5*. Rockville, MD: National Institute on Alcohol Abuse and Alcoholism.

Miller, W. R., & Marlatt, G. A. (1984). *Manual for the comprehensive drinker profile*. Odessa, FL: Psychological Assessment Resources.

Miller, W. R., & Rollnick, S. (1991). Using assessment results. In W. R. Miller and S. Rollnick (Eds.), *Motivational interviewing* (pp. 89–99). New York: Guilford Press.

Miller, W. R., & Tonigan, J. S. (1996). Assessing drinkers' motivation for change: The Stages of Change Readiness and Treatment Eagerness Scale (SOCRATES). *Psychology of Addictive Behaviors, 10*(2), 81–89.

Miller, W. R., Tonigan, J. S., & Longabaugh, R. (1995). *The Drinker Inventory of Consequences (DrInC)*. Bethesda, MD: National Institutes of Health.

NIAAA. (1995). *The physicians' guide to helping patients with alcohol problems*. Washington, DC: National Institute of Health.

Prochaska, J. O., DiClemente, C. C., & Norcross, J. C. (1992). In search of how people change: Applications to addictive behaviors. *American Psychologist, 47*, 1102–1114.

Raistrick, D., Dunbar, G., & Davidson, R. (1983). Development of a questionnaire to measure alcohol dependence. *British Journal of Addiction, 78*, 89–95.

Robins, L. N., Helzer, J. E., Cottler, L. B., & Goldring, E. (1998). *The Diagnostic Interview Schedule, Version IV.* St. Louis, MO.

Rollnick, S., Heather, N., Gold, R., & Hall, W. (1992). Development of a short "Readiness to Change" questionnaire for use in brief opportunistic interventions. *British Journal of Addiction, 87*, 743–754.

Rosenberg, H. (1993). Prediction of controlled drinking by alcoholics and problem drinkers. *Psychological Bulletin, 113*, 129–139.

Russell, M., Martier, S. S., Sokol, R. J., Mudar, P., Bottoms, S., Jacobson, S., & Jacobson, J. (1994). Screening for pregnancy risk-drinking. *Alcoholism: Clinical and Experimental Research, 18*, 1156–1161.

Schuckit, M. A. (2000). *Drug and alcohol abuse: A clinical guide to diagnosis and treatment* (5th ed.). New York: Kluwer Academic.

Selzer, M. L. (1971). The Michigan Alcoholism Screening Test: The quest for a new diagnostic instrument. *American Journal of Psychiatry, 127*, 1653–1658.

Selzer, M. L., Vinoker, A., & van Rooijen, L. (1975). The 13-item Short MAST (SMAST). *Journal of Studies on Alcohol, 36*, 117–126.

Skinner, H. A., & Allen, B. A. (1982). Alcohol dependence syndrome: Measurement and validation. *Journal of Abnormal Psychology, 91*, 199–209.

Skinner, H. A., & Sheu, W. J. (1982). Reliability of alcohol use indices: The lifetime drinking history and the MAST. *Journal of Studies on Alcohol, 43*, 1157–1170.

Sobell, L. C., & Sobell, M. B. (1992). Timeline Followback: A technique for assessing self-reported ethanol consumption. In J. Allen & R. Z. Litten (Eds.), *Measuring alcohol consumption: Psychosocial and biological methods* (pp. 41–72). Totowa, NJ: Humana Press.

Sobell, L. C., Sobell, M. B., & Nirenberg, T. D. (1988). Behavioral assessment and treatment planning with alcohol and drug abusers: A review with an emphasis on clinical application. *Clinical Psychology Review, 8*, 19–54.

Spitzer, R. L., Williams, J. B. W., Kroenke, K., Linzer, M., deGruy, F. V., Hahn, S. R., Brody, D., & Johnson, J. G. (1994). Utility of a new procedure for diagnosing mental disorders in primary care. The PRIME MD 1000 Study. *Journal of the American Medical Association, 272*, 1749–1756.

Surawicz, F. G. (1980). Alcoholic hallucinosis: A missed diagnosis. *Canadian Journal of Psychiatry, 25*, 57–63.

Tonigan, J. S., Miller, W. R., & Brown, J. M. (1997). The reliability of Form 90: An instrument for assessing alcohol treatment outcome. *Journal of Studies on Alcohol, 58*, 358–364.

United States Department of Health and Human Services, Substance Abuse and Mental Health Services Administration (n. d.). *Summary of findings from the 2000 National Household Survey on Drug Abuse.* Retrieved October 28, 2000, from http://www.samhsa.gov/oas/NHSDA/ 2kNHSDA/ chapter3.htm. Tables retrieved January 16, 2002, from http://www.samhsa.gov/oas/ nhsda/2kdetailedtabs/Vol_1_Part_2/sect2v1.htm.

Winokur, G., & Black, D. W. (1987). Psychiatric and medical diagnoses as risk factors for mortality in psychiatric patients: A case–control study. *American Journal of Psychiatry, 144*, 208–211.

World Health Organization. (1997). *The Composite International Diagnostic Interview—Version 2.1.* Geneva: Author.

10

Drug Abuse

Jennifer Antick and Kim Goodale

Description of the Problem

The 1950s ad slogan "better living through chemistry" provides an interesting starting point for this chapter on drug abuse assessment. It is particularly fitting in a time when public sentiment about substance use has never been more ambivalent. At once, society both looks for chemical cures for problems and at the same time tries to eradicate "drug culture." The substances that we often turn to for help, healing, and stress relief are increasingly themselves problematic. Substance use touches all of us because although drug abuse may involve illegal behavior, many substances of abuse are covertly sanctioned and promoted and others are both legal and openly promoted for controlled use in our society (Goldstein, 2001). These contradictions may contribute to the confusion so many mental health practitioners appear to experience over the assessment of substance use and abuse. In this arena, as much as any other set of disorders, it is particularly important to remain cognizant of the ambivalence we may experience as participants in our own cultural and personal contexts. It is with this in mind that the reader is invited to consider the artificial nature of distinctions between legal, illegal, over the counter, and prescription substances. This chapter concerns substances of abuse other than alcohol, which is addressed in a separate chapter. The present chapter discusses drugs of abuse, their costs, common terms, recent use statistics, diagnostic criteria, a case illustration, procedures for gathering information, commonly used standardized interview formats and tools, and "dos and don'ts" to keep in mind in the diagnostic interview.

Some of the most commonly abused drugs, according to Julien (1997) and the National Institute on Drug Abuse (NIDA, 1998a, 1998b, 1999, 2000a, 2000b, 2000c), include:

1. Cannabinoids: hashish and marijuana.

Jennifer Antick and Kim Goodale • School of Professional Psychology, Pacific University, Forest Grove, Oregon 97116.

2. Central nervous system depressants (the traditional sedative-hypnotic drugs and antiepileptic drugs): barbiturates, benzodiazepines, gamma hydroxybutyrate (GHB), and methaqualone.
3. Dissociative anesthetics: ketamine, phencyclidine (PCP), and analogs.
4. Hallucinogens/psychedelics: lysergic acid diethylamide (LSD), mescaline, psilocybin.
5. Opioids, morphine derivatives, and synthetic opiates: codeine, fentanyl, heroin, morphine, opium, Demerol, oxycodone, Oxycontin.
6. Stimulants: amphetamine, cocaine, methamphetamine, methylene-dioxymethamphetamine (MDMA), methylphenidate, and nicotine.
7. Anabolic-andronergic steroids: oxymetholone, nandrolone phenproprionate.
8. Inhalants: volatile solvents (paint thinners, gasoline, glues, aerosol spray paint, hair spray, vegetable oil spray for cooking), gases (ether, chloroform, nitrous oxide), and nitrites (amyl nitrite, butyl nitrite).
9. "Club drugs": drugs from other categories that are grouped by use patterns such as MDMA, LSD, GHB, ketamine, rohypnol, and methamphetamine.

Drug, alcohol, and tobacco use are reported to cause more deaths, illnesses, and disabilities than any other preventable health condition (Robert Wood Johnson Foundation, 2001). One of the most recent figures estimates the cost of alcohol, and illicit drug abuse in the United States for 1998 was $143.4 billion. Projected overall costs of drug abuse for the year 2000 (still being tabulated) were $160.7 billion, with $110.5 billion of this figure representing lost productivity (Office of National Drug Control Policy [ONDCP], 2001). These figures also include the costs of premature death, institutionalization, short- and long-term hospitalization, and productivity loss for victims of drug/alcohol abuse-related crime. In addition, the figures account for federal spending attempts to reduce the supply of illegal drugs, social welfare costs, and the costs of running of the justice system and correctional facilities, which are increasingly occupied with drug-related crimes and their adjudicated offenders (ONDCP, 2001). These figures do not include the substantial cost to the private sector, such as privately funded legal defense, property damage for victims of crime, private or public costs of treatment, or private costs in maintaining a substance use disorder (NIDA, 1999). Other considerations include those medical conditions directly caused by use as well as the contributions of drug use to the development, exacerbation, or complication of other illnesses or injuries that require their own specific treatment or significantly longer lengths of hospitalization. For example, individuals who use drugs are at higher risk for contracting and spreading HIV/AIDS, hepatitis B and C, and tuberculosis (ONDCP, 2001; Spittal & Schechter, 2001). Prevalence of medical disorders is high among substance abuse patients and includes hypertension, coronary heart disease, chronic liver disease, and as stated above, hepatitis C (Weisner, Mertens, Parthasarathy, Moore, & Lu, 2001). Stimulant abuse, such as amphetamine, cocaine, or MDMA (Ecstasy), is also considered one of the most common causes of stroke in young adults (McEvoy, Kitchen, & Thomas, 1998).

Terms commonly used when addressing substance use include (American Psychiatric Association [APA], 2000; Julien, 1997; Substance Abuse and Mental Health Services Administration [SAMHSA], 2000):

1. Addiction: A chronic, relapsing disease, characterized by compulsive drug-seeking and drug use and by neurochemical and molecular changes in the brain.
2. Comorbid disorders: Psychiatric disorders that coexist with a second psychiatric disorder.
3. Cross-tolerance: A condition in which a drug can prevent the withdrawal symptoms associated with physical dependence on a different drug.
4. Current use: Use of a drug at once in the past 30 days.
5. Drugs: Chemical substances use for their effects on bodily processes.
6. Drug interactions: Modifications of the action of one drug by the concurrent or prior administration of another drug.
7. Drug misuse: Use of any drug for a medical or recreational purpose when other alternatives are available, practical, or warranted, or when drug use endangers either the user or others with whom he or she may interact.
8. Drug tolerance: A state of progressively decreasing responsiveness to a drug.
9. Heavy use: The use of a drug on five or more occasions in the past 30 days.
10. Intoxication: Development of a reversible condition after recent ingestion of a psychoactive substance.
11. Physical dependence: A state in which use of a substance is required for a person to function normally. Note that a person may be physically dependent on a substance without meeting criteria for addiction or dependence.
12. Psychoactive drugs: Chemical substances that alter mood or behavior as a result of alterations in the functioning of the brain.
13. Psychological dependence: Compulsion to use a drug for its pleasurable effects. Such dependence may lead to a compulsion to misuse a drug.
14. Routes of administration: The ways drugs can be taken into the body. These are oral, intravenous, intramuscular, topical, subcutaneous, intranasal, or inhaled dose. The method of ingestion affects how the drug is broken down in the body and how long the chemical has a psychoactive effect.
15. Substance abuse: A maladaptive pattern of substance use leading to a clinically significant impairment or distress.
16. Substance use: Ingestion of a drug or drugs without the experience of any negative consequences.
17. Withdrawal: A substance-specific state that is reached on cessation or reduction of substance use that has been heavy or prolonged.

Symptoms

In general, substance use disorders are characterized by cognitive, behavioral, and physiological symptoms indicating that the individual continues use of a substance despite significant substance-related problems. In many cases, use of these substances develops into a pattern of repeated self-administration that results in tolerance, withdrawal and compulsive drug-taking behavior (APA, 2000). The most recent National Household Survey of Drug Abuse (NHSDA; SAMHSA, 1999, 2000) estimated that 14 million Americans are current illicit drug users (approximately 6.3% of the population in the United States 12 years or older). The survey suggested that more men than women use illicit drugs. However, rates of nonmedical use of pain relievers, tranquilizers, stimulants, and sedatives were similar between men and women. Among adolescents between 12 and 17, 9.7% admitted to having used an illicit drug within 30 days before the interview. Adults between 18 and 25 consistently use more drugs more often than any other age group. NIDA recently suggested that the most accurate number estimating prescription drug misuse is somewhere between the 4 million estimated by NIDA and the 9.3 million estimated by the NHSDA (Vastag, 2001). Illicit drug use is highly correlated with educational status, with those who had not completed high school reflecting the highest rates and college graduates with the lowest rates of use compared with other educational groupings. This is particularly useful information in light of the data suggesting that young adults at different educational levels are equally likely to have tried illicit drugs in their lifetimes. Importance of these data for the business community is also clear when one considers that out of 11.8 million American adults using illicit drugs, 9.1 million are employed either part or full time. This same set of data suggest that approximately 3.5 million Americans aged 12 and older meet full diagnostic criteria for substance dependence on illicit drugs (SAMHSA, 1999, 2000).

Leshner (1999) suggests that there are two general categories that describe people who use drugs. He further asserts that these two groups of people present different clinical pictures. One category is the "sensation seekers." These people probably begin their use for the positive sensory experiences the substances can produce. They may also use to feel accepted by peers. Eventually, their use begins to interfere with daily functioning. Leshner notes that this picture is most consistent with adolescence and young adulthood. The second category he discusses is the person who uses substances in order to mediate negative emotional states. Individuals in this group are also theorized to have other mental health problems in addition to their use. The "self-medication" hypothesis is often used to explain what prolonged drug use and exacerbations of the psychological symptoms come from extended use. Regardless of the reasons for use or reasons for continuing to use, the common feature of all addiction is an "uncontrollable compulsion to seek and use drugs" (Leshner, 1999). Most of the problems that develop in individuals with substance use disorders begin with such uncontrollable compulsion, and follow with inappropriate or illegal behaviors to satisfy the compulsion. It is this pattern of uncontrollable compulsions and their concomitant compensatory behaviors that we refer to as addiction. Severity of the clinical picture then varies by the number of risk factors the person has, the age of onset, specific consequences of use, physical response to the substance(s), psychological rewards of use, and the psychosocial support for use. Most people with addiction will experience a chronic, relapsing disorder in which multiple treatment episodes are likely to be required over their life span (Minkoff, 1998, 2000).

There are substantive differences in use patterns and types of comorbidity, as well as treatment needs that vary by the age and gender of the person needing treatment (Ott, Tarter, & Ammerman, 1999). There also are important considerations for people from various cultural, ethnic, and religious backgrounds who have different norms and mores for substance use, beliefs about seeking help "outside" the group, values about family involvement, and norms about the pace at which new relationships (like therapist–client relationships) proceed. Clinicians should be prepared to make accommodations for individuals who need special physical assistance, help with reading or writing or communicating, transportation coordination, and translation or interpretations services for those individuals for whom English is not their primary language (Fisher & Harrison, 2000; Gordon, 1994; Riehman, Hser, & Zeller, 2000).

Diagnostic Considerations

Diagnostic and Statistical Manual of Mental Disorder, Fourth Edition, Text Revision. The *DSM-IV-TR* (APA, 2000) is the most prominent method of classifying the behaviors and consequences of substance use.

The *DSM-IV-TR* diagnostic criteria for Substance Abuse are:

A. Maladaptive pattern of substance use leading to clinically significant impairment or distress, as manifested by one (or more) of the following, occurring within a 12-month period:
   (1) Recurrent substance use resulting in a failure to fulfill major role obligations at work, school, or home (e.g., repeated absences or poor work performance related to substance use; substance-related absences, suspensions or expulsions from school; neglect of children or household).
   (2) Recurrent substance use in situations in which it is physically hazardous (e.g., driving an automobile and operating a machine when impaired by substance use).
   (3) Recurrent substance-related legal problems (e.g., arrests for substance-related disorderly conduct).
   (4) Continued substance use despite having persistent or recurrent social or interpersonal problems caused or exacerbated by the effects of the substance (e.g., arguments with spouse about consequences of intoxication, physical fights).
B. The symptoms have never met the criteria for Substance Dependence for the class of substance.

The diagnosis of Substance Abuse may be applied to alcohol, amphetamines, cannabis, cocaine, hallucinogens, inhalants, opioids, phencyclidine, sedatives, hypnotics, or anxiolytics, and other or unknown substances.

The diagnostic criteria for substance dependence are:

A. Maladaptive pattern of substance use, leading to clinically significant impairment or distress, as manifested by three (or more) of the following, occurring at any time in the same 12-month period:
   (1) Tolerance, as defined by either of the following:
       (a) A need for markedly increased amounts of the substance to achieve intoxication or desired effect.
           or
       (b) Markedly diminished effect with continued use of the same amount of the substance.
   (2) Withdrawal, as manifested by either of the following:
       (a) The characteristic withdrawal syndrome for the substance
           or
       (b) The same (or a closely related) substance is taken to relieve or avoid withdrawal symptoms.
   (3) The substance is often taken in larger amounts or over a longer period than was intended.
   (4) There is a persistent desire or unsuccessful efforts to cut down or control substance use.
   (5) A great deal of time is spent in activities necessary to obtain the substance (e.g., visiting multiple doctors or driving long distances), use the substance (e.g., chain-smoking), or recover from its effects.
   (6) Important social, occupational, or recreational activities are given up or reduced because of substance use.
   (7) The substance use is continued despite knowledge of having a persistent or recurrent physical or psychological problem that is likely to have been caused or exacerbated by the substance (e.g., current cocaine use despite recognition of cocaine-induced depression, or continued drinking despite recognition that an ulcer was made worse by alcohol consumption).

The clinician should specify if a person presents with evidence of tolerance or withdrawal by indicating, "With Physiological Dependence," or if not, "Without Physiological Dependence." In addition, course specifiers include:

- Early Full Remission
- Early Partial Remission
- Sustained Full Remission
- Sustained Partial Remission
- On Agonist Therapy
- In a Controlled Environment.

The Substance Dependence diagnosis may be applied to all of the drugs specified for inclusion in Substance Abuse, with the additions of Nicotine and Polysubstance Dependence. The Polysubstance Dependence diagnosis is used when a person repeatedly uses at least three groups of substances (not including caffeine and nicotine), but no single substance predominated, and when Dependence criteria were met for substances as a group but not for the specific substances (APA, 2000). Each of the *DSM* diagnoses for each class of substances requires the ruling out of the symptoms as occurring due to a general medical condition or better accounted for by another mental health disorder.

Additional considerations include the challenges of assessing and diagnosing individuals who present with both mental health and substance use problems. Assessment under these conditions can be particularly challenging as psychoactive substances, by definition, produce changes in the mental, emotional, and physiological state of the individual, often mimicking or masking coexisting mental health problems. Alternatively, most major mental health problems can make the diagnosis of substance use disorders more complicated (Brady et al., 1996). Minkoff (1998, 2000) suggests adopting a "welcoming expectation" and assuming that any client is likely to have a comorbid condition. Assuming this, one should be prepared to assess for both mental health and substance use disorders with all clients.

PROCEDURES FOR GATHERING INFORMATION

The American Society of Addiction Medicine (ASAM) has established a rigorous set of criteria for patient placement decisions based upon assessment. The ASAM Patient Placement Criteria—Revised (PPC-2R; ASAM, 2001; Center for Substance Abuse Treatment [CSAT], 2001) requires assessment in six areas of an individual's life:

- Dimension 1: Acute intoxication and withdrawal potential
- Dimension 2: Biomedical conditions and complications
- Dimension 3: Emotional, behavioral, or cognitive conditions and complications
- Dimension 4: Readiness to change
- Dimension 5: Relapse, continued use, or continued problem potential
- Dimension 6: Recovery/living environment

Each of the above dimensions is reflective of the multidimensional nature of addiction and the multilevel assessment and treatment planning that is required in response. The ASAM criteria lend consistency to the weight placed on specific aspects of an individual's impairment and the best placement or intensity of treatment for his or her individual clinical picture.

For most clinical researchers, assessment and goal-setting for treatment are not separate but related processes. Assessment begins with the very first clinical contact, interview, or screening and continues throughout the treatment process. Because individuals presenting for treatment frequently report that they were able to establish brief periods of pretreatment or between-treatment abstinence, clinicians must be prepared to assess for past successes in addition to the person's difficulties. Even very short periods of abstinence reveal clients' skills, resources, and coping strategies that are useful in designing treatment (APA, 2000; ASAM, 2001; Miller & Berg, 1992).

Motivational interviewing or MI (CSAT, 1999; Miller & Rollnick, 1991) origi-nally developed as an assessment strategy and later was determined to be useful as a treatment methodology. A major premise of motivational interviewing is that ambivalence is required for change to take place and that ambivalence about mak-ing large-scale changes is completely normal. Further, motivational interviewing presupposes that ambivalence is part of the process of recovery as opposed to an obstacle for recovery. Reflective listening in conjunction with an empathic, support-ive, and directive counseling style is said to provide conditions in which change can occur. One of the goals of MI is to create a collaborative partnership between therapist and client, one to which each brings important expertise. A successful interview is characterized by the development and amplification of discrepancy between the client's goals, values, and current behavior; "rolling" with resistance (rather than opposing it); and support for the client's self-efficacy and optimism by focusing on the client's strengths instead of his or her failures or problems. This helps to foster the hope and expectancy for positive change the client needs to make and the difficult changes he or she is challenged to make.

A complementary model is that of Prochaska and DiClemente's Stages of Change (Prochaska & DiClemente, 1991; Prochaska, DiClemente, & Norcross, 1992). This model, like motivational interviewing, can be applied to any situation in which a change in human behavior is desired, including substance use. Application of the model helps to identify client readiness to accept different types of treatment, measure clients' progress in treatment, and provide a founda-tion for both client and treatment provider in understanding the client's strengths as well as difficulties.

The five Stages of Change are:

1. Precontemplation: The person is not yet considering treatment and may be "in denial" of a substance use problem.
2. Contemplation: In this stage, the individual acknowledges having a prob-lem but is not yet ready to make specific behavioral changes.
3. Preparation: Planning for change takes place in this stage.
4. Action: The person begins to modify his or her behavior, environment, or experiences to overcome his or her problems.
5. Maintenance: The person works to maintain the gains and prevent relapse in this stage.

There are several compelling reasons for the interviewer to integrate Motivational Interviewing skills as well the Stages of Change into their repertoire. First, they are transtheoretical by design, so they can be used by individuals from very different theoretical orientations including cognitive, behavioral, psychody-namic, or modified 12-step approaches. Second, these approaches can help to create a common language for interdisciplinary staff, reducing "translation" time and simplifying what is often rhetoric to clients. Lastly, even one session of Motivational Interviewing informed by the Stages of Change improves treatment outcomes, even when Motivational Interviewing methods do not continue during treatment (Miller & Rollnick, 1991; Prochaska & DiClemente, 1991; Prochaska et al., 1992; SAMHSA, 1999).

Case Illustration

Joan is a 34-year-old, single, Caucasian woman with three elementary school age children and a live-in boyfriend of several years. She presented for treatment for depressive symptoms and unremitting headache pain. A recent medical examination had prompted the referral when her medical practitioner was unable to help her with her headaches and major medical concerns were ruled out. She had reportedly already been stabilized on antidepressants prior to her referral to the therapist, but she noted that her depressive symptoms had been worsening lately and her prescribed medication was no longer sufficient to help her. The medical practitioner wanted a consultation to her diagnosis and recommendations for treatment. Joan revealed very early in the assessment that she had been having headaches because she had been "sick" from her "medicine." She further revealed that her medicine was Oxycontin, that it was not prescribed, and that she was given such pills by her ex-boyfriend with whom she had regular contact. She reported that she had been very afraid of telling her medical practitioner about such illegal use and was concerned that she would lose her medical care. She stated that she was "getting sick" when trying to cut down or stop using altogether, which she had been attempting for the past year off and on. Joan reported nausea, vomiting, and unremitting pounding headaches during these times. She indicated that feelings of sickness were debilitating and interfering more with her role fulfillment than the drugs. She noted that when she resumed taking her pills, these unpleasant symptoms would resolve and she could function in her daily responsibilities once again. She reported that even though she had a great "sense of well-being" from the pills, she also wanted to stop using. She stated that she wanted to quit because it was illegal, that it kept her "tied" to her ex-boyfriend in an "unhealthy" way, and that she was worried that she was not as good a mother as she wanted to be to her children. Risk issues to the children were ruled out, as were risk of harm to herself and to others. She denied using alcohol to excess, misusing any over-the-counter medications or supplements, or using any other drugs. She described depressive symptoms consistent with dysthymic disorder, denied a history of sexual or physical abuse, denied any legal concerns or occupational problems. She noted that she had been diagnosed with depression 3 years prior to taking her first Oxycontin and noted that it also helped her manage her depressive symptoms and that her depressive symptoms were worse when she was off the medication for more than 1 day. She noted that the longest she had been able to go without the pills was $2\frac{1}{2}$ days before the symptoms (withdrawal) were intolerable. Joan revealed all of this in the context of a structured interview format. No further testing was completed as the client had already identified for herself a problem and for the clinician the criteria for substance dependence, with physiological dependence. Joan had not considered that significant depressive symptoms and "sickness" she experienced were part of the withdrawal pattern for opiates. In addition, her symptoms only remitted after taking more of the substance. Dependence on the substance is exemplified by the pattern of her behavior in use: a persistent desire to cut down or stop abusing the substance with numerous unsuccessful attempts, the damage to important relationships from her continued use, risk of significant legal ramifications, and time spent in pursuit of obtaining medications. She was clearly moving between preparation and action stages of change, and her ambivalence was clearly articulated as well. Motivational Interviewing methods were carried out to complete the diagnostic interview and gather sufficient information to begin treatment planning in conjunction with the client's readiness to change. In this particular case, additional instruments and structure were not necessary. However, most individuals present at earlier stages of readiness to change and may need multiple contacts for engagement in the assessment and treatment planning process to occur.

STANDARDIZED INTERVIEW FORMAT

Since the assessment interview lays the groundwork for treatment, obtaining relevant information is still one of the main strategies. Because most clients have had experience making changes in some area of their lives, it can be very helpful to learn from them what they already know about their problems, as well as what they have done in the past that has worked for them. It is also very important to determine what healthy efforts are already being implemented (Rosengren, Downey, & Donovan, 2000). Some basic questions that may be helpful include:

- Has your substance use ever changed?
- Is this a slip from a previous sobriety? (Follow-up: How did you manage to stay clean for that length of time?)
- Is this new behavior?
- Is this situation-specific?
- Is this in response to a new stressor at home, school, or with family? (Follow-up: What other things are you doing to cope that are even slightly effective?)
- When are you able to refuse use even when substances are available? (Follow-up: How do you accomplish that?)
- Who else might notice that you have been making an effort?

INFORMATION CRITICAL TO MAKING THE DIAGNOSIS

Brief screenings may also be a very useful way for busy clinicians to begin the assessment process. They include a sampling of items that are consistent with problematic substance use (Bastiens, Francis, & Lewis, 2000; Cooney, Zweben, & Fleming, 1995). Questions should begin with general questions about caffeine intake, diet, and then move into tobacco screening.

1. Do you smoke?
   If yes, ask:
   - How much do you smoke? (amount, frequency)
   - For how long have you smoked?
   - Have you ever tried to quit?
   - What are your obstacles to quitting?
   - What has helped you in the past to decrease or quit smoking for periods of time?
2. Have you ever smoked in the past?
   If yes, ask:
   - When did you quit?
   - How long did you smoke?
   - How much did you smoke?
   - How hard was it to quit?
   - How many times have you quit?
   - What helped/How did you do it?

3. Then ask:
   - Have you had any alcohol in the past year?
   - Have you used any drugs in the past year? (Make sure to ask about misuse of over-the-counter and prescription medications.)
4. If the answer is no to both the questions in 3, ask:
   - Have you ever used alcohol or drugs?
     – How long ago?
   - Are you in recovery from alcohol or drugs?
   - Please describe your past use of alcohol or drugs.
   - Do you have a family history of alcohol or drug use?
5. If the answers to both the questions in 3 are yes, follow the age- and gender-appropriate screens listed below.
6. For late adolescents and young adults consider using the RAFFT screen:
   - Do you use to relax?
   - Do you use when alone?
   - How many of your friends use?
   - Is there a history of substance abuse in the family?
   - Have you gotten into trouble because of your use?
7. For adult men, use the CAGE screen:
   - Have you ever thought about cutting down on your drinking or drug use?
   - Have you ever been annoyed by people's criticism of your drinking/drug use?
   - Have you ever felt guilty about your drinking/drug use?
   - Have you ever used alcohol or drugs to get you going in the morning? (eye-opener)
8. For women, use the TACE screen:
   - How many drinks (much of the drug) does it take for you to feel high?
   - Have you ever been annoyed by people's criticism of your drinking/drug use?
   - Have you ever thought about cutting down on your drinking or drug use?
   - Have you ever used alcohol or drugs to get you going in the morning? (eye-opener)
9. For elders, use the CHARMM screen:
   - Have you ever thought about cutting down? Do you have rules about drinking or drug use?
   - Has your pattern of use changed recently? (how)
   - Has anyone expressed concern about your alcohol or drug use?
   - What role does alcohol or drugs play in your life?
   - Have you ever used alcohol or drugs more than you intended?
   - Have you ever had problems with your medications or taken more than prescribed?

For all screens, any yes answer should be investigated further. Two or more "yes" answers suggest that the person may benefit from further assessment in this area. Minimal follow-up should include drug(s) used, method of use, amount and frequency of use, duration of use, periods of abstinence, role of alcohol/drugs in the person's life, consequences of use, additional coping strategies, and support systems that are consistent with changes in use. Consistent with ASAM criteria, it is recommended that the clinician also include questions about physical health, suicidal or aggressive ideation intent or plan, family and social relations, including sexual activity; physical and sexual abuse; school and work; and financial or legal problems, including driving while intoxicated or any arrests. It is also advisable to complete a thorough mental status examination (Northwest Frontier Addiction Technology Transfer Center [NFATTC], 2001).

There are many tools available for the assessment of substance use disorders. A select few are highlighted here. The most useful assessment instruments are valid, reliable, and provide information about drugs and alcohol as well as mental health symptoms.

1. The Addiction Severity Index is a structured interview designed to assess problem severity in seven of the areas of life commonly affected by drug abuse: medical condition, employment, drug use, alcohol use, illegal activity (separate from those related to the procurement or possession of illicit drugs), family relationships, and psychiatric condition (McLellan et al., 1992; McLellan, Luborsky, Woody, & O'Brien, 1980).

2. The Drug Use Screening Inventory—Revised (DUSI-R) is an instrument created to assess the multiple problems of individuals who abuse alcohol and other drugs. The DUSI-R is a multidimensional screening tool, assessing disturbances in the following 10 domains: substance use, behavior patterns, health status, psychiatric disorders, social competency, family system, school performance/adjustment, work adjustment, peer relationships, and leisure/recreation. The relative severity of each of these problem domains is rank ordered, helping in prioritizing treatment targets. It may then be useful in monitoring treatment progress (Tarter, 1990; Tarter and Hegedus, 1991).

3. The Substance Abuse Subtle Screening Inventory-3 (SASSI-3; Miller, 1997) is a brief assessment tool that is intended to differentiate between use, abuse, and dependence in clients. It addresses issues of validity encountered by other instruments and earlier versions of the SASSI and is easy to score and use with clients.

4. The Structured Clinical Interview for *DSM* (First, Spitzer, Gibbon, & Williams, 1997) is important to consider as well. It is thorough and completely compatible with the diagnostic system. It is very useful in ensuring consistency in diagnoses and problem identification and, with proper training and supervision, can be administered by staff of various levels of training.

5. There are also several questionnaires consistent with the Motivational Interviewing and Stages of Change models. For more information, see SAMHSA Treatment Improvement Protocol Series No. 35 (CSAT, 1999).

The individual tools discussed above are recommended for use within the context of a complete biopsychosocial evaluation. However, they can be useful in determining the need for further assessment.

Dos and Don'ts

Dos

- Practice reflective listening
- Ask about previous successes no matter how small
- Acknowledge and attend to specific strengths and abilities that the client can bring to bear on the problem area
- Express respect and genuine empathy
- If your personal ambivalence is in the way, seek consultation
- Acknowledge how hard it is to make large-scale behavioral changes
- Validate the person's efforts
- Learn from the client
- Integrate motivational interviewing skills into your repertoire.

Don'ts

- Don't label
- Don't judge
- Don't assume
- Don't jump to conclusions.

Summary

Diagnostic interviewing requires a complex set of skills; not the least of which is rapport building. It is incumbent upon the diagnostician to combine technical information gathering skills with respect and empathy for the client's very personal challenges. The technical aspects of assessing for substance use disorders include integration of age- and gender-appropriate screens, mastery of structured interviewing methods, and appropriate use of standardized assessment tools. In addition, attending to readiness for any particular change as well as that person's ambivalence is likely to improve the outcome of the assessment.

References

American Psychiatric Association. (2000). *Diagnostic and statistical manual of mental disorders* (4th ed., text rev.). Washington, DC: Author.

American Society of Addiction Medicine. (2001). *Patient placement criteria for the treatment of substance-related disorders, Second Edition—Revised (ASAM PPC-2R)*. Washington, DC: Author.

Bastiens, L., Francis, G., & Lewis, K. (2000). The RAFFT as a screening tool for adolescent substance use disorders. *American Journal on Addictions, 9*, 10–16.

Brady, S., Hiam, C. M., Saemann, R., Humbert, L., Fleming, M. Z., & Dawkins-Brickhouse, K. (1996). Dual-diagnosis: A treatment model for substance abuse and major mental illness. *Community Mental Health Journal, 32*, 573–578.

Center for Substance Abuse Treatment. (1999). *Enhancing motivation for change in substance abuse treatment* (Treatment Improvement Protocol [TIP] Series). Washington, DC: U.S. Government Printing Office.

Center for Substance Abuse Treatment. (2001). *The role and current status of patient placement criteria in the treatment of substance use disorders* (Treatment Improvement Protocol [TIP] Series). Washington, DC: U.S. Government Printing Office.

Cooney, N. L., Zweben, A., & Fleming, M. F. (1995). Screening for alcohol problems and at-risk drinking in health-care settings. In R. K. Hester & W. R. Miller (Eds.), *Handbook of alcoholism treatment approaches: Effective approaches* (2nd ed., pp. 45–60). Boston: Allyn & Bacon.

First, M. B., Spitzer, R. L., Gibbon, M., & Williams, J. B. W. (1997). *User's guide to the Structured Clinical Interview for DSM-IV Axis I Disorders: Clinician Version* (SCID-CV). Washington, DC: American Psychiatric Press.

Fisher, G. L., & Harrison, T. C. (2000). *Substance abuse: Information for school counselors, social workers, therapists, and counselors* (2nd ed.). Boston: Allyn & Bacon.

Goldstein, A. (2001). *Addiction: From biology to drug policy* (2nd ed.). New York: Oxford University Press.

Gordon, J. U. (Ed.). (1994). *Managing multiculturalism in substance abuse services.* Thousand Oaks, CA: Sage.

Julien, R. M. (1997). *A primer of drug action: A concise, nontechnical guide to the actions, uses, and side effects of psychoactive drugs* (8th ed.). New York: Freeman.

Leshner, A. I. (1999). Science-based views of drug addiction treatment. *Journal of the American Medical Association, 282*, 1314–1316.

McEvoy, A. W., Kitchen, N. D., & Thomas, D. G. T. (1998). Intracerebral hemorrhage caused by drug abuse. *Lancet, 351*, 1029–1030.

McLellan, A. T., Kushner, H., Metzger, D., Peters, R., Smith, I., Grissom, G., et al. (1992). The Addiction Severity Index (5th ed.). *Journal of Substance Abuse Treatment, 9*, 199–213.

McLellan, A. T., Luborsky, L., Woody, G. E., & O'Brien, C. P. (1980). An improved diagnostic evaluation instrument for substance abuse patients: The Addiction Severity Index. *Journal of Nervous and Mental Diseases, 168*, 26–33.

Miller, G. A. (1997). *The Substance Abuse Subtle Screening Inventory-3 manual.* Spencer, IN: Spencer Evening World.

Miller, S. D., & Berg, I. K. (1992). *Working with the problem drinker.* New York: Norton.

Miller, W. R., & Rollnick, S. (1991). *Motivational interviewing: Preparing people to change addictive behavior.* New York: Guilford Press.

Minkoff, K. (1998). *Individuals with co-occurring psychiatric and substance disorders in managed care systems: Standards of care, practice guidelines, workforce competencies and training curricula.* University of Pennsylvania Center for Mental Health Policy and Services Research. Available from www.upenn.edu/cmhpsr.

Minkoff, K. (2000). *State of Arizona service planning guidelines: Co-occurring psychiatric and substance disorders* (edited version). Acton, MA: Author.

National Institute on Drug Abuse. (1998a). *Methamphetamine abuse and addiction.* National Institute on Drug Abuse Research Report Series (NIH Publication No. 98-4210). Washington, DC: U.S. Department of Health and Human Services.

National Institute on Drug Abuse. (1998b). *Nicotine addiction.* National Institute on Drug Abuse Research Report Series (NIH Publication No. 98-4342). Washington, DC: U.S. Department of Health and Human Services.

National Institute on Drug Abuse. (1999). *Cocaine abuse and addiction.* National Institute on Drug Abuse Research Report Series (NIH Publication No. 99-4342). Washington, DC: U.S. Department of Health and Human Services.

National Institute on Drug Abuse. (2000a). *Anabolic steroid abuse.* National Institute on Drug Abuse Research Report Series (NIH Publication No. 00-3721). Washington, DC: U.S. Department of Health and Human Services.

National Institute on Drug Abuse. (2000b). *Heroin abuse and addiction.* National Institute on Drug Abuse Research Report Series (NIH Publication No. 00-4165). Washington, DC: U.S. Department of Health and Human Services.

National Institute on Drug Abuse. (2000c). *Inhalant abuse.* National Institute on Drug Abuse Research Report Series (NIH Publication No. 00-3818). Washington, DC: U.S. Department of Health and Human Services.

Northwest Frontier Addiction Technology Transfer Center. (2001). *Performance assessment rubrics for the addiction counseling competencies* (Oregon Office of Alcohol and Drug Abuse Programs). Salem: Author.

Office of National Drug Control Policy. (2001). *The economic costs of drug abuse in the United States, 1992–1998* (Publication No. NCJ-190636). Washington, DC: Executive Office of the President.

Ott, P. J., Tarter, R. E., & Ammerman, R. T. (1999). *Sourcebook on substance abuse: Etiology, epidemiology, assessment, and treatment.* Boston: Allyn & Bacon.

Prochaska, J. O., & DiClemente, C. C. (1991). Stages of change in the modification of problem behaviors. In M. Hersen, R. M. Eisler, & P. M. Miller (Eds.), *Progress in behavior modification* (Vol. 27, pp. 184–214). Newbury Park, CA: Sage.

Prochaska, J. O., DiClemente, C. C., & Norcross, J. C. (1992). In search of how people change: Applications to addictive behaviors. *American Psychologist, 47,* 1102–1114.

Riehman, K. S., Hser, Y.-I., & Zeller, M. (2000). Gender differences in how intimate partners influence drug treatment motivation. *Journal of Drug Issues, 30,* 823–839.

Robert Wood Johnson Foundation. (2001). *Substance abuse: The nation's number one health problem: Key indicators for policy.* Princeton, NJ: Author.

Rosengren, D. B., Downey, L., & Donovan, D. M. (2000). I already stopped: Abstinence prior to treatment. *Addiction, 95,* 65–77.

Spittal, P. M., & Schechter, M. T. (2001). Injection drug use and despair through the lens of gender. *Canadian Medical Association Journal, 164,* 802–804.

Substance Abuse and Mental Health Services Administration. (1999). *National Household Survey on Drug Abuse: Population estimates, 1999.* Retrieved May 13, 2002, from www.samhsa.gov/OAS/NHSDA/tobacco/highlights.htm.

Substance Abuse and Mental Health Services Administration. (2000). *National Household Survey on Drug Abuse: Population estimates, 2000.* Retrieved May 13, 2002, from www.samhsa.gov/oas/NHSDA/2kNHSDA/highlights.htm.

Tarter, R. E. (1990). Evaluation and treatment of adolescent substance abuse: A decision tree method. *American Journal of Drug and Alcohol Abuse, 16,* 1–46.

Tarter, R. E., & Hegedus, A. M. (1991). The Drug Use Screening Inventory. *Alcohol Health and Research World, 15,* 65–76.

Vastag, B. (2001). Mixed message on prescription drug abuse. *Journal of the American Medical Association, 285,* 2183–2184.

Weisner, C., Mertens, J., Parthasarathy, S., Moore, C., & Lu, Y. (2001). Integrating primary care with addiction treatment: A randomized controlled trial. *Journal of the American Medical Association, 286,* 1715–1723.

11

Sexual Dysfunctions and Deviations

Nathaniel McConaghy

Description of the Disorders

The descriptions of mental disorders provided by the *Diagnostic and Statistical Manual of Mental Disorders*, Fourth Edition (*DSM-IV*; American Psychiatric Association [APA], 1994) are those currently most widely used in the scientific literature. Development of the *DSM* beginning with the third version was strongly influenced by the criticism of previous diagnostic procedures which allowed clinicians considerable latitude in determining the features on which they based their diagnoses. As a result the diagnoses made on the same patients by different clinicians could vary considerably, that is, they lacked reliability. Matarazzo (1983) emphasized that these levels could be as low as 49–63% for specific psychiatric diagnoses. To minimize this cause of reduced diagnostic reliability, criteria were defined in recent versions of the *DSM* for most mental disorders. The aim was that the definitions would be sufficiently precise that different interviewers would experience no uncertainty as to whether the criteria were present or absent in a particular patient. Ideally the definitions were those termed operational, in that each operation involved in reaching the diagnosis was defined so completely that no subjective judgment was necessary by the interviewer. Though succeeding editions of the *DSM* have attempted to provide such operationally defined criteria for mental disorders, many of the attempts still remain unsuccessful, perhaps more for sexual dysfunctions and deviations than other conditions. Criticisms of the *DSM-IV* diagnostic criteria, terminologies, and omissions for the sexual dysfunctions and deviations continue to be made in the clinical and research literature.

Nathaniel McConaghy • School of Psychiatry, University of New South Wales, Paddington, N.S.W. 2021, Australia.

SEXUAL DYSFUNCTIONS

DSM-IV described sexual dysfunctions as characterized by disturbance in sexual desire and in the psychophysiological changes that characterize the sexual response cycle. It detailed diagnostic features for four groups of sexual dysfunctions. Sexual desire disorders included hypoactive sexual desire, deficiency or absence of sexual fantasies and desire for sexual activity, and sexual aversion disorder, aversion to and active avoidance of genital sexual contact with a sexual partner. Sexual arousal disorders included female sexual arousal disorder, persistent or recurrent inability to attain, or to maintain until completion of the sexual activity, an adequate lubrication-swelling response of sexual excitement; and male erectile disorder, a similar inability in relation to adequate erection. Orgasm disorders included female and male orgasmic disorders, persistent or recurrent delay in, or absence of, orgasm following a normal sexual excitement phase; and premature ejaculation, persistent or recurrent onset of orgasm and ejaculation with minimal sexual stimulation before, on, or shortly after penetration and before the person wishes.

To diagnose hypoactive sexual desire, arousal, and orgasmic disorders, *DSM-IV* stated the clinician should take into account such factors as the subject's age, sexual experience, adequacy of sexual stimulation, novelty of the sexual partner, and frequency of sexual activity. It did not give operational criteria on which the clinician could base decisions concerning these factors. Some researchers individually developed such criteria. Rowland, Cooper, and Schneider (2001) reviewed attempts to provide them for premature ejaculation and suggested use of a flowchart as a solution. Kelly, Strassberg, and Kircher (1990) provided operational criteria for the diagnosis of female orgasmic disorder. It was to be diagnosed as present in women if they reported that orgasm resulted from 5% or less of all sexual activities with their partners and absent if it resulted from 70% or more of such activities. The *DSM-IV* group of sexual pain disorders included dyspareunia, recurrent or persistent genital pain associated with sexual intercourse in either a male or a female; and vaginismus, recurrent or persistent involuntary spasm of the musculature of the outer third of the vagina when penetration with penis, finger, tampon, or speculum is attempted.

To receive a *DSM-IV* diagnosis of sexual disorder in the above four categories, the condition must cause marked distress or interpersonal difficulty. This allowed absence of orgasmic capacity not to be considered a dysfunction in the significant percentage of women who report they enjoy intercourse although they do not reach orgasm (McConaghy, 1993). If any sexual dysfunctions are better accounted for by another Axis I disorder (except another sexual dysfunction) they do not receive the diagnosis. Those due to the direct physiological effect of a substance (e.g., a drug of abuse or a medication) or a general medical condition are categorized separately. Diseases causing pain, debility, anxiety, or depression may impair sexual desire, arousal, and orgasm, as may drugs of abuse and a wide range of medications. These include antihypertensive agents, antiarrhythmics, diuretics, vasodilators, and psychiatric and anticonvulsant drugs (Schiavi & Segraves, 1995; The Process of Care Consensus Panel, 1999). The final category, sexual dysfunctions not otherwise specified, included those which do not meet the criteria of specific dysfunctions, such as when the clinician cannot determine if the dysfunction was primary or due to a medical condition or substance. In investigating sexual dysfunctions in patients with panic disorder and social phobia, Figueira, Possidente, Marques, and Hayes (2001) excluded the *DSM-IV* criterion for sexual dysfunctions, which stated that the diagnosis should not be given to those conditions which were better accounted for by another Axis I disorder. They did so because they considered this criterion prevents awareness of the impact of anxiety disorders on sexuality.

An important omission in the *DSM-IV* may have resulted from its basis in the medical model. It ignored aspects of sexual behaviors that are common and important in determining the sexual satisfaction of couples, or at least of middle-class couples who are mainly the subjects of research. Frank, Anderson, and Rubinstein (1978) investigated the presence in 100 predominantly White, well-educated, happily married couples not only of sexual dysfunctions, problems of performance, but also what they termed sexual difficulties, problems resulting from the emotional tone of sexual relations. The most common difficulties reported by the women were inability to relax, too little foreplay before intercourse, disinterest, and the partner choosing an inconvenient time. The most common reported by the men were attraction to persons other than their spouses, too little foreplay before intercourse, too little tenderness after intercourse, and the partner choosing an inconvenient time. Not only were difficulties more commonly reported by men and women than were dysfunctions, their presence correlated more strongly with reduced sexual satisfaction than did dysfunctions. In men, the correlation between presence of dysfunctions and reduced sexual satisfaction was insignificant. Similar findings were reported in a study of couples seeking treatment for lack of sexual satisfaction (Snyder & Berg, 1983). Sexual dissatisfaction in women did not correlate with the presence of dysfunctions, and in men only with the uncommon dysfunction of failure to ejaculate in intercourse. Sexual dissatisfaction in both sexes correlated strongly with the partner's lack of response to sexual requests, and the frequency of intercourse being too low. The nature of sexual difficulties suggests that they result from poor communication in couples concerning their sexual wishes and needs.

SEXUAL DEVIATION: PARAPHILIAS AND GENDER IDENTITY DISORDERS

The terms "paraphilias" and "gender identity disorders" are used in the *DSM-IV* for conditions previously referred to as sexual deviations; behaviors seen as deviating from those currently considered socially acceptable. The essential features of paraphilias were stated to be recurrent, intense sexually arousing fantasies, sexual urges, or behaviors generally involving (1) nonhuman objects, (2) the suffering or humiliation of oneself or one's partner, or (3) children or other nonconsenting persons, that occur over a period of at least six months. The fantasies or urges do not have to be carried out, but as with the behaviors, must cause significant distress or impairment in social, occupational, or other important areas of functioning. This and the criterion requiring their presence over at least 6 months are those which have made the *DSM-IV* classification of paraphilias unacceptable to many researchers and clinicians. O'Donohue, Regev, and Hagstrom (2000) detailed their objections in relation to the diagnosis of pedophilia. The comment of Marshall and Eccles (1991) regarding the earlier version of the *DSM* classification remains relevant to the *DSM-IV*. This was that many rapists, incest offenders, exhibitionists, and a substantial number of non-familial child molesters, do not display or report deviant sexual urges yet they persistently engage in sexually offensive behaviors, so that most clinicians tend to ignore *DSM* disorders. The subjects who carry out these behaviors are commonly called sex offenders, a term requiring legal rather than mental disorder criteria.

DSM-IV provided brief descriptions for some commoner paraphilias. These include exhibitionism, exposure of one's genitals to an unsuspecting stranger; fetishism, use of nonliving objects (e.g., female undergarments); voyeurism, the act of observing an unsuspecting person who is naked, in the process of disrobing, or engaged in sexual activity; and frotteurism, touching and rubbing against a nonconsenting person. Pedophilia, defined as sexual activity with a prepubesent child or children (generally aged 13 years or younger) by a person who is at least 16 years and 5 years older, was included. Hebephilia, sexual attraction of older persons to pubertal or immediately postpubertal subjects, was not. It is mainly experienced or expressed by men toward young males and has similar characteristics to male homosexual pedophilia in that its subjects are commonly not sexually attracted to or interested in social relationships with adults, making both conditions resistant to treatment.

Another significant omission from the *DSM-IV* classification of paraphilias was sexual assault. Involvement in sexual masochism and/or sadism was included and related to torture, mutilation, or killing. The evidence from investigations of men and women who belong to clubs for sado-masochists indicates that their behaviors rarely involve significant trauma or causes significant distress or impairment in social, occupational, or other important areas of functioning (McConaghy, 1993). The *DSM-IV* descriptions were that sexual masochism involved the act (real, not simulated) of being humiliated, beaten, bound, or otherwise made to suffer. Sexual sadism involved acts (real, not simulated) in which the psychological or physical suffering (including humiliation) of the victim is sexually exciting. Telephone scatologia (obscene phone calls), necrophilia (corpses), partialism (exclusive focus on part of the body), zoophilia (animals), coprophilia (feces), klismaphilia (enemas), and urophilia (urine) were listed as examples of paraphilias not otherwise specified.

Changes in the *DSM-IV* classification of cross-dressing behaviors including abandonment of the terms transvestism and transsexualism created considerable confusion. Transvestic fetishism was classified as a paraphilia occurring in heterosexual men, distinguished from the sexual use of female clothes in fetishism by the clothes being used for cross-dressing. It included the wearing of female clothes to produce sexual arousal accompanying masturbation, the form found most commonly in adolescent boys. Their need to obtain female clothes secretly may lead them to steal from clotheslines or from neighboring houses, leading to criminal charges. An unknown percentage of adolescent boys with transvestic fetishism develop the adult form, previously termed transvestism. It is characterized by reported reduction or loss of sexual arousal with cross-dressing as it increasingly produces feelings of relaxation, relief from responsibility, and/or of sensuality, elegance, and beauty (McConaghy, 1993). There are no reports of women periodically cross-dressing to enjoy feeling masculine when alone. Person, Terestman, Myers, Goldberg, and Salvadori (1989) found that a percentage of female university students experienced fetishistic transvestism similar to that of adolescent males. Men who in adulthood experience the change in motivation for cross-dressing often join social clubs organized by men with the condition. As most stress that the sexual arousal associated with their cross-dressing is no longer of significance, their *DSM-IV* classification as transvestic fetishists rather than transvestites is unacceptable to them and therefore seems inappropriate. The *DSM-IV* classification has led to controversy in relation to its statement that the disorder had been described only in heterosexual men (Bullough & Bullough, 1997; Zucker, 1997).

A percentage of male transvestites, who in adolescence experienced sexual arousal to cross-dressing, seek sex-conversion in adulthood, usually as they approach middle age. The majority of men seeking sex-conversion do so in early adulthood and report they cross-dressed since childhood without sexual arousal, to conform with feelings that they really belonged to the opposite sex. Women seeking sex-conversion do so over a wider age range but otherwise give a similar history, never having experienced sexual arousal with cross-dressing. Many clinicians continue to term these women and both groups of men who seek sex-conversion, transsexuals, rather than as having gender identity disorder, the diagnosis given them in the *DSM-IV*. Its primary criterion for the diagnosis was a strong and persistent cross-gender identity. In adolescents and adults, this was manifested by the stated desire to be, to live, or to be treated as of the opposite sex; frequent passing as the other sex; or the conviction they had the typical feelings and reactions of the other sex. Additional criteria were (1) persistent discomfort or sense of inappropriateness with their sex, (2) the disturbance was not concurrent with a physical intersex condition, and (3) it caused clinically significant distress or impairment in social, occupational, or other important areas of functioning. The *DSM-IV* also gave the diagnosis of gender identity disorder to male and female children who showed marked opposite-sex type behaviors, who were termed homosexual by pediatricians in the 1940s and 1950s (Bender & Paster, 1941). *DSM-IV* stated gender identity disorder was manifested in children by four or more of the features: (1) desire to be, or the insistence that one is, of the other sex; (2) cross-dressing; (3) preference for cross-sex roles in play or fantasy; (4) intense desire to participate in opposite-sex games and pastimes; and (5) strong preference for opposite sex playmates. The majority of these children identify as homosexual in adulthood, and a few identify as transsexual. The former are, of course, not classified in the *DSM-IV* as having a mental disorder, while the latter are diagnosed as having gender identity disorder. Green and Young (2001) retained the term transsexuals for the men and women they diagnosed using the criteria of the *DSM-IV* for gender identity disorder.

Sexual disorders not otherwise specified include distress about a pattern of repeated sexual relationships involving a succession of lovers who are experienced by the individual only as things to be used, and persistent and marked distress about sexual orientation.

Procedures for Gathering Information

The Clinical Interview

Though little research has investigated how the majority of clinicians obtain information about the sexual disorders of patients who seek treatment, it appears that the major method remains the clinical interview. The Process of Care Consensus Panel (1999) concluded that taking a comprehensive sexual, medical, and psychosocial history was the essential first step in the management of erectile dysfunction. The Panel was established with the support of a grant from the Sexual Function Health Council to develop a model for evaluation and treatment of erectile dysfunction. It consisted of 11 U.S. multidisciplinary specialists who were recognized authorities in the treatment of male sexual dysfunction. The core positions of the Panel were developed in a three-stage process, which included (1) an initial consensus conference, (2) focus group discussion with primary care practitioners, and (3) expert panel review and formulation of clinical guidelines. Marshall (1999) in his review of current North American treatment programs for sexual offenders considered eight areas of functioning that were typically assessed by interviews, self-report questionnaires, and physiological procedures. Most programs operated on a limited budget, and if a fully comprehensive assessment package was employed, there would be little time or resource left to do treatment. Under these conditions, interviews should provide most of the information along with a limited set of self-report measures. Andrews, a major researcher of diagnostic procedures, stated that physicians in clinical practice make diagnoses by listening to the patient and, after a few minutes, formulating a hypothesis as to the probable diagnosis. They then listen further and ask additional questions as a means of checking the validity of their original hypothesis (Andrews & Peters, 1998). My own practice varies to the extent that after formulating a diagnostic hypothesis I ask further questions to attempt to invalidate that hypothesis by excluding possible alternative diagnoses.

It is likely the clinical interview remains the major diagnostic tool of clinicians because of its flexibility, which is reduced in semistructured and totally lacking in structured interviews, discussed subsequently. Following the introduction of the latter interviews, the clinical interview was frequently termed unstructured. This term is misleading as the clinical interview does have a structure in the sense that it investigates specified domains, though not necessarily in a specific order. Marshall (1999) listed the appropriate domains for interviewing sex offenders as sexual behavior, social functioning, life history, cognitive processes, personality, substance abuse, physical problems, and relapse-related issues. As pointed out in the *Maudsley Handbook of Practical Psychiatry* (Goldberg, 1997), the clinical interview, rather than systematically checking a symptom inventory, starts with investigation of the patients' presenting condition. It proceeds to assess their mental state from their appearance and general behavior, talk, mood, attention and thought content, evidence of abnormal beliefs or interpretations of experiences or bodily sensations, and cognitive status in terms of memory, orientation, and general knowledge. In training students to use a clinical interview, they are commonly encouraged to keep a list of such domains by them to ensure they are all investigated.

The clinical interview enables the clinician to frame questions so that they are understandable and acceptable to the patients. If while investigating the presenting sexual problem the clinician gains the impression that it is secondary to more generalized emotional and relationship difficulties, these can be explored, as they may require priority in treatment. The clinical interview allows the specific inquiries to be made which are necessary to establish the presence of sexual dysfunctions and difficulties in patients who do not spontaneously report them. Several studies have established that such patients make up the majority of those with these conditions (McConaghy, 1993). The interviewer can vary the nature and order of questions in the light of the patient's responses and behavior. They can decide, possibly intuitively more than consciously, the persona to adopt which is most likely to elicit the patient's trust and enable him or her to feel at ease. This requires taking into account the patient's sex, age, appearance, dress, socioeconomic background, intelligence, vocabulary, level of education, ethnic origin, and moral, ethical, and sexual attitudes and values. There is little research-based information concerning how different interviewers conduct clinical interviews. When observed in training and peer-review procedures, they vary markedly in the extent to which they modify their personalities including their vocabulary, assertiveness, and apparent ethical structure and social status to become the person they believe the patient would relate to best.

If patients show signs of guilt, embarrassment, or reluctance to talk when particular topics are introduced, clinicians can respond with encouragement and support. They can thus elicit crucial information, which may not be obtained with the rigid format of a structured interview or questionnaire. Patients are unlikely to reveal such information unless the clinician establishes a relationship with them, which makes them confident it will not be disclosed, deliberately or inadvertently, without their permission. Relevant information from patients who are developmentally delayed, brain damaged, severely depressed, markedly though disordered, confused, or under the influence of substances can often only be obtained by the appropriate modification of questioning which is possible with the clinical interview, unlike more structured procedures. It is generally accepted that these procedures are not suitable for patients who cannot give coherent responses to questions or maintain attention for periods of 30 min or more. In a validity study of the widely used structured Composite International Diagnostic Interview (CIDI) in patients with schizophrenia (Cooper, Peters, & Andrews, 1998), patients who could not do so were excluded. Some patients with severe depression, confusion, brain-damage, developmental delay, or under the influence of substances also cannot meet these criteria. Establishing and maintaining a relationship with these patients in which adequate information can be obtained requires the more flexible approach of the clinical interview. Also, these patients are rarely able or motivated to complete self-rating scales or questionnaires. This is particularly relevant in the assessment of sex offenders, a percentage of whom are intellectually impaired, brain-damaged, or psychotic (McConaghy, 1993).

Clinicians need to determine the policy to adopt concerning behaviors, which it is legally mandatory that they report. Finkelhor (1984) estimated that 36% of caseworkers in Boston did not report their last case of child sexual abuse. Berlin, Malin, and Dean (1991) advanced evidence that the introduction of mandatory reporting of such abuse in Maryland deterred undetected adult abusers from entering treatment and patients disclosing abuse that occurred during treatment. It failed to increase the number of abused children identified. Presumably, clinicians who routinely report such behaviors inform their patients concerning this policy at the beginning of the interview.

Directivity of the Interview

The interviewer may regularly modify the directivity of the clinical interview, enabling information not investigated in structured diagnostic interviews to be obtained. Commonly, the clinician commences the interview nondirectively, adopting a listening approach and asking a minimum of questions, so giving the patient the opportunity to take charge. This allows assessment of such aspects of patients' personality as their confidence, verbal ability, assertiveness, and dominance. If, as the interview progresses in a nondirective mode, the patient ceases to provide relevant information, the clinician can become more directive. The assumption of a more directive role needs to be done in a manner that does not threaten or antagonize assertive patients, or allow obsessional or paranoid patients who commonly provide excessive details, to consider that the clinician is dismissing information they consider highly relevant.

Content of the Interview

As pointed out above, the clinical interview is usually commenced by asking patients the nature of their problem or why they have sought help. While assessing how the patient responds to this opportunity to take charge of the interview, it usually is possible also to obtain much of the information required to establish the nature of their presenting complaint. Additional necessary information can be obtained after the clinician becomes directive in questioning. This information usually includes any past history of similar problems, other illnesses, previous treatment, childhood and adolescent relationships with parents and siblings, social and sexual relationships and practices including fantasies, unwanted sexual experiences, coercive acts carried out, and history of contraceptive use where appropriate. Educational and work history, current domestic, social, sexual, and occupational situations, including the nature and extent of recreational interests and activities, use of recreational drugs, including alcohol and tobacco as well as any medications, and any past criminal offenses also need to be determined. If the patient's presentation of his/her history, and/or their vocabulary, suggest the presence of memory or intellectual impairment, this will require specific investigation. Severity of depression requires assessment if there is evidence of reduced enjoyment of life events or of appetite or sleep disturbance. If the patient has had previous treatment or been charged or convicted with criminal offenses, records of such treatment or charges should be obtained where possible.

Investigation of some sexual experiences poses special problems. Wyatt and Peters (1986) considered that multiple probing questions needed to be asked about specific types of abusive sexual behaviors by interviewers given special training in ideologically correct attitudes to identify women who had been sexually abused in childhood. Studies using this methodology found much higher prevalence rates than did studies not using them. At the same time it is necessary to avoid influencing the patient by suggestion to develop false memories of coercion. Damages have been awarded against therapists on the basis that they implanted false memories of child sexual abuse in patients (Arndt, 1994).

Interview with the Partner

In view of the importance of couples' communication of sexual feelings and wishes to their sexual satisfaction, the relationship of patients with sexual difficulties or dysfunctions with their partners should be assessed by interviewing the couple. Interviews of partners may also be indicated for patients with other sexual disorders, particularly if the presence of personality disorders is suspected. These interviews may be carried out after the initial assessment of the patients or, where appropriate, delayed until treatment is initiated. The nature of the couple's relationship is most commonly made intuitively from observation of their interaction in the interview, interpreted in the light of both partners' account of their present and previous relationships. In addition to verbal expressions indicative of affection or hostility, or indeed of both, the couple's body language including supportive touching usually gives the interviewer insight into the nature of their relationship. If the presenting person questions the need for the partner to be interviewed as he or she and not the partner has the sexual problem, the possible importance of the information the partner can supply when interviewed, initially alone and then with the patient, should be emphasized.

Establishment of the Therapeutic Relationship

It is my practice to attempt to formulate hypotheses concerning the nature of the patient's condition and personality within a few minutes of initiating the interview and, in the light of these hypotheses, to commence to consider the treatment most likely to be effective with which the patient will comply. The rest of the interview is then used to obtain data to support or reject these hypotheses. Other clinicians may prefer to continue to collect information without the need of such hypotheses. It is important to remain aware from the beginning of the clinical interview that while one is obtaining the information considered relevant, one is also commencing the process of treatment by establishing a relationship with the patient which will maximize his or her confidence and trust in one's abilities.

The degree to which this is done successfully not only will increase the nonspecific effects of the treatment instituted but the likelihood the patient will continue
to comply with it. Reported dropout rates from treatment for sexual dysfunctions
and deviations vary remarkably (McConaghy, 1993). It is likely that this in part
reflects the varying abilities of clinicians to establish appropriate relationships
with their patients.

Personality Assessment

Determination of the presence of significant personality disorders in patients
seeking treatment for sexual disorders is of major importance clinically because
personality disorders markedly influence patients' ability to provide accurate
information, their motivation to change their behaviors, and the nature of the relationship they attempt to establish with the clinician. If this relationship is handled
inappropriately, lack of compliance with, or major disruption of the treatment
plan can result, so that the patient is not helped or indeed may be harmed, and
the clinician may also suffer considerable distress. The personality features I have
found most important to detect in diagnostic interviewing of patients with sexual
disorders are those indicative of antisocial, borderline, and dependent personality
disorders. *DSM-IV* pointed out that although antisocial and borderline personality are both characterized by manipulative behavior, individuals with antisocial
disorder are manipulative to gain profit, power, or some other material gratification, whereas the goal in borderline personality disorder is directed more toward
gaining the concern of caretakers. The *DSM-IV* further pointed out that the essential feature of dependent personality disorder is a pervasive and excessive need to
be taken care of. To gratify their needs for power, concern, or care, patients with
these personality disorders attempt, possibly largely unconsciously, to make inappropriate relationships with the therapist. Early identification of the disorders will
alert the therapist to the likelihood of these attempts being made so that they can
be immediately dealt with appropriately.

Antisocial personality was one of the variables which significantly predicted
recidivism in the meta-analysis by Hanson and Bussiere (1998) of the findings of
61 sex offender recidivism studies. A further reason to recognize antisocial traits
is, as pointed out in *DSM-IV*, that patients who show them are frequently deceitful. They are likely to distort their account of their behavior, possibly in part
unconsciously, minimizing features, which show them in a bad light. It is therefore important where possible to check the reliability of the history they give
when interviewing partners or acquaintances, and by obtaining records of any
earlier treatments. Antisocial personality is more prevalent in male than female
patients (*DSM-IV*). Its presence may be suggested early in the interview by the
patients' air of confidence, at times reflected in his use without requesting
permission, of the first name of the interviewer. When he discusses behaviors or
sexual problems which could have harmful effects on others, particularly those
emotionally involved with him, he will usually show little evidence of ethical
concern or empathy if the interviewer maintains a neutral attitude and shows
no evidence of disapproval. Directive questioning is likely to reveal that he

commonly truanted in childhood and adolescence, abused drugs, and showed other delinquent behaviors. His subsequent record of educational, occupational, social, and sexual activities demonstrated an ability to easily form relationships and impress others with his qualities but an inability to persist once the activities or relationships become demanding or boring.

Antisocial patients are likely to comply poorly with treatment and frequently miss appointments. Consistent with their tendency to be deceitful, they may deny having carried out offenses of which they have been convicted. Many sex offender treatment programs will not accept subjects who deny their offenses. Maletzky (1996) criticized this approach. Impressed that sexual offenders mandated into treatment did as well as those who entered voluntarily, he followed up offenders who maintained denial at entry to his program. Sixty percent admitted something by the end of a cognitive behavioral program. Also, the vast majority of those who completed the program while continuing to maintain denial, did not relapse. They were markedly safer to be in the community than were those who admitted their offenses but did not complete treatment. Schlank and Shaw (1996) involved men who denied carrying out the sex offense of which they were convicted in a victim empathy module. The men were referred by their probation officers after failing to be accepted into therapy programs due to denial. Though their denial was not directly challenged, they were informed that the treatment module aimed at reducing it and so prepare them for a regular treatment program. If they were no longer in denial by the end of the module, they would not be required to undertake physiological evaluations and would be refunded the payment they had contributed for them. Fifty percent admitted their offenses by the end of the module. In my experience, if antisocial patients can be maintained in treatment by attempting to establish a relationship with them on the basis of their own values, this at times benefits both them and the society. With this approach, I stress the value of therapy in increasing their life satisfaction or enabling them to avoid unpleasant social consequences or incarceration. I find evidence of disapproval from the therapist results in these patients being less likely to report behaviors, which they sense will elicit further disapproval.

Borderline personality disorder though occurring in some men, is more likely to be shown by women (*DSM-IV*). As pointed out earlier, *DSM-IV* stated that patients with this disorder are driven to gain the concern of caretakers. Its recognition early in the interview is important so that the therapist can be alerted to the need to set appropriate limits to deal with the possibility of some borderline patients' potential seductiveness. Its presence may be indicated by the patients' expressions of intense gratitude, stating that for the first time in their lives they have encountered someone who is really concerned for them, who truly understands them, and to whom they have revealed information they have told no one else. The inexperienced therapist may accept these statements at face value rather than seeing them as possible indications that the patients have unconscious wishes to establish a special intimate relationship, so they will be treated differently from the therapist's other patients. Other forms of presentation of these subjects can also result in the therapist becoming over-involved and losing objectivity. They may show an initial apathy and withdrawal which the therapist feels challenged to overcome. They may give a distressed recital of overwhelmingly tragic life events, so eliciting the therapist's sympathy. They may report impulses to carry out aggressive or sexual attacks on children and at times imply they have acted on such impulses, so that the therapist reacts with shock and alarm. The potential danger of failure of the therapist to deal appropriately with these patients' needs for concern is highlighted by the finding that sexual involvement of therapists with patients, which occurs at a disturbingly high frequency, is most likely to be reported by patients with borderline personalities (Gutheil, 1989).

Appropriate questioning usually will reveal that, like subjects with antisocial personality disorder, those with borderline personality disorder abused drugs or showed other delinquent behaviors in childhood and adolescence. They commonly were involved in sexual relationships they experienced as destructive due to their transience, their association with emotional turbulence or aggression, and/or their resulting in pregnancy. They frequently report being victims of child sexual abuse, often in the form of incest. Suicidal attempts, or self-mutilative acts, such as cutting arms or legs, are often repeated, consistent with the low self-esteem basic to this personality disorder. Once alerted to the possible presence of borderline personality features in the patient, the therapist needs to be aware of the importance of establishing a relationship in which the patient will improve and the therapist remains comfortable. In dealing with the patient's needs for concern, the therapist should show the same level as she or he does with other patients.

Treatment of these patients is likely to be long and involved, often with an initial honeymoon period when they appear to respond and their relationship to the therapist is positive, followed by relapse and requests for more time and attention. This second stage may prove threatening to the therapist who initially became over-involved in response to the patients' mode of presentation, and so gave them a great deal of attention and time. When therapists become aware of patients with borderline features, they should inform the patients that they will continue to see them for as long as is necessary and define the amount of time they can give to this. With this procedure, there is no danger of the therapists giving more time in the initial stages of treatment than they can maintain indefinitely. It enables the therapist to continue to see the patient irrespective of their behavior within the limits established at the commencement of therapy.

Dependent personality disorder is associated with either an inability to tolerate normal anxiety and depression produced by inevitable life stresses, or a tendency to react to these stresses with above-average levels of these emotions. It will be suggested in the interview by the patients' lack of confidence, evident anxiety or depression, and excessive requests for help. Its diagnosis is supported by evidence of their past inability to cope with the stresses which were a part of their education, employment, and emotional relationships. People with this personality will give a history of having performed poorly at school, as they found examinations stressful, and often avoided them. They are likely to have had several jobs, leaving one after another as they encountered difficulties. The *DSM-IV* description points out that they tend to allow other people (often a single other person) to take the initiative and assume responsibility for most major areas of their lives. In my experience the people who assume this responsibility are commonly supportive or controlling in personality and consciously or unconsciously prefer relationships with dependent persons. Like the patients they may resist the therapist's attempts to change the nature of the patients' dependent relationships.

In the diagnostic interview of patients with dependent personalities, the clinician needs to be sufficiently supportive to engage these patients while encouraging the maximum independence of which they are capable. Particular attention needs to be given to discovering activities which they are likely to enjoy but require some independence. If the patients can be persuaded to carry them out, they will reinforce the behavioral changes the therapist wishes to produce. The activities could include physically sensual activities such as massages or warm baths for patients with hypoactive sexual desire. Their partners or other important acquaintances should be encouraged to gradually cease rewarding with sympathy the symptoms shown by the patient to elicit caring responses, and commence rewarding healthy behaviors with encouragement and praise. Without this change, dependent patients are likely to remain unmotivated to cooperate with the therapist's treatment plan.

When it is suspected that patients have significant personality disorders, it is more imperative that attempts be made to corroborate their history by interviewing relatives and contacts. It is not unusual for patients with antisocial or borderline personalities to try to prevent this, saying, for example, that they dislike their relatives too much to allow any contact. If it is considered sufficiently important, it may be necessary to make treatment conditional on their giving permission for such interviews.

Termination of the Interview

Toward the end of the diagnostic interview, the clinician should be planning its termination and must allow sufficient time for this. Without this, patients can leave feeling they have been asked a lot of questions or been allowed to talk freely but have been given no answers. It is my practice at this stage to present the patient either with a treatment plan or an explanation why further information is required before this can be done. Other therapists prefer to interview the patient on a number of occasions before making a decision about treatment. When a treatment plan is proposed, the clinician should ensure that patients are fully aware of what it entails, including its likely cost, and why it, rather than alternatives, has been selected. Any reservations patients have concerning the plan should be fully dealt with, so that following its discussion they commit themselves either to accepting the plan, or to make a decision concerning this within the next week, possibly in consultation with the person who referred them.

Validity of the Clinical Interview

Research evaluating the validity of diagnostic interviewing has largely been limited to investigating structured and semistructured procedures. It will be discussed in relation to them. From an experiential perspective, the accuracy of the information obtained in a clinical interview depends on the ability of the clinician to correctly assess to what extent the patient's self-report can be accepted without modification and to what extent it should be regarded as distorted and in need of further confirmation. Determination of the patient's personality is of value in this regard. Patients who are attention-seeking are likely to exaggerate their symptoms, those with antisocial personalities may lie concerning them, and those who are depressed or have the high ethical standards commonly associated with obsessional features may present them in a somewhat negative light. Though most clinicians feel confident of their ability to utilize the clinical interview to obtain information, which is at least sufficiently accurate for them to effectively treat their patients, little research has been carried out to justify this confidence. Furthermore, in their own practice, clinicians tend to modify the diagnostic categories they were taught to use during their apprenticeship with their teachers. This tendency for the diagnoses of clinicians to be somewhat idiosyncratic probably may not significantly alter the type of treatment all but a few patients receive. However, in the few where it does, it could be expected that the clinician believes the treatment indicated by his or her diagnosis will be more effective than the alternative treatment his colleagues making a different diagnosis would use. At times they may be correct. In relation to therapists using the same form of treatment, Guthrie (2000) considered it well established that some produce consistently better outcomes than others.

Observational Assessment

Intuitive interpretation of observations of subjects' nonverbal behaviors plays a major role in assessment in the clinical interview. As a separate assessment procedure, observations of sexual behaviors either directly or by videotape were briefly popular in the more permissive climate of the 1970s (LoPiccolo, 1990). LoPiccolo considered there were convincing arguments against their employment. These included that the effect of observation on patients with sexual dysfunctions would make it unlikely that their observed behaviors would be similar to their private behaviors, that the procedure would be unacceptable to the majority of couples, and that it allowed the exploitation of patients by the therapist. These issues were certainly relevant to the "sexological exam," described by LoPiccolo, in which sex therapists stimulated the breasts and genitals of the opposite sex partner to assess and demonstrate physiological responsiveness. However, it would seem possible to provide adequate ethical safeguards to allow videotaped observational assessment of couples' sexual interactions. With the use of preliminary sessions to allow the couples to adjust to the procedure, it would seem possible their observed behavior would be sufficiently related to their private behavior for its assessment to be of value. This is accepted to be the case with the observational assessment of non-sexual behaviors such as phobias, and the physiological assessment of genital arousal to sexual stimuli, both of which remain widely used. It is likely that taboos concerning sexuality remain the major obstacle to observational assessment of sexual activity. Such taboos contributed to the abandonment of surrogate sex therapy, in which such assessment played a major role. Observational assessment along with physical testing to determine the adequacy of erections was introduced for those occurring during sleep or produced by masturbation (Karacan, 1978). It remains an accepted practice in relation to erections produced by sildenafil citrate (Viagra), intracavernosal injection of prostaglandin E1 or other substances, or an external vacuum device.

Maletzky (1980) used observational assessment of treated exhibitionists. A comely actress, unknown to them, placed herself in situations in which they had previously frequently offended. The subjects had been informed that experimental and unusual procedures would be used. Observational assessments of the effeminate behavior of boys were made by clinicians (Rekers & Lovaas, 1974), teachers (Kagan & Moss, 1962), or parents (Bates, Bentler, & Thompson, 1973). The therapists observed boys playing with boys' and girls' toys through a one-way mirror. The teachers and parents were requested to complete inventories reporting the effeminate behaviors shown by their pupils or sons. A scale for rating behaviors observed in adult men, which were considered effeminate, was developed by Schatzberg, Westfall, Blumetti, and Birk (1975). It has not been used widely, possibly because of its complexity as well as the lack of attention given such behaviors in men as compared with the equivalent behaviors in boys. The *DSM-IV* discussed the differential diagnosis of what it termed sissy behavior in boys with gender identity disorder. It did not refer to effeminate behavior in men, however.

CASE ILLUSTRATIONS

A Sex Offender with Dependent Personality Disorder

The psychiatrist's letter concerning Mr. K. P., a 39-year-old man, stated he was referred for assistance with pedophilia. He was currently facing charges arising out of this problem. He was convicted of a similar offense in his early adult life for which he had been treated by a psychologist. He had been seeing the psychiatrist for some years for pain management related to a work accident. The psychiatrist added that the patient was a rather helpless personality with a history of poor psychosocial skills. Mr. K. P. was currently taking Prozac 40 mg. I also received a letter from his general practitioner, stating that Mr. K. P. said he was under the influence of alcohol when he carried out an indecent assault on a young boy. The doctor said Mr. K. P. was adopted and was repeatedly sexually assaulted when young by a neighbor who rewarded him with toys. The doctor considered the two issues that dominated the patient's life—chronic neck pain and the indifference of his wife. He was a very passive individual and expected others to solve his problems for him. He had received extensive counseling over the years to change aspects of his life without success. Both the psychiatrist and general practitioner referred to Mr. K. P. by his first name throughout their letters, suggesting they adopted a paternalistic attitude to him.

Prior to his appointment I received two letters from Mr. K. P. In one he stated he was abused as a child and had been adopted as his natural mother was addicted to drugs and could not look after him. His adopted parents never taught him about sex and used to control his life. He was on a disability pension and asked if I would consider reducing the fees for his treatment. His letter was accompanied by a certificate dated some months previously, stating he was on a disability pension and his wife was receiving a wife's pension and also a child disability allowance for their son. His other letter contained two psychological test results, but no attached letter from a psychologist. One was an 18 page Adult Clinical Interpretive Report titled "MMPI-2 and the Minnesota Report." It pointed out he felt socially inadequate, had poor social skills, avoided close relationships, was introverted, and viewed others as unfriendly or threatening. It concluded the most likely diagnosis was schizophrenia, possibly paranoid type, or a paranoid disorder, but that the information in the report should most appropriately be used by a trained, qualified interpreter. The second was a Myer–Briggs Type indicator, Form G, a self-scorable answer booklet. It informed Mr. K. P. he was an ISFJ type, a particularly dependable personality, sympathetic, tactful, kind, and genuinely concerned, and supportive to people. It continued in this positive vein, and concluded he was highly valued in the workplace and at home, and along with the extravert of his type, was the feeling backbone of our society. The 40 page "Introduction to Type" which accompanied it revealed that ISFJ was an Introverted Sensing with Extraverted Feeling type.

In my experience it is rare for patients to communicate with me prior to the initial interview, and those who do, unless they want specific relevant information, usually have a particular agenda. In the discussion of the clinical interview, I stated that within the first few minutes I attempted to develop hypotheses concerning the nature of the patient's condition and personality, which I then attempted to confirm or reject. In Mr. K. P.'s case, I developed such an hypothesis prior to the initial interview, based on the content of his clinicians' letters, and his expectation that I would be willing without payment to devote the time to read the extensive material he had sent prior to the initial interview. The hypothesis was that he had marked dependency needs and felt entitled to be given special consideration by others. As many people would not give him this special consideration, he was likely to feel aggrieved that he had not been treated fairly in his life. In relation to the psychological test results, I thought, in view of the information in his therapists' letters, that the personality description in the MMPI was likely to be accurate, but not the probable diagnoses of schizophrenia, though he may have some paranoid features.

In the initial interview Mr. K. P. reported he was charged with two sexual assaults on a boy aged 7. He was pleading guilty to the charges and was very anxious to receive treatment for sexual interest in children of which he was aware. He was seeing his referring psychiatrist every few weeks, a psychologist weekly, and his referring general practitioner at least monthly. The general practitioner had prescribed the antidepressant Prozac. He was in the process of seeking treatment from a religious institution, which provided treatment for sex offenders. It was very expensive and he was attempting to arrange for his church to pay for the program.

The history he gave was that he was adopted as a baby and raised as an only child by parents who though loving were very strict, and prevented him from having contact with other children. When aged 8, he was sexually assaulted on a number of occasions by a male neighbor, but did not report the behavior as he was happy to receive toys as an inducement. He was nervous at school, had no close friends, and was called a "poofter" (homosexual), possibly because he was poor at sport. He was aware of sexual attraction to boys who were usually a few years younger, but never acted on this. After he left school he obtained a clerical position. His first heterosexual experience was with a single mother when he was 22. Their relationship lasted a year, and he said he enjoyed her company but was not comfortable with their sexual activity as he did not find her attractive.

Due to his parents limiting his friendships and his staying out at night, he then shifted to another city where he did similar work. He felt lonely living on his own in a strange city, and went to a local swimming pool to meet people. He said some boys, whom he revealed on questioning to be aged 10, approached him for money and he did touch some of the boys, but the police bashed him up on several occasions, so that he agreed to everything they suggested to him. He pleaded guilty to the charges and was given a 3-year bond to accept treatment. As he described it, the treatment appeared to be cognitive–behavioral combined with a medication, which reduced his sexual urges. After it was ceased, he continued to be unaware of sexual attraction to boys. He subsequently had a sexual encounter with an adult man but did not enjoy it and did not repeat the experience. He then commenced a relationship with a woman colleague. However, he felt lacking in confidence in their sexual activity, often not being aroused or ejaculating prematurely, and they agreed to separate.

On a holiday in Thailand with the help of Thai friends, he met a number of women. After his return he wrote to some of them and then arranged for one to come to this country to marry him when he was aged 32. He was initially nervous in their sexual activity but later enjoyed it and thought his wife did also. They had two children, a girl aged 3 and a boy aged 6, who was treated for hyperactivity. About 4 years ago, he had a car accident driving to work, which resulted in severe back and neck pain which prevented him from working. He has remained on a disability pension and continues to have regular physiotherapy and oral medication and at times injections for pain.

His wife had been in clerical employment from soon after her arrival in Australia. I did not question why a few months previously she was receiving a wife's pension and a child disability allowance for their son. I thought if I did, this might make him suspicious that I was not sufficiently concerned for him. He might then withhold information about which he sensed I could be judgmental. He resented his wife keeping the money she earned for herself or to send to her parents in Thailand. In the last few years, she had sex with him only when he pleaded with her until refusing his requests for over a year. She now showed no affection to him and rejected any physical contact. He has not asked her why her feelings changed but suspected she might be involved with another man, as she spent a lot of time in social functions connected with her work, which she did not allow him to attend. She expected him to be totally responsible for looking after the children, and doing the shopping and housework, so that most of his days were taken up by these activities. What little social life he had was with Thai friends of his wife. Since the assault, he had been rejected by the Thai community. He did not usually drink alcohol or take other substances and had a strong involvement in the Anglican church.

In answer to direct questioning, he said he had started to become aware of sexual interest in young boys in the past few years when the sexual relationship with his wife deteriorated. The two sexual assaults with which he was charged took place when he was attending a party with his Thai wife and her friends and had drank almost a whole bottle of Asian rum which he said was not available in this country and contained 80% alcohol. He touched the penis over the clothes of the son of a family present at the party. He said this occurred when the boy was jumping on him. He followed the boy into a bedroom, performed fellatio on him, and was observed. Though he expressed marked regret for the sexual assaults, he did not appear depressed in mood, and his sleep pattern and appetite were unchanged. The main affect he expressed was a sense that he had been unfairly treated throughout his life.

My diagnostic assessment was that he suffered from homosexual pedophilia, a sex offense with a high risk of recidivism (McConaghy, 1993). His personality would constitute a barrier to treatment and would be resistant to change. It was likely he would seek supportive treatment from a number of therapists and would consider any attempts to limit this and confront his dependency needs to be unfair and lacking in concern for him. He would expect considerable time and attention from therapists without payment, an expectation some therapists would not be prepared to fulfil indefinitely. Their failure to do so would provoke resentment, which he would be unable to express openly, but would add to his sense of unfair treatment. While he remained in this psychological state, he would not be able to develop an appropriate sense of responsibility for his behavior.

A Patient with Sexual Aversion and Schizophrenia

Ms. S. V., aged 34, was referred for help with a complaint of sexual frustration associated with persistently elevated sexual arousal. On interview, she reported she had sexual urges all the time, which put her in a bad mood. She felt the urges in the genital area. She had never had a sexual partner and stated that she didn't trust men. She had formed a friendship with a man a few years ago and enjoyed his company at first. After a few months, she stopped seeing him as he wanted a more physical relationship. She would tolerate her hand being held but not kissing or cuddling. When asked if masturbation relieved the sexual urge, she said she rarely masturbated as she did not enjoy it. She then volunteered that when she was adolescent she had masturbated and enjoyed the associated feeling of sexual arousal. The feeling of sexual frustration commenced when she was aged 20. She agreed that her negative feeling to sexual arousal commenced at the same time, adding that she hated feeling aroused. When she was 22, a male friend kissed her and put his tongue in her mouth, which made her feel violated and she left, and stopped seeing him. She had no sexual contact with men since. She had fantasies of intercourse with them but felt bad that she experienced sexual arousal.

She gave a history of a happy childhood, feeling loved by her parents and close to her two older brothers. She enjoyed school and did well scholastically, studying accountancy at university. She had a close male friend there but did not kiss or cuddle as he had a girl friend. She thought that otherwise she could have wanted a sexual relationship with him. At age 20, she commenced to develop paranoid delusions, was suicidal, and was hospitalized for treatment of schizophrenia. Since then she was treated with a number of antipsychotic medications, responding initially, but then relapsing, so that she continued to be regularly hospitalized. There were periods when she was able to do clerical work and the feeling of sexual frustration was under control. She attributed this to an antidepressant being added to the antipsychotic medication. However the feeling would return, while she remained on the medication. From the age of 24, when she was out of hospital, she lived on her own, as she felt distressed when she felt sexually aroused with other people present. In her last employment about 18 months ago, she felt attracted to a male colleague but learned he had a partner. Her mental state then deteriorated severely with severe thought disorder and feelings of panic associated with the belief people were coming into the unit where she lived. She was again hospitalized. For the first time, she agreed to take clozapine. It was combined with the antidepressant, Prozac, and she improved markedly. She was able to return to live alone on a disability pension but continued to have some paranoid delusions from time to time. She spent most of her time at home, watching television. She felt her concentration was not sufficiently good for her to read.

As Ms. S. V. had remained emotionally appropriate and clear thinking to this point in the interview, I thought it was appropriate to discuss the possibility of adding cognitive behavioral management to her current therapy to reduce the feeling she labeled sexual frustration. I suggested it could result from normal sexual feelings which she experienced as negative. If she could be helped to replace this negative response with a positive one, this could lead to her expressing sexual feelings in behavior, and so lose the feeling of frustration. She showed marked rejection when I raised the possibility of her accepting these feelings, turning her head away and saying "I don't want to be sexually aroused, its disgusting." She added that a feeling of being watched made her dislike of being sexually aroused worse. She wanted a change of medication to relieve her of sexual feelings.

In view of her negative reaction I suggested that she might be more comfortable discussing the treatment I suggested with the psychiatrist who referred her. I could inform him concerning it. She then became angry and said that she would not get involved with the doctor who tried to help her accept her feelings of sexual arousal and that she would rather die than deal with it. Her angry feelings increased and she said challengingly "Why should I have to feel good about sex." I asked could she accept being helped to feel indifferent to sexual feelings. She then said "I'm being made to do this by others." As her level of anger continued to increase I considered that the stress of my suggestion was causing her to regress into a more paranoid state and that I should terminate the interview before she lost emotional control. I emphasized that it was entirely her decision concerning any treatment I had suggested and I would make this point when I communicated with her psychiatrist. She left at this point still obviously angry.

My assessment was that her schizophrenia was not sufficiently under control for her to be able to discuss calmly the use of a behavioral approach to her feelings of sexual frustration, at least with a psychiatrist who had not built up a positive relationship with her over time. It was possible that her negative feelings to sexual arousal resulted from a paranoid belief that people were aware when she felt sexually aroused, and so were due to schizophrenia rather than sexual aversion. This could be clarified if her schizophrenic symptoms responded to further treatment.

STANDARDIZED INTERVIEW FORMATS

The Structured Interview

In response to the evidence of the low reliability of diagnoses based on clinical interviews, researchers, particularly those involved in epidemiological studies, devoted considerable attention to attempts to improve it. Improved reliability, of course, does not guarantee improved validity, an issue which is only recently receiving adequate attention. The major issue for clinicians involved in patient treatment is whether adopting procedures which focus on increasing reliability will improve patient outcome. No attempts have been made to investigate what was termed by Nelson and Hayes (1981) the treatment validity of diagnoses reached by different clinicians or procedures. Treatment validity of a diagnosis measures the outcome with the treatment selected on the basis of that diagnosis. Clearly, improvement of this aspect of diagnoses would be of value to clinicians.

Increasing the reliability of diagnoses was accomplished in two ways. First, the criteria for making the diagnosis were standardized, as in the *DSM-IV*, and attempts were made to operationalize the definitions of the criteria, to limit differences in their interpretation by different interviewers. The second method to improve reliability was development of structured or semistructured interviews. With structured interviews, the interviewers ask the same questions in the same order and manner, usually after training to ensure they do so. Provided the patient answered the questions in the same way in interviews by two different interviewers, the diagnoses made by the two based on the patients' answers, and interpreted by the same operationally defined diagnostic criteria, should be the same, that is, their reliability would be perfect. Semistructured interviews allowed the interviewer, again usually following training, to depart to some extent from the structured set of questions. Structured and semistructured interviews unlike clinical interviews investigate only the patient's symptomatology, not other aspects of their life history.

The most widely used structured and semistructured interviews have not included modules for diagnosing sexual disorders. Clinicians treating these disorders have, therefore, to rely on evidence of the value of these interview formats from their use in other conditions, to determine if they should attempt to develop them for sexual disorders. First, they need to know if structured and semistructured interviews have meaningfully improved the reliability of diagnoses over those made in clinical interviews.

Relative Reliability of Clinical and Structured Interviews

Evidence of the low reliability of diagnoses based on clinical interviews, which is still cited, was found in studies in the 1970s and 1980s (Matarazzo, 1983). These compared the diagnoses made on the same patients by different clinicians, using their personal interview procedures and diagnostic criteria. At that time little attention was given to development of consistent diagnostic criteria. Currently most clinicians largely accept standardized criteria such as those of the DSM-IV. It is likely that similar studies of diagnoses made in clinical interviews would now find higher reliability. This was the case for the only such study which has been conducted, discussed subsequently (Peters & Andrews, 1995). As stated earlier, research has largely been limited to investigating the reliability and validity of structured interviews. However, no studies have investigated their reliability using the methodology of the 1970s and 1980s studies of clinical interviews. These would require comparison of diagnoses reached using different structured or semistructured interviews and also different accepted diagnostic criteria. Studies doing one of these two things have been carried out and found levels of reliability which were not superior to those of the earlier clinical interviews.

van den Brink et al. (1989) interviewed 175 nonpsychotic, nonaddicted psychiatric outpatients with the Present State Examination. Diagnoses were obtained using both the CATEGO computer program (Wing & Sturt, 1978) and DSM-III criteria (American Psychiatric Association, 1987). Agreement between the diagnoses made by the two diagnostic systems was 58% for cases of depression and 46% for cases of anxiety, comparable with the 49–63% for diagnoses made by different clinicians using clinical interviews in the earlier studies (Matarazzo, 1983). Using the opposite procedure of comparing diagnoses made with different structured and semistructured interviews using the same diagnostic criteria, Andrews, Peters, Guzman, and Bird (1995) also found similar low levels of reliability. Their study was the first to compare the widely used structured CIDI and the semistructured Schedules for Clinical Assessment in Neuropsychiatry (SCAN). Both were administered by trained interviewers in counterbalanced order to diagnose 101 patients. Scoring algorithms were developed, in consultation with the developers of the instruments, to allow DSM-III diagnoses to be made for agoraphobia/panic, social phobia, obsessive compulsive disorder, and depression from both interviews. The kappa values indicated that the concordance between the

CIDI and the SCAN diagnoses was at best fair, with the overall kappa for the diagnoses for the current period being 0.41 and for the lifetime period being 0.39.

Relative Validity of Clinical and Structured Interviews

Peters and Andrews (1995) pointed out that to assess the validity of diagnoses made using structured interviews such as the CIDI, they needed to be compared with diagnoses of established validity, yet such diagnoses were lacking. They commented that it was the lack of faith in the reliability and validity of the clinical interview that instigated the move to develop structured interviews. A single clinical interview was therefore not an appropriate "gold standard" against which to assess the CIDI. In the absence of such a standard, Spitzer (1983) suggested use of a clinical standard, which he termed a LEAD standard. This acronym referred to the three requirements for this standard diagnosis: (1) It should be based on Longitudinal information, obtained not in one evaluation, but at several points in time. (2) It should be a consensus diagnosis made by at least two Experts after they independently evaluate the patient. (3) All Data available for the patient except that from the instrument being assessed, should be taken into account in reaching the diagnosis. This could include questionnaire data, previous clinical information, and information from contacts. The advantage of the LEAD procedure was considered to be the fact that it emulated actual clinical practice. Peters and Andrews (1995) found it was not until the 1990s that studies examined the reliability and validity of LEAD diagnoses. They cited studies finding that these diagnoses were stable over a 6-month period, and that their interrater reliability was as good as that of diagnoses made using structured and semistructured interviews.

Peters and Andrews concluded that the LEAD standard proved a useful and robust procedure against which to test other diagnostic procedures. They used it to assess the validity of the CIDI-Auto to provide *DSM-III-R* diagnoses of seven categories of anxiety disorders in the diagnosis of 98 consecutive patients accepted for treatment at an Anxiety Disorders Unit. The CIDI-Auto is the World Health Organization (WHO, 1993) approved computerized version of the pencil-and-paper CIDI. The experts making the LEAD diagnosis were eight experienced clinicians at the unit. Each patient was interviewed in routine clinical fashion, without the use of checklists, by two of the experts. They independently made *DSM-III-R* diagnoses based on the information obtained at the interview, questionnaire data routinely collected at the unit, and any information supplied by clinicians who knew the patients, including that obtained during the period of 2–10 months the patients were treated. LEAD standard diagnoses were defined as the diagnoses on which there was consensus between the two experts at post-treatment or on which they could reach consensus after reconsideration. Consensus was reached by the experts for all patients. There were a total of 153 LEAD diagnoses and 298 CIDI-Auto diagnoses for the 98 patients, so that the CIDI-Auto produced about twice as many diagnoses per patient as did the LEAD procedure. Agreement for particular diagnostic categories was poor, with only two diagnoses having a kappa greater than 0.4. The greater number of diagnoses made by the CIDI-Auto compared to those made in the clinical interview was reflected in the pattern of sensitivity and specificity values, with the CIDI-Auto showing high sensitivity but low specificity. That is to say, the CIDI-Auto was unlikely to diagnose ill subjects as well, but to diagnose many well subjects as ill. Peters and Andrews (1995) concluded that in an epidemiological survey, where the aim is to determine the prevalence of disorders, the specificity of the CIDI-Auto will need to be improved, perhaps by altering the questions about severity to increase the threshold for diagnosis.

Cooper and Singh (2000) pointed out concern over similar findings of high prevalence of mental illness found in community surveys using structured interviews, and standardized diagnostic criteria were being expressed by workers who themselves were involved in planning the surveys. They reviewed the changes in prevalence of mental illness found over three periods in which structured interviews and standardized diagnostic criteria were developed. Prior World War II, the handful of studies based on clinical interviews by psychiatrists found mean prevalence estimates of under 4%. In the following period until around 1980 standardized interviews such as the Present State Examination were developed for use by psychiatrists and were found to provide good inter-rater agreement. Surveys using these procedures found the average prevalence of mental disorders to be around 20%. In the next two decades there was a shift from the use of semi-structured interviews by experienced clinicians to tightly structured schedules administered by trained lay interviewers and clinical evaluation by computerized diagnosis. Cooper and Singh 2000 pointed out that assessment of large population samples must, by virtue of the interviewer's lack of experience, omit the flexible probing and clinical judgment previously thought necessary for diagnosis. This contrasted with the intention of the developers of the widely used CIDI, which they stated, was to provide an instrument, which would as closely as possible replicate a psychiatrist's diagnosis in situations where diagnosis by clinicians was not feasible.

Cooper and Singh cited the review of Regier et al. (1998) of two large-scale estimates of the prevalence of mental disorders in the United States, the Epidemiological Catchment Area studies (ECA: Robins & Regier, 1991) and the National Comorbidity Survey (NCS: Kessler et al., 1994). Apart from marked differences in the mean prevalence rates of individual diagnoses, indicating poor reliability, the total prevalence rates were deemed too high to provide useful guidance to the extent of need. One year prevalence was 20%, and lifetime prevalence was 32% in the ECA first wave, and 29% and 48%, respectively, in the single-wave NCS. All these rates were considered so much higher than the annual estimate of 2.8% for severe mental disorder in the United States (National Advisory Mental Health Council, 1993) as to raise doubts about the relevance of such data in gauging service needs. Regier et al. (1998) considered that many people receiving diagnoses with structured interviews who did not come to medical attention may be having appropriate homeostatic responses that are neither pathological or in need of treatment. Alternatively the high rates of syndromes could be due to inclusion of mild forms of true psychopathological disorders. In either case they considered severity, impairment, comorbidity, and duration criteria additional to those in the

DSM-IV were required for relevant assessment of prevalence of mental disorders. They recommended that the deficits in compatibility between the Diagnostic Interview Schedule, the CIDI, and variants of the CIDI now being used in various parts of the world will need to be made explicit and reduced to have a cumulative science in which successive versions in instrument development produce increasing reliability and validity in estimating prevalence rates.

Cooper and Singh (2000) pointed out that reliance on fully structured survey techniques has not settled the question of diagnostic validity. They considered it was not generally appreciated how far most standardized interviews have diverged from the clinical case-taking methods, quoting Goldberg's (1997) description of these referred to earlier. They recommended that clinical judgment be restored to diagnosis of mental disorders. In this respect, they cited Regier et al.'s (1998) recommendation that as self-reported symptoms alone were inadequate for diagnosis, they should be supplemented by data on illness severity and duration and associated functional impairment. They considered that if these could be rated reliably at a single interview, this would constitute a real advance in public-health knowledge. They did not point out that such an interview would seem more equivalent to the traditional clinical interviews, which unlike standardized interviews, are not limited to investigation of patients' symptomatology.

Training in Clinical Interviewing

In the light of the evidence discussed, there would seem to have been an unfortunate lack of balance in attempts to improve diagnostic interviewing. Extensive resources have been devoted to the development of structured interviews to be administered by trained lay persons for use in epidemiological research, with the expectation that they would provide reliable and valid diagnoses. Meanwhile, little attention has been given to evaluating and, if necessary, attempting to improve the reliability and treatment validity of the clinical interview which appears to remain the most widely used procedure for making diagnoses for treatment purposes by clinicians. An incidental finding of the study of Peters and Andrews (1995), which attempted to validate the Auto-CIDI by comparison with LEAD diagnoses, indicated that the reliability of clinical interviews made by psychologists and psychiatrists working in the same treatment unit was high, as was their validity assessed against LEAD diagnoses. They found that the agreement between the diagnoses made by two interviewers following independent initial routine clinical interviews was excellent (kappa = 0.93). When the initial diagnoses were compared with the LEAD diagnoses made after 2–10 months, they were identical for 86 of the 98 patients. This finding suggests that diagnostic interviewing may be improved by devoting resources to evaluating the methods in which clinicians in their professional education are trained to use the clinical interview. The findings of Peters and Andrews (1995) indicate it should be possible to ensure that with appropriate training, clinicians will be able to make diagnoses using it which have high levels of reliability and validity comparable to those reported in their study.

However, the divergence in interest of clinicians and researchers seems such that there is little indication that researchers will adopt this approach rather than the current one of attempting to improve the reliability and validity of structured procedures by modifying diagnostic criteria to make them less liable to diagnose illness in well people. Adoption of this procedure in relation to the *DSM-IV* has been done in a manner which also seems to reflect the lack of interaction between experts who make these changes and experienced clinicians. Slade and Andrews (2002) pointed out that in response to criticisms that diagnoses reached with structured interviews were identifying symptoms considered not severe enough to warrant treatment, a diagnostic criterion for clinical significance was added to approximately half the diagnostic categories in *DSM-IV*. The symptoms were required to cause clinically significant distress or impairment in social, occupational (academic), or other important areas of functioning. Spitzer and Wakefield (1999) recommended that the clinical significance criterion should be evaluated separately for each disorder and, if shown redundant, removed. Sexual disorders were not examined in the surveys finding the high prevalences of mental disorders, so there would seem no indication to add this criterion to the *DSM-IV* criteria for sexual disorders. Nevertheless it was added, making the criteria for diagnosis of paraphilias unacceptable to many researchers and clinicians. Also, there is no empirical information on the reliability or validity of *DSM-IV* diagnoses of sexual disorders generally, due to their being ignored in *DSM* field trials (O'Donohue, Regev, & Hagstrom, 2000).

Clearly, diagnostic procedures established to be of high reliability are necessary for researchers to be confident that the patients who received a particular diagnosis in different studies suffered from the same defined group of symptoms. In view of the lack of development of standardized structured interviews for diagnosis of *DSM-IV* sexual disorders, some sexuality researchers developed their own procedures. Raymond, Coleman, Ohlerking, Christenson, and Miner (1999) designed a semistructured interview to evaluate the presence or absence of all *DSM-IV* sexual disorders. It followed the format used in the Structured Clinical Interview for *DSM-IV* Axis I Disorders—Patient Edition (SCID-P: First, Spitzer, Gibbon, & Williams, 1995). van Lankveld and Grotjohann (2000) used the structured CIDI (WHO, 1992) to evaluate *DSM-III-R* criteria for psychiatric disorders in heterosexual couples with sexual dysfunctions. As the interview did not investigate sexual disorders, they created a structured interview to diagnose them according to *DSM-IV* criteria. Figueira et al. (2001) employed the SCID-P to diagnose social phobia and panic disorder. As it did not diagnose sexual disorder, they developed what they termed a semistructured anamnesis for this purpose. The reliability and validity of diagnoses made by these individually designed procedures was usually unestablished. van Lankveld and Grotjohann supported the validity of the diagnoses made by their interview by comparing them with the subjects' responses to the Golombok Rust Inventory of Sexual Satisfaction (GRISS: Rust & Golombok, 1986).

Knowing that the diagnostic procedures they use are of high reliability in relation to those used by researchers would be of value to clinicians. They could apply the results of studies to their patients knowing that those they diagnosed with the same condition were comparable to those investigated in the studies. There is unfortunately no indication that such improvement in reliability and treatment validity of diagnosis will be made by improved training in clinician interviewing. Rather, as stated above, the current trend is likely to continue of modifying structured interviewing procedures and diagnostic criteria. If so, the suggestions being made that such interviews investigate aspects of the patient's condition additional to their symptomatology should be followed. Before adopting such structured interviews, clinicians will need to be reassured that the impersonality and lack of flexibility imposed on the interviewer by the structured procedure does not reduce the likelihood of engagement necessary for the patient to remain in treatment. Loss of patients is more important to clinicians whose income is dependent on the success of their practice, than for researchers. Indeed the latter could benefit from the loss of less compliant patients from their studies. This loss could contribute to the subjects of research studies not being representative of those treated by clinicians (Guthrie, 2000). As yet, the value of flexibility has been demonstrated in relation to treatment rather than interview procedures (Jacobson, Schmaling, & Holtzworth-Munroe, 1989). In the immediate future it would seem clinicians will continue to use the clinical interview as their major diagnostic procedure. Hopefully some researchers will follow Peters and Andrews (1995) in investigating the reliability and validity of diagnoses made with its current use.

QUESTIONNAIRE AND RATING SCALE INVESTIGATIONS

With the emergence of behaviorism as a major influence on clinical practice in the 1960s, the validity of data obtained in interviews was treated with suspicion as based on self-report rather than observation of behavior. As evidence demonstrated the limited validity and relevance of widely used behavioral observations in research, self-report as a source of information was rehabilitated (McConaghy, 1993). Some behaviorally oriented researchers preferred that subjects' self-reports were elicited by questionnaires or rating scales completed by patients rather than clinical interviews, expecting that this would increase the reliability of the information obtained. Also the former procedures were considered to have the added advantage of being less influenced by the interviewer. Findings of earlier studies were overlooked which suggested that the possible increase in reliability and apparent objectivity obtained may be at the sacrifice of some degree of validity. These studies investigated the accuracy of psychiatrists' assessments of patients' clinical response to treatment made in clinical interviews. The psychiatrists were required to determine which patients were treated with placebo and which with active medication. Their global judgments proved highly valid in comparison to the objective methods of assessing treatment response employed, which included psychological tests, rating scales, and physiological measures (Lipman, Cole, Park, & Rickels, 1965; Paredes, Baumgold, Pugh, & Ragland, 1966). Paredes et al. pointed out that in making global assessments in clinical interviews, clinicians were sensitive to a multitude of factors. When they were limited to rating behavior on scales, they narrowed their perspective, reducing their ability to make valid intuitive judgments.

A similar narrowing of perspective may occur with patients' assessments of their own responses. Women reported increased satisfaction in their sexual relationship on a sexual history form but decreased satisfaction with specific activities, determined by the Sexual Interaction Inventory (De Amicis, Goldberg, LoPiccolo, Friedman, & Davies, 1985). The authors suggested that the difference resulted from whether a global emotional response or attitude was assessed or a specific reaction to a given behavior or activity. They concluded sex therapy may have been more effective in improving the way clients felt about their sexuality than in reversing specific presenting symptoms. Rating scales are not necessarily immune from influence of the expectations of persons conducting the study. AuBuchon and Calhoun (1985) asked 18 women to record their mood on a 16-item adjective checklist twice weekly for 8 weeks. Nine were randomly selected and informed that the study was investigating a possible relationship of mood with their menstrual cycles. Their self-report scales demonstrated a negative relationship. The scales of those not so informed did not. The authors attributed the relationship found to the social expectancy and demand characteristics resulting from the information.

The validity of data collected by interview or questionnaire can vary depending on the sexual behavior and the subjects investigated, so that the validity of the questionnaire or rating scale needs to be established for the particular behavior and type of subjects investigated. Solstad and Hertoft (1993) interviewed a hundred Danish middle-aged men who had previously completed a questionnaire containing 46 questions about sexuality. In their questionnaire responses, none reported erectile dysfunction in the last year and four reported they had previously sought treatment because of problems in their sexual life. In the interview seven reported they suffered from erectile dysfunction more than occasionally in the last year and eleven reported that they had previously sought treatment for sexual problems. Durant and Carey (2000) compared the test–retest reliability over an 8-week period of data collected by interview compared to self-administered questionnaire, investigating the sexual behaviors of women psychology students. The students also completed daily diary cards during the period, reporting whether they had carried out the behaviors. The test–retest reliability for both interview and questionnaire data was high, but the frequency of vaginal intercourse with a condom reported in the interview was lower than that recorded in the diary. Also the discrepancy between the data obtained in both procedures and by diary was greater the more frequent the behaviors. Durand and Carey considered it was of significance that these young well-educated women underreported in interviews their practice of safer sex compared to riskier activities. The finding contrasted with those of studies of community samples of men and women who had homosexual, bisexual, or sex-worker partners.

Records in diaries that behaviors were carried out on a particular date may not have been made on that date, but subsequently, casting doubt on their accuracy. Taylor, Agras, Schneider, and Allen (1983) asked patients to record on diary cards their home use of relaxation audiotapes. Their use of the tapes was independently monitored without the patients' knowledge, by incorporation of electronic devices in the tape players with which they were provided. Comparison of the diary cards and monitoring devices revealed that 32% of patients falsely reported their use of the tapes on the cards. Reporting of failure to use a relaxation tape may not be comparable to reporting sexual behaviors. The latter may therefore be more commonly reported on the date stated in the diary. Use of an electronic diary incorporating a similar device could assess this but would infringe current consent requirements that patients be informed in advance of all details of investigations.

Holland, Zolondek, Abel, Jordan, and Becker (2000) stated that use of self-report questionnaires has become an integral part of assessing sexual interest in sex offenders, as it was sometimes easier for offenders to admit deviant thoughts and behaviors on self-report questionnaires. They advanced evidence that the Sexual Interest Cardsort Questionnaire had high internal consistency and correlated well with clinical classification. They emphasized it should be used only as part of a broad assessment, including clinical interview. Catania, Gibson, Chitwood, and Coates (1990a) found that telephone surveys were rapidly becoming the mainstay of AIDS-related sexual behavioral assessment, though drug users and street youth were unlikely to have residential telephones. They considered that depending on the sensitivity of the topic, measurement error might be less or greater than with face-to-face interviews, but there were indications that socially undesirable behaviors were less likely to be underreported in telephone interviews.

Lewontin (1995) questioned the validity of the data provided by self-reported questionnaire in the study by Laumann, Gagnon, Michael, and Michaels (1994), one of the first to provide comprehensive information concerning the sexual behavior of a representative sample of U.S. citizens. He focussed on the finding that men reported 75% more sexual partners in the most recent 5 years than did women, whereas the average number of sex partners reported by men and women should, discounting homosexual partners, be equivalent. Laumann et al. attributed the discrepancy largely to men exaggerating or women understating the number of their partners, leading Lewontin to comment that in the single case where one can actually test the truth, the investigators themselves think it most likely that people are telling themselves and others enormous lies.

Before this is accepted, other explanations for this commonly reported discrepancy between the reports of men and women need to be excluded (McConaghy, 1999). Studies reporting the discrepancy did not include female prostitutes who would have large numbers of male partners. Most investigated only heterosexual intercourse, raising the issue of how men and women who have had sexual intercourse with same sex partners react to such questions. Laumann et al. (1994) found that 9% of men and 5% of women had same sex partners. The majority of these men and women identified as heterosexual. The mean numbers of their partners compared to those of the remaining men and women were for men, 44.3 versus 15.7, and for women, 19.7 versus 4.9. It is possible that some of the men and women with same sex partners may report the number of these partners as if they were of the opposite sex, regarding questionnaires investigating only opposite sex relationships as homophobic. In a study of medical students, 17% of men and 9% of women experienced a person of the opposite sex being so sexually aroused they felt it useless to stop them when they themselves did not want sexual intercourse. Four percent of men reported they were so sexually aroused they could not stop themselves when the partner of the opposite did not want intercourse (McConaghy & Zamir, 1995). Women have consistently been found to consider the emotional component of sexual intercourse much more important than do men (McConaghy, 1993). It is possible that sexually coerced or coercive men as compared with women are more likely to include the perpetrator or victim in the number of their sexual partners. The finding that men report having more sexual partners that do women may be evidence not so much of lack of validity of their report of their sexual behaviors as of deficiencies in methodology of the investigations.

A number of studies have demonstrated the validity of self-reports for particular sexual behaviors. Degree of reduction in sex offenders' deviant sexual urges correlated with the medroxyprogesterone-produced reduction in their levels of testosterone, to which they were blind (McConaghy, Blaszczynski, & Kidson, 1988). Incidence of HIV seroconversion was predicted from risk indices based on self-reported sexual behaviors (Catania, Gibson, Marin, Coates, & Greenblatt, 1990b). Reported increase in safe-sex behaviors correlated with fall in prevalence of sexually transmitted diseases (McConaghy, 1993). Men's reports of their sexual orientation correlated with their penile volume responses (McConaghy, 1993). Men but not women who identify as homosexual as compared to heterosexual were consistently found to have more older brothers (Blanchard, 1997). Men and women who anonymously reported by questionnaire that they had a degree of homosexual feelings had more older brothers than those who reported no homosexual feelings (McConaghy et al., in press).

Both structured and clinical interviews can produce invalid data as compared with anonymous questionnaires due to the reluctance of subjects to report sexual behaviors about which they feel embarrassed. A series of studies using anonymous questionnaires found at least 20% of men and women reported ever having had homosexual feelings and/or activities. Less than 10% report them in interviews (McConaghy et al., in press). The validity of the anonymous reports was supported by their correlation with the subjects' reported opposite sex-linked behaviors and the number of their older brothers. Adolescents are more reluctant than adults to report socially unaccepted sexual feelings or behaviors. This reluctance resulted in experienced sex researchers accepting the statements of adolescents exposed to increased opposite sex hormone levels prenatally and their matched controls that virtually none had experienced such feelings or behaviors. The finding was ignored that the highest percentages of homosexual feelings or behaviors reported anonymously by adults were experienced in adolescence. At least one in five of the adolescents studied would be expected to have had homosexual feelings and/or behaviors (McConaghy, 1993).

In research studies of particular sexual behaviors, the use of questionnaires completed by the patient or the interviewer can be essential in ensuring that the relevant information concerning the behaviors is obtained from all subjects investigated. When the emphasis is on patient treatment, it is necessary to be aware that the use of structured procedures additional to the diagnostic interview can reduce patient compliance with treatment. Reading (1983) randomly allocated paid male volunteers to report details of their sexual behavior either by interview after 1 and 3 months; by interview after 1, 2, and 3 months; or by the latter procedure plus diary cards completed daily and returned every 3 days. Thirty-four percent allocated to the last form of assessment discontinued it, as compared to fourteen percent with the first, and sixteen percent with the second. Another three subjects dropped out from the diary card assessment prior to first month, considering it was causing them difficulty maintaining their sexual potency.

Wincze and Carey (1991) pointed out that though patient-completed questionnaires provided extensive information at little cost, they had not been widely used in clinical practice. They considered this was due to their administration being time-consuming and inconvenient in a busy practice and their clinical utility being limited as most were developed for specific purposes in research studies. Nevertheless they reported that in assessing patients with sexual dysfunctions they used a number of self-report questionnaires and suggested sources of other measures which could be useful. One of these, the compendium of Davis, Yarber, Bauserman, Schreer, and Davis, was updated in 1998. An example of limited clinical utility of questionnaires was reported by Andersen and Broffitt (1988). The Sexual Experience Scale of the Derogatis Sexual Functioning Inventory was not able to identify women subjects with sexual dysfunctions. They considered this was due to its providing a meaningful assessment of the occurrence of sexual behaviors but not their frequency. As an assessment of self-reported sexual behavior of sexually active heterosexual individuals, they considered that simple alternative could be self-reports of intercourse frequency. They found this frequency to be stably reported by healthy subjects over four occasions at four monthly intervals.

INFORMATION CRITICAL TO MAKING THE DIAGNOSIS

In diagnosing sexual disorders, as the earlier discussion of the validity of structured interview diagnoses has made clear, not only is it necessary to obtain information concerning the exact nature of dysfunctional, paraphilic, or gender identity disordered behaviors but to determine the significance to attach to it. The *DSM-IV* provided no operational definitions for many of the criteria necessary to make this determination, including the frequency which justifies the disorders being considered persistent. Sixty-three percent of the women and forty percent of the men in the predominantly White, well-educated, happily married couples investigated by Frank et al. (1978) experienced sexual dysfunctions at times. The most common in women were difficulty getting excited and/or reaching orgasm, and in men, ejaculating too quickly and difficulty getting or maintaining an erection. Irrespective of their persistence, their occurrence would attract *DSM-IV* diagnoses in only a minority, in view of the criterion requiring that they cause marked distress or interpersonal difficulty. Eighty-five percent of the couples stated that their sexual relations were very or moderately satisfying.

Seeking treatment for symptoms of sexual dysfunctions would seem an indication that they are causing marked distress or interpersonal difficulty. However, failure to seek treatment does not mean that the symptoms are not causing these problems, so they could still meet this *DSM-IV* criterion. The number of men and women who seek treatment for sexual problems is a small percentage of those identified both among patients reporting other illnesses and in community studies, as having the symptoms of sexual dysfunctions (McConaghy, 1993). Some may decide against treatment as they consider it will be too demanding, in terms of time or psychological effort, too expensive, or unlikely to be effective. To decide if the symptoms of sexual dysfunction justify a *DSM-IV* diagnosis in subjects who do not seek treatment, it is therefore necessary to establish the reasons for their decision. Knowledge of the development of effective physical treatments for erectile dysfunction, of which the first were penile prostheses and intracavernous injections, significantly increased the number of men seeking treatment for this disorder as compared to those for which there were no widely known equally effective procedures. Since its approval by the U.S. Food and Drug Administration in March 1998, sildenafil citrate (Viagra) has been used by millions of men for the treatment of erectile dysfunction (Boyce & Umland, 2001).

It is also important in making a diagnosis to establish the reason why subjects who report symptoms of sexual dysfunction do seek treatment. Women may do so for failure to achieve orgasm sufficiently frequently, not because they are dissatisfied, but because their partners are. It would seem inappropriate to immediately diagnose such women as suffering from orgasmic dysfunction and proceed to treat them for this condition. That a significant number of men communicate dissatisfaction to their partners concerning the partners' failure to achieve orgasm is suggested by the finding that over 50% of women report having faked orgasms with intercourse (McConaghy, 1993). The diagnosis of a communication problem should be considered, and if confirmed, treatment should be directed to correcting this. This diagnosis would also seem appropriate for many patients who seek treatment for sexual difficulties, problems related to the emotional tone of the patients' relationships, which are more important determinants of their sexual satisfaction than their dysfunctions, the problems of performance (Frank et al., 1978; Snyder & Berg, 1983). Communication problems related to male expectations of sexual performance can also be responsible for some men seeking treatment for what they consider is premature ejaculation when they ejaculate several minutes after penetration but before their partner reaches orgasm.

When it is concluded that the patient has a sexual dysfunction, it may be necessary to determine the possible contribution of organic causes by physical investigation. It is usually required for older men with erectile problems. If men give a history of situational erectile dysfunction in that they obtain adequate erections in private masturbation, organic factors can usually be excluded. Men with hypoactive sexual desire and those whose erectile disorder is not situational require physical examination to exclude such conditions as hypertension and hypogonadism, and blood and urine screening to exclude diabetes, hyperprolactinemia (raised levels of the pituitary hormone prolactin), and hyper- and hypothyroidism. The Process of Care Consensus Panel (1999) recommended in evaluating erectile dysfunction that testosterone assay should be carried out, and in addition standard serum chemistries, blood cell count and lipid profiles, if these had not been done in the past year. It is likely sildenafil or intracavernous injection of vasodilating chemicals are prescribed by most medical practitioners for erectile dysfunction without other investigations than physical examination, exclusion of diabetes, and possibly testosterone level estimation. If these treatments fail to produce erections adequate for intercourse, the patient is likely to be referred to clinicians specializing in the treatment of erectile dysfunction.

These clinicians may use nocturnal penile tumescence assessment with the aim of differentiating psychogenic and organic causes. Meisler and Carey (1990) considered a conservative appraisal to be the assessment misdiagnosed in as many as 20% of the men investigated. It is advisable for medicolegal purposes in assessment of patients complaining of erectile disorder secondary to compensatible accidents or injuries. Impairment of penile blood flow as a cause of erectile dysfunction is assessed by determination of the penile-brachial index. This is the ratio of the blood pressure in the penile arteries, commonly measured by Doppler ultrasound probe, and conventionally measured blood pressure in the brachial artery in the arm. When its reduction is sufficient to suggest the presence of vascular pathology, further physical investigations are carried out if it is necessary to determine the nature of the pathology. Assessment of neurogenic factors producing impotence is indicated if the patient has a history of diabetes, pelvic pathology, or radical prostatectomy, or if physical examination reveals the absence of the cremasteric or bulbocavernosal reflex or reduced lower limb reflexes.

Physical and laboratory examinations are more rarely carried out on women with sexual dysfunctions. As with men it is necessary to exclude illness, medications, or substances as responsible for reduced sexual interest or ability to reach orgasm. The effects of neurological and vascular diseases on the sexuality of women are much more poorly documented than their effects on men. They are commencing to receive more attention (Goldstein & Berman, 1998). Physical examination is necessary to investigate dyspareunia, but hormone studies are not routine in the investigation of sexually dysfunctional women, in the absence of evidence of hormonal imbalance such as excessive hirsutism. The significant hormonal fluctuations that occur throughout the menstrual cycle have not been demonstrated to be accompanied by consistent fluctuations in sexual behaviors (McConaghy, 1993).

In diagnosing paraphilias it is necessary to determine whether the subject has deviant sexual fantasies, and if so, the degree of distress they cause, and the likelihood of their being acted upon. Such fantasies are common in both men and women, and isolated sexually deviant acts are carried out by the majority of adolescent males (McConaghy, 1993). About 15% of male and 2% of female university students in the United States and Australia reported some likelihood of having sexual activity with a prepubertal child if they could do so without risk (Malamuth, 1989; McConaghy, Zamir, & Manicavasagar, 1993). A significant percentage of apparently otherwise normal men show penile volume evidence of arousal to pictures of nude girl children (Freund, McKnight, Langevin, & Cibiri, 1972). Freund et al. concluded that for the non-deviant adult male, the female child—at least from her sixth year—was biologically a more appropriate surrogate sexual object than a male person. They believed that many heterosexual pedophilic offences were carried out by men who are not truly pedophilic in their sexual preference. Over 30% of men reported sexual fantasies of tying up and of raping a woman, and 10–20% of torturing or beating up a woman

(Crepault & Couture, 1980; Person et al., 1989). If deviant fantasies, like paraphilic behaviors, are reported to clinicians, they must distress the subject and be persistent to receive a *DSM-IV* diagnosis of paraphilia. Most clinicians consider that with or without distress concerning persistent or non-persistent fantasies of sexual activity with children, any possibility of the subject acting upon them justifies the diagnosis of pedophilia and indicates a need for treatment. Similar considerations apply to the diagnosis as paraphilias of sexual fantasies of harming adolescents or adults.

Early studies reported that, as groups, pedophiles and rapists could be distinguished from control subjects by their penile circumference responses to audio- or videotaped descriptions of sexual activities or pictures of male and female nudes of various ages. This encouraged the widespread use of these responses both in diagnosis and assessment of outcome with treatment of individual pedophiles and rapists. Subsequent studies showed inconsistent results (McConaghy, 1993). Factors contributing to this inconsistency include that penile circumference responses do not immediately reflect penile volume responses. In a number of men, while the penile volume increases, the circumference initially decreases. Only after a delay of up to 2 min does the circumference commence to increase in parallel with the volume increase. Penile volume response assessment was the method originally introduced to measure men's sexual arousal. Following its validation for this purpose, it was replaced by circumference assessment, as this was assumed without investigation to be equivalent to volume assessment. Volume assessment requires the subject to view the evoking stimulus for 10 s, whereas circumference assessment requires him to view it for up to 2 min. With the latter procedure, the man has much more time to modify his response by fantasying alternative stimuli. In addition, the ability of both assessment procedures to discriminate pedophiles and rapists from normal controls is limited by the fact that a significant percentage of controls shows evidence of arousal to stimuli of children or acts of sexual aggression. Meta-analysis of studies using penile circumference assessment demonstrated that it discriminated rapists from non-rapists, as groups (Lalumiere & Quinsey, 1994). The fact that it was necessary to combine the results of several studies by meta-analysis to obtain convincing statistical evidence that the assessment discriminated the two groups would seem evidence that it should be used only to investigate groups, not individuals. Nevertheless the authors concluded that the result supported its use to identify individual offenders' treatment needs and risk of recidivism.

In the meta-analysis of Hanson and Bussiere (1998) of studies of recidivism, phallometric assessment of sexual interest in children was the strongest predictor of recidivism; the assessment of sexual interest in rape was unrelated. The authors made no distinction between use of penile volume or circumference as assessments. Penile circumference assessment is as yet unstandardized and the method used may be chosen from several after initial results are examined, increasing the likelihood of false positive errors. Though Marshall (1996) suggested that the wisest course of action may be to withdraw clinical use of penile circumference assessment of paraphilic interest until more adequate data are available, it continues to be widely used for this purpose.

DOS AND DON'TS

Do continuously hold in mind that when assessing patients, you are also establishing a relationship with them. An appropriate relationship will ensure their continued attendance and compliance with treatment. Maintain an attitude of warmth and involvement rather than detached inquiry.

Do ask all patients if they have any sexual problems, whatever their presenting complaint. The majority of patients with these problems will not report them unless asked (McConaghy, 1993). Their reluctance to report them is paralleled by that of many clinicians to inquire concerning them. Seidman and Rieder (1994) cited a 1990 report of the Department of Health and Human Services which charged all health care providers to take a complete sexual and drug use history with all adolescent and adult patients and to give advise and counseling concerning strategies for avoiding infection and unwanted pregnancies. Studies indicated that only 11–37% of primary care physicians routinely took a sexual history from new patients. They considered that many psychiatrists (and presumably psychologists) were ill at ease with explicit sexual history taking.

Do ask partners how they communicate their sexual feelings and wishes to each other, and encourage them to do so verbally. The importance of communication in relation to sexual satisfaction was discussed earlier. Lack of verbal communication is common. Psychology student couples reported that their commonest initiation of sexual activity was nonverbal, as were the majority of positive responses (Byers & Heinlein, 1989). Sixty percent of rejections were verbal, and verbal as compared to nonverbal rejections were resolved more satisfactorily.

Do ask about sexual fantasies. Many patients are disturbed about fantasies of what are considered deviant behaviors, and may need reassurance that they are experienced by a significant percentage of the normal population (McConaghy, 1993). At the same time, investigate whether the patient has urges to carry out the behaviors fantasized.

Do remain aware that most adolescents will not readily reveal sexual activities or feelings considered deviant, an awareness not always shown, even by experienced sexuality researchers (McConaghy, 1993). In addition, evidence has been advanced that many adolescents not only experience such feelings but express them in behaviors (Person et al., 1989; Templeman & Stinnett, 1991).

Do inquire about sexual behaviors that increase the risk of obtaining or transmitting sexual infections. Seidman and Rieder (1994) in reviewing studies of sexual behavior in the United States found that most 18–24-year-olds had multiple, serial sex partners and did not consistently use condoms. They pointed out that male-to-female transmission of HIV was five times as likely with anal as with vaginal intercourse. Anal intercourse was rarely discussed in the medical literature and was apparently a topic of extreme sensitivity for many individuals, including physicians. It was reported to occur in the last year in 9% of women with opposite sex partners; 1.2% stated it occurred in their last sexual experience (Laumann et al., 1994). Suarez and Miller (2001) found that recent data indicated increased risk behavior both in the United States and abroad, accompanied by increased rates of sexually transmitted diseases and possibly of HIV. Oncale and

King (2001) found that 30% of men and 41% of women undergraduates reported that a sexual partner had tried to dissuade them from using a condom and concluded that perceived decrease in physical pleasure posed a particular problem for sex and health educators. Where appropriate, immunization against hepatitis A and B should be recommended.

Do include alcohol and tobacco use in the drugs of abuse you ask if patients are using. Apart from the possible contribution of both to sexual dysfunctions, use of alcohol has a strong association with sex offending behaviors in adolescent and adult men (Johnson & Knight, 2000; Firestone et al., 2000).

Do ask patients on medications if there are sexual side-effects.

Do establish that women are having regular mammography and Pap smears and that older men are being regularly investigated for prostate enlargement and cancer. It is now established that screening for prostate cancer improves outcome (Litwin, 1999).

Do keep complete written records of your interviews with patients. Legal actions based on claims of your failure to have given necessary information or advice can be avoided if you recorded at the time that you had done so.

Don't be inhibited if due to lack of experience you feel somewhat diffident or embarrassed when questioning patients about the details of their sexual activity, normal and deviant. Most patients will not react negatively if you show some signs of this diffidence. Many of them will also be diffident and may feel more comfortable with a therapist who is not a model of total assurance.

Don't let feelings of discomfort due to lack of experience prevent you from asking all the appropriate questions or cause you to use technical language rather than words you can be sure the patient will understand. For some patients, these will be the colloquial words that other patients would regard as crude or obscene.

Don't provide patients with the information you are trying to elicit, particularly if there is evidence that they may be motivated to distort their history. If the interviewer asks a series of leading questions, this can encourage suggestible patients or those who wish to provide evidence that they suffer from a significant disorder to confirm the suggestions implicit in such questions.

Don't assume older patients are not sexually active. As they are aware of the still prevalent belief that older people don't or shouldn't have any sexual activity, many are reluctant to seek help if they are having sexual problems. Brecher (1984) found that men and women aged 50 to over 70 considered the belief widespread that few if any older people continue sexual activity. The belief was evident in Lewontin's (1995) scorn of Laumann et al.'s (1994) acceptance "without the academic equivalent of a snicker" that 45% of men aged 80–84 still have sex with a partner. Findings supporting the validity of their acceptance were cited by McConaghy (1998).

Don't focus on sexual dysfunctions in isolation from couples' emotional relationship. LoPiccolo (1992) in developing a postmodern sex therapy emphasized that sexual dysfunctions may play an adaptive role in maintaining couples' equilibrium and the therapist should remain alert to this possibility.

Don't allow the presence of other Axis I disorders to prevent you from seeking evidence of symptoms of sexual dysfunctions that are commonly also present.

These can be due to medication for schizophrenic or manic-depressive symptoms. However, Figueira et al. (2001) found that 75% of patients with panic disorder and 33% of those with social phobias had the symptoms of *DSM-IV* sexual dysfunctions. Ninety-three percent of male pedophiles met the *DSM-IV* criteria for other Axis I disorders which in twenty-four percent was a sexual dysfunction (Raymond et al., 1999).

Don't allow your sympathy for subjects reporting sexual victimization to cause you to treat them as special patients so that you depart from your usual practice. Your usual practice is the result of your training and experience. Any departure from it is likely to produce a less satisfactory result. Treating victims as requiring extra concern can convey the message that their competence to cope with the trauma is suspect, so that they require more than your usual attention. In particular it is important while being supportive of appropriate distress, not to reinforce illness behaviors such as regression, as McCombie and Arons (1980) pointed out in regard to the counseling of victims of sexual assault. Concern for patients must be accompanied by awareness that ultimately if they are to enjoy life again they must cease to be victims. Therapist must not over-react to the possibility or the reality of their patients' past traumatic experiences but rather award them the respect for their ability to survive, a respect which will enable them to recover from the effects of the experiences.

SUMMARY

In diagnostic interviews of patients with sexual dysfunctions, it is necessary also to investigate sexual difficulties, the problems resulting from the emotional tone of their relationships, as these are more important in determining sexual dissatisfaction. Subjects can be reassured about the relative commonness of deviant sexual fantasies unless they report any likelihood of expressing them in coercive or other inappropriate behaviors. The relevant information to diagnose sexual disorders is obtained by most therapists in a clinical interview. It also allows investigation of the presence of personality disorders and the establishment of relationships with patients which will maximize the likelihood of their remaining in and complying with treatment. Case illustrations are given outlining difficulties in managing patients with dual diagnoses. The increasing concern that structured interviews diagnose too many apparently well subjects as ill makes it unlikely they will replace the clinical interview to diagnose sexual disorders by clinicians, at least until their validity is markedly improved. It is suggested that improved training of professionals in use of the clinical interview may enable them to make highly reliable and valid diagnoses with its use. Hopefully input from clinicians will stimulate more effective operationalization of diagnostic criteria for sexual disorder in the next version of the *DSM*. The high prevalence of symptoms of sexual dysfunctions and deviations makes their diagnosis dependent not so much on their presence as their persistence and intensity and the degree to which they distress the subject. The reluctance of patients to reveal sexual problems to their clinicians and of clinicians to inquire concerning them needs correction. Organic causes require investigation, particularly in sexual dysfunctions in the middle-aged and elderly.

REFERENCES

American Psychiatric Association. (1987). *Diagnostic and statistical manual of mental disorders* (3rd ed., revised, pp. 467–481). Washington, DC: Author.

American Psychiatric Association. (1994). *Diagnostic and statistical manual of mental disorders* (4th ed.). Washington, DC: Author.

Andersen, B. L., & Broffitt, B. (1988). Is there a reliable and valid self-report measure of sexual behavior? *Archives of Sexual Behavior, 17*, 509–525.

Andrews, G., & Peters, L. (1998). The psychometric properties of the composite international diagnostic interview. *Social Psychiatry and Psychiatric Epidemiology, 33*, 80–88.

Andrews, G., Peters, L., Guzman, A.-M., & Bird, K. (1995). A comparison of two structured diagnostic interviews: CIDI and SCAN. *Australian and New Zealand of Psychiatry, 29*, 124–132.

Arndt, B. (1994, May 28–29). An abuse of trust. *The Weekend Australian*, 23.

AuBuchon, P. G., & Calhoun, K. S. (1985). Menstrual cycle symptomatology: The role of social expectancy and experimental demand characteristics. *Psychosomatic Medicine, 47*, 35–45.

Bates, J. E., Bentler, P. M., & Thompson, S. K. (1973). Measurement of deviant gender development in boys. *Child Development, 44*, 591–598.

Bender, L., & Paster, S. (1941). Homosexual trends in children. *American Journal of Orthopsychiatry, 11*, 730–743.

Berlin, F. S., Malin, H. M., & Dean, S. (1991). Effect of statutes requiring psychiatrists to report suspected sexual abuse of children. *American Journal of Psychiatry, 148*, 449–453.

Blanchard, R. (1997). Birth order and sibling sex ratio in homosexual versus heterosexual males and females. *Annual Review of Sex Research, 8*, 27–67.

Boyce, E. G., & Umland, E. M. (2001). Sildenafil citrate: A therapeutic update. *Clinical Therapeutics, 23*, 2–23.

Brecher, E. M. (1984). *Love, sex and aging*. Boston: Little, Brown and Co.

Bullough, B., & Bullough, V. (1997). Are transvestites necessarily heterosexual? *Archives of Sexual Behavior, 26*, 1–12.

Byers, E. S., & Heinlein, L. (1989). Predicting initiations and refusals of sexual activity in married and cohabitating heterosexual couples. *Journal of Sex Research, 26*, 210–231.

Catania, J. A., Gibson, D. R., Chitwood, D. D., & Coates, T. J. (1990a). Methodological problems in AIDS behavioral research: Influences on measurement error and participation bias in studies of sexual behavior. *Psychological Bulletin, 108*, 339–362.

Catania, J. A., Gibson, D. R., Marin, B., Coates, T. J., & Greenblatt, R. M. (1990b). Response bias in assessing sexual behaviors relevant to HIV transmission. *Evaluation and Program Planning, 13*, 19–29.

Cooper, B., & Singh, B. (2000). Population research and mental health policy (Editorial). *British Journal of Psychiatry, 176*, 407–411.

Cooper, L., Peters, L., & Andrews, G. (1998). Validity of the Composite Diagnostic Interview (CIDI) psychosis module in a psychiatric setting. *Journal of Psychiatric Research, 32*, 361–368.

Crepault, C., & Couture, M. (1980). Men's erotic fantasies. *Archives of Sexual Behavior, 9*, 565–581.

Davis, C. M., Yarber, W. L., Bauserman, R., Schreer, G., & Davis, S. L. (1998). *Handbook of sexuality-related measures*. Thousand Oaks, CA: Sage.

De Amicis, L. A., Goldberg, D. C., LoPiccolo, J., Friedman, J., & Davies, L. (1985). Clinical follow-up of couples treated for sexual dysfunction. *Archives of Sexual Behavior, 14*, 467–489.

Durant, L. E., & Carey, M. P. (2000). Self-administered questionnaires versus face-to-face interviews in assessing sexual behavior in young women. *Archives of Sexual Behavior, 29*, 309–322.

Figueira, M. D., Possidente, E., Marques, C., & Hayes, K. (2001). Sexual dysfunction: A neglected complication of panic disorder and social phobia. *Archives of Sexual Behavior, 26*, 369–377.

Finkelhor, D. (1984). *Child sexual abuse new theory and research*. New York: The Free Press.

Firestone, P., Bradford, J. M., McCoy, M., Greenberg, D., Curry, S., & Larose, M. R. (2000). Prediction of recidivism in extrafamilial child molesters based on court-related assessments. *Sexual Abuse: A Journal of Research and Treatment, 12,* 203–221.

First, M. B., Spitzer, R. L., Gibbon, M., & Williams, J. B. W. (1995). *Structured clinical interview for DSM-IV axis I disorders—patient edition.* New York: New York State Psychiatric Institute.

Frank, E., Anderson, B., & Rubinstein, D. (1978). Frequency of sexual dysfunction in "normal" couples. *New England Journal of Medicine, 299,* 111–115.

Freund, K., McKnight, C. K., Langevin, R., & Cibiri, S. (1972). The female child as a surrogate object. *Archives of Sexual Behavior, 2,* 119–133.

Goldberg, D. (1997). *The Maudsley handbook of practical psychiatry.* Oxford: Oxford University Press.

Goldstein, I., & Berman, J. (1998). Vasculogenic female sexual dysfunction: Vaginal engorgement and clitoral erectile insufficiency syndrome. *International Journal of Impotence Research, 10,* S84–S90.

Green, R., & Young, R. (2001). Hand preference, sexual preference, and transsexualism. *Archives of Sexual Behavior, 30,* 565–574.

Gutheil, T. G. (1989). Borderline personality disorder, boundary violations, and patient–therapist sex: Medicolegal pitfalls. *American Journal of Psychiatry, 146,* 597–602.

Guthrie, E. (2000). Psychotherapy for patients with complex disorders and chronic symptoms. *British Journal of Psychiatry, 177,* 131–137.

Hanson, R. K., & Bussiere, M. T. (1998). Predicting relapse: A meta-analysis of sexual offender recidivism studies. *Journal of Consulting and Clinical Psychology, 66,* 348–362.

Holland, L. A., Zolondek, S. C, Abel, G. G., Jordan, A. D., & Becker, J. V. (2000). Psychometric analysis of the sexual interest cardsort questionnaire. *Sexual Abuse: A Journal of Research and Treatment, 12,* 107–122.

Jacobson, N. S., Schmaling, K. B., & Holtzworth-Munroe, A. (1989). Research-structured vs. clinical flexible versions of social learning-based marital therapy. *Behavior Research and Therapy, 27,* 173–180.

Johnson, G. M., & Knight, R. A. (2000). Developmental antecedents of sexual coercion in juvenile sexual offenders. *Sexual Abuse: A Journal of Research and Treatment, 12,* 165–178.

Kagan, J., & Moss, H. A. (1962). *Birth to maturity.* New York: Wiley & Sons.

Karacan, I. (1978). Advances in the psychophysiological evaluation of male erectile impotence. In J. LoPiccolo & L. LoPiccolo (Eds.), *Handbook of sex therapy* (pp. 137–145). New York: Plenum Press.

Kelly, M. P., Strassberg, D. S., & Kircher, J. R. (1990). Attitudinal and experiential correlates of anorgasmia. *Archives of Sexual Behavior, 19,* 165–177.

Kessler, R. C., McGonagle, K. A., Zhao, S., Nelson, C. B., Hughes, M., Eshleman, S., Wittchen, H. U., & Kendler, K. S. (1994). Lifetime and 12-month prevalence of DSM-III-R psychiatric disorders in the United States: Results from the National Comorbidity Survey. *Archives of General Psychiatry, 51,* 8–19.

Lalumiere, M. L., & Quinsey, V. L. (1994). The discriminability of rapists from non-sex offenders using phallometric measures. A meta-analysis. *Criminal Justice and Behavior, 21,* 150–175.

Laumann, E. O., Gagnon, J. H., Michael, R. T., & Michaels, S. (1994). *The social organization of sexuality.* Chicago: University of Chicago Press.

Lewontin, R. C. (1995, April 20). Sex, lies, and social science. *The New York Review,* 24–29.

Lipman, R. S., Cole, J. O., Park, L. C., & Rickels, K. (1965). Sensitivity of symptom and nonsymptom-focused criteria of outpatient drug efficacy. *American Journal of Psychiatry, 122,* 24–27.

Litwin, M. S. (1999). Urology. *Journal of the American Medical Association, 281,* 495–496.

LoPiccolo, J. (1990). Sexual dysfunction. In A. S. Bellack, M. Hersen, & A. E. Kazdin (Eds.), *International handbook of behavior therapy and modification* (2nd ed., pp. 547–564). New York: Plenum Press.

LoPiccolo, J. (1992). Postmodern sex therapy for erectile failure. In R. C. Rosen & S. R. Leiblum (Eds.), *Erectile disorders assessment and treatment* (pp. 171–197). New York: Guilford.

Malamuth, N. M. (1989). The attraction to sexual aggression scale: Part two. *Journal of Sex Research, 26,* 324–354.

Maletzky, B. M. (1980). Assisted covert sensitization. In D. J. Cox & R. J. Daitzman (Eds.), *Exhibitionism: Description, assessment, and treatment* (pp. 289–293). New York: Garland STPM Press.

Maletzky, B. M. (1996). Denial of treatment or treatment of denial? *Sexual Abuse: A Journal of Research and Therapy, 8,* 1–5.

Marshall, W. L. (1996). Assessment, treatment and theorizing about sex offenders. *Criminal Justice and Behavior, 23*, 162–199.

Marshall, W. L. (1999). Current status of North American assessment and treatment programs for sexual offenders. *Journal of Interpersonal Violence, 14*, 221–239.

Marshall, W. L., & Eccles, A. (1991). Issues in clinical practice with sex offenders. *Journal of Interpersonal Violence, 6*, 68–93.

Matarazzo, J. D. (1983). The reliability of psychiatric and psychological diagnosis. *Clinical Psychology Review, 3*, 103–145.

McCombie, S. L., & Arons, J. H. (1980). Counselling rape victims. In S. L. McCombie (Ed.), *The rape crisis intervention handbook* (pp. 145–171). New York: Plenum Press.

McConaghy, N. (1993). *Sexual behavior, problems, and management.* New York: Plenum Press.

McConaghy, N. (1998). Sexual dysfunction. In M. Hersen & V. B. Van Hasselt (Eds.), *Handbook of clinical geropsychology* (pp. 239–271). New York: Plenum Press.

McConaghy, N. (1999). Unresolved issues in scientific sexology. *Archives of Sexual Behavior, 28*, 285–318.

McConaghy, N., & Zamir, R. (1995). Heterosexual and homosexual coercion, sexual orientation and sexual roles in medical students. *Archives of Sexual Behavior, 24*, 489–502.

McConaghy, N., Blaszczynski, A., & Kidson, W. (1988). Treatment of sex offenders with imaginal desensitization and/or medroxyprogesterone. *Acta Psychiatrica Scandinavica, 77*, 199–206.

McConaghy, N., Zamir, R., & Manicavasagar, V. (1993). Non-sexist sexual experiences survey and scale of attraction to sexual aggression. *Australian and New Zealand Journal of Psychiatry, 27*, 686–693.

McConaghy, N., Hadzi-Pavlovic, D., Stevens, C., Manicavasagar, V., Buhrich, N., & Vollmer-Conna, U. (in press). Fraternal birth order and ratio of heterosexual/homosexual feelings in women and men.

Meisler, A. W., & Carey, M. P. (1990). A critical reevaluation of nocturnal penile tumescence monitoring in the diagnosis of erectile disorder. *Journal of Nervous and Mental Disease, 178*, 78–89.

National Advisory Mental Health Council. (1993). Health care reform for Americans with severe mental illnesses. *American Journal of Psychiatry, 150*, 1447–1465.

Nelson, R. O., & Hayes, S. C. (1981). Nature of behavioral assessment. In A. S. Bellack & M. Hersen (Eds.), *Behavioral assessment* (2nd ed., pp. 3–37). New York: Pergamon Press.

O'Donohue, W., Regev, L. G., & Hagstrom, A. (2000). Problems with the DSM-IV diagnosis of pedophilia. *Sexual Abuse: A Journal of Research and Treatment, 12*, 95–105.

Oncale, R. M., & King, B. M. (2001). Comparison of men's and women's attempts to dissuade sexual partners from the couple using condoms. *Archives of Sexual Behavior, 30*, 379–391.

Paredes, A., Baumgold, J., Pugh, L. A., & Ragland, R. (1966). Clinical judgment in the assessment of psychopharmacological effects. *Journal of Nervous and Mental Disease, 142*, 153–160.

Person, E. S., Terestman, N., Myers, W. A., Goldberg, E. L., & Salvadori, C. (1989). Gender differences in sexual behaviors and fantasies in a college population. *Journal of Sex and Marital Therapy, 15*, 187–198.

Peters, L., & Andrews, G. (1995). Procedural validity of the computerized version of the Composite International Diagnostic Interview (CIDI-Auto) in the anxiety disorders. *Psychological Medicine, 25*, 1269–1280.

Raymond, N. C., Coleman, E., Ohlerking, F., Christenson, G. A., & Miner, M. (1999). Psychiatric comorbidity in pedophilic sex offenders. *American Journal of Psychiatry, 156*, 786–788.

Reading, A. E. (1983). A comparison of the accuracy and reactivity of methods of monitoring male sexual behavior. *Journal of Behavioral Assessment, 5*, 11–23.

Regier, D. A., Kaelber, C. T., Rae, D. S., Farmer, M. E., Knauper, B., Kessler, R. C., & Norquist, G. S. (1998). Limitations of diagnostic criteria and assessment instruments for mental disorders. *Archives of General Psychiatry, 55*, 109–115.

Rekers, G. A., & Lovaas, O. I. (1974). Behavioral treatment of deviant sex-role behavior in a male child. *Journal of Applied Behavior Analysis, 7*, 173–190.

Robins, L. N., & Regier, D. A. (1991). *Psychiatric disorders in America.* New York: Free Press.

Rowland, D. L., Cooper, S. E., & Schneider, M. (2001). Defining premature ejaculation for experimental and clinical investigations. *Archives of Sexual Behavior, 30*, 235–253.

Rust, J., & Golombok, S. (1986). The GRISS: A psychometric instrument for the assessment of sexual dysfunction. *Archives of Sexual Behavior, 15*, 157–165.

Schatzberg, A. F., Westfall, M. P., Blumetti, A. B., & Birk, C. L. (1975). Effeminacy 1: A quantitative rating scale. *Archives of Sexual Behavior, 4*, 31–41.

Schiavi, R. C., & Segraves, R. T. (1995). The biology of sexual function. *Psychiatric Clinics of North America, 18*, 7–23.

Schlank, A. M., & Shaw, T. (1996). Treating sexual offenders who deny their guilt: A pilot study. *Sexual Abuse: A Journal of Research and Treatment, 8*, 17–23.

Seidman, S. N., & Rieder, R. O. (1994). A review of sexual behavior in the United States. *American Journal of Psychiatry, 151*, 330–341.

Slade, T., & Andrews, G. (2002). Empirical impact of DSM-IV diagnostic criterion for clinical significance. *Journal of Nervous and Mental Disease, 190*, 334–337.

Snyder, D. K., & Berg, P. (1983). Determinants of sexual dissatisfaction in sexually distressed couples. *Archives of Sexual Behavior, 12*, 237–246.

Solstad, K., & Hertoft, P. (1993). Frequency of sexual problems and sexual dysfunction in middle-aged Danish males. *Archives of Sexual Behavior, 22*, 51–58.

Spitzer, R. L. (1983). Psychiatric diagnosis: Are clinicians still necessary? *Comprehensive Psychiatry, 24*, 399–411.

Spitzer, R. L., & Wakefield, J. C. (1999). DSM-IV diagnostic criterion for clinical significance: Does it help solve the false positives problem? *American Journal of Psychiatry, 156*, 1856–1864.

Suarez, T., & Miller, J. (2001). Negotiating risks in context: A perspective on unprotected anal intercourse and barebacking among men who have sex with men—Where do we go from here? *Archives of Sexual Behavior, 30*, 287–300.

Taylor, C. B., Agras, W. S., Schneider, J. A., & Allen, R. A. (1983). Adherence to instructions to practice relaxation exercises. *Journal of Consulting and Clinical Psychology, 51*, 952–953.

Templeman, T. L., & Stinnett, R. D. (1991). Patterns of sexual arousal and history in a "normal" sample of young men. *Archives of Sexual Behavior, 20*, 137–150.

The Process of Care Consensus Panel. (1999). The process of care model for evaluation and treatment of erectile dysfunction. *International Journal of Impotence Research, 11*, 59–74.

van den Brink, W., Koeter, M. W. J., Ormel, J., Dijkstra, W., Giel, R., Slooff, C. J., & Wohlfarth, T. D. (1989). Psychiatric diagnosis in an outpatient population. *Archives of General Psychiatry, 46*, 369–372.

van Lankveld, J. J. D. M., & Grotjohann, Y. (2000). Psychiatric comorbidity in heterosexual couples with sexual dysfunction assessed with the Composite International Diagnostic Interview. *Archives of Sexual Behavior, 29*, 479–498.

Wincze, J. P., & Carey, M. P. (1991). *Sexual dysfunction*. New York: Guilford Press.

Wing, J. K., & Sturt, E. (1978). *The PSE-ID-Catego system: Supplementary manual*. London: MRC Social Psychiatry Unit.

World Health Organization. (1992). *Composite international diagnostic interview. Version 1.1*. Geneva: WHO, Division of Mental Health.

World Health Organization (1993). *CIDI-Auto version 1: Administrator's guide*. Sydney: Training and Reference Centre for WHO CIDI.

Wyatt, G. E., & Peters, S. D. (1986). Issues in the definition of child sexual abuse in prevalence research. *Child Abuse and Neglect, 10*, 231–240.

Zucker, K. J. (1997). Letter to the Editor. *Archives of Sexual Behavior, 26*, 671–672.

12

Eating Disorders

Risa J. Stein, Shani Stewart, G. Ken Goodrick,
Walker S. C. Poston, and John P. Foreyt

Anorexia nervosa, bulimia nervosa, and binge eating disorder (BED) all involve observable eating, and often purging, behaviors. However, in order to develop a complete conceptual picture of each disorder, additional sociocultural, behavioral, cognitive, and emotional processes must be considered. To complicate matters, altered physiological functioning may result from as well as cause emotional and cognitive dysfunction. Thus, although interviewers will want to uncover diagnostic criteria, they should keep in mind the dynamics of the disorder so that the behavioral, cognitive, affective, and social manifestations can be put into a conceptual whole.

Prevalence of anorexia nervosa among adolescent females is estimated to be 0.5–1%. Bulimia, which according to research is a more common eating disorder when compared to anorexia nervosa, is estimated to occur in 1–5% of college age women and 1–3% among adolescent girls and young women (Harris & Kuba, 1997). Approximately 15–50% of patients in weight-control programs experience BED while estimates for community samples range from 1% to 4% (Goldfein, Devlin, & Spitzer, 2000).

Anorexia Nervosa

Of the three disorders described in this chapter, anorexia nervosa is the one most noted for its severe course and consequences. It is the eating disorder most likely to result in death, most often from the complications arising from the state of starvation. Anorexia nervosa is a perplexing condition, for its most notable

Risa J. Stein • Department of Psychology, Rockhurst University, Kansas City, Missouri 64110. Shani Stewart and Walker S. C. Poston • Department of Psychology, University of Missouri-Kansas City, Kansas City, Missouri 64110. G. Ken Goodrick • Department of Family and Community Medicine, Baylor College of Medicine, Houston, Texas 77030. John P. Foreyt • Nutrition Research Clinic, Baylor College of Medicine, Houston, Texas 77030.

characteristic is self-imposed starvation in a country and culture blessed with an abundance of food. However, for anorectics, the apparent illogic of their actions is overridden by a psychological framework ruled by two powerful contingencies: the reward of weight loss and a morbid fear of fatness (Garner, Garfinkel, & Bemis, 1982).

The *Diagnostic and Statistical Manual for Mental Disorders*, Fourth Edition (*DSM-IV*) (American Psychiatric Association [APA], 1994) diagnostic criteria for anorexia nervosa are presented in Table 1. Anorectics of the binge eating/purging type tend to be heavier, with more lability of mood, impulsivity, and drug abuse. It is notable that 95% of anorectics are females (APA, 1987). Such disproportionate representation of females likely indicates the strong cultural influences in its etiology (Brownell, 1991). In the United States and many of the other Western nations, slenderness has become synonymous with attractiveness, and it is apparent that the achievement of both is an expectation more of women than of men.

Physical symptomatology includes low metabolic rate, low blood pressure, cold intolerance, insomnia, bradycardia, pathological EEG patterns, alopecia, and dry skin (Bemis, 1978; Williamson, 1990). There is also an increased comorbidity of the affective and anxiety disorders with anorexia nervosa, and alcoholism and other psychiatric diagnoses including eating disorders are more likely in first-degree relatives (Halmi et al., 1991).

A number of psychological traits characterize the anorectic, including shyness, anxiety, and obsessive–compulsive behaviors (Bemis, 1978). These characteristics, although the source of much inner turmoil, are frequently manifested in outward behaviors viewed positively by family and friends. In many families, the presymptomatic anorexic child is frequently perceived as the pride and joy of the brood, often characterized by parents as being well behaved, high achieving,

---

TABLE 1. *DSM-IV* Diagnostic Criteria for Anorexia Nervosa[a]

A. Refusal to maintain body weight at or above a minimally normal weight for age and height (e.g., weight loss leading to maintenance of body weight less than 85% of that expected; or failure to make expected weight gain during period of growth, leading to body weight less than 85% of that expected).
B. Intense fear of gaining weight or becoming fat, even though underweight.
C. Disturbance in the way in which one's body weight or shape is experienced; undue influence of body weight or shape on self-evaluation, or denial of the seriousness of the current low body weight.
D. In postmenarchal females, amenorrhea, that is, the absence of at least three consecutive menstrual cycles. (A woman is considered to have amenorrhea if her periods occur only following hormone, e.g., estrogen, administration.)

Specify type
   Restricting type: During the episode of anorexia nervosa, the person does not regularly engage in binge eating or purging behavior (i.e., self-induced vomiting or the misuse of laxatives or diuretics).
   Binge eating/purging type: During the episode of anorexia nervosa, the person regularly engages in binge eating or purging behavior (i.e., self-induced vomiting or the misuse of laxatives or diuretics).

[a]From American Psychiatric Association (1993).

and perfectionistic (Halmi, Goldberg, Eckert, Casper, & Davis, 1977). Some authors (e.g., Bruch, 1978; Rosman, Minuchin, Baker, & Liebman, 1977), however, suggest that many of the anorectic traits are engendered by the particular interactional patterns and values of the families involved. Bruch (1977) noted that among anorectic families, parents tended to be overprotective, overconcerned, and overambitious with expectations of obedience and superior performance of the children.

BULIMIA NERVOSA

In recent years, bulimia nervosa has gained increasing attention as the extent of its occurrence and the severity of its symptomatology have become known. Although bulimia is literally translated to mean "ox hunger," for most who have this condition, eating has little association with the fulfillment of normal biological hunger. Binge eating may be more a result of voluntary dietary restriction, distorted perceptions of body size, and the need to achieve an ideal body. The purging behavior is learned as a way to rid the body of excess calories from a binge; however, purging and subsequent dietary restriction lead to the next binge, thus continuing the cycle.

The *DSM-IV* (APA, 1993) diagnostic criteria for bulimia nervosa are presented in Table 2.

Data from the available literature and a survey of professionals concerned with eating disorders failed to show a requirement that the binge consist of a large

TABLE 2. *DSM-IV* Diagnostic Criteria for Bulimia Nervosa[a]

A. An episode of binge eating is characterized by both of the following:
    (1) Eating, in a discrete period of time (e.g., within any 2-hr period), an amount of food that is definitely larger than most people would eat during a similar period of time and under similar circumstances.
    (2) A sense of lack of control over eating during the episode (e.g., a feeling that one cannot stop eating or control what or how much one is eating).
B. Recurrent inappropriate compensatory behavior in order to prevent weight gain, such as self-induced vomiting; misuse of laxatives, diuretics, enemas, or other medications; fasting; or excessive exercise.
C. The binge eating and compensatory behaviors both occur, on average, at least twice a week for 3 months.
D. Self-evaluation is unduly influenced by body shape and weight.
E. The disturbance does not occur exclusively during episodes of Anorexia Nervosa.

Specify type
    Purging type: During the current episode of bulimia nervosa, the person has regularly engaged in self-induced vomiting or the misuse of laxatives, diuretics, or enemas.
    Nonpurging type: During the current episode of bulimia nervosa, the person has used other compensatory behaviors, such as fasting or excessive exercise, but has not regularly engaged in self-induced vomiting or the misuse of laxatives, diuretics, or enemas.

---

[a]From American Psychiatric Association (1993).

amount of food, or that the minimal binge frequency in criterion C (Table 2) be met before a diagnosis of bulimia nervosa is made (Wilson, 1992). Thus, bulimics may binge slowly, a binge may consist of only a few potato chips, and binging may occur as infrequently as once per week. The important psychological factors of feeling that the eating is out of control, that the food is "forbidden," and the resulting purging response seem to be the critical features for the diagnosis. Variations of bulimia nervosa are listed under "Eating disorders not otherwise specified" in *DSM-IV* (APA, 1993).

There is controversy as to whether the modality of purging is more important diagnostically than the psychological motivation to rid one's body of calories. For example, a patient of ours habitually "corrected" her binge episodes with 20-mile bike rides. The excursions were marked by their compulsive and urgent quality; they sometimes occurred at odd hours in the morning, during inclement weather, or even during the course of a social gathering. This patient was repulsed by the idea of vomiting, but she nevertheless had an extreme purgative reaction to binging.

The physical toll taken by the practice of bulimia is not so great as the one experienced by the anorexic; however, it can be severe. Among the physical sequelae are esophageal rupture and hiatal hernias from frequent vomiting, urinary infections, impaired kidney function, irregular menstrual cycles, dental problems, electrolyte disturbances, and metabolic and endocrine changes (Mitchell, Specker, & de Zwann, 1991; Neuman & Halvorson, 1983). Because many bulimics maintain a normal weight and appear healthy, the damage done by their compulsion often goes unrecognized, even by the closest of contacts, until medical intervention is required.

For most bulimics, there is a psychological cost of their practice that parallels the physical ones. Our culture promotes standards of acceptable behavior concerning ingestion and elimination (including vomiting). Bulimic behavior, with its sometimes prodigious consumption and forced elimination, crosses the boundaries of acceptability. Most who engage in this practice are exceedingly aware of its unacceptability, and some are ashamed of it. Such awareness is associated with the low self-esteem, feelings of inadequacy, and self-derogation observed among many bulimics. The shame that accompanies this practice is probably the primary reason this problem remained in the closet for so long and continues to remain there for many sufferers.

BINGE EATING DISORDER

Some individuals have problems with recurrent binge eating, but do not engage in compensatory vomiting or use of laxatives. In recognition of this disorder, the *DSM-IV* (APA, 1993) criteria include BED as an eating disorder deserving of further study (Table 3). BED, as proposed, includes the following criteria: recurrent episodes of binge eating in the absence of the inappropriate compensatory behaviors characteristic of bulimia nervosa, lack of a feeling of control over eating, and distress over binge eating.

TABLE 3. Research Criteria for Binge Eating Disorder[a]

A. Recurrent episodes of binge eating. An episode of binge eating is characterized by both of the following:
   (1) Eating, in a discrete period of time (e.g., within any 2-hr period), an amount of food that is definitely larger than most people would eat in a similar period under similar circumstances.
   (2) A sense of lack of control over eating during the episode (e.g., a feeling that one cannot stop eating or control what or how much one is eating).
B. The binge eating episodes are associated with three (or more) of the following:
   (1) Eating much more rapidly than normal
   (2) Eating until feeling uncomfortably full
   (3) Eating large amounts of food when not feeling physically hungry
   (4) Eating alone because of being embarrassed by how much one is eating
   (5) Feeling disgusted with oneself, depressed, or very guilty after overeating
C. Marked distress regarding binge eating is present.
D. The binge eating occurs, on average, at least 2 days a week for 6 months.
   Note: The method of determining frequency differs from that used by bulimia nervosa; future research should address whether the preferred method of setting a frequency threshold is counting the number of days on which binges occur or counting the episodes of binge eating.
E. The binge eating is not associated with the regular use of inappropriate compensatory behaviors (e.g., purging, fasting, excessive exercise) and does not occur exclusively during the course of anorexia nervosa or bulimia nervosa.

---

[a]From American Psychiatric Association (1993).

BED is more common in women than in men and present in about 2% of the general population and about one third of those presenting for weight control treatment (Spitzer et al., 1992). The diagnostic criteria indicate that this disorder shares the same dynamics found in bulimia nervosa, including binge eating and increased rates of psychopathology. However, although bulimics are often of average weight, binge eating is positively related to body mass index (BMI). Many of the strategies involved in treatment of binge eating have evolved from those proven efficacious for bulimia. These include antidepressant medication, cognitive–behavioral therapy, interpersonal therapy, and self-help strategies.

The assessment of binge eating should address the role of stress in the binge eater's life. Recent research suggests that binge eating intensifies as a result of perceived daily hassles (Crowther, Sanftner, Bonifazi, & Shepherd, 2001). As stress increases, the likelihood of a binge episode increases as do the total number of calories consumed during the binge. Similarly, stress may also negatively impact treatment outcome. For example, Pendleton and colleagues (2001) found that the mean binge days/week was 3.3 times greater among BED patients experiencing high levels of negative stress at treatment commencement than among those reporting low levels at the 16-month follow-up.

OVERVIEW OF CONDITIONS

The diagnostic interview process should address the specific criteria set forth in the DSM-IV to achieve an official diagnosis. While probing for specifics, the interviewer should keep in mind psychological themes often occurring with eating disorders. These themes may involve:

1. The extreme fear of being fat, or the disgust at being fat.
2. Low self-esteem exacerbated by a hypercritical body image, and failure to control eating habits and weight.
3. The belief that self-worth hinges on bodily appearance.
4. The perceived blocks to developing interpersonal relationships due to negative self-image and the feeling of isolation associated with eating disorders.
5. The intrapunitive nature of exercise and other abusive purging techniques as well as the feeling that self-punishment is deserved for failure to control eating or weight.

PROCEDURES FOR GATHERING INFORMATION

Our procedure for gathering information is generally to incorporate this process into treatment as naturally and comfortably as possible. The initial meeting has more of the elements of an interview than subsequent ones. Issues suspected to have relevance to the client's eating problem are explored and investigated. Their validity is determined by the manner in which the client is affected (i.e., "treatment validity"); if they bring insight or change or both, then relevance is verified.

The multifactorial etiology of eating disorders often requires a multidisciplinary approach to treatment. In such cases, it is important for the therapist to be aware of the diagnoses of the other caregivers involved, as they may have relevance. For example, in anorexia nervosa, weight must be returned to a medically determined minimum before effective work can begin on the psychological issues (Bruch, 1973; Goldner & Birmingham, 1994). In cases of bulimia, the client may seek psychotherapeutic help without prior consultation with a physician. It is incumbent on the therapist to insist on medical examination early in treatment as well as during its course if any form of purging is involved. As indicated previously, the continual practice of vomiting and abuse of diuretics or laxatives can lead to serious physical consequences. Our experience has been that the participation of a physician and dietitian is essential in the treatment of an eating disorder. An exercise physiologist is also needed to prescribe sensible exercise.

It is not our expectation that the initial diagnostic meeting (usually the first treatment session) will reveal much of the client's difficulties. Eating disorders and the associated practices (e.g., vomiting) are considered aberrant in our society, and most clients are acutely aware of this proscription. Thus, it is common for information to be purposely withheld, "forgotten," or distorted in the early interviews. This pattern is especially typical of anorectics, who frequently deny the existence of a problem and do not see the necessity for their presence in treatment. Obtaining accurate information is a *process* based on many of the factors that make for effective treatment: a good therapeutic relationship, trust, and the client's sense that the therapist is working with and for his or her benefit. We find that as our relationship with the client solidifies, the diagnostic picture becomes concurrently richer.

Considering the shame involved in these disorders, it may be helpful with a female patient if the interviewer is a female who has had personal experience with eating disorders and can self-disclose that fact. At least the interviewer can reveal that she has at times overeaten after being on a diet and felt somewhat out of control at times. She might also discuss how vomiting brings a feeling of relief in the case of stomach flu, and how she can understand how this can become a habit.

Sensitivity is another important aspect of the process of diagnosis. The therapist needs to be aware of the client's sensitive areas in probing for information and, at times, be willing to delay seeking the information until readiness on the client's part is apparent. A good example of this necessity occurs with the use of food records. Although we find records to be invaluable tools for diagnosis and treatment, some react to our use of them with considerable resistance. Food records require individuals to document patterns that they have frequently denied or suppressed. Their accurate utilization would be tantamount to a personal confrontation with the problem. The therapist needs to be aware of the client's readiness for such confrontation in suggesting the use of food records.

A particularly sensitive area for many patients is that of the effect their disturbed eating patterns and real or imagined body image have on their sexual relations. A recent patient of ours, Beth, had lost a substantial amount of weight in treatment and found that one of its concomitants was a deteriorating relationship with her husband. Symptomatic of this deterioration was his growing sexual impotence. This problem, needless to say, created stress in both parties. With regard to Beth and her treatment, these occurrences were viewed in terms of their possible utilization as a rationale for returning to the prior state (i.e., overweight and disordered eating). From the standpoint of diagnosis, Beth revealed these problems and saw their possible pertinence to treatment.

CASE ILLUSTRATIONS

Case 1

Linda is an attractive, normal-weight 32-year-old female employed at a temporary services agency. She is living with her husband Bill, an accountant who has little understanding of or tolerance for the psychology of eating disorders. He apparently has no ability to express warmth or sympathy for her problem. When Linda came to her first session, she was binging and purging about 5 times per week. Binges were quite variable in amount, and purging consisted of vomiting, taking 10 or more laxative and stool softener pills each day, and engaging in at least 2 hours a day of intense aerobic exercise and swimming.

Linda's father was an alcoholic who verbally abused her. She had very traumatic dating experiences in high school and had dabbled in drugs and alcohol after graduating. Her self-esteem was near zero. She had two small children and felt very guilty about being an inadequate mother.

The following are excerpts from her initial interviews:

T: What is the main reason you have come to this clinic?

P: Well, I guess it's because I'm too fat.

T: What parts of your body are too fat?

P: My legs are really too thick. I am wearing loose pants. If you could see my legs, you would see the legs of an elephant. [Her legs appear normal.]

T: How did your legs get thick? Have they always been thick? [Therapist leads the patient to elaborate on body image distortion.]

P: Ever since I was a teenager. They got thick because I eat too much. I can't stop eating.

T: What do you mean, you can't stop eating? [Explore sense of lack of control.]

P: Well, when I am home by myself I get to eating whatever I can find. Like a bag of potato chips or any leftover food in the fridge. Once I get going, I really look for all the food I can find that can be eaten.

T: Don't you stop eating when you are full?

P: I really don't realize I am full, my eating just keeps going until I just can't eat any more. I worry about choking to death.

T: What do you do after you eat all you can?

P: For a few minutes, I just seem to blank out mentally. Then I go to the bathroom.

T: What do you do in the bathroom?

P: You know, I get rid of it.

T: Get rid of the food? [Not probing for intimate details of method at this early stage.]

P: Yes.

T: How do you feel then?

P: I feel weak, but I'm glad the food didn't stay in my body.

T: So without getting rid of the food you would be fat, given the amount of food you eat?

P: I can't imagine how fat I would be. Like the fat lady of the circus.

T: But you feel your legs are too fat? [Probe for body image]

P: Yes. I wish I could just take a knife and carve them down to decent size. They have fat surgery now for that, don't they?

* * *

T: Tell me about your last problem with food.

P: I was at a restaurant. I was having a salad with nonfat dressing since I really can't eat any fat in my food [dietary rigidity]. My neighbor was with me and she told me to try a bite of her apple turnover because she said it was so good. So I did.

T: What happened then?

P: I started to feel nauseous right away. I could feel the fat from that turnover inside my throat and I could see in my mind's eye the fatty food in my stomach. It was like I swallowed a spider, something I wanted to get rid of right away, so I went to the restroom and did it.

T: Did you feel O.K. after getting rid of it?

P: No, of course not. I knew I was getting out of control in my eating since I had eaten the turnover. So I went home and jogged slowly in the park for about 1 hour. I think the calories from 1 hour of jogging would burn up the turnover. I need to jog to get back into control.

T: You must be in really good shape to be able to jog for an hour.

P: I guess so. But I plan to increase my jogs to 2 hours on weekends because I think that will help burn up the fat on my legs. I see marathon runners and they have nice legs, I mean the women who run all the time.

Case 2

Karen is a 24-year-old female who came into treatment for bulimia. She had been married for 2 years to Dennis, a 27-year-old attorney. Her bulimia had become increasingly worse during the past year, and she had become frightened. Her husband called to make the appointment and accompanied her to the first session. Karen was later seen individually in therapy, and a pattern became increasingly clear. After graduating from college, Karen took a job as a filing clerk at a large oil company at her father's insistence. She was still in the same job when we began meeting. She was clearly overqualified, hated it, but she had not attempted to leave. Second, Karen had been a skilled organist at her local church, where she was respected and in great demand on Sundays and for special occasions. She also had many close friends there. When she married, her husband insisted that she join his church, one of Houston's largest, where he was deacon and active on many church committees. Because the church had many talented organists, she played only once there in almost 2 years. Third, Dennis's mother, who lived close by, called or visited daily. Her calls were frequently like, "Put Channel 13 on right now. There's a program I want you to see," or "Look at the advertisement on page 6 of today's paper. There is a dress there you should buy."

T: These examples we have been discussing over the past few sessions seem to be related.
P: I have not seen the connection previously, but it is as if I do not have any control over my life any more.
T: Tell me more about that.
P: Well, my father got me my job, which I cannot stand, but I seem to be afraid to leave. I attend my husband's church and no longer play the organ, which I love to do. My husband's mother tells me what I should watch, read, and wear. Who is running my life? About the only part of my life I control is my weight, by binging and purging.

Through problem-solving and some assertiveness training, Karen decided to change jobs, attend her husband's church once a month with him and play the organ at her church the rest of the time, and take a more direct stance with her mother-in-law. With the control shifted to Karen, her bulimia decreased dramatically.

STANDARDIZED INTERVIEW FORMATS

Structured interview formats ensure that all diagnostic criteria are covered in an orderly fashion during the interview process. This structure is important for research projects and for clinics as well.

The Eating Disorder Inventory (EDI) and the EDI-2 are assessment devices created to measure psychological characteristics and maladaptive behaviors common to anorexia nervosa and bulimia nervosa (Williamson, Anderson, Jackman, & Jackson, 1995). The 64-item EDI has eight subscales. The subscales Drive for Thinness, Bulimia, and Body Dissatisfaction were created in order to assess an individual's attitude toward their body shape, weight, and eating habits (Picard, 1999). The other five subscales: Ineffectiveness, Perfection, Interpersonal Distrust, Interoceptive Awareness, and Maturity Fears examine psychological characteristics similar to those endorsed by individuals with an eating disorder (Pickard, 1999). The EDI-2, a revised version of the EDI, has the same features and items as the EDI with the addition of 27 items forming the three subscales of Asceticism, Impulse Regulation, and Social Insecurity. Because the EDI and EDI-2 are so closely related, many of the psychometric properties that were established for the EDI are relevant for the EDI-2 as well (Pickard, 1999).

Much of the normative data available for the EDI and the new subscales of the EDI-2 were based on both male and female clinical and non-clinical college samples (Williamson et al., 1995). Internal consistency is fairly high for the EDI and EDI-2. With the exception of the Maturity Fears subscale (0.65), the alpha coefficients for the EDI scale range from 0.69 to 0.93. However, these coefficients are a product of a sample of 11–18-year-olds (Williamson et al., 1995). In addition, the alpha coefficients for the EDI-2 range from 0.70 to 0.80, with the exception of the Asceticism subscale (0.40). These coefficients were produced with a group of non-clinical subjects (Williamson et al., 1995). The test–retest reliability was assessed at three different intervals: 1-week test–retest reliability ranged from 0.67 to 0.95; 3-week test-retest reliability ranged from 0.65 to 0.92; and 1-year test–retest reliability ranged from 0.41 to 0.75.

Concurrent, predictive, and discriminant validity have each been established for the EDI and EDI-2. During a 1- and 2-year follow-up, the EDI accurately predicted the presence of binge eating using the Bulimia scale (Williamson et al., 1995). In addition, the EDI subscales, Drive for Thinness, Bulimia, and Body Dissatisfaction, demonstrated expected correlations with measures assessing eating and dieting behaviors and not with general psychopathology measures (Williamson et al., 1995). An inverse relationship was demonstrated for the remaining subscales (Ineffectiveness, Perfection, Interpersonal Distrust, Maturity Fears, and Interoceptive Awareness). These subscales were highly correlated with general psychopathology measures rather than with measures assessing eating and dieting behaviors. Finally, the EDI was able to accurately classify 85% of participants into subtypes of anorexia nervosa (Williamson et al., 1995).

Overall, the EDI and EDI-2 are useful measures for diagnosing eating disorders. Furthermore, the EDI and EDI-2 can be used as treatment outcome measures (Williamson et al., 1995). Both measures are simple to administer and require approximately 20 min. However, there are several concerns regarding the use of these measures. For example, because these measures are self-report inventories, there is the possibility that an individual can over- or under-report symptomatology. Furthermore, because the EDI and EDI-2 are general eating disorder assessment devices, it may be inappropriate to use them when working with particular populations (i.e., female athletes and handicapped individuals).

The commonly used Eating Disorders Examination (EDE; Cooper & Fairburn, 1987) consists of 62 items assessing symptoms of bulimia over the 4-week period preceding the interview. The instrument was designed more for assessing therapeutic progress than for detailed initial diagnosis. The EDE consists of four subscales (Shape Concern, Weight Concern, Dietary Restraint, and Eating Concern) and several individual items assessing frequency of binge eating in a semistructured interview format (Pike, Loeb, & Walsh, 1995). EDE questions are designed to differentiate among three types of overeating: objective bulimic episodes, objective overeating, and subjective bulimic episodes. The EDE regards consumption of large amounts of food and loss of control as criteria for a binge episode. The presence or absence of these criteria distinguishes the previously mentioned categories of overeating. For instance subjective bulimic episode is characterized by the absence of consuming large amounts of food and the presence of loss of control while objective overeating involves the inverse. Objective bulimic episode is characterized by the presence of both criteria (Pike et al., 1995). As part of the EDE's examination of the frequency of overeating and purging, the patient is asked to keep a food diary for 4 weeks (Pike et al., 1995).

Beumont, Kopec-Schrader, Talbot, and Touyz (1992), found that each of the subscales in the EDE demonstrate acceptable internal consistency (alpha ranging from 0.68 to 0.78). Several studies have assessed the interrater reliability of the EDE. Cooper and Fairburn (1987) reported perfect correlations between raters on 27 out of 62 items on the EDE. The remaining items had correlation coefficients ranging from 0.69 to 1.00. Because the EDE is administered in an interview format by interviewers trained in the assessment of eating disorders, the measure is less vulnerable to false information than self-report measures. The EDE also has been found to discriminate between anorexia nervosa and bulimia nervosa as well as bulimia nervosa and restrained eaters (Pike et al., 1995).

The Interview for Diagnosis of Eating Disorders (IDED; Williamson, 1990) was designed to evaluate the core psychopathology of bulimia nervosa, anorexia nervosa, and obesity. It also assesses diagnostic criteria proposed by Williamson (1990) for "compulsive overeating," which is similar to BED. This instrument covers historical, medical, and family information as well as current behavior and cognitions regarding eating and food. The IDED has rating scales for each disorder, which allow the evaluator to rate each *DSM-IV* symptom on a 7-point scale.

INFORMATION CRITICAL TO MAKING THE DIAGNOSIS

Strong evidence suggests that eating disorders are influenced by physiological factors, familial food habits, sociocultural influences, self-perception, familial interaction patterns, and emotional status. The following discussion highlights information that we, from our research and experience, consider important in the diagnosis of eating disorders. This information is applicable to all the eating disorders, though the extent of applicability may differ with the disorder and individual.

Prior to an elaboration of *what* is required for a diagnosis, a reiteration of the *how* of this process is important. For some patients, there is considerable shame, guilt, and pain associated with their problem. In this regard, the revelation of the particulars of their difficulty is often an emotionally trying task. Hence, we feel that sensitivity and tentativeness are essential in obtaining information. No information is worth risking the impairment of the therapeutic relationship. Information is obtained most readily and comfortably when it is obtained in the context of therapy, and not apart from it, that is, inquiries regarding behavior, interpersonal relationships, and feelings are made as part of a treatment session when appropriateness is obvious and the client is judged ready.

Medical and Physical Status

For almost all the eating disorders, the point of departure for treatment is information concerning the state of the client's physical health. As noted earlier, the practices regularly engaged in by some clients can cause varying degrees of physical damage and even death. Therefore, medical assessment is a necessary first step to ensure the client's physical welfare. In cases in which the disorder has severe physical ramifications, it is highly recommended that periodic medical evaluation be incorporated into the treatment plan. It should be noted that the individual's physical appearance may belie the physiological imbalances that are not always obvious. Many bulimics maintain a normal weight while in the throes of extensive purging practices. The electrolyte imbalances that result from this behavior may not become observable until clients have fallen into a severe state of distress.

A BMI of 16 or less is indicative of anorexia nervosa (LoBuono, 2001). The client's physical condition is sometimes intimately associated with readiness for therapy. If the disorder has progressed to its more advanced stages, the consequences of the starvation will make any attempt at therapy fruitless. Such clients must achieve a medically prescribed weight and strength before such efforts can begin (Goldner & Birmingham, 1994).

Because of the potentially severe consequences of anorexia, we suggest that treatment of a client begin even if all the diagnostic criteria have not been met. In particular, the criterion of 15% below expected weight (APA, 1987) must be viewed with flexibility. For some clients, original body weight represents a degree of overweight; for others, normal or even underweight. In the latter cases, 15–20% weight loss may yield severe emaciation.

Who Wants the Treatment?

This question is an important one in processes that require personal change. When treatment has been sought by the client, the motivation implied provides the basis for effective therapeutic work. On the other hand, when the impetus for treatment derives from another, greater difficulties can be expected. This difficulty is typified in anorexia, in which it is frequently the case that the client is brought to treatment by concerned parents. The client is generally unable to comprehend the existence of a problem and is therefore disinclined to enter treatment.

The matter of who wants the treatment is also problematic in cases of BED with obesity. We occasionally find that a client has come for treatment because of the insistence or at least strong encouragement of another. The source of this encouragement is often the family physician, spouse, or close relative. In such instances, the matter of client motivation is explored in detail at the beginning of treatment. If it is apparent that the client does not desire treatment, it is usually recommended that treatment be delayed until a more appropriate time.

BEHAVIOR

Behaviors are the external manifestation of the eating disorder; their nature and frequency largely define the severity of the problem. Examples of these behaviors include binge eating, vomiting, limited food intake, excessive exercise, and strange food-related rituals (e.g., order of food consumption, insistence on a specific place setting, lists of forbidden foods, and regular departures to the bathroom after meals). It is helpful for both diagnosis and treatment that such behaviors be quantified. By so doing, the client and therapist have a baseline with which to compare later progress.

For the nonhospitialized client, self-report is the only practical way to obtain information on behavior. Self-reporting can be accomplished through use of either food records or short-term dietary and behavioral recall. It is our preference to use food records, though both techniques have value. Because of the sensitive nature of these behaviors, we place no insistence on these records if the client shows resistance to their completion.

The client's behavioral patterns may assist in the development of a more specific definition of the disorder and enhance the possibility of using appropriate interventions. The usefulness of behavioral patterns is exemplified by the bulimic and nonbulimic variations of anorexia. Some investigators define a bulimic anorectic as an anorectic who purges. Strober (1981), however, studied the etiology of bulimia in anorexia nervosa and found significant differences. Primarily, his results indicated that the family life of the bulimic anorexic is more tumultuous, conflict-ridden, and negative in comparison to that of the nonbulimic. Bulimics also seem to have greater tendencies to engage in impulsive behaviors: drug use, alcoholism, stealing, self-mutilation, and suicide (Casper, Eckert, Halmi, Goldberg, & Davis, 1980; Garfinkel, Moldofsky, & Garner, 1980; LoBuono, 2001; Wilson, 1991). In contrast to the typical view of the anorectic as introverted, the bulimic variation is likely to be more socially and sexually active (Casper et al., 1980; Johnson, 1982; Russell, 1979). The symptom complexes that differentiate the bulimic and nonbulimic anorectic suggest disorders of substantially different etiological and psychological nature.

There appears to be a significant comorbidity of the affective and anxiety disorders with anorexia nervosa (Halmi et al., 1991). Although personality disorders, especially borderline personality disorder, have been thought to be associated with bulimia nervosa, the relationship is not clear (Ames-Frankel et al., 1992). Low frustration tolerance and low self-esteem are also frequently noted psychological correlates (Foreyt, Poston, Winebarger, & McGavin, 1998).

Cognitive and Emotional Factors

Examples of cognitive distortions have been reported for anorexia nervosa (Garner et al., 1982), binge eating (Loro & Orleans, 1981), and obesity

(Mahoney & Mahoney, 1976). We have found that certain of these distortions are present in all eating disorders, indicating the possibility of a cultural pattern gone awry. In some, for example, staunch perfectionism is the cause of much distress and sometimes failure. These individuals proceed with substantial success on a diet until the first infraction occurs, no matter how minor. The inability to maintain a perfect record sends many into a binge that ends with self-recrimination and guilt. Emotional factors such as being teased about weight and shape, and other factors such as body dissatisfaction, dietary restraint, weight cycling, and negative affect were found to be significant predictors for binge eating in obese women and men (Womble et al., 2001).

Psychological characteristics associated with anorexia included distorted thoughts and beliefs (Garner et al., 1982), distorted body image (Crisp & Kalucy, 1974), and fears about matters of self-control (Bruch, 1977). Perfectionism in the anorectic takes on an extreme form. The anorectic perceives her body as too large regardless of how thin she becomes (Warah, 1989). Some carry this trait in all aspects of their life as well as in their anorexia.

Familial Factors

The eating disorders are the products of multiple influences. One of the most important influences is the family, for it has an impact on the individual's development of self-concept, values, food and eating patterns, and personal standards. Specific ways in which the family may impact eating disorders have been suggested by various clinicians and theorists (e.g., Bruch, 1973, 1977; Rosman et al., 1977; White & Boskind-White, 1981; Pike & Rodin, 1991).

The therapist should assess for familial patterns of interactions and behaviors related to the client's difficulties. The works of Bruch (1973) and Rosman et al. (1977) provide insight into the characteristics of the obese and anorexic families. Of the two, the latter has been the subject of more research, and therefore more is known. Research on the familial factors associated with bulimia has been sparse. In a clinical investigation, Strober (1981) reported a number of significant differences between families of bulimic and nonbulimic anorectics. Families of bulimics, in comparison to those of nonbulimics, were found to have less structure, less cohesion, and more conflict and negativity.

In cases in which the client remains in the care of the parents, diagnosis and treatment of the entire family is frequently necessary. In particular, young adolescents with anorexia nervosa or bulimia nervosa may be able to maintain their weight gain and improve their psychosocial adjustment when both parents and adolescent are involved in therapy within family-based treatment programs (Ghaderi, 2001). Overall, family therapy is typically viewed as an important therapeutic component (Goldner & Birmingham, 1994).

There have been mixed results regarding the association between sexual abuse and eating disorders. However, it is generally accepted that sexual abuse is a common theme among anorectics (Thompson, 1994; Wonderlich, Brewerton, Jocic, Dansky, & Abbott, 1997). Tripp and Petrie (2001) found that women who were sexually abused reported feelings of shame and guilt resulting in body disparagement they hypothesize may play a role in the subsequent development of eating disorders.

Social Factors

For many with eating disorders, social factors are pertinent to both the etiology and maintenance of their disorder. From a sociocultural perspective, eating disorders are likely to be a product of contemporary American society (i.e., a society that places inordinate value on slimness while simultaneously emphasizing the consumption of an abundant food supply).

Bulimia, like anorexia nervosa, is a problem primarily of young women. In this regard, it is probable that some of the sociocultural pressures that result in anorexia operate to influence the onset of bulimia, as well. White and Boskind-White (1981) theorized that this condition occurs because of the need for some women to fit into the role of "stereotyped femininity." In fulfilling this stereotyping, these researchers suggest, the basis for bulimia is also developed and reinforced; this basis includes a need to please others, tendencies toward passivity, and an excessive concern for appearance and thinness.

In many cases of bulimia, for example, the notion of purging is obtained from an acquaintance or friend as an alternative to the consequences of excessive eating. For the suggestive, purging begins as a logical and apparently socially acceptable way to consume voraciously without substantial weight gain. Unfortunately, a rather innocent induction can progress into a disturbing, all-encompassing compulsion. For anorectics, it is not unusual to find that their social activities, work, or both impact the development of their disorder. Those involved in ballet, gymnastics, modeling, or cheerleading seem to have particular pressures to maintain sylphlike figures. High schools, for example, often have eligibility requirements for the cheerleading squad that include rather stringent height–weight standards.

One phenomena frequently observed in individuals suffering from eating disorders is difficulty with interpersonal relationships. Among bulimics, problems in this area are the frequent cause of a binge. Obese children are often social outcasts discriminated against to the point that their social development is impeded. Lacking the rewards of social interaction, some may seek solace through eating. The ways in which social factors may contribute to an eating disorder are varied and often complex. Discerning them is an important part of the diagnostic process.

Racial Differences

For many years it had been assumed that eating disorders occurred almost solely among European and European American women; particularly, in the upper class. Thus, investigations into eating disorders among women of color had been sadly neglected. However, new research has shown that women of color are not exempt from developing eating disorders. It is estimated that 1–4% of women of color suffer from anorexia nervosa and/or bulimia nervosa (Miller & Pumariega, 2001). Moreover, research has shown that BED is common among women of color, particularly among African-American women ranging in age from 45 to 54 years (Harris & Kuba, 2001). However, due to a paucity of research in this particular area, diagnostic criteria and therapeutic approaches useful with women of color are lacking.

According to several studies, there are a variety of factors leading to the development of eating disorders in women of color. Factors such as acculturation, peer group identification, and family situations are known to impact the prevalence of eating disturbances among African American women. For example, studies have shown that there is a positive correlation between eating disorders and the separation from one's ethnic culture to the dominant culture (Harris & Kuba, 1997). For example, some cultures such as African American and Latin American, demonstrate greater acceptance of a fuller body. But, when the dominant culture suggests a thin ideal body type, conflicts can result between the two cultures, which foster an identity crisis for the individual. When this conflict is internalized, it may lead to the development of an eating disorder (Harris & Kuba, 1997).

Other factors, including socioeconomic status (SES), have also been shown to affect eating patterns in women of color. For example, some studies have shown that differences in SES could predict anorectic and bulimic behaviors among African-American and Latin American adolescents. Like their Caucasian counterparts, African-American women who attained a higher education level and social status were at a higher risk for developing anorectic and bulimic behaviors than African American women who were not as affluent socially and economically (Harris & Kuba, 2001).

Racial differences between Black and White women have also been noted using the EDE. Although no distinctions are seen between healthy females of both racial groups, assessment of clinical samples suggests that Black women with BED are less concerned with body weight and shape than are their White counterparts. Moreover, Black women evidence higher body weight and more frequent binging than White women. Finally, White women with BED are more likely to have a positive history of bulimia nervosa than are Black women with BED (Pike, Dohm, Striegel-Moore, Wilfley, & Fairburn, 2001). Thus, the clinical picture for White and Black female binge eaters may be very dissimilar.

Overall, an assumption on the part of the interviewer of a low prevalence of eating disorders in women of color may produce an inaccurate diagnosis. Moreover, women of color may evidence eating pathologies that do not entirely overlap with the eating disorder symptomatology presented in the *DSM-IV*, thus complicating the process of making a valid eating disorder diagnosis. Due to the potential for diagnostic problems, Harris and Kuba (1997) have proposed guidelines for increasing the accuracy of diagnosing eating disorders in women of color (Table 4).

GENDER DIFFERENCES

Although a higher percentage of women suffer from eating disorders, studies have shown that men are affected by eating disorders as well, and that these

TABLE 4. Guidelines for Accurately Diagnosing Eating Disorders in Women of Color[a]

A. Explore the history of eating patterns in the client's family and culture while considering the pattern of differentiation or rejection of the culture by the woman with an eating disorder.
B. Consider the deviation of the client's current eating habits from those expected within her culture, and evaluate diagnostically using the cultural expectations as a standard.
C. Be prepared to diagnose specific pathological eating patterns that are self-destructive but are not described by the *DSM-IV*. These might include ritual dieting binge eating episodes.
D. Examine the client's concept of beauty. Has it changed? When did this change occur? Is this concept congruent with the ethnoculture of origin, or is it primarily related to the expectations of a more oppressive ethnocultural image?
E. Examine self-hatred in relation to ethnoculture. This self-hatred may be expressed metaphorically through the use of food. For example, self-loathing may appear as restricted food intake. Consider that classic symptoms may be modified in women of color who have eating disorders or may appear in entirely different clusters (Lee et al., 1989).
F. Be willing to use the *DSM-IV* diagnostic category of "Eating Disorder Not Otherwise Specified," giving enough specificity to justify insurance coverage for clients with atypical symptoms.

[a]From Harris and Kuba (1997).

illnesses are similar in both males and females (Woodside et al., 2001). In all likelihood, men are underdiagnosed for eating disorders because many studies involve clinically referred rather than community samples. For instance, Anderson (2001) examined the prevalence rates for anorexia in clinical and community samples of males and reported rates of 5–10% and 16%, respectively.

Studies of individuals involved in weight-control programs have demonstrated that women are 1.5 times more likely than men to have BED. Male binge eaters tend to evidence a higher BMI and are more likely to be classified as obese while their female counterparts experience greater body dissatisfaction. Males in this group also report a greater frequency of drug abuse (Barry, Grilo, & Masheb, 2001).

Physiological Factors

Recent research has suggested that serotonin may play a role in the development of eating disorders in certain individuals. For example, perhaps in an effort to compensate for low serotonin levels, bulimics and binge eaters may consume high quantities of carbohydrates or foods high in tryptophan and low in protein (Foreyt et al., 1998). It also has been noted that medication in the form of antidepressants, which help to produce higher levels of serotonin, given to bulimic patients help to control their bulimic behaviors. The opposite may hold true for anorexic patients. Overly high levels of serotonin are thought to inhibit appetite and thus reduce food intake subsequently resulting in weight loss. However, this hypothesis is based, in part, on the observation that medications which act to increase serotonin are ineffective for anorexics (Foreyt et al., 1998).

Other studies also have observed serotonin levels along with additional neurochemical changes. For example, while bulimic women with and without childhood abuse evidenced low serotonin levels, those with an abusive history also had relatively lower cortisol levels (Steiger et al., 2001). Furthermore, the same study also found a reduced platelet paroxetine binding in women suffering from bulimia nervosa. Although studies like these suggest that physiological conditions may explain symptoms and behaviors in eating disorders, it is still noted that these neurochemical changes may not cause eating disorders. For example, physiological changes may be due to the behaviors demonstrated in eating disorders, rather than vice versa (Foreyt et al., 1998).

DOS AND DON'TS

Do try to lessen the stigma of eating disorders so that the patient may be more willing to disclose symptomatology. This can be accomplished by explaining the prevalence of eating disorders in the population, by explaining how eating disorders are caused by unrealistic cultural norms for body shape and size, the mistaken idea that diets are effective in weight management, and by self-disclosure. For example:

T: I understand that you are here because you feel out of control in your eating. How do you feel about this problem?

P: I guess I have an addictive personality. I am the kind of person who can't control myself.

T: Almost every patient tells me what you have just said. But I want you to know that there are hundreds of thousands of people in this country who have exactly the same problem that you have. The problem is caused by the body's natural response to dieting. If you try to breathe really shallowly for a long time, soon you will be gasping uncontrollably for air. Would you blame yourself or feel like you had an "air addiction?"

P: You mean if I gasped for air after breathing shallowly?

T: Yes.

P: No, I guess not, since anybody would gasp for air.

T: O.K. So you shouldn't blame yourself for "gasping for food" after being on a diet, right?

P: I guess not.

T: One thing you need to realize is that you dieted because there is a widespread belief that dieting works to control weight. So you shouldn't blame yourself for dieting. I mean, everybody does it. But now we know that almost everyone who develops an eating disorder, a problem with controlled eating, has a history of serious dieting. Scientists are fairly sure that this is caused by physiological processes, not psychological. In other words you shouldn't blame yourself for your eating-control problems. Now our task is to find out all about your eating control problems so that we can help you do what you need to do to change those physiological processes so you can eat normally.

* * *

T: I should tell you that I have never been officially diagnosed with an eating disorder, but I can tell you that sometimes when I have to skip breakfast and have a hectic day at work, that sometimes when I go home I really pig out on bad stuff, like pizza and chips. And I should know better, since I am a doctor! So perhaps I have some of the symptoms of eating disorders, but not quite as serious as most people who come in to the clinic. But I can identify with what you are going through. I mean, I am like you in some ways. You know, we're all in the same boat as women trying to cope with the weird ideas about what we should look like and what we should eat in this society!

Don't imply that the patient may have an eating disorder because of some unresolved past sexual trauma, such as incest. There is no evidence for such a direct causality (Pope & Hudson, 1992; Waller, 1991), and bringing up such subjects in the evaluation phase may only add to the patient's burden of guilt and shame associated with eating disorders. It may be best to stick to cultural/physiological explanations of eating disorders and let patients reveal any history of abuse later in therapy.

Don't reinforce the notion that the patient has a disease and that family members will be consulted to help the patient. In eating disorders, it may be best to explain the problem as a cultural/physiological problem in which the patient and family members are equally involved as victims.

SUMMARY

The diagnosis of eating disorders is far more complex than simply checking the criteria listed in the DSM. Their complex nature, multiple etiologies, family dynamics, and highly refractory nature make them exceedingly challenging clinical problems.

ACKNOWLEDGMENT. Preparation of this manuscript was supported in part by Grant 1RO1 DK43109–01A1 from the National Institutes of Diabetes and Digestive and Kidney Diseases.

REFERENCES

American Psychiatric Association. (1987). *Diagnostic and statistical manual of mental disorders* (3rd ed., Revised). Washington, DC: Author.

American Psychiatric Association. (1994). *Diagnostic and statistical manual of mental disorders* (4th ed., draft criteria). Washington, DC: Author.

Ames-Frankel, J., Devlin, M. J., Walsh, B. T., Strasser, T. J., Sadik, C., Oldham, J. M., & Roose, S. P. (1992). Personality disorder diagnoses in patients with bulimia nervosa: Clinical correlates and changes with treatment. *Journal of Clinical Psychology, 53*, 90–96.

Anderson, A. E. (2001). Progress in eating disorders research. *American Journal of Psychiatry, 158*(4), 515–517.

Barry, D. T., Grilo, C. M., & Masheb, R. M. (2001). Gender differences in patients with binge eating disorder. *International Journal of Eating Disorders, 31*, 63–70.

Bemis, K. M. (1978). Current approaches to the etiology and treatment of anorexia nervosa. *Psychological Bulletin, 85*, 593–617.

Beumont, P. V. J., Kopec-Schrader, E. M., Talbot, P., & Touyz, S. W. (1992). *Measuring the specific psychopathology of eating disorder patients.* Unpublished manuscript.

Brownell, K. D. (1991). Dieting and the search for the perfect body: Where physiology and culture collide. *Behavior Therapy, 22*, 1–12.

Bruch, H. (1973). *Eating disorders.* New York: Basic Books.

Bruch, H. (1977). Psychological antecedents of anorexia nervosa. In R. A. Vigersky (Ed.), *Anorexia nervosa* (pp. 1–10). New York: Raven Press.

Bruch, H. (1978). *The golden cage.* Cambridge, MA: Harvard University Press.

Casper, R. C., Eckert, E. D., Halmi, K. A., Goldberg, S. C., & Davis, J. M. (1980). Bulimia: Its incidence and clinical importance in patients with anorexia nervosa. *Archives of General Psychiatry, 37*, 1030–1035.

Cooper, Z., & Fairburn, C. G. (1987). The eating disorder examination: A semistructured interview for the assessment of the specific psychopathology of eating disorders. *International Journal of Eating Disorders, 6*, 1–8.

Crisp, A. H., & Kalucy, R. S. (1974). Aspects of the perceptual disorder in anorexia nervosa. *British Journal of Medical Psychology, 47*, 349–361.

Crowther, J. H., Sanftner, J., Bonifazi, & Shepherd, K. L. (2001). The role of daily hassles in binge eating. *International Journal of Eating Disorders, 29*, 449–454.

Eliot, A. O., & Wood-Baker, C. (2001). Eating disordered adolescent males. *Adolescence, 36*(143), 535–543.

Foreyt, J. P., Poston, W. S. C., Winebarger, A. A., & McGavin, J. K. (1998). Anorexia nervosa and bulimia nervosa. In E. J. Mash & R. A. Barkley (Eds.), *Treatment of childhood disorders* (pp. 647–691). New York, NY: The Guilford Press.

Garfinkel, P. E., Moldofsky, H., & Garner, D. M. (1980). The heterogeneity of anorexia nervosa: Bulimia as a distinct subgroup. *Archives of General Psychiatry, 37*, 1036–1040.

Garner, D. M., Garfinkel, P. E., & Bemis, K. M. (1982). A multidimensional psychotherapy for anorexia nervosa. *International Journal of Eating Disorders, 1*, 3–46.

Ghaderi, A. (2001). Review of risk factors for eating disorders: Implications for primary prevention and cognitive behavioural therapy. *Scandinavian Journal of Behavior Therapy, 30*(2), 57–74.

Goldfein, J. A., Devlin, M. J., & Spitzer, R. L. (2000). Cognitive behavioral therapy for the treatment of binge eating disorder: What constitutes success? *American Journal of Psychiatry, 157*(7), 1051–1056.

Goldner, E. M., & Birmingham, C. L. (1994). Anorexia nervosa: Methods of treatment. In L. Alexander-Mott & D. B. Lumsden (Eds.), *Understanding eating disorders: Anorexia nervosa, bulimia nervosa, and obesity* (pp. 135–157). Washington, DC: Taylor & Francis.

Halmi, K. A., Eckert, E., Marchi, P., Sampugnaro, V., Apple, R., & Cohen, J. (1991). Comorbidity of psychiatric diagnoses in anorexia. *Archives of General Psychiatry, 48*, 712–718.

Halmi, K. A., Goldberg, S. C., Eckert, E., Casper, R., & Davis, J. P. (1977). Pretreatment evaluation in anorexia nervosa. In R. A. Vigersky (Ed.), *Anorexia nervosa* (pp. 43–54). New York: Raven Press.

Harris, D. J., & Kuba, S. A. (1997). Ethnocultural identity and eating disorders in women of color. *Professional Psychology: Research and Practice, 28*(4), 341–347.

Harris, D. J., & Kuba, S. A. (2001). Eating disturbances in women of color: An exploratory study of contextual factors in the development of disordered eating in Mexican-American women. *Health Care for Women International, 22*, 281–298.

Johnson, C. (1982). Anorexia nervosa and bulimia. In T. J. Coates, A. C. Peterson, & C. Perry (Eds.), *Promoting adolescent health: A dialogue on research and practice* (pp. 397–412). New York: Academic Press.

Lee, S., Chiu, H. F. K., & Chen, C. N. (1989). Anorexia nervosa in Hong Kong—Why not more in Chinese? *British Journal of Psychiatry, 154*, 683–688.

LoBuono, C. (2001). Identifying and managing eating disorders. *Patient Care, 35*(22), 25–39.

Loro, A. D., & Orleans, C. S. (1981). Binge eating is obesity: Preliminary findings and guidelines for behavioral analysis and treatment. *Addictive Behaviors, 6*, 155–166.

Mahoney, M. J., & Mahoney, K. (1976). *Permanent weight control.* New York: W.W. Norton.

Miller, M. N., & Pumariega, A. J. (2001). Culture and eating disorders: A historical and cross-cultural review. *Psychiatry, 64*(2), 93–110.

Mitchell, J., Specker, S., & de Zwaan, M. (1991). Comorbidity and medical complications of bulimia nervosa. *Journal of Clinical Psychiatry, 52*, 13–20.

Neuman, P. A., & Halvorson, P. A. (1983). *Anorexia nervosa and bulimia: A handbook for counselors and therapists.* New York: Von Nostrand Reinhold.

Pendleton, V. P., Willems, E., Swank, P., Poston, W. S. C., Goodrick, G. K., Reeves, R. S., & Foreyt, J. P. (2001). Negative stress and the outcome of treatment for binge eating. *Eating Disorders: The Journal of Treatment and Prevention, 9*, 351–360.

Picard, C. L. (1999). The level of competition as a factor for the development of eating disorders in female collegiate athletes. *Journal of Youth and Adolescence, 28*(5), 583–594.

Pike, K. M., Dohm, F. A., Striegel-Moore, R., Wilfley, D. E., & Fairburn, C. G. (2001). A comparison of black and white women with binge eating disorder. *The American Journal of Psychiatry, 158*, 1455–1460.

Pike, K. M., Loeb, K., & Walsh, B. T. (1995). Binge eating and purging. In D. B. Allison (Ed.), *Handbook of assessment methods for eating behaviors and weight-related problems: Measures, theory, and research* (pp. 303–346). Thousand Oaks, CA: Sage.

Pike, K. M., & Rodin, J. (1991). Mothers, daughters, and disordered eating. *Journal of Abnormal Psychology, 100*, 198–204.

Pope, H. G., & Hudson, J. I. (1992). Is childhood sexual abuse a risk factor for bulimia nervosa? *American Journal of Psychiatry, 149*, 455–463.

Rosman, B. L., Minuchin, S., Baker, L., & Liebman, R. (1977). A family approach to anorexia nervosa: Study, treatment, and outcome. In R. A. Vigersky (Ed.), *Anorexia nervosa* (pp. 341–348). New York: Raven Press.

Russell, G. F. M. (1979). Bulimia nervosa: An ominous variant of anorexia nervosa. *Psychological Medicine, 9*, 429–448.

Spitzer, R. L., Devlin, M., Walsh, B. T., Hasin, D., Wing, R., Marcus, M., Stunkard, A., Wadden, T., Yanovski, S., Agras, S., Mitchell, J., & Nonas, C. (1992). Binge eating disorder: A multisite field trial of the diagnostic criteria. *International Journal of Eating Disorders, 11*, 191–203.

Steiger, H., Gauvin, L., Israel, M., Koerner, N., Ng Ying Kin, N. M. K., Paris, J., & Young, S. N. (2001). Association of serotonin and cortisol indices with childhood abuse in bulimia nervosa. *Archives of General Psychiatry, 58*(9), 837–843.

Strober, M. (1981). A comparative analysis of personality organization in juvenile anorexia nervosa. *Journal of Youth and Adolescence, 10*, 285–295.

Thompson, B. W. (1994). *A hunger so wide and so deep: American women speak out on eating problems.* Minneapolis: Minnesota Press.

Tripp, M. M., & Petrie, T. A. (2001). Sexual abuse and eating disorders: A test of a conceptual model. *Sex Roles, 44*(1/2), 17–32.

Waller, G. (1991). Sexual abuse as a factor in eating disorders. *British Journal of Psychiatry, 159*, 664–671.

Warah, A. (1989). Body image disturbance in anorexia nervosa: Beyond body image. *Canadian Journal of Psychiatry, 34*, 898–905.

White, W. C., & Boskind-White, M. (1981). An experiential-behavioral approach to the treatment of bulimarexia. *Psychotherapy: Theory, Research and Practice, 18*, 501–507.

Williamson, D. A. (1990). *Assessment of eating disorders: Obesity, anorexia, and bulimia nervosa.* New York: Pergamon Press.

Williamson, D. A., Anderson, D. A., Jackman, L. P., & Jackson, S. R. (1995). Assessment of eating disordered thoughts, feelings, and behaviors. In D. B. Allison (Ed.), *Handbook of assessment methods for eating behaviors and weight-related problems: Measures, theory, and research* (pp. 347–386). Thousand Oaks, CA: Sage.

Wilson, G. T. (1991). The addiction model of eating disorders: A critical analysis. *Advances in Behavioral Research and Therapy, 13*, 27–72.

Wilson, G. T. (1992). Diagnostic criteria for bulimia nervosa. *International Journal of Eating Disorders, 11*, 315–319.

Womble, L. G., Williamson, D. A., Martin, C. K., Zucker, N. L., Thaw, J. M., Netemeyer, R., Lovejoy, J. C., & Greenway, F. L. (2001). Psychosocial variables associated with binge eating in obese males and females. *International Journal of Eating Disorders, 30*(2), 217–221.

Wonderlich, S. A., Brewerton, T. D., Jocic, Z., Dansky, B. S., & Abbott, D. W. (1997). Relationships of childhood sexual abuse and eating disorders. *Journal of the American Academy of Child and Adolescent Psychiatry, 36*, 1107–1113.

Woodside, D. B., Garfinkel, P. E., Lin, E., Goering, P., Kaplan, A. S., Goldbloom, D. S., & Kennedy, S. H. (2001). Comparisons of men with full or partial eating disorders, men without eating disorders, and women with eating disorders in the community. *American Journal of Psychiatry, 158*(4), 570–574.

13

Psychophysiological Disorders

ELLIE T. STURGIS

The conditions identified as psychophysiological disorders have had an interesting history. It is as if one is involved in a game of hide and seek: now you see them; now you do not. This history is reflective of the changes in the understanding of medical and psychological disorders over the past century. Early in the century, a dualistic model pervaded in which the mind and body were considered separate entities. Any influence of one upon the other was hypothesized as unidirectional. The discipline of health psychology emerged in the late 1970s and included psychologists of varied disciplinary persuasions and methodologies who shared common interests in health and illness (Revenson & Baum, 2000). A non-dualistic understanding of behavior emerged—the biopsychosocial model (Engel, 1977; Schwartz, 1982). This approach viewed health and illness as an integration of physiological, psychological, and social factors with no single system being primary. Each part of the symptom affected and was affected by each other component. Proponents of this model argued that disorders or diseases were not caused by single agents or factors, that is, the reciprocal interaction of varied factors resulted in the manifestation of the symptoms (Revenson & Baum, 2000).

Research in the biopsychosocial model stimulated more effective theories and research designs and facilitated multidisciplinary thinking. Most important, the model proposed a multicause, multieffect approach to health and behavior. Individuals began to examine responses at different levels. Not only could we assess observable behavior, but we were also able to examine cognitive variables such as schemas, expectancies, perceived control; psychophysiological activity (e.g., electromyographic, electrodermal, cardiovascular, electroencephalogic patterns); biochemical functioning; cortical structure (computer tomography [CT] scan, magnetic resonance imaging [MRI]); and cortical activity (positron-emission tomography [PET] scans). The ability to examine a phenomenon at multiple levels of analysis was enlightening and revealed further evidence of the reciprocal interactions among biological, psychological, and social factors in creating conditions of health and illness (Revenson & Baum, 2000).

ELLIE T. STURGIS • Counseling Associates of Southwest Virginia, Blacksburg, Virginia 24060.

The classification of psychophysiological disorders has reflected changes in the conception of the disorders. In the first and second volumes of the Diagnostic and Statistical Manual of Mental Disorders ((*DSM-I* and *II*) American Psychiatric Association [APA], 1952, 1968), the diagnostic codes generally exemplified concepts of mind–body dualism; that is, disorders were caused by biological mechanisms or psychological mechanisms. The *DSM-I* and *II* classified physical conditions deemed as being primarily functional in nature, that is, caused by psychological factors, as Psychophysiologic Disorders and included codes for skin, musculoskeletal, respiratory, cardiovascular, hemic and lymphatic, gastrointestinal (GI), genitourinary, endocrine, nervous system (neurasthenic neurosis in *DSM-II*) disorders, and reactions of organs of special senses.

The *DSM-III* and *DSM-III-R* reflected the emerging biopsychosocial model of psychosomatic illness. These systems dropped the classification of psychophysiological disorders per se, establishing a more inclusive categorization of mental disorder named Psychological Factors Affecting Physical Condition. This category was used to describe any physical condition to which psychological factors were judged to be contributory; it described disorders previously diagnosed as psychosomatic or psychophysiologic (APA, 1980, 1987). Common examples for the category included obesity, headaches, pain (angina pectoris, menstruation, sacroiliac, rheumatoid arthritis), cardiovascular problems (tachycardia, arrhythmia, cardiospasm), GI disorders (gastric and duodenal ulcers, pylorospasm, nausea and vomiting, regional enteritis, and ulcerative colitis), and frequent micturition.

In developing the *DSM-IV*, the authors increasingly relied on data from previous research and empirical field trials to develop the diagnostic categories. Stoudemire et al. (1996) conducted an extensive literature review and supported the idea that psychological variables affect many physical conditions. The Task Force on *DSM-IV* examined this extensive literature and consulted with primary care physicians and consultation psychiatrists. It determined that the conditions represented by the diagnosis did not constitute mental disorders but were physical disorders. The category ceased to exist as a mental disorder but was moved to another section of the *DSM-IV*, "Other Conditions That May Be a Focus of Clinical Attention." The disorder continues to be coded on Axis I with the relevant medical condition coded on Axis III.

Research related to the psychophysiological disorders has steadily increased over the past few decades despite fluctuations in the nomenclature used to represent the disorders. In preparing this chapter, I examined research patterns among the most commonly diagnosed psychophysiological disorders using *PsychInfo*, the online version of *Psychological Abstracts*. Searches were conducted using several diagnoses as keywords. The numbers of articles published in each decade for each designation are summarized in Table 1.

A review of the table indicates several points. First, research is generally reported for specific disorders, not for the generic term psychophysiological. Second, there is significant growth in published research into disorders historically considered as psychophysiological. During the 1950s, *PsychInfo* yielded no hits for such research whereas the 1990s show considerable activity. Research efforts have examined many facets of the varied disorders including etiology,

TABLE 1. Summary of Publications on Common Psychophysiological Disorders

Keyword	1950–1959	1960–1969	1970–1979	1980–1989	1990–1999
Psychophysiological disorders	0	5	25	38	50
Chronic pain[a]	0	0	36	1,168	3,014
Irritable bowel syndrome	0	0	0	5	155
Hypertension[b]	0	0	65	195	107
Headaches[c]	0	1	212	860	1,379
Ulcers[d]	0	12	150	250	160
Total	0	19	890	3,610	6,484

Values represent entries with multiple categories.
[a]Chronic, somatoform, back, myofacial pain, and pain management.
[b]Hypertension and essential hypertension.
[c]Headache, migraine headache, and tension headache.
[d]Ulcer and GI ulcer.

assessment, contributing factors, treatment, and evaluation. It is interesting to note the two areas in which a decrease in research activity was observed in the 1990s. In both cases, significant medical and pharmacological advances occurred. In the case of peptic ulcer disease, medical thinking shifted away from a psychosomatic orientation, as the roles of bacterial flora (i.e., *Helicobacter pylori*) and the immune systems in the etiology of ulcers were elucidated and it became possible to eradicate this bacteria using antibiotics (National Institutes of Health Consensus Development Panel on *Helicobacter pylori* in Peptic Ulcer Disease, 1994; Rauws & Tytgat, 1990). During the ensuing decade, research into the nonbiological aspects of peptic ulcer disease decreased markedly; however, there has been some resurgence in interest in the biopsychosocial aspects of the disorder. Current research shows that many ulcers occur in the absence of the bacterium and that eradication of the bacterium with antibiotics can sometimes fail to cure symptoms or prevent recurrence (Levenstein, 2002).

Psychological research on migraine headaches showed a decline following the introduction of two serotonin D1 agonists that targeted the nerves and cranial blood vessels involved in headache onset. Despite the potential for serious side effects in some patients, use of these medications resulted in a reliable constriction of the cerebral blood vessels and in many cases, terminated the headache almost immediately, thus reducing the motivation of clients to engage in more time demanding intervention procedures. As in the case with peptic ulcers, however, these medicines are not effective for all individuals. There continues to be a role for psychosocial interventions.

Increased understanding seldom simplifies the conceptual process. Such is the case in the diagnosis and treatment of psychophysiological disorders or those medical conditions complicated by psychological factors. In the ensuing chapter, implications of the biopsychosocial approach to the evaluation of two particular disorders will be considered. Although the principles discussed will have relevance to many disorders, their importance in the diagnosis and formulation of treatment plans for irritable bowel syndrome (IBS) and chronic pain will be highlighted.

IRRITABLE BOWEL SYNDROME

Description of the Disorder

IBS (previously known as irritable colon, spastic colon, mucous colitis, and spastic colitis) is a term used to refer to abdominal pain and changed bowel habits not explained by another disease process such as bacterial infection, lactose deficiency, or inflammatory bowel disease (Blanchard, 2001; Thompson, Creed, Drossman, Heaton, Mazzacca, 1992). The disorder affects 9–22% of the North American population and accounts for 12% of all visits to general practitioners and 28% of visits to gastroenterologists (Toner, Segal, Emmott, & Myran, 2000). Prospective follow-up studies have indicated that the symptoms of IBS do not typically remit spontaneously over time. In a review of 6 studies, Blanchard (2001) found that 24–57% of IBS patients were unchanged or worse 5 years later.

Despite the high utilization of health care providers by individuals with IBS, Whitehead, Bosmajian, Zonderman, Costa, and Schuster (1988) found that most sufferers do not seek medical attention. Estimates of the prevalence of IBS indicate that rates are approximately twice as great for women than men, with three times as many women seeking care for the disorder from a general practitioner. In tertiary health centers, female clients are 4–5 times more prevalent than male patients. In contrast to most medical disorders, most IBS researchers use only women in their samples (Toner et al., 2000).

The gastroenterology community has specified the criteria for the disorder, with the most current revision being labeled the Rome II criteria (Thompson et al., 1999). According to this conceptualization, the disorder is diagnosed if an individual exhibits the following symptoms for at least 12 weeks (not necessarily continuous) during the past 12 months. The person experiences abdominal pain or discomfort and two of the following apply: (1) the pain is relieved by defecation, (2) its onset is associated with a change in the frequency or consistency of the stool, and (3) its onset is associated with a change in the form or appearance of the stool. Other symptoms supportive of the diagnosis are: (1) the occurrence of fewer than three bowel movements a week or more than three movements in a day; (2) the presence of hard or lumpy stools; (3) the presence of loose or watery stools; (4) feelings of urgency to have a bowel movement; (5) the need to strain while having a movement; (6) feelings of having an incomplete bowel movement; (7) passing mucus during a bowel movement; and (8) feelings of abdominal fullness, bloating, or swelling.

While numerous studies have shown that people with IBS who do not seek health care do not differ from healthy controls on a number of variables (Drossman et al., 1988; Welch, Hillman, and Pomare, 1985; Whitehead et al., 1988), research among those who do seek medical attention has revealed a number of contributors to the disorder. Research investigating clients diagnosed with psychiatric disorders and investigations of psychopathology in IBS patients have revealed that IBS patients show concomitant mood (Dewsnap, Gomborone, Libby, & Farthing, 1996; Lydiard, 1992; Walker et al., 1990), panic (Lydiard, 1992; Noyes, Cook et al., 1990; Walker et al., 1990), general anxiety (Blanchard, 2001; Lydiard, 1992; Tollefson,

Tollefson, Pederson, Luxenberg, & Dunsmore, 1991), post-traumatic stress (Irwin et al., 1996), and social phobic disorders (Blanchard, 2001). Several studies have shown a higher exposure rates to early physical and sexual abuse among individuals with IBS (Leserman et al., 1996; Walker, Katon, Roy-Byrne, Jemelka, & Russo, 1993) with the severity of the symptoms increasing with higher levels of sexual abuse (Drossman, Talley, Leserman, Olden, & Barreiro, 1995). The cognitions of patients with IBS have been found to differ from non-patients as they show higher levels of fear of disease (Toner et al., 1999), selective attention to GI sensations (Whitehead & Pallson, 1998), and higher levels of self-blame and self-silencing (Ali & Toner, 1996; Toner et al., 2000).

Procedures for Gathering Information

Unfortunately, there are no definitive tests for IBS (Blanchard, 2001). Because symptoms of IBS can mimic signs of other GI pathophysiology, a complete examination by a physician is indicated. Medical conditions to be ruled out through such a medical evaluation include inflammatory bowel disease, intestinal parasites, and lactose intolerance (Toner et al., 2000). A recent position paper for the American Gastroenterological Association recommended that routine evaluations for IBS should include a physical examination; complete blood count with sedimentation rate; a biochemical analysis of the stool for the presence of ova, parasites, and blood; and either a flexible sigmoidoscopy or colonoscopy (Drossman, Whitehead, & Camilleri, 1997).

In addition to a medical evaluation, the interview should obtain a narrative history of the disorder including its onset and the presence of relevant psychosocial events surrounding the initiation and continuation of symptoms. In addition, the clinician will want to learn about the patient's perceptions of the course of the illness as well as the impact of the symptoms on relationships, daily activities, and the quality of life. The therapist should also note the presence of other physical problems, as a long history of multiple physical symptoms, high rates of disability, multiple diagnostic procedures, or poorly explained medical problems can alert the therapist to possible somatic patterns of expression of illnesses. The interview can also be used to gather information about a client's openness to assumptions underlying a cognitive or cognitive–behavioral model of treatment by examining whether symptoms are triggered by factors such as fatigue, diet, work pressures, family pressures, etc. (Toner et al., 2000).

Any comprehensive assessment will also include completion of a daily symptom diary used to evaluate the frequency of bowel movements, associated symptoms, food avoidance, activity avoidance, and medication usage (Blanchard, 2001). Data from a 1–2 week period is helpful in establishing a definitive diagnosis of the disorder.

Given the higher incidence of psychiatric comorbidity in IBS patients in tertiary medical settings, the current and lifetime prevalence of psychiatric disorders should be assessed, with particular emphasis on anxiety, mood, and somatoform disorders. This is particularly important in treatment planning, as it may be necessary to treat the coexisting disorder in addition to the IBS (Toner et al., 2000).

As is the case with other medical disorders with significant psychological components, it is important to assess the social context of the individual including gender role expectations, social supports, stressors, cognitive expectancies, and coping style. Toner et al. (2000) provide an excellent discussion of social and cognitive factors affecting the course of IBS.

Case Illustration

The patient is a 33-year-old, Caucasian female referred to the author by her physician. The patient is an associate at a prestigious law firm and a decision regarding partnership is expected this year. She reports a 10-year history of GI pain and symptoms beginning in law school. A physical examination and a panel of tests revealed no significant organic pathology. The interview questions are adapted from the Albany IBS History (Blanchard, 2001). Because of space limitations only portions of the interview are reproduced below.

T: I am interested in learning more about your current medical condition. How would you describe the problem?

C: I have a lot of abdominal pain, diarrhea, and bloating. I need to go to the bathroom three or four times a day to have a bowel movement. Going to the bathroom usually relieves the pain.

T: Any bleeding or dark, tarry stools?

C: Not really; occasionally after I have gone over and over, I'll have some traces of blood on the toilet paper, but the doctor says that is from the irritation of wiping.

T: When did your GI distress become a problem?

C: About 10 years ago, when I was in the first year of law school.

T: I know that you have seen Dr. X for your problems. When did you first seek medical treatment for your symptoms?

C: About 4 years after they initially occurred, once I had real insurance coverage. I've had all kinds of tests—blood work, stool samples, a sigmoidoscopy, a colonoscopy; nothing showed up even though they have been repeated.

T: What, if any, medications have you taken for your symptoms?

C: Let me see … seems like I've been on everything in the book over time: Bentyl, Donnatal (antispasmotics), Ativan and Klonopin (anxiolytics), Welbutrin (antidepressant), Lomotil (antispasmodic), Reglan (motility stimulant), Metamucil, and Citracil (fiber). I am still taking Ativan, Welbutrin, and Citracil. I know there are more but I can't remember them. They should be listed in my records.

T: Have any of these medications led to significant improvement?

C: Not really, the symptoms may improve for a bit, but they don't help over time. I didn't like the effects of some of them; they took me off my game.

T: Tell me about the pain. Do you frequently have pain in the abdominal area?

C: Yes, most days of the week.

T: What, if anything, relieves the pain?

C: It generally gets better if I can go to the bathroom and have a bowel movement, but there are times when that doesn't help.

T: Do you ever notice that you may need to have several bowel movements to relieve the pain?

C: Yes

T: When you have a bowel movement that relieves pain, what it its consistency?

C: Usually loose and watery; occasionally like small hard peas. Sometimes there is a mucous-like substance mixed in.

T: Is your abdominal pain at all related to your menstrual cycle?

C: I generally have more frequent and painful episodes around the time of my period. I get cramps, but this pain is different.

T: Does the pain usually occur in a specific location? If so, can you show me where it generally occurs?

C: It is usually about here (points to left lower quadrant).

T: When the pain first began, did you notice any change in bowel habits?

C: I began to have frequent bowel movements and diarrhea, often three or four times a day. Occasionally I have periods of constipation, but generally diarrhea.

T: Are there certain kinds of situations or actions that seem to trigger the pain?

C: Eating, being in a long meeting, appearing in court, time pressures, social functions.

T: Does the condition ever cause you to avoid activities?

C: I can't really avoid anything work-related, but I do get anxious when I think I may have an episode. Whenever I can avoid it, I don't go to social functions. If I do go, I try to arrive early and leave as soon as is gracefully possible.

T: Have you ever had an accident where you soiled your underclothes because you were unable to make it to the bathroom on time?

C: No, but I worry about that a lot. I have had a lot of very close calls. I don't eat before going to court or to a long meeting. I probably know where every restroom in town is and what condition it is in. I find that that is one of the first things I check out when I go somewhere new. I always choose the aisle seat on a plane or when buying tickets to anything, and I generally sit near the back of the plane or near the exit in an auditorium.

T: You mentioned you worry about having an accident. Can you tell me more about that?

C: Sure. I guess I am really scared what would happen if I did have an accident. After all, in my profession, it is incredibly important that I seem in control at all times. People rely on me to keep them out of trouble. I work in a firm of mostly men; there is one female, but she has been a partner for a long time. She came up when it was really hard to be in law and a female. I have never seen her show any weakness. As a matter of fact, everyone I work with seems to have it all together. I can think of nothing worse than having an accident in front of them. I think it may be worse this year as I am being considered for partnership. My work stands for itself; I have an excellent track record and put in more billable hours than any of the other associates, but I never feel confident enough. I'm not sure they will want me to be a permanent part of the firm.

T: That must be pretty stressful. Let me shift a bit. I'm interested in your understanding of your disorder. What do you think is causing it?

C: I've been told numerous times that I don't have cancer or some other life-threatening condition; I guess I believe it, but I do worry about it at times. I know stress makes my condition worse, but I know the diarrhea is real and the pain feels pretty real too. I'm not sure exactly what I believe is going on.

T: Are you involved in a particular relationship at present?

C: No; with my work involvement and with this problem, I don't have much extra energy for a social life.

T: Who knows about your condition?

C: I've told my mother; she has a similar condition. A couple of my girlfriends know something is wrong; I often have to escape to the bathroom while we are out to eat. I've wondered if they think I have an eating disorder, but I have avoided bringing it up. I don't think I've told anyone else.

T: So there really isn't anyone in your life who gives you much support about your bowel problem?

C: No.

T: What about in other areas of your life; how do you let people know you need or would like support?

C: I don't do that much. If I'm feeling down, I may give someone a call and see if they want to do something. If they specifically ask what is going on in my life, I might talk about things, but I generally tell people I'm fine. It is hard for me to ask for help or support.

T: Is that because you predict nobody would support you?

C: I'm not sure; I've always been pretty self-reliant.

T: Tell me a little about your early life.

C: I was one of two children. My father was a successful businessman but was probably an alcoholic. He drank every night and his behavior was pretty erratic. My mother was the perfect housewife; always making sure things went well. The house was perfect and she was the typical June Cleaver when Dad came home.

T: Much chaos?

C: A lot of tension but there was little fighting. I'm not sure Mom was very happy, but she never talked about her feelings much. Dad left her when I was 11. I haven't had much to do with him since; actually, he hasn't had much to do with any of us. Mom eventually went to work in a bank; I went to college on scholarship. I really don't remember that much about growing up. I've just known I need to take care of myself if I'm going to be safe in life.

T: You mentioned feeling down. Have you been having problems with your mood?

C: Yes, I've been diagnosed as having depression. (Further screening indicates the client meets criteria for Major Depression).

Standardized Interview Formats

Blanchard and his associates have published the only standardized interview for IBS (Blanchard, 2001). This inventory has been the primary diagnostic tool in their IBS treatment program. The inventory has three parts. The first part includes a format for obtaining a detailed history and description of GI symptoms. Care is taken to obtain a comprehensive description of each symptom along with a behavioral analysis of the antecedents and consequences of the symptom. The second section includes a psychosocial history, a current description of psychological functioning, and a delineation of potential problem areas. This section also includes a history of GI symptoms and diseases in the extended family and potential problems in the patient's life. Data from the first two sections can be used in treatment planning for the client. The third section includes a mental status examination. The interview typically takes about 45 min if the standardized form is used.

Information Critical to Making the Diagnosis

As a medical disorder, the diagnosis of IBS needs to be made by a physician. However, my review of the medical records indicates that all of the recommended tests were done and yielded negative results. The symptoms consistent with a diagnosis of IBS are the presence of abdominal pain relieved by defecation, the diarrhea, the change in form of the stool, and the change in frequency of bowel habits. Other factors supportive of the IBS diagnosis are the frequency of symptoms, the consistency of the stools, the presence of mucous, and the feelings of urgency. The interview also revealed a number of factors common to the disorder that may be a focus of treatment including fears of losing control of the bowels, fear of disease, hypersensitivity to GI sensations, difficulty accessing social supports, avoidance of activities, and depression. Given the account of her early family life, this area should be examined further.

CHRONIC PAIN

Description of the Disorder

Researchers and clinicians now agree that pain is a perceptual experience that is influenced by a number of factors: biological, emotions, social and environmental context, sociocultural background, meaning, beliefs, attitudes, and expectations (Turk & Okifuji, 2002). The sensory component of pain is termed nociception; however, the experience of the individual is a perceptual one.

Primary models to define pain have used a categorical approach, with duration or diagnosis forming its basis (Turk & Melzack, 2001c). Acute pain is pain associated with tissue damage, inflammation, or a disease process that is of relatively brief duration (e.g., hours to weeks), regardless of the cause or intensity. Pain that accompanies a disease or injury that does not resolve within the expected time frame (e.g., months or years) is termed chronic pain. Intermittent, recurring pain or episodes of acute pain that are interspersed with pain-free intervals are termed intermittent pain (e.g., migraine headaches and sickle cell crises). The term chronic progressive pain is used to describe the pain associated with progressive disease states such as metastatic cancer or chronic obstructive pulmonary disease. Other classification systems emphasize the diagnosis associated with the pain (e.g., migraine headache, low back, temporamandibular joint, or neuropathic pain. (Turk & Melzack, 2001c).

Pain is the primary symptom prompting people to seek medical attention. Research has shown that uncontrolled and prolonged pain can alter both the peripheral and central nervous systems through the processes of neural plasticity and central sensitization. Consequently, pain can become a disease in and of itself. Recognition of the significance of pain has become an increasingly important feature of health care. Indeed, there is a movement in the United States to consider pain as a fifth vital sign along with blood pressure, temperature, heart rate, and respiration. Pain control is now considered an integral part of a patient's rights (Turk & Melzack, 2001b).

The experience of pain is influenced by many factors including physical pathology (Polatin & Mayer, 2001; Robinson, 2001), psychiatric comorbidity (Sullivan, 2001), cultural background (Craig et al., 2001; Craig & Wyckoff, 1987), past experience (Block et al., 1980; Haber and Roos, 1985), meaning of the experience (Flor & Turk, 1988; Gil, Williams, Keefe, & Beckham, 1990; Turk & Rudy, 1991, 1992; Turk & Okifuji, 1997), personality variables (Turk & Okifuji, 2001), and reinforcement contingencies (Block et al., 1980; Flor, Kerns, & Turk, 1987).

Procedures for Gathering Information

Patients with chronic pain generally present with a fairly complex picture and there are many procedures for gathering information. Indeed, Turk and Melzack (2001a) published a major work outlining the varied assessment processes. Before seeing a mental health clinician, most patients have been seen by physicians and physical therapists and have had extensive medical evaluation including physical examinations, X-rays, evaluations of body mechanics, pressure point sensitivity, electromyographic (EMG) studies, MRIs, and varied functional workups. If the client has not had a thorough workup, referral to a physician is important before a more psychosocial intervention is initiated.

The diagnostic interview comprises the backbone of the psychosocial assessment. In addition, the clinician will want to assess pain behavior (Keefe, Williams, & Smith, 2001), the pain diary (Jensen & Karoly, 2001), and measures of the pain experience such as the McGill Pain Questionnaire (Melzack, 1975) or the West Haven-Yale Multidimensional Pain Inventory (WHYMPI) (Kerns, Turk, and Rudy, 1985). The latter has been found to be useful in the matching of patients to treatment approaches (Turk & Okifuji, 2001). It might be noted that a recent study by Burns, Kubilus, Bruehl, and Harden (2001) suggests an addition to the WHYMPI that may further augment the patient-treatment matching process.

Given the comorbidity of chronic pain with psychiatric disorders, an evaluation is made of the current and lifetime prevalence of psychiatric disorders, with particular attention to depression, panic and post-traumatic stress disorder, substance abuse and dependence, somatoform disorder, and conversion disorder (Sullivan, 2001). Researchers have used diagnostic interviews and standardized tests commonly used in clinical settings.

The assessment of pain beliefs and coping techniques is particularly important in the evaluation and treatment of chronic pain patients. Instruments with good psychometric characteristics and utility with chronic pain patients are the brief form of the Survey of Pain Attitudes (Tait & Chibnall, 1997), the Pain Beliefs and Perceptions Inventory (Williams & Thorn, 1989), The Pain Stages of Pain Questionnaire (Kerns, Rosenberg, Jamison, Caudill, & Haythornthwaite, 1997), and the Coping Strategies Questionnaire (Rosenstiel & Keefe, 1983).

Case Illustration

The client is a 49-year-old male who has a 2-year history of back pain. He is currently out of work and filing for disability. He is married with two children. Previous medical evaluation revealed no significant organic pathology except some pressure point sensitivity. Questions come from a variety of sources including the Psychosocial Pain Inventory (Heaton et al., 1982), the McGill Comprehensive Pain Questionnaire (Melzack, 1975; Melzack et al., 1981), and the WHYMPQ (Kerns et al., 1985). The objectives of the interview are to: (1) obtain a "pain history," (2) identify events that precede exacerbations in the patient's pain perceptions or pain behavior, (3) clarify how persons in the patient's environment react to the pain, (4) evaluate daily activities, (5) identify whether the patient has any relatives or friends who suffer from disability, and (6) evaluate significant stressors in the patient's past and present. As before, only excerpts of the interview are presented here.

T: Let me start by getting an idea about your current pain. Where does it hurt (one may want to provide a drawing to help the patient explain where it hurts)?

C: See, it starts here just below the waist, travels down my left hip and leg, and goes to my foot.

T: What is the pain like?

C: Mostly a dull ache, like a toothache. Sometimes it burns. If it gets really bad, it stabs.

T: When did you first notice the pain?

C: About June 15, 2 years ago. I was working in the yard. I bent over to pull some weeds and I heard something snap. The pain was intense—I fell to my knees. My wife had to help me into the house and into the recliner.

T: What did you do about the pain?

C: I waited until Monday and then went to see my doctor. He did an exam and gave me some muscle relaxants and sent me home to bed.

T: How did that work?

C: I was fine while in bed; whenever I got up and started moving around, it got worse.

T: On a level of 1–10 with 10 being the most intense pain you can imagine, what is your pain level now?

C: About an 8 (Note: the patient seems to be comfortable in the seated position. He is smiling).

T: Does it get better than that?

C: When I am sitting in the recliner or lying down it sometimes drops to a 7 or so. When it is bad, it gets up to a 10.

T: What do you do to control the pain?

C: I use a heating pad and my wife rubs it. I take Darvocet and Soma every 4 hr. One Darvocet is prescribed, but on bad days I will take two or three at a time.

T: What happens if you run out of medication?

C: My doctor writes the prescription so I have some extras to get me over tough times. I also take Goody powders to help out.

T: On days that it isn't too bad, what is different?

C: Generally the wife is at home, and we can do some things together. It doesn't bother me as much when I'm really interested in what is going on with TV. It gets better during football season when the Hokies are doing well. That Michael Vick is something!

T: What makes it worse?

C: Lifting, moving around a lot, and being tired.

T: What do you think causes the pain?

C: The doctor doesn't agree, but I think I snapped or tore something when I hurt it. He says he can't find anything wrong, but I know how it feels. Suddenly, it just gave out. I also think I must have arthritis or something the way it aches and gets stiff.

T: How do you sleep?

C: Not well; I wake up at least three times a night and have trouble getting back to sleep.

T: What do you do if you wake up?

C: I'll take something for pain if it is about time. If I can't get back to sleep I go to the kitchen and make coffee and then lie down on the recliner and try to go back to sleep.

T: How does that work?

C: Sometimes good; sometimes not.

T: Were you having any difficulty with pain before that day in the yard?

C: Some, particularly after a long day at work. You can't lift and move things all the time at my age and not feel something.

T: Tell me a little about what was going on in your life about the time you hurt your back.

C: I was working at the plant in the warehouse. I helped to pack and load the boxes. Business wasn't real good then, and they were considering laying some of us off. My wife had gotten a job to help out with the money. We were having problems making ends meet. The kids were out of school.

T: So it was kind of a tense time with the job and all.

C: Yeah, I guess so. The plant actually laid off 50 workers two weeks later and many haven't been asked back yet.

T: Have you done any other work?

C: I can't work. You see, I can't lift the boxes. I want to go back to work; we are really strapped, but I can't. I've considered a different kind of job, but I never finished high school. I'm not sure what I would do.

T: Tell me about a typical day.

C: I get up and have breakfast with my wife before she leaves for work. I spend most of the day in the recliner watching TV. You don't know how boring that is. I try to straighten up the kitchen and put clothes into the washer for the wife. Once they are wet it hurts too much to reach down and move them to the dryer but I do help with the washing. I heat up leftovers from the night before for lunch. If she tells me what to do, I get stuff out to defrost for dinner then I am whipped; I lay down with the heating pad or sit in the recliner. I'm there when the kids get home from work and listen out for them. The wife gets home about six and I usually sit in the kitchen with her when she cooks dinner. At night we watch TV, then I go to bed. Not much of a life is it?

T: It does seem pretty limited. How does your wife react to your pain?

C: She worries about me a lot. She rubs my back in the evening with Ben-Gay. She goes with me to the doctor and is as frustrated as I am that I'm not getting better. Luckily she has insurance and has me covered, so I can still get care. She used to want to have sex, but she now understands that I really want to, but that I'm afraid it will hurt my back more. She doesn't push it. She's a real jewel.

T: Tell me about some of your other habits. How much coffee do you drink a day?

C: I usually go through three pots a day.

T: I notice cigarettes in your pocket. So you smoke?

C: Yeah; I had tried to quit before I hurt my back but I started back. It calms my nerves. My wife doesn't like me to smoke in the house, so I try to go outside to the deck to smoke.

She understands if I am hurting too much to go outside. She bought an air freshening machine for the den.

T: How many cigarettes do you smoke a day?

C: I'm down to a pack a day. I used to smoke 2 packs when I was working but that is too expensive.

T: What about alcohol?

C: Money is tight so I have really cut down. I usually drink about a six pack in the late afternoon and evening to help the pain. It really dulls it better than the pills do, I think.

T: You indicate you have cut down. If there was more beer there, would you drink more?

C: Yes; my wife limits me here; I can only drink what is in the house.

T: What kinds of things do you do outside the house?

C: I'm not driving much. I sometimes have to run out for cigarettes or emergencies. I go to the doctor and therapist, but my wife drives when she can. I've had to quit going to church and to the Mason's. I just can't sit that long. I hate to shop but occasionally I go with my wife if I am getting stir crazy. I like to go to the grocery with her—they have one of those carts I can ride in and we get better food when I go along.

T: You used to do the yard work; who is doing it now?

C: Luckily Charlie is getting old enough. I go out to the deck to supervise, but he does most of the work.

T: How are things going financially?

C: It is really tight. We were able to refinance the house and that helped. I've applied for disability and gotten turned down twice. I now have an attorney and he thinks with my good work record, I have a good chance.

T: Tell me about your work history.

C: Thirty years with the same company. I started working for them when I dropped out of high school. A good worker. Never missed a day unless I had the flu or something. I was known as a hard worker; showed up, put in my hours.

T: Tell me a little about your early life.

C: I was the oldest of four boys. No sisters.

T: What were your mother and father like?

C: Mom—she was a saint. Always doing for other people. She was a real loving person. She could squeeze the buffalo off a nickel. She always made ends meet and got a good meal on the table. We didn't have any extra, but we were OK.

T: And your father?

C: He was a real tough guy. He came up hard and lived hard. He worked hard when he worked, but every now and then he just went on a toot and didn't work for a while.

T: What did he do?

C: Manual labor—building and painting mostly. I started working with him when I was about 11. He had been drinking one night and lost control of the truck and was killed when I was 17. I quit school then and went to work at the furniture plant. I needed to help Mom support the family.

T: How was discipline handled at home?

C: Mom would talk to us. Dad would whale us half to death. Mom tried to handle things so Dad wouldn't get involved.

T: When did you marry your wife?

C: Fifteen years ago.

T: You've been seeing the doctor and physical therapist for some time. Why did you call to see me?

C: Dr. S seemed to think you could teach me some ways to live with the pain better. It isn't getting better with anything he tries. I think my wife has been begging him to try something else. One of the people at the store where she worked went through the treatment here and told her she is better, so I thought it was worth a try. The church has been praying for me too. Maybe this is some form of answer. I can't lose anything.

Standardized Interview Formats

Given the extensive history of treatment for chronic pain, there are a number of accepted structured and semistructured interviews. Primary ones are the Psychosocial Pain Inventory (Heaton et al., 1982) and the McGill Pain Questionnaire (Melzack, 1975). Karoly and Jensen (1989), Phillips (1988), and Gatchel (2000) also include models of interviews in their texts.

Information Critical to Making the Diagnosis

The duration of the back pain and nonresponsiveness to treatment indicate that this client meets criteria for chronic low back pain. The results of the physical examination are consistent with the diagnosis. Other characteristics consistent with the diagnosis are the high level of perceived pain which does not vary much his pain behaviors including reduced activity level, avoidance of physical activity, and pattern of alcohol and drug use. His wife appears to reinforce pain activity by assuming more responsibilities around the house, attending to his pain, rubbing his back, and reducing sexual demands. His report of his father's disciplinary actions is consistent with the literature. It is also noteworthy that the onset of pain coincided with a time of work insecurity. It is possible that the pain condition allowed him to avoid the loss of status that might have occurred if he had been laid off. He was also reaching the stage in life that continued physical work would have been increasingly challenging. He is an individual who started working early in life and has worked steadily primarily at a single job since then. Given his education and job history, chances for a job other than manual labor were slim, thus the injury allowed him an honorable way to avoid the negative prospects facing him. Other factors that could contribute to the pain problem are his caffeine and nicotine use and drug and alcohol use. An assessment of possible comorbid psychiatric difficulties is indicated. The client appears amenable to trying a different approach to treatment.

DOS AND DON'TS

The assessment and treatment of psychophysiological disorders presents a unique opportunity to the clinician. Patients with these disorders often present to the mental health system in a negative fashion. They have been described by the acronym SHAFT. These are often *s*ad, *h*ostile, *a*nxious, *f*rustrated individuals who have *t*enaciously held onto the medical establishment. When they perceive symptoms as being disregarded, they *t*ry, try again to convince the health care professional of the legitimacy of the systems, thus the manifestations of the discomfort sometimes appear to be extreme. The clients often don't understand a biopsychosocial approach to illness and perceive their referral to the clinician as a sign the physician believes the complaints are imaginary. The initial interview is an excellent opportunity to begin to break down this resistance. A number of the suggested Dos and Don'ts can assist this process.

- Do: Take time to establish rapport with the client. Talk about the referral and her perceptions of what it means. Spend some time, even in the first interview, explaining how biological, psychological, and social factors interact to influence illness. It can be helpful to use examples of disorders accepted as being physical (diabetes is a convenient one) and talk about how stress can affect the symptoms of the disorder.
- Don't: Ignore signs of resistance. It will save time in the long run.
- Do: Use the interview to establish possible links between cognitions, relationships, and actions and the disorder.
- Don't: Squander the interview opportunity and use it only to make a differential diagnosis.
- Do: Be judicious in the selection of assessment instruments for completion, particularly in the clinical setting. Use only those measures needed to provide information that will be useful in treatment planning and outcome evaluation. Most clients are resistant to excessive testing unless they are engaged in a research project. Incorporate the themes into the interview process and use an additional pen-and-pencil measure if the results will directly affect the treatment process. Explain how you will use any information provided by the instrument.
- Don't: Chase the client away from treatment before he gives it a chance.
- Do: Approach the client as a collaborator. Her insights and actions are critical if treatment is to be effective. However, she is likely used to a much more passive role.
- Don't: Present as the expert who can cure the disorder. All cognitive and behavioral interventions will require work on the part of the client.
- Do: Share your formulation of the case with the client and solicit input. This input may help to make necessary alterations in the treatment process.
- Don't: Assume the client understands why you are approaching treatment the way you are.
- Do: Maintain contact with the referring physician or health care professionals.
- Don't: Hesitate to ask for additional medical evaluation if you think it is indicated. Be prepared to give your rationale for the request, often discussing other patients for whom such information was important in the treatment planning process.
- Do: Use questioning as a way to help translate cognitive beliefs into tentative hypotheses that can be tested.

- Don't: Assume clients will automatically accept the therapist's assertions and explanations.
- Do: Stay focused on the here and now in treatment.
- Don't: Assume discussing past events will affect current symptoms. If the past is discussed, as it sometimes must be, it should be framed in a way to emphasize what the client can do in the present to move beyond the past.
- Do: Use homework assignments and always review the results with the client. During the assessment, diaries can provide important diagnostic information. During treatment, homework can help the client to incorporate the principles of treatment into their daily lives.
- Don't: Forget to reinforce the importance of homework by showing the client how his collaboration affects the treatment process.
- Do: Anticipate setbacks and work through them to inform the treatment process and make necessary modifications.
- Don't: Assume that a one-size-fits-all approach will work in all cases.
- Do: Include significant others in the assessment and treatment process, as appropriate. It is helpful later if some contact is established initially, provided the client is amenable to such inclusion.
- Don't: Ignore the power of others' influence on the client's symptoms and reactions.

SUMMARY

Mental health clinicians have a great deal to offer in the assessment and treatment of psychophysiological disorders. The biopsychosocial model provides a valuable heuristic in understanding the development and change of such conditions. This chapter briefly reviewed two disorders as representative of the host of such disorders. Although the interview is less important to the diagnosis of these conditions, it is of paramount importance in understanding the manifestation of the disorder in a particular individual and helping the client to buy into the treatment process. The interview actually begins the treatment process as it allows the clinician to educate the client regarding her disorder. The principles discussed for interviewing clients with IBS and chronic pain can be applied to other disorders.

REFERENCES

Ali, A., & Toner, B. B. (1996). Sexual abuse and self-blame in women with irritable bowel syndrome. *Psychosomatic Medicine, 58,* 66.
American Psychiatric Association. (1952). *Diagnostic and statistical manual of mental disorders.* Washington, DC: Author.
American Psychiatric Association. (1968). *Diagnostic and statistical manual of mental disorders* (2nd ed.). Washington, DC: Author.
American Psychiatric Association. (1980). *Diagnostic and statistical manual of mental disorders* (3rd ed.). Washington, DC: Author.

American Psychiatric Association. (1987). *Diagnostic and statistical manual of mental disorders* (3rd ed., rev. ed.). Washington, DC: Author.

American Psychiatric Association. (1994). *Diagnostic and statistical manual of mental disorders* (4th ed.). Washington, DC: Author.

Blanchard, E. B. (2001). *Irritable bowel syndrome: Psychosocial assessment and treatment*. Washington, DC: American Psychological Association.

Block, A. R., Kremer, E. F., & Gaylor, M. (1980). Behavioral treatment of chronic pain: Variables affecting treatment efficacy. *Pain, 8*, 367–371.

Burns, J. W., Kubilus, A., Bruehl, S., & Harden, R. N. (2001). A fourth empirically derived cluster of chronic pain patients based on the Multidimensional Pain Inventory: Evidence for repression within the dysfunctional group. *Journal of Consulting and Clinical Psychology, 69*, 663–673.

Craig, K. D., Prkachin, K. M., & Grunau, R. E. (2001). The facial expression of pain. In D. C. Turk & R. Melzack (Eds.), *Handbook of pain assessment* (2nd ed., pp.153–169). New York: Guilford Press.

Craig, K. D., & Wyckoff, M. (1987). Cultural factors in chronic pain management. In G. D. Burrows, D. Elton, & G. Stanley, (Eds.), *Handbook of chronic pain management* (pp. 99–108), Amsterdam: Elsevier.

DeGood, D. E., & Tait, R. C. (2001). Assessment of pain beliefs and pain coping. In D. C. Turk and R. Melzack (Eds.), *Handbook of pain assessment* (2nd ed., pp. 320–345). New York: Guilford Press.

Dewsnap, P., Gomborone, J., Libby, G., & Farthing, M. (1996). The prevalence of symptoms of irritable bowel syndrome among acute psychiatric inpatients with an affective diagnosis. *Psychosomatics, 37*, 385–389.

Drossman, D. A. (1996). Gastrointestinal illness and the biopsychosocial model [Editorial]. *Journal of Clinical Gastroenterology, 22*, 252–254.

Drossman, D. A., McKee, D. C., Sandler, R. S., Mitchell, C. M., Cramer, E. M., Lowman, B. C. et al. (1988). Psychosocial factors in the irritable bowel syndrome: A multivariate study of patients and non-patients with irritable bowel syndrome. *Gastroenterology, 95*, 701–708.

Drossman, D. A., Talley, N. J., Leserman, J., Olden, K. W., & Barreiro, M. A. (1995). Sexual and physical abuse and gastrointestinal illness. *Annals of Internal Medicine, 123*, 782–794.

Drossman, D. A., Whitehead, W. E., & Camilleri, M. (1997). Medical position statement: Irritable bowel syndrome. *Gastroenterology, 112*, 2118–2119.

Engel, G. (1977). The need for a new medical model: A challenge for biomedicine. *Science, 196*, 129–136.

Flor, H., Kerns, R. D., & Turk, D. C. (1987). The role of the spouse, reinforcement, perceived pain, and activity levels of chronic pain patients. *Journal of Psychosomatic Research, 31*, 251–259.

Flor, H., & Turk, D. C. (1988). Chronic back pain and rheumatoid arthritis: Relationship of pain-related cognitions, pain severity, and pain behaviors. *Journal of Behavioral Medicine, 11*, 251–265.

Gatchel, R. J. (2000). How practitioners should evaluate personality to help manage patients with chronic pain. In R. J. Gatchell & J. N. Weisberg (Eds.), *Personality characteristics of patients with pain* (pp. 241–257). Washington: American Psychological Association.

Gil, K. M., Williams, D. A., Keefe, F. J., & Beckham, J. C. (1990). The relationship of negative thoughts to pain and psychological distress. *Behavior Therapy, 21*, 349–352.

Haber, J. D., & Roos, C. (1985). Effects of spouse abuse and/or sexual abuse in the development and maintenance of chronic pain in women. *Advances in Pain Research and Therapy, 9*, 889–895.

Heaton, R. K., Getto, C. J., Lehman, R. A. W., Fordyce, W. E., Brauer, E., & Groban, S. E. (1982). A standardized evaluation of psychosocial factors in chronic pain. *Pain, 12*, 165–174.

Irwin, C., Falsetti, S. A., Lydiard, R. B., Ballenger, J. C., Brock, C. D., & Brener, W. (1996). Comorbidity of posttraumatic stress disorder and irritable bowel syndrome. *Journal of Clinical Psychiatry, 57*, 576–578.

Jensen, M. P., & Karoly, P. (2001). Self-report scales and procedures for assessing pain in adults. In D. C. Turk & R. Melzack (Eds.), *Handbook of pain assessment* (2nd ed., pp. 15–34). New York: Guilford Press.

Karoly, P., & Jensen, M. P. (1989). *Multimethod assessment of chronic pain*. New York: Pergamon Press.

Keefe, F. J., Williams, D. A., & Smith, D. A. (2001). Assessment of pain behaviors. In D. C. Turk & R. Melzack (Eds.), *Handbook of pain assessment* (2nd ed., pp. 170–187). New York: Guilford Press.

Kerns, R. D., Rosenberg, R., Jamison, R. N., Caudill, M. A., & Haythornthwaite, J. (1997). Readiness to adopt a self-management approach to chronic pain: The Pain Stages of Change Questionnaire (PSOCQ). *Pain, 72*, 227–234.

Kerns, R. D., Turk, D. C., & Rudy, T. E. (1985). The West Haven-Yale Multidimensional Pain Inventory (WHYMPI). *Pain, 23*, 345–356.

Leserman, J., Drossman, D. A., Li, Z., Toomey, T. C., Nachman, G., & Glogau, L. (1996). Sexual and physical abuse history in gastroenterology practice: How types of abuse impact health status. *Psychosomatic Medicine, 58*, 4–15.

Levenstein, S. (2002). Psychosocial factors in peptic ulcer and inflammatory bowel disease. *Journal of Clinical and Consulting Psychology, 70*, 739–750.

Lydiard, R. B. (1992). Anxiety and the irritable bowel syndrome. *Psychiatric Annals, 22*, 612–618.

Melzack, R. (1975). The McGill Pain Questionnaire: Major properties and scoring methods. *Pain, 1*, 277–299.

Melzack, A. R., Taenzer, P., Feldman, P., & Kinch, R. A. (1981). Labour is still painful after prepared childbirth. *Canadian Medical Association Journal, 125*, 357–363.

National Institutes of Health Consensus Development Panel on *Helicobacter pylori* in Peptic Ulcer Disease (1994). *Helicobacter pylori* in peptic ulcer disease. *Journal of the American Medical Association, 272*, 65–69.

Noyes, Jr., R., Cook, B., Garvey, M., & Summers, R. (1990). Reductions of gastrointestinal symptoms following treatment for panic disorder, *Psychosomatics, 31*, 75–79.

Phillips, H. C. (1988). *The psychological management of chronic pain: A treatment manual.* New York: Springer.

Polatin, P. B., & Mayer, T. G. (2001). Quantification of function in chronic low back pain. In D. C. Turk & R. Melzack (Eds.), *Handbook of pain assessment* (2nd ed., pp. 191–203). New York: Guilford Press.

Rauws, E. A. J., & Tytgat, G. N. J. (1990). Cure of duodenal ulcer associated with eradication of *Helicobacter pylori. Lancet, 335*, 1233–1235.

Revenson, T. A., & Baum, A. (2000). Introduction. In A. Baum, T. A. Revenson, & J. E. Singer (Eds.), *Handbook of health psychology.* Mahwah, NJ: Lawrence Erlbaum Associates.

Robinson, J. P. (2001). Disability evaluation in painful conditions. In D. C. Turk & R. Melzack (Eds.), *Handbook of pain assessment* (2nd ed., pp. 248–272). New York: Guilford Press.

Rosenstiel, A. K., & Keefe, F. J. (1983). The use of coping strategies in chronic low back pain patients: Relationship to patient characteristics and current adjustment. *Pain, 17*, 33–44.

Schwartz, G. (1982). Testing the biopsychosocial model: The ultimate challenge facing behavioral medicine? *Journal of Consulting and Clinical Psychology, 50*, 1040–1053.

Stoudemire, A., Beardsley, G., Folks, D. G., Goldstein, M. G., Levenson, J., McNamara, M. E. et al., (1996). Psychological factors affecting physical condition (PFAPC). In T. A. Widiger, A. J. Frances, H. A. Pincus, R. Ross, & W. W. Davis (Eds.), *DSM-IV Sourcebook* (Vol. 2, pp. 1051–1078).Washington, DC: American Psychiatric Association.

Sullivan, M. D. (2001). Assessment of psychiatric disorders. In D. C. Turk & R. Melzack (Eds.), *Handbook of pain assessment* (2nd ed., pp. 275–291). New York: Guilford Press.

Tait, R. C., & Chibnall, J. T. (1997). Development of a brief version of the Survey of Pain Attitudes, *Pain, 70*, 229–235.

Thompson, W. G., Creed, F., Drossman, D.A., Heaton, K. W., & Mazzacca, G. (1992). Functional bowel disease and functional abdominal pain. *Gastroenterology International, 5*, 75–91.

Thompson, W. G., Longstreth, G. F., Drossman, D. A., Heaton, K. W., Irvine, E. J., & Muller-Lissner, S. A. (1999). Functional bowel disorders and functional abdominal pain. *Gut, 45*, 1143–1147.

Tollesfson, G. D., Tollefson, S. L., Pederson, M., Luxenberg, M., & Dunsmore, G. (1991). Comorbid irritable bowel syndrome in patients with generalized anxiety and major depression. *Annals of Clinical Psychiatry, 3*, 215–222.

Toner, B. B., Segal, Z. V., Emmott, S. D., & Myran, D. (2000). *Cognitive–behavioral treatment of irritable bowel syndrome: The brain–gut connection.* New York: Guilford.

Toner, B. B., Ali, A., Stuckless, N., Weaver, H., Ackman, D. E., Tang, T. N. et al. (1999, August). *Development of a gender role socialization scale for women.* Paper presented at the Annual Meeting of the American Psychological Association, Boston.

Turk, D. C., & Melzack, R. (2001a). *Handbook of pain assessment* (2nd ed.), New York: Guilford Press.

Turk, D. C., & Melzack, R. (2001b). Preface. In D. C. Turk and R. Melzack (Eds.), *Handbook of pain assessment* (2nd ed., pp. xiii–xvi). New York: Guilford Press.

Turk, D. C., & Melzack, R. (2001c). The measurement of pain and the assessment of people experiencing pain. In D. C. Turk and R. Melzack (Eds.), *Handbook of pain assessment* (2nd ed., pp. 3–11). New York: Guilford Press.

Turk, D. C., & Okifuji, A. (1997). What factors affect physicians' decisions to prescribe opioids for chronic non-cancer pain patients? *Clinical Journal of Pain, 13,* 330–336.

Turk, D. C., & Okifuji, A. (2001). Measuring treatment to assessment of patients with chronic pain. In D. C. Turk & R. Melzack (Eds.), *Handbook of pain assessment* (2nd ed., pp. 400–413). New York: Guilford Press.

Turk, D. C., & Okifuji, A. (2002). Psychological factors in chronic pain: Evolution and revolution. *Journal of Consulting and Clinical Psychology, 70,* 678–690.

Turk, D. C., & Rudy, T. E. (1991). Chronic pain and the injured worker: Integrating physical, psychosocial, and behavioral factors. *Journal of Occupational Rehabilitation, 1,* 159–179.

Turk, D. C., & Rudy, T. E. (1992). Cognitive factors and persistent pain: A glimpse into Pandora's box. *Cognitive Therapy and Research, 16,* 99–122.

Walker, E. A., Roy-Byrne, P. P., & Katon, W. J. (1990). Irritable bowel syndrome and psychiatric illness. *American Journal of Psychiatry, 147,* 565–572.

Walker, E. A., Katon, W. J., Roy-Byrne, P. P., Jemelka, R. P., & Russo, J. (1993). Histories of sexual victimization in patients with irritable bowel syndrome or inflammatory bowel disease. *American Journal of Psychiatry, 150,* 1502–1506.

Welch, G. W., Hillman, L. C., & Pomare, E. W. (1985). Psychoneurotic symptomatology in the irritable bowel syndrome: A study of reporters and non-reporters. *British Medical Journal, 291,* 1382–1384).

Whitehead, W. E., Bosmajian, L., Zonderman, A. B., Costa, Jr., P. T., & Schuster, M. M. (1988). Symptoms of psychologic distress associated with irritable bowel syndrome: Comparison of community and medical clinic samples. *Gastroenterology, 95,* 709–714.

Whitehead, W. E., & Palsson, O. S. (1988). Is rectal pain sensitivity a biological marker for irritable bowel syndrome? Psychological influences on pain perception. *Gastroenterology, 115,* 1263–1271.

Williams, D A., & Thorn, B. E. (1989). An empirical assessment of pain beliefs. *Pain, 36,* 351–358.

14

Post-Traumatic Stress Disorder (Combat)

B. Christopher Frueh, Jon D. Elhai, and Mark B. Hamner

Description of the Disorder

The Clinical Syndrome of PTSD

In 1980, the American Psychiatric Association's (APA) *Diagnostic and Statistical Manual of Mental Disorder (DSM)* nosologic system formally defined and recognized the cluster of acute, and potentially chronic, symptoms often seen in victims of traumatic events (e.g., combat, sexual, and physical assault), naming this condition post-traumatic stress disorder (PTSD; APA, 1994). Since *DSM-IV* (APA, 1994), the disorder has been classified as an "anxiety" disorder and is defined by six basic criteria: (1) the historical antecedent of a traumatic event that involves both actual or threatened death or serious injury, and an intense response of fear, helplessness, or horror; (2) persistently re-experiencing the traumatic event through intrusive memories, dissociative flashbacks, recurrent distressing dreams, and/or psychological or physiological reactivity upon exposure to associated cues; (3) avoidance of stimuli associated with the event, or a numbing of general responsiveness, including efforts to avoid thoughts and feelings related to the trauma, efforts to avoid activities or situations that arouse recollections of the trauma, loss of interest in significant activities, social detachment, and/or reduced affect; (4) existence of persistent symptoms of increased arousal such as hypervigilance, sleep disturbance, irritability or outbursts of anger, impaired concentration, and/or exaggerated startle response; (5) duration of the disturbance for at least one month; (6) the pervasive effects of the disturbance causing clinically significant distress or impairment in social, occupational, or other important areas of functioning.

B. Christopher Frueh, Jon D. Elhai, and Mark B. Hamner • Veterans Affairs Medical Center, Charleston, South Carolina 29401.

There also is emerging evidence of neurobiological markers (e.g., changes in the hypothalamic–pituitary–adrenal axis, noradrenergic, and serotonergic function) that differentiate PTSD from other affective and anxiety disorders (e.g., Bremner et al., 1999; Rasmusson et al., 2000; Southwick et al., 1999; Yehuda, Boisoneau, Lowery, & Giller, 1995); and data from studies examining psychophysiological responding support prominence of autonomic symptoms and heightened reactivity (Keane et al., 1998).

Complicating the syndrome is the fact that PTSD is typically accompanied by multiple comorbid Axis I and II disorders, including major depression, substance abuse, panic attacks, and psychotic symptoms (Hamner et al., 2000; Keane & Wolfe, 1990; Kilpatrick et al., 2000), poor quality of life (Zatzick et al., 1997), medical illness comorbidity (Schnurr, Spiro, & Paris, 2000; Wagner, Wolfe, Rotnitsky, Proctor, & Erickson, 2000), and extreme social maladjustment (Frueh, Turner, Beidel, & Cahill, 2001; MacDonald, Chamberlain, Long, Nigel, & Flett, 1999). In fact, it is notable that a majority (69%) of veterans evaluated within Veterans Affairs (VA) Medical Center PTSD clinics seek disability payments for their debilitating social and occupational impairment (Frueh, Gold, & de Arellano, 1997).

Finally, PTSD is highly prevalent throughout American society, including VA Medical Centers. Epidemiological estimates of PTSD put the current prevalence at 8–14% in the general population (APA, 1994; Kaplan, Sadock, & Greb, 1994; Kessler, Sonnega, Bromet, Hughes, & Nelson, 1995), with higher rates of current (up to 15%) and lifetime (up to 31%) prevalence for veterans exposed to war zone trauma (Card, 1987; Center for Disease Control, 1988; Kulka et al., 1990). Preliminary data from a recently funded VA project indicate that prevalence of PTSD among those treated within VA primary care clinics is 9–12% (Magruder et al., 2002). Other studies suggest that prevalence in VA primary care is even higher, at 20% (Hankin, Spiro, Miller, & Kazis, 1999). Among certain disadvantaged groups, history of trauma exposure and PTSD rates may be higher still (Mueser et al., 1998). For example, in an urban mental health center it was found that 94% of patients had a history of trauma exposure and 42% had diagnoses of PTSD (Switzer et al., 1999). In addition, PTSD is often chronic and many combat veterans still suffer severe symptoms from wars fought 30 (e.g., Vietnam) or 50 (World War II) years ago (Gold et al., 2000; Sutker, Winstead, Galina, & Allain, 1990). A striking example of this is that PTSD prevalence among World War II veterans remains high (12%) some 50 years after the combat has ended, with many veterans still suffering in their late 70s (Spiro, Schnurr, & Aldwin, 1994). Thus, it is evident that millions of traumatized Americans (veterans and civilians) suffer PTSD or symptoms characteristic of PTSD. Given that there are over 5 million surviving American veterans of foreign wars, the potential number of veterans currently with PTSD is well above the half million mark. The VA medical system carries the burden of providing mental health, medical, social, and disability services to a large number of persons with severe PTSD and other associated mental illnesses.

Taken together, data indicate that PTSD is a severe, chronic, and prevalent psychiatric disorder resulting in considerable emotional distress and social disruption. The full clinical syndrome of combat-related PTSD often presents as a complex clinical picture and constitutes a significant diagnostic and treatment challenge.

The VA Disability Evaluation Process

Because it is important to consider the context within which diagnostic evaluations are conducted, some discussion of the VA disability evaluation process is germane to this chapter, as many veterans evaluated for PTSD are seeking disability at the time of their evaluation. People who suffer from severe mental illnesses often experience occupational impairment and related financial hardships (Drake et al., 1999; Kouzis & Eaton, 2000). Military veterans may apply for service-connected disability payments for any physical or psychiatric condition, including PTSD, that was initiated during or caused by their military service, and which impairs their ability to earn a living. There is a growing trend in the VA system for veterans to seek these funds. Recent data show that Gulf War veterans draw disability compensation at a much higher rate (16%) than veterans of any previous conflict, and almost twice the current rate (8.6%) of World War II veterans (*Wall Street Journal*, 1999). Furthermore, 69–94% of veterans seeking treatment for PTSD within the VA system apply for psychiatric disability (Fontana & Rosenheck, 1998; Frueh et al., 1997; Frueh, Smith, & Barker, 1996a).

In 1996 total compensation and pension expenditures for the VA were estimated to be just over $18 billion, with 2.2 million of the surviving 25.4 million veterans (8.9%) receiving some level of service-connected disability benefits (Oboler, 2000). If granted, a rating of disability severity is made on a 0–100% basis. The relationship between disability payments and disability ratings (on 0–100% basis) is curvilinear, and many benefits (e.g., some medical/dental coverage) do not begin until a rating of 100% is awarded. Even veterans who are rated as 90% disabled stand to benefit significantly from an increase to 100%. When claims are denied, or only partially granted, veterans may appeal the decision an indefinite number of times. Such repeat claims outnumber original claims almost three to one and dominate the VA adjudication and appeals system. For veterans who are granted disability compensation there is a continuing disability review, usually every other year, to determine whether they remain eligible for disability payments. For many chronically ill veterans, the process of obtaining and maintaining disability payments is a protracted struggle. However, the financial incentives are significant. For example, in South Carolina, where per capita income is about $17,000 before taxes (Bureau of Economic Analysis), a single veteran without dependents who was 100% service connected in 1999 received an annual tax-free income of $23,868, in addition to other benefits. See review by Oboler (2000) for more description of the VA's disability evaluation process.

Symptom Reporting Patterns among Veterans

One difficulty often faced in diagnostic evaluations for PTSD with veterans is that symptom reports often seem grossly unrealistic or inconsistent. Research studies consistently demonstrate that combat veterans evaluated for PTSD within the VA exhibit: extreme and diffuse levels of psychopathology across instruments measuring different domains of mental illness, and extreme elevations on the validity scales of the Minnesota Multiphasic Personality Inventory-2 (MMPI-2) in a "fake-bad" or overreporting direction (Fairbank, Keane, & Malloy, 1983; Frueh, Hamner, Cahill, Gold, & Hamlin, 2000). These validity scales (e.g., the $F–K$ index) take advantage of the stereotypes held by many lay people who assume that serious mental illnesses involve a large number of bizarre symptoms, such that high scores indicate endorsement of items rarely endorsed by even the most severely mentally ill persons. Combat veterans also are prone to inflate their reports of combat exposure over time (Southwick, Morgan, Nicolaou, & Charney, 1997). This general reporting pattern significantly complicates accurate diagnostic decision-making and frequently casts doubt on the credibility of symptom reports (Frueh et al., 2000).

Compensation-Seeking and Symptom Reporting Patterns

Some researchers have speculated that the phenomenon of apparent symptom overreporting may reflect motivation of veterans to present as severely disabled in order to obtain disability compensation (Atkinson, Henderson, Sparr, & Deale, 1982; Lees-Haley, 1989). Several studies have examined the influence of compensation-seeking status on symptom reporting patterns using self-report measures of psychopathology. Although results from two early studies were mixed (Jordan, Nunley, & Cook, 1992; Schneider, 1979), conclusions were limited by the manner in which compensation-seeking was defined and in how subjects were grouped for analyses. Two studies (Frueh et al., 1996a, 1997) examined this issue by differentiating veterans on the basis of financial incentive, such that veterans were classified into two groups at the time of evaluation. "Compensation-seeking" veterans were those currently seeking, or planning to seek, VA disability compensation or increases in existing disability payments for PTSD. "Non-compensation-seeking" veterans were those *not* intending to seek VA disability compensation for their symptoms of PTSD. The percentage of veterans classified as "compensation-seeking" in each of these two studies was identical (69%). Compensation-seeking veterans produced significantly more pathological scores on clinical measures and obtained much higher elevations on MMPI-2 validity scales (e.g., $F–K$) associated with symptom exaggeration and malingering than did "non-compensation-seeking" veterans. These results were obtained despite the fact that the two groups did not differ in frequency of PTSD diagnoses. Furthermore, differences on most indices exceeded effect sizes of 1.0, even when the effects of income, global assessment of functioning (GAF), and clinician-rated severity of PTSD were controlled for.

There also is evidence to suggest that the MMPI-2 validity scales can be used as a screening instrument to identify veterans who may be exaggerating their psychopathology in order to gain disability compensation. Specifically, while compensation-seeking was not statistically over-represented among veterans with $F–K$ indices of ≥ 13 (Smith & Frueh, 1996), veterans with $F–K$ indices of ≥ 22 were much more likely to be compensation-seeking, and scored much higher on self-report measures of psychopathology, despite having lower rates of PTSD diagnoses and similar rates of other comorbid diagnoses (Gold & Frueh, 1999). These data suggest that availability of disability benefits influences the way in which veterans present their difficulties. This is consistent with evidence that individuals from other compensation-seeking populations (e.g., injury and pain litigants) also tend to overreport symptoms (Rothke et al., 1994).

Implications of Compensation-Seeking and Symptom Reporting Patterns

The specter of disability payments and symptom overreporting patterns may complicate diagnostic decision-making regarding PTSD criteria and differential diagnosis. Experience suggests that many patients acknowledge using evaluations as a means of documenting, through clinicians' reports, psychiatric difficulties to bolster disability claims. It is important that clinicians in VA practice settings should expect that many veterans will present with unrealistic symptom pictures, but these should not necessarily be taken as evidence of malingering. In fact, in most cases with this population validity scale, elevations are more likely to be due to extreme psychological distress than feigning (Franklin, Repasky, Thompson, Shelton, & Uddo, 2002). If the MMPI-2 is used, traditional validity scale cut points ($F-K > 12$) may not be appropriate. Instead, population specific cut points ($F-K > 22$, $F(p) > 8$) should be considered (Gold & Frueh, 1999). In addition, a new MMPI-2 validity scale offers promise for detecting those veterans who are distorting their symptom reports (Elhai et al., 2002). The Infrequency-Post-Traumatic Stress Disorder scale (*Fptsd*) was created from MMPI-2 items that were infrequently endorsed by nearly 1,000 PTSD-diagnosed male combat veterans presenting for treatment at VA Medical Center PTSD clinics. The validity of *Fptsd* has been preliminarily established, and it appears significantly less related to psychopathology and distress than previously established MMPI-2 validity scales among veterans evaluated for PTSD, while better at discriminating simulated from genuinely reported PTSD. On the other hand, careful follow-up evaluation of overreporting veterans is warranted, including careful examination of military documentation, structured interviews, behavioral assessments, and perhaps even psychophysiological assessment. In the sections that follow we describe the evaluation procedures and instruments in more detail, including case illustrations, information critical to making the diagnosis, and diagnostic assessment "Dos and Don'ts."

PROCEDURES FOR GATHERING INFORMATION

There are a number of strategies for gathering relevant information in the diagnostic assessment of veterans with symptoms of PTSD. Perhaps more so than for most other psychiatric disorders, broadly based assessment strategies are needed to fully capture the complexity and severity of combat-related PTSD (Frueh et al., 2001). In the section that follows we provide an overview of the assessment modalities that have been used to evaluate combat veterans. In addition to a careful psychosocial history and Mental Status Exam, we recommend the following assessment strategies.

Structured Interviews

The structured interview is the most frequently used assessment strategy for evaluating veterans. Interviews provide a strategy for assessing for a range of relevant experiences and symptoms. They allow the clinician to query the veteran (and sometimes collateral sources) about functioning across a number of relevant areas and to make clinical ratings based not only on patient report, but also on behavioral observations. They also allow for standardized assessment and generally offer known reliability and validity coefficients. Interviews also have one important limitation with regard to their application in the assessment of combat veterans: they may be vulnerable to the same type of negative reporting bias that affects self-report inventories in this population. This bias may be a result of the inherent retrospective nature of the assessment and the influence of a variety of other economic or systemic forces (e.g., disability compensation incentives). Structured interviews can be used to obtain information regarding lifetime exposure to traumatic experiences, PTSD symptoms, and other psychiatric symptoms. We will discuss structured interviews in more detail in the next section of this chapter.

Self-Report Inventories

A number of general (e.g., MMPI-2) and specific self-report inventories are widely used in the assessment of combat-related PTSD. Examples of the latter include the *Mississippi Scale for Combat Related PTSD* (Keane, Caddell, & Taylor, 1988), *Impact of Event Scale* (Horowitz, Wilner, & Alvarez, 1979), and the *PTSD Checklist* (PCL; Blanchard, Jones, Buckley, & Forneris, 1996), which provide reliable and valid measures of PTSD symptoms and are highly correlated with diagnostic interviews for PTSD. Several other measures also exist. Objective psychometric inventories have a number of general strengths: they are usually easy to administer; do not require a great deal of time to score or interpret; allow for standardized assessment procedures across multiple patients and sites; allow for comparison of individual veterans to other veteran groups or clinical populations; offer known, and usually adequate, reliability and validity coefficients; and allow veterans to complete the testing procedures at their own pace and represent their affective experience without influence from examiners.

There are also several general drawbacks in the use of self-report inventories with this population. As noted earlier there is the widely demonstrated finding that combat veterans evaluated for PTSD tend to exhibit (1) extreme and diffuse levels of psychopathology across instruments measuring different domains of mental illness, and (2) extreme elevations on the validity scales of the MMPI-2 in a "fake-bad" or unrealistic direction (see Frueh et al., 2000). An additional limitation of self-report measures in general is that the consolidation of a number of items into one scale means that equivalent scores (by two different respondents) may be achieved for very different reasons. Scale scores on self-report inventories may call attention to a general domain, but more specific assessment of actual behaviors, antecedent situations, and the function of the behavior may be more relevant information. Thus, the global assessment provided by self-report inventories may be helpful in identifying general domains of relative psychopathology, but more specific behavioral assessments are likely required to develop treatment plans aimed at targeting specific areas of concern. This also points toward the importance of examination of "critical items" in making interpretations of general scale scores.

Psychophysiological Assessment

There is a wide body of literature demonstrating the utility of psychophysiological measures (e.g, heart rate, blood pressure) in the assessment of PTSD (e.g., Blanchard, Kolb, & Prins, 1991), and there is evidence suggesting that reduced physiological reactivity is associated with improvements in both PTSD symptoms and areas of social adjustment (Boudewyns & Hyer, 1990). The prominence of autonomic symptoms in combat veterans with PTSD has been consistently documented via studies of psychophysiological responding, which show clear evidence of heightened reactivity in combat veterans with PTSD (e.g., Keane et al., 1998). In these studies, standardized combat-related cues (e.g., combat sounds and pictures) or individually developed scripts are presented while physiological reactivity is measured via blood pressure, heart rate, forehead electromyogram (EMG), or galvanic skin response (GSR). Combat veterans with PTSD have significantly larger blood pressure and heart rate responses during traumatic cue exposure than do combat veterans without PTSD, although EMG and GSR have proven to be less reliable for purposes of differentiation (e.g., Orr et al., 1990). Sensitivity and specificity for the studies cited above ranged from 0.70 to 0.90 and 0.80 to 1.00, respectively. Furthermore, psychophysiological reactivity may provide relatively good discrimination even when individuals are attempting to exaggerate or disguise their responses (Gerardi, Blanchard, & Kolb, 1989). Thus, this assessment modality is less susceptible to the negative reporting bias (conscious or unconscious) potentially found with self-report measures.

Patient Ratings

Obtaining daily patient ratings of relevant social behaviors, activities, and problems represents a strategy to collect data that is linked to specific and quantifiable behaviors and events. It has an inherent advantage because it is not retrospective in nature, and should not be vulnerable to the same biases that influence responding on more global self-report measures. It also provides data over a specified period of time (e.g., a week or month), rather than providing only cross-sectional data, as do self-report inventories and structured interviews. Patient ratings can also be developed for just about any behavior, and therefore can be tailored to an individual's needs. In other words, assessments are not limited to targets that are represented by nomothetically derived instruments. Furthermore, they can be expanded to include relevant antecedents, cognitions, and consequences of behaviors, so as to provide more information about symptoms and social functioning. Patient ratings have provided valuable information on treatment outcome in several studies with veterans (e.g., Frueh, Turner, Beidel, Mirabella, & Jones, 1996b).

One limitation of patient ratings is that because of their nature and the period of time involved, they generally do not contribute much toward making initial diagnoses. An additional limitation of patient ratings is that they require patient compliance with a procedure that asks them to spend about 2–5 min a day making relevant ratings. Therefore, they do not provide immediate information, and are subject to the compliance of each individual patient. However, compliance may be encouraged by making sure that patients understand the rationale for the assessment and by establishing regular joint reviews of patient ratings with the clinician. Our experience is that patients are generally likely to comply with such procedures when they see that the results are actually incorporated into the development and implementation of ongoing treatment plans. In this way, the role of the procedure is complicated because it may serve as both an assessment tool and part of an intervention when used during the course of treatment.

Behavioral Assessments

Behavioral assessment can be multifaceted, including a variety of other strategies, and may be used to evaluate both psychiatric symptoms and social functioning along the full range of difficulties associated with the clinical syndrome of combat-related PTSD. One strategy requires patients to respond to a variety of role-played social situations while the clinician makes ratings on the quality of social skills exhibited across a number of potentially problematic situations (e.g., expression of disapproval or criticism, assertiveness, confrontation and anger expression, receiving compliments). Although this does not provide information about how well or how often an individual uses appropriate social behaviors outside of the clinic setting, it does allow for assessment of an individual's repertoire of social behaviors (e.g., skill deficits and strengths). A functional analysis conducted with veterans and/or collateral others can provide valuable information regarding specific symptoms and problem areas. These strategies may require more time and resources than are available for most clinical evaluations, and they do not provide a good diagnostic aid, but they can serve as a valuable basis for the development of behavioral treatment plans to address other specific symptoms and problem areas.

Summary

Given the complexities of assessment with combat veterans evaluated for PTSD (e.g., symptom overreporting, symptom severity), clinicians should not rely only on self-report measures because they may be the most vulnerable to negative reporting biases. Furthermore, because the syndrome of PTSD in veterans comprises a complex set of multidimensional domains, it seems improbable that any single measure will be sufficient to provide a comprehensive evaluation. Thus, an array of different assessment strategies, including behavioral measures, may be necessary. Where resources permit, comprehensive assessment of this population should consist of a multi-method approach, including structured interviews and self-report measures. Other assessment strategies, such as psychophysiological assessment, patient ratings, and behavioral assessments, may prove helpful to address specific questions. Clinicians might consider relying on the "funnel" metaphor of assessment (see Hawkins, 1979): the global assessment provided by structured interviews and self-report inventories may be helpful in identifying general domains of relative psychopathology and interpersonal maladjustment, but more specific functional (behavioral) assessments and patient ratings are then necessary to identify specific behaviors, antecedents, and functions of the behaviors.

CASE ILLUSTRATION

"Mr. Smith" is a 52-year-old African-American male, who was referred for evaluation by his primary care physician after the patient revealed during a routine physical examination that he frequently suffered from combat-related nightmares and difficulty sleeping. With no previous psychiatric treatment history, this evaluation was the first time he ever met with a mental health professional. The evaluation procedures included a psychosocial history interview, two trauma interviews (Combat Exposure Scale, Trauma Assessment for Adults), psychiatric interviews (Structured Clinical Interview for *DSM-IV* [SCID], Clinical-Administered PTSD Scale [CAPS]), and self-report instruments (MMPI-2, Mississippi PTSD Scale, Beck Depression Inventory [BDI]). Also, his VA medical record and military Form DD-214 were reviewed, with additional information elicited from his wife, Mrs. Smith, who accompanied him to this appointment.

At the time of his evaluation, Mr. Smith reported living with his wife and two teenage children in the quiet suburbs of a medium-sized metropolitan city. He reported being married to his wife for the past 20 years. The veteran stated that while he gets along with his wife and children, most of the time "I just want them to leave me alone." When asked about his family of origin, Mr. Smith stated that he was close to his family when growing up, but does not talk to his family members often now.

In terms of education, Mr. Smith reported attaining a college education after serving in the military, majoring in accounting. He has had his own accounting firm for 15 years, where he currently works full-time. He employs several secretaries and additional accountants, with whom he does not associate, preferring to work alone in his office with the door closed. However, he often stares into space in his office, without accomplishing the work he had set out to do. A veteran friend of his talked Mr. Smith into applying for PTSD-related disability compensation. Although Mr. Smith claimed that he does not feel like he needs disability compensation (and does not know enough about PTSD to know if he has it), he reported that sometimes his decreased work productivity makes him think that perhaps he should apply.

Mr. Smith indicated that he received basic training at Ft. Jackson, South Carolina, and later received advanced infantry training. He was shipped to Vietnam in 1968 and served a 1-year tour of duty in the Army, after which he served in the Army reserves in the United States for an additional year. Although much of his Vietnam tour was uneventful, the patient's time there was significant for specific incidents of combat exposure. Serving during a time of numerous enemy attacks in South Vietnam, known as the "Tet Offensive," he reported going on several combat patrols, and receiving incoming enemy fire on a number of occasions. The patient alleged that several men in his platoon were killed in action, and in one case, one of the men died within 5 feet of the patient. Mr. Smith also reported receiving enemy and sniper fire on a few occasions, and witnessed a truck within his combat convoy hit a land mine, with a man sustaining serious injuries. Mr. Smith further stated that as a result of these traumatic events, he became extremely fearful during his tour of duty in Vietnam. Review of his Form DD214 supported his self-reported military history. He denied other lifetime trauma exposure.

After returning from Vietnam, Mr. Smith started drinking 4–7 cans of beer every night. His alcohol use did not appear to get in the way of his work but seemed to interfere at times with his relationship with his family, with repeated familial attempts to get him to stop drinking. About one year ago, his physician told him that continuing to drink would be detrimental to his health, since he recently developed adult-onset diabetes. It was at this time, when he decreased his alcohol use, that his symptoms of nightmares, sleep disturbance, and social withdrawal became much worse.

Based on the CAPS interview, Mr. Smith appears to suffer from numerous symptoms of PTSD. He reported several reexperiencing symptoms, including experiencing unwanted memories of his traumatic experiences from Vietnam on a weekly basis. On rare occasions, these unwanted memories felt so vivid that to some extent Mr. Smith lost touch with his current surroundings. The veteran's nightmares of Vietnam reportedly happened several nights per week, after which he would not be able to return to bed for 1–2 hr, impairing his sleep schedule and increasing his fatigue during the day. Numerous environmental cues similar to those from Vietnam, including the sounds of helicopters, driving by the beach, and viewing news reports about the U.S. war on terrorism, remind Mr. Smith of his traumatic events and trigger psychological and physical distress several times a month.

Mr. Smith also claimed to suffer from a variety of avoidance/numbing PTSD symptoms. For example, he routinely attempts to avoid thinking about the traumatic events he experienced and often goes out of his way to avoid activities that might remind him of Vietnam (i.e., the beach, the evening TV news, etc.). While he used to enjoy numerous sports and hobbies and spending time with friends and relatives, he now prefers to be alone most of the time, lacking enjoyment in any work or recreational activities. As implied earlier, the patient feels strongly cut off from most people in his life. He also acknowledged feeling emotionally empty, without currently experiencing any intense emotions like love, happiness, or pleasure. For example, he reported feeling unemotional at the recent funeral of a close friend, and reported feeling "flat" at his own birthday party earlier in the year.

Symptoms of hyperarousal were also present for the veteran. He acknowledged spending a large amount of time trying to safeguard his family and home, by routinely inspecting all doors and windows. Most of the time Mr. Smith avoids crowds, and in rare instances when he is forced to be in a crowd, he always positions himself so that he has a good view without blind spots, feeling more protected this way. When a loud noise or something unexpected (i.e., a car backfiring) occurs outside of his home or workplace, he becomes "jumpy" and remains anxious for several hours afterward.

Results from the SCID indicate that Mr. Smith also suffers from Major Depressive Disorder. Specifically, in the past year, he has become more depressed, feeling tired much of the time, with trouble concentrating, decreased appetite, and fleeting thoughts of suicide. Although some of these symptoms conceptually overlap with PTSD, it appears that Mr. Smith meets criteria for both disorders. He also meets criteria for alcohol abuse in partial remission.

Interestingly, a number of Mr. Smith's symptoms may appear to be psychotic in nature. For example, his hypervigilance in crowds may seem like paranoia. His vivid reexperiencing ("flashbacks") resembles visual hallucinations seen in psychotic-disordered individuals. Additionally, his avoidance of people and emotional numbness could be confused with the negative symptoms of schizophrenia. However, these psychotic-like symptoms are often found in PTSD patients, and it was decided that these symptoms better reflect PTSD symptoms than psychotic experiences. This differential diagnostic decision was based on the qualitative nature of these symptom reports and the finding that he did not display gross impairment in reality testing. For example, his unusual perceptual experiences were virtually all related to combat-related images/sounds, and he easily recognized that they were fleeting "nightmares" or "flashbacks."

Mr. Smith's MMPI-2 was interpreted to be valid and suggested that he is in significant distress. In fact, his L and K scores were below a T score of 45, with an F score of about 95. Although an F score of that magnitude is often seen in individuals overreporting their psychiatric symptoms, it is quite typical of highly distressed PTSD patients; furthermore, his $F-K$ index was well below 22, and neither his $F(p)$ or $Fptsd$ scales were elevated. Thus, he was considered to be responding in a relatively open and honest manner. His highest clinical scale scores were on scales 2 and 8, with additional elevations on scales 6 and 7, overall indicating significant levels of depression, thinking and concentration problems, as well as suspiciousness and sensitivity, anxiety and rumination. The MMPI-2's PTSD scales were also very elevated. Similarly, his Mississippi PTSD scale score of 115 suggests significant combat-related PTSD symptomatology. His BDI score of 38 is further evidence of his depressive symptoms. Overall, this profile on self-report measures is typical of those seen in combat veterans with severe PTSD.

Mr. Smith's wife corroborated her husband's report of difficulties. She acknowledged that he had appeared to be sad and withdrawn, especially in the past year or so. She has awakened at night several times, to find her husband throwing punches in the air while asleep, not being able to return to sleep afterward. Because Mr. Smith has insisted on avoiding social activities, Mrs. Smith has felt more and more isolated from her friends and family members.

In terms of behavioral observations, Mr. Smith was well groomed and cooperative with the evaluation. He positioned his chair in a corner of the office, reportedly not wanting anyone or anything to surprise him from behind. He made occasional eye contact with the examiner, but slightly less than what would be considered appropriate. At first, he seemed somewhat uncomfortable and reluctant to talk about his emotional problems. Through the course of the evaluation, however, he seemed to warm up to the examiner. Mr. Smith became very anxious and tearful at times when discussing traumatic experiences from the war, seeming to try hard to push back his tears.

In combination, the data described above were used to assign diagnoses of PTSD and Major Depression and to begin appropriate treatment planning with Mr. Smith.

STANDARDIZED INTERVIEW FORMATS

Relevant standardized interview formats for evaluating veterans for combat-related PTSD fall into three general categories, including interviews that assess for (1) trauma exposure, (2) PTSD symptoms, and (3) other psychiatric conditions. We will address each of these categories, with most emphasis on the first two since the latter is discussed in great detail elsewhere.

Trauma Exposure

Prior to conducting an assessment of PTSD symptoms per se, it is important to establish that a history of traumatic exposure is present (e.g., Criterion A for a

DSM-based diagnosis of PTSD). In fact, it is worth noting that PTSD is the only psychiatric disorder with a historical antecedent (i.e., trauma) included in the formal diagnostic criteria. We recommend using separate interviews to assess general lifetime traumatic experiences and level of combat exposure. The former is important because research shows that many combat veterans with PTSD also endorse childhood histories of abuse, as well as histories of violent behaviors and victimization after their combat experiences (Smith, Frueh, Sawchuck, & Johnson, 1999); the latter is important for gaining a more thorough understanding of each veteran's combat experiences.

Trauma Assessment for Adults—Interview Version (Resnick et al., 1996). This 17-item instrument assesses for lifetime history of traumatic events, including combat experiences, physical abuse and assault, sexual assault, homicide of a close friend or family member, natural disaster, serious accidents, exposure to health threatening chemicals, witnessing someone being seriously injured or killed, and other situations that involved fear of being killed or seriously injured, or in which serious injury did take place. Age of first and most recent occurrence is determined for multiple incidents of a given type, and follow-up questions are included to assess perceived life threat. This instrument has been demonstrated to have strong psychometric properties and has been widely used in clinical practice and research on trauma exposure in adults (Resnick, 1996).

Other reliable and valid measures for assessing lifetime trauma history exist; including the *Trauma History Questionnaire* (Green, 1995) and the *Revised Conflict Tactics Scale* (Straus et al., 1996); and the *Childhood Trauma Questionnaire* (Bernstein et al., 1994) may be administered to adults in order to learn about childhood abuse and neglect (Sher, Stein, Asmundson, McCreary, & Forde, 2001). Each measure uses behaviorally specific language to elicit traumatic experiences and yields other relevant information about traumatic experiences, such as number of events, ages of event occurrence, and physical injuries that may have occurred.

Combat Exposure Scale (CES; Keane et al., 1989). The CES is a seven-item self-report questionnaire measuring the extent of exposure to military combat-related traumatic events. The CES takes approximately 5 min to administer, and was developed for use in psychiatric settings. Good internal consistency (0.85), and excellent test–retest reliability (0.97) have been reported for the CES by its authors.

There is evidence that veterans may fabricate their military history or reports of combat exposure with some regularity (Burkett & Whitley, 1998; McGrath & Frueh, 2002), and there is evidence that many veterans' reports of combat exposure become exaggerated over time (Southwick et al., 1997). Therefore, in addition to administering the CES, it is also important to obtain objective documentation of veterans' military service and experiences by reviewing their Form DD214. This form is a one-page summary that all military veterans receive at discharge. Although it is not a comprehensive description of their activities or overseas duty postings, and it may be easily forged, it does provide a starting point for verification of military service, era served, and medals received. Because this is an important document necessary to obtain many veteran benefits, be skeptical of any veteran who claims not to have his/her copy of Form DD214, or who claims that his combat experiences are not evident or cannot be reported because they were "classified" (Burkett & Whitley, 1998). In the rare instances where this happens or where other doubts persist, additional investigation is warranted before proceeding with evaluation or treatment. Clinicians may request to review the veteran's VA "C-File," and supporting military documentation can be received through the National Personnel Records Center via the Freedom of Information Act by writing National Personnel Records Center, Army (Air Force or Navy) Records Center, 9700 Page Boulevard, St. Louis, MO, 63132, or by visiting http://www.usdoj.gov/04foia/index.html.

Post-Traumatic Stress Disorder

CAPS (Blake et al., 1990; Weathers & Litz, 1994; Weathers, Ruscio, & Keane, 1999). The CAPS is a 17-item structured interview that assesses both frequency and intensity of PTSD symptoms according to *DSM-IV* (APA, 1994) criteria. It provides both a dichotomous index for PTSD diagnosis and a continuous index of PTSD symptom severity. The scale has been shown to have robust psychometric properties, including strong interrater reliability (0.92–0.99), high internal consistency (0.73–0.85), and high convergent validity (Weathers & Litz, 1994; Weathers, Keane, & Davidson, 2001). It is a highly regarded instrument because it provides information on both symptom intensity and frequency, has clear behavioral anchors, and possesses excellent psychometric properties. An additional strength of the CAPS is that it is widely used throughout VA Medical Centers and Vet Centers across the country, and a VA-sponsored CD-ROM instructional program is available at most VA facilities to help train interviewers. Therefore, it has been the subject of rigorous research and is considered by many to be the gold-standard instrument for making a diagnostic decision regarding PTSD among combat veterans (Weathers et al., 2001).

Although the instrument does not include standardized or objective items for assessing malingering or symptom overreporting, each item does include a space for circling "QV" for "questionable validity." Interviewers are encouraged to probe for detailed descriptions of symptoms, to look for inconsistencies or unlikely descriptions of symptom reports, and to incorporate behavioral observations into their ratings. In other words, interviewers are required to use some degree of clinical judgment in making symptom ratings and to note those instances for which they suspect symptom reports are of questionable validity. Thus, clinicians should look for congruence between symptom reports of exaggerated startle response and behavioral reactions to loud, sudden noises (e.g., do they "jump" when a door slams?); reports of cued reactivity and affective response to discussing traumatic events (e.g., do they appear anxious, distressed, or avoidant when recounting combat experiences?); claims of hypervigilance and comfort with the interview situation (e.g., do they sit easily with their back to the door, or do they reposition the chair?); descriptions of flat affect and observable behavioral evidence (e.g., do they appear animated and interested vs. flat and detached?); and many other possibilities.

While the CAPS is probably the most widely used interview for combat-related PTSD in both clinical settings and research studies, there are other structured interviews for PTSD. These include: the *Structured Interview for PTSD* (Davidson, Malik, & Travers, 1997), *PTSD Symptom Scale Interview* (Foa, Riggs, Dancu, & Rothbaum, 1993), and the PTSD modules of comprehensive psychiatric interviews such as the SCID (Spitzer, Williams, Gibbon, & First, 1997), *Diagnostic Interview Schedule* (Robins, Helzer, Croughan, & Ratliff, 1981), *Mini-International Neuropsychiatric Interview* (MINI; Sheehan et al., 1998), and *Anxiety Disorders Interview Schedule—Revised* (DiNardo, Moras, Barlow, Rapee, & Brown, 1993) among others. All of these measures have shown reasonably good psychometric properties and have features to recommend their use (see comprehensive review by Newman, Kaloupek, & Keane, 1996).

Other Psychiatric Conditions

Because virtually all combat veterans with PTSD are expected to have other concurrent psychiatric disorders (Keane & Wolfe, 1990) it is important to conduct a thorough assessment of other psychiatric conditions. A number of reliable and valid structured interviews currently exist for making Axis I psychiatric diagnoses. The most widely used of all these is probably the SCID (Spitzer, Williams, Gibbon, & First, 1997). The SCID is a comprehensive, highly structured psychiatric interview that generally takes between 45 min and 2 hr to administer, depending on the number and nature of symptoms endorsed. It uses decision tree logic to assess the major adult Axis I disorders in *DSM-IV* and ICD-10. It has been demonstrated to have good psychometric properties in the evaluation of persons with serious mental illness. Another psychometrically strong measure is the MINI (Sheehan et al., 1998). Similar in structure and psychometric properties to the SCID, the MINI is an abbreviated interview that takes approximately 10–30 min to complete. It elicits all the symptoms listed in the symptom criteria for *DSM-IV* and ICD-10 for 15 major Axis I categories, and one Axis II disorder. Part of its appeal is that it can be administered in a relatively brief period of time and requires less training than the SCID. Both of these measures have been widely used with combat veterans evaluated for PTSD.

In addition to diagnosing Axis I disorders apart from PTSD, it may be helpful to evaluate a number of other related psychiatric dimensions. The *Structured Clinical Interview for DSM-IV Axis II: Personality Disorders* (First, Gibbon, Spitzer, Williams, & Benjamin, 1997) is a useful, reliable, and valid measure for making diagnostic decisions regarding Axis II personality disorders. To further evaluate symptom severity among relevant identified domains we recommend: the *Hamilton Rating Scales for Anxiety and Depression* (Hamilton, 1959) for assessing severity of anxiety and depressive symptoms, the *Positive and Negative Syndrome Scale* for schizophrenia (PANSS; Kay, Fiszbein, & Opler, 1987) for measuring severity of psychotic features, and the *Addiction Severity Index* (ASI; McLellan, Luborsky, Woody, & O'Brien, 1980) for measuring substance abuse and dependence variables. Additionally, the *Clinical Global Impressions Scale* (CGI; Guy, 1976) provides Severity and Global Improvement Subscales to measure overall severity of psychiatric illness and then improvement over time. These are 7-point scales, which are part of the ECDEU Assessment Manual for Psychopharmacology.

This is not intended to be a complete list of instruments, and other excellent measures exist for assessing domains of psychopathology relevant to PTSD in combat veterans.

INFORMATION CRITICAL TO MAKING THE DIAGNOSIS

According to the APA's *DSM* nosologic system, six categories of experiences or symptom clusters are required in order to make a formal diagnosis of PTSD (APA, 1994). In addition, there are other pieces of clinical information that are critical to making accurate diagnoses among combat veterans. In combination, these are:

1. *Establishing the historical antecedent of a traumatic event (Criterion A).* This is best accomplished through structured trauma interviews and review of military documents (e.g., Form DD214) to verify combat exposure reports.

2. *Evaluating frequency and severity of "reexperiencing" symptoms, such as intrusive memories, dissociative episodes, nightmares, and cued reactivity to trauma cues (Criterion B).* This is best accomplished through structured interviews (e.g., CAPS), with supporting evidence from self-report measures (e.g., Mississippi Scale, PCL). Interviews with collateral others, patients ratings, and behavioral assessments may also provide valuable information.

3. *Evaluating "avoidance" and "numbing" symptoms, including avoidance of stimuli/ thoughts/feelings/activities associated with the trauma, numbing of general responsiveness, loss of interest in significant activities, social detachment, and/or reduced affect (Criterion C).* This is best accomplished through structured interviews (e.g., CAPS), with supporting evidence from self-report measures (e.g., Mississippi Scale, PCL). Interviews with collateral others, patients ratings, and behavioral assessments may also provide valuable information.

4. *Evaluating the "arousal" symptoms, including hypervigilance, sleep disturbance, irritability or outbursts of anger, impaired concentration, and/or exaggerated startle response (Criterion D).* This is best accomplished through structured interviews (e.g., CAPS), with supporting evidence from self-report measures (e.g., Mississippi Scale, PCL). Psychophysiological assessment, interviews with collateral others, patients ratings, and behavioral assessments may also provide valuable information.

5. *Evaluating whether the duration of the disturbance exceeds one month (Criterion E).* This is best accomplished not only by the patient's self-report but also by the report of collateral others.

6. *Determining whether the trauma-related symptoms cause significant distress or impairment in social, occupational, or other important areas of functioning (Criterion F).* This is best accomplished through structured interviews (e.g., CAPS, SCID, MINI), clinical ratings (e.g., CGI, Hamilton Rating Scales), review of psychosocial history (e.g., employment and marital status, history of legal involvement), and self-report measures that assess other domains (e.g., MMPI-2, BDI). Interviews with collateral others, patients ratings, and behavioral assessments may also provide valuable information.

7. *Determining the nature and severity of psychiatric symptoms for other concurrent Axis I and II disorders*. This is best accomplished through general structured psychiatric interviews (e.g., SCID, MINI), clinical ratings (e.g., CGI, Hamilton Rating Scales, PANSS, ASI), and self-report measures that assess other domains (e.g., MMPI-2, Beck Inventories).

8. *Determining the authenticity of the trauma and symptom reports*. Use of MMPI-2 validity scales can provide a useful screening instrument for detecting exaggerated or feigned symptom reports. Structured interviews, psychophysiological assessment, and review of military and VA records (e.g., Form DD214, VA C-file) should provide information valuable to making this evaluation.

DOS AND DON'TS

Do: Conduct a thorough assessment of each veteran's trauma history, symptoms of PTSD, and symptoms of other concurrent Axis I and II features. Careful diagnostic assessment will be an invaluable guide to treatment planning and will help lay the foundation for building a therapeutic alliance. Veterans are often pleasantly surprised and appreciative when clinicians demonstrate their understanding and expertise by "asking the right questions." Although initially time-consuming, this careful assessment will pay enormous dividends in the long run by helping to target appropriate clinical interventions. It will also help to provide strong documentation, via reports filed in VA medical records, of veterans' difficulties, which may head-off later requests for assessment related to veterans' disability claims.

Don't: Do not overwhelm veterans with an assessment process that is so lengthy or tedious that it pushes them away from treatment. We have found it helpful to break the assessment process up into two or three sessions of several hours each. Typically we ask veterans to complete self-report instruments (e.g., MMPI-2) on a separate occasion from the psychiatric interviews. When doing this it is important to schedule all sessions within a fairly short window of time (e.g., 1–3 weeks) so that veterans do not become impatient or frustrated with this process.

Do: Provide a careful explanation for the purpose of the evaluation. Many veterans are mistrustful of the VA and/or impatient with regard to receiving clinical services. Therefore, it is important that they understand the need for such careful (and potentially time-consuming) evaluation procedures. If they understand that the assessment is critical to develop the most appropriate treatment plan and to accurately document their psychiatric difficulties in the medical record, they are usually willing to cooperate fully with the assessment procedures.

Don't: Be apologetic about the assessment procedures or create the impression that they are just part of the VA's bureaucratic "red tape" that must be endured prior to receiving clinical services.

Do: Do reassure veterans that they can exercise control of the interview procedures and may stop or pause the interviews whenever they choose.

Don't: Allow veterans to bully you or other staff, "bend" clinic rules, or circumvent routine evaluation procedures in such a way that they gain special or preferential treatment not accorded to other veterans. To maximize the therapeutic alliance it will be important to set firm boundaries with patients from the outset.

Do: Inquire about veterans' disability status and disability-seeking plans. This provides important contextual information for interpreting results of evaluation procedures. We recommend that the following questions be asked via a self-report questionnaire: (1) Do you currently have a VA service-connected disability? (2) If so, for what conditions and at what percent? (3) Do you currently have any disability claims or appeals pending with the VA? (4) If so, for what conditions? (5) Do you plan to file any disability claims or appeals in the near future? (6) If so, for what conditions? These questions can be embedded in a self-report instrument that includes other types of relevant questions (e.g., employment and legal status).

Don't: Assume that just because a veteran is seeking VA disability compensation for PTSD that s/he is an unreliable historian or prone to exaggerate or feign psychopathology. In fact, most (e.g., approximately 70%) veterans seeking treatment for PTSD also seek disability. Therefore, it is important to use such information cautiously.

Do: Exhibit sensitivity during the trauma interview. For persons with PTSD, this may be an extremely difficult, anxiety-provoking aspect of the evaluation. Thus, it is important to conduct element with the utmost sensitivity and care. Be prepared for some veterans to respond with tears, agitation, anger, physiological symptoms, or other signs of extreme anxiety. In some cases it may be necessary to give veterans breaks or pauses to recollect their composure; certainly they should be reassured that they are in control of the interview and can stop it or pause it whenever they choose to.

Don't: Do not be apologetic about this aspect of the evaluation or assume that veterans will be unable to tolerate it. In other words, don't send any signals regarding demand characteristics about how you expect a patient to react. It is best to be "matter-of-fact" and straightforward, providing a brief introduction and rationale before proceeding with the interview.

Do: Make an effort to obtain all relevant details about each veteran's lifetime trauma history.

Don't: Do not pressure or coerce veterans into revealing all details about their trauma history, especially at this early stage of their engagement in treatment. In fact, upon occasion it may be clinically indicated to discontinue a trauma interview altogether once the presence of Criterion A events has been established and move on to other aspects of the evaluation. It is not necessary to obtain all details in order to establish whether an individual meets *DSM* criteria. Furthermore, inquiring about the specific details, such as thoughts, feelings, and reactions that accompanied traumatic events, that may be important for treatment can be conducted at a later stage when trust and rapport have had a chance to develop.

Do: Conduct diagnostic assessments via a multidisciplinary effort. Most specialty PTSD clinics in VA Medical Centers consist of some combination of psychiatrists, psychologists, social workers, and/or nurses. Each of these disciplines has expertise to offer and using a team approach to evaluations offers several benefits, including allowing diagnostic decisions to be made by a consensus of expert opinion and setting the stage for multidisciplinary treatment efforts.

Don't: Do not overwhelm veterans with an assessment process that is redundant. It is important to approach each evaluation with a well-coordinated plan about who will do what. Specifically, do not have two interviewers conducting identical or similar interviews on the same content area.

Do: Collect, review, and integrate data from sources other than structured psychiatric interviews, such as appropriate self-report questionnaires (e.g., MMPI-2, Mississippi Scale for PTSD, BDI), psychophysiological assessment (e.g., pulse and heart rate reactivity to trauma cues), collateral-other reports, and behavioral assessments. Data from these other sources may prove especially helpful in cases where there is conflicting or ambiguous evidence, or in cases of suspected symptom exaggeration or malingering.

Don't: Do not overwhelm veterans with an assessment process that is unnecessarily complicated. We recommend using a relatively concise set of standard evaluation instruments and procedures to be used with all patients, reserving other specific measures for addressing specific questions on a case-by-case basis. For example, psychophysiological assessment is probably not feasible or necessary for all evaluations. However, because it is not susceptible to faking, in cases of suspected malingering, it may prove extremely useful to address the specific question of whether the symptom of cued reactivity is present.

Do: Use the MMPI-2 appropriately to provide additional data regarding personality features, symptom acuity, and evaluation response set or style. In particular, the MMPI-2 can serve as a screening measure for symptom exaggeration or malingering, so long as population-specific cutoffs are used, rather than traditional cutoffs. For example, rather than using an $F–K$ index score of ≥ 12, we recommend a cutoff of ≥ 22; for the $F(p)$ scale a score of ≥ 8. When exceeded, this screening cutoff score should indicate the need for additional focused evaluation (e.g., psychophysiological assessment) to rule out malingering.

Don't: Do not rely on the MMPI-2 as a diagnostic tool, and do not use the MMPI-2 alone to make diagnoses of malingering. Furthermore, do not rely on traditional MMPI-2 validity scale cutoffs for invalid responding, as these scales have proven to be highly vulnerable to genuine psychological distress in this population.

Do: Provide patients with thoughtful feedback regarding the results of their evaluation. It is important to be straightforward and honest with this information. This provides patients important information about themselves, sends the message that the evaluation results have been carefully considered and constitutes an important element of clinical care, helps with treatment planning, and may assist in establishing a therapeutic alliance. If a multidisciplinary team conducted the evaluation, it may prove valuable to provide patient feedback with the entire team present.

Don't: Do not provide feedback to veterans using too much technical jargon or professional terminology. While in most cases it is important to provide the specific *DSM* diagnoses, it is also important to focus on describing these in ways that patients can understand and allowing them to ask questions about anything they do not understand.

Do: Write careful and thoughtful reports that integrate all evaluation data. Be sure to remember that these reports are likely to be used by the veteran as supporting documentation in VA disability claims rulings; remember also that veterans served within the VA system have the right to review documents in their medical record, and most will eventually read their reports.

Don't: Do not write anything in your reports that you will not feel comfortable explaining or discussing with the patient concerned.

Do: Use diagnostic assessments and all data from the evaluation procedures as a foundation for treatment planning. This information should have clear implications for developing and implementing appropriate interventions. The evaluation and feedback process should serve as a stage of treatment in such a way that patients perceive subsequent interventions as logical extensions of the assessment.

Don't: Do not neglect to implement targeted evaluation strategies throughout treatment to help measure therapeutic progress and fine-tune treatment approaches.

SUMMARY

The clinical syndrome of combat-related PTSD is a severe, chronic, and prevalent psychiatric disorder resulting in considerable emotional distress and social disruption, and often constitutes a significant diagnostic challenge. Studies consistently demonstrate that combat veterans evaluated for PTSD within the VA exhibit extreme and diffuse levels of psychopathology across different domains of mental illness, and extreme elevations on validity scales of the MMPI-2 in a "fake-bad" or overreporting direction. This overreporting response style may be at least partially caused by the specter of disability payments, which many veterans apply for. Furthermore, exaggeration of symptom reports obviously complicates diagnostic decision-making regarding PTSD criteria, differential diagnosis, and development of appropriate treatment plans. There are a number of strategies for gathering relevant information in the diagnostic assessment of veterans with symptoms of PTSD, including structured interviews, self-report measures, psychophysiological assessment, patient ratings, and behavioral assessments. In particular, structured interviews are crucial for making accurate diagnoses, and should include interviews to evaluate lifetime and combat trauma history, PTSD symptoms according to *DSM* criteria (e.g., CAPS), and symptoms of other psychiatric conditions. Throughout this chapter we discuss a number of assessment strategies for reducing susceptibility to malingering and symptom overreporting. In addition, we present a case illustration, list information critical to making the diagnosis, and address assessment "Dos and Don'ts" to provide a thorough picture of the diagnostic assessment of PTSD among combat veterans.

REFERENCES

American Psychiatric Association. (1994). *Diagnostic and statistical manual of mental disorders* (4th ed.). Washington, DC, Author.

Atkinson, R. M., Henderson, R. G., Sparr, L. F., & Deale, S. (1982). Assessment of Vietnam veterans for posttraumatic stress disorder in veterans administration disability claims. *American Journal of Psychiatry, 139,* 1118–1121.

Berndt, E. R., Koran, L. M., Finkelstein, S. N., Gelenberg, A. J., Kornstein, S. G., Miller, I. M., Thase, M. E., Trapp, G. A., & Keller, M. B. (2000). Lost human capital from early-onset chronic depression. *American Journal of Psychiatry, 157,* 940–947.

Bernstein, D. P., Fink, L., Handelsman, L., Foote, J., Lovejoy, M., Wenzel, K., Sapareto, E., & Ruggiero, J. (1994). Initial reliability and validity of a new retrospective measure of child abuse and neglect. *American Journal of Psychiatry, 151,* 1132–1136.

Blake, D. D., Weathers, F. W., Nagy, L. N., Kaloupek, D. G., Klauminzer, G., Charney, D. S., & Keane, T. M. (1990). A clinician rating scale for assessing current and lifetime PTSD: The CAPS-1. *The Behavior Therapist, 18,* 187–188.

Blanchard, E. B., Jones, A. J., Buckley, T. C., & Forneris, C. A. (1996). Psychometric properties of the PTSD Checklist (PCL). *Behaviour Research and Therapy, 34,* 669–673.

Blanchard, E. B., Kolb, L. C., & Prins, A. (1991). Psychophysiological responses in the diagnosis of post-traumatic stress disorder in Vietnam veterans. *Journal of Nervous and Mental Disease, 179,* 99–103.

Boudewyns, P. A., & Hyer, L. (1990). Physiological response to combat memories and preliminary treatment outcome in Vietnam veteran PTSD patients treated with direct therapeutic exposure. *Behavior Therapy, 21,* 63–87.

Bremner, J. D., Staib, L. H., Kaloupek, D., Southwick, S. M., Soufer, R., & Charney, D. S. (1999). Neural correlates of exposure to traumatic pictures and sound in Vietnam combat veterans with and without posttraumatic stress disorder: A positron emission tomography study. *Biological Psychiatry, 45,* 806–816.

Burkett, B. G., & Whitley, G. (1998). *Stolen valor: How the Vietnam generation was robbed of its heroes and history.* Dallas, TX: Verity Press.

Card, J. J. (1987). Epidemiology of PTSD in a national cohort of Vietnam veterans. *Journal of Clinical Psychology, 43,* 6–17.

Center for Disease Control. (1988). Health status of Vietnam veterans. *Journal of the American Medical Association, 259,* 2701–2724.

Davidson, J. R. T., Malik, M. A., & Travers, J. (1997). Structured interview for PTSD (SIP): Psychometric validation for *DSM-IV* criteria. *Depression and Anxiety, 5,* 127–129.

DiNardo, P. A., Moras, K., Barlow, D. H., Rapee, R. M., & Brown, T. A. (1993). Reliability of *DSM-III-R* anxiety disorder categories: Using the Anxiety Disorders Interview Schedule—Revised (ADIS-R). *Archives of General Psychiatry, 50,* 251–256.

Drake, R. E., McHugo, G. J., Bebout, R. R., Becker, D. R., Harris M., Bond, G. R., & Quimby, E. (1999). A randomized clinical trial of supported employment for inner-city patients with severe mental disorders. *Archives of General Psychiatry, 56,* 627–633.

Elhai, J. D., Frueh, B. C., Gold, P. B., Gold, S. N., & Hamner, M. B. (2000b). Clinical presentations of posttraumatic stress disorder across trauma populations: A comparison of MMPI-2 profiles of combat veterans and adult survivors of child sexual abuse. *Journal of Nervous and Mental Disease, 188,* 708–713.

Elhai, J. D., Ruggerio, K. J., Frueh, B. C., Beckham, J. C., Gold, P. B., & Feldman, M. E. (2002). The infrequency-posttraumatic stress disorder scale (*Fptsd*) for the MMPI-2: Development and initial validation with veterans presenting with combat-related PTSD. *Journal of Personality Assessment, 79,* 531–549.

Fairbank, J. A., Keane, T. M., & Malloy, P. F. (1983). Some preliminary data on the psychological characteristics of Vietnam veterans with posttraumatic stress disorder. *Journal of Consulting and Clinical Psychology, 51,* 912–919.

First, M. B., Gibbon, M., Spitzer, R. L., Williams, J. B., & Benjamin, L. S. (1997). *Structured Clinical Interview for DSM-IV Axis II: Personality Disorders.* Washington, DC: American Psychiatric Press.

Foa, E. B., Riggs, D. S., Dancu, C. V., & Rothbaum, B. O. (1993). Reliability and validity of a brief instrument for assessing post-traumatic stress disorder. *Journal of Traumatic Stress, 6,* 459–474.

Fontana, A., & Rosenheck, R. (1998). Effects of compensation seeking on treatment outcomes among veterans with posttraumatic stress disorder. *Journal of Nervous and Mental Disease, 186,* 223–230.

Franklin, C. L., Repasky, S. A., Thompson, K. E., Shelton, S. A., & Uddo, M. (2002). Differentiation over-reporting and extreme distress: MMPI-2 use with compensation-seeking veterans with PTSD. *Journal of Personality Assessment, 79,* 274–285.

Frueh, B. C., Gold, P. B., & de Arellano, M. A. (1997). Symptom overreporting in combat veterans evaluated for PTSD: Differentiation on the basis of compensation seeking status. *Journal of Personality Assessment, 68*, 369–384.

Frueh, B. C., Hamner, M. B., Cahill, S. P., Gold, P. B., & Hamlin K. (2000). Apparent symptom overreporting among combat veterans evaluated for PTSD. *Clinical Psychology Review, 20*, 853–885.

Frueh, B. C., Smith, D. W., & Barker, S. E. (1996a). Compensation seeking status and psychometric assessment of combat veterans seeking treatment for PTSD. *Journal of Traumatic Stress, 9*, 427–439.

Frueh, B. C., Turner, S. M., Beidel, D. C., Mirabella, R. F., & Jones, W. J. (1996b). Trauma Management Therapy: A preliminary evaluation of a multicomponent behavioral treatment for chronic combat-related PTSD. *Behaviour Research and Therapy, 34*, 533–543.

Frueh, B. C., Turner, S. M., Beidel, D. C., & Cahill, S. P. (2001). Assessment of social functioning in combat veterans with PTSD. *Aggression and Violent Behavior, 6*, 79–90.

Gerardi, R. J., Blanchard, E. B., & Kolb, L. C. (1989). Ability of Vietnam veterans to dissimulate a psychophysiological assessment for post-traumatic stress disorder. *Behavior Therapy, 20*, 229–243.

Gold, P. B., Engdahl, B. E., Eberly, R. E., Blake, R. J., Page, W. F., & Frueh, B. C. (2000). Trauma exposure, resilience, social support, and PTSD construct validity among former prisoners of war. *Social Psychiatry and Psychiatric Epidemiology, 35*, 36–42.

Gold, P. B., & Frueh, B. C. (1999). Compensation-seeking and extreme exaggeration of psychopathology among combat veterans evaluated for PTSD. *Journal of Nervous and Mental Disease, 187*, 680–684.

Green, B. (1995). Trauma History Questionnaire. Unpublished instrument and data.

Guy, W. (1976). *ECDEU assessment manual for psychopharmacology*. Washington DC: DHEW.

Hamilton, M. (1959). The assessment of anxiety states by rating. *British Journal of Medical Psychology, 32*, 50–55.

Hamner, M. B., Frueh, B. C., Ulmer, H. G., Huber, M. G., Twomey, T. J., Tyson, C. T., & Arana, G. W. (2000). Psychotic features in chronic PTSD and schizophrenia: Comparative severity. *Journal of Nervous and Mental Disease, 188*, 217–221.

Hankin, C. S., Spiro, A., Miller, D. R., & Kazis L. (1999). Mental disorders and mental health treatment among U. S. Department of Veterans Affairs outpatients: The Veterans Health Study. *American Journal of Psychiatry, 156*, 1924–1930.

Hawkins, R. P. (1979). The functions of assessment: Implications for selection and development of devices for assessing repertoires in clinical, educational, and other settings. *Journal of Applied Behavior Analysis, 12*, 501–516.

Horowitz, M. J., Wilner, N. R., & Alvarez, W. (1979). Impact of event scale: A measure of subjective distress. *Psychosomatic Medicine, 41*, 208–218.

Jordan, R. G., Nunley, T. V., & Cook, R. R. (1992). Symptom exaggeration in a PTSD inpatient population: Response set or claim for compensation. *Journal of Traumatic Stress, 5*, 633–642.

Kaplan, H. I., Sadock, B. J., & Grebb, J. A. (1994). *Synopsis of psychiatry: Behavioral sciences, clinical psychiatry* (7th ed.). Baltimore: Williams & Watkins.

Kay, S. R., Fiszbein, A., & Opler, L. A. (1987). The positive and negative syndrome scale (PANSS) for schizophrenia. *Schizophrenia Bulletin, 13*, 261–276.

Keane, T. M., Caddell, J. M., & Taylor, K. L. (1988). Mississippi scale for combat-related posttraumatic stress disorder: Three studies in reliability and validity. *Journal of Consulting and Clinical Psychology, 56*, 85–90.

Keane, T. M., Fairbank, J. A., Caddell, J. M., Zimering, R. T., Taylor, K. L., & Mora, C. A. (1989). Clinical evaluation of a measure to assess combat exposure. *Psychological Assessment, 1*, 53–55.

Keane, T. M., Kolb, L. C., Kaloupek, D. G., Orr, S. P., Blanchard, E. B., Thomas, R. G., Hsieh, F. Y., & Lavori, P. W. (1998). Utility of psychophysiological measurement in the diagnosis of posttraumatic stress disorder: Results for a Department of Veterans Affairs cooperative study. *Journal of Consulting and Clinical Psychology, 66*, 914–923.

Keane, T. M., & Wolfe, J. (1990). Comorbidity in Post-Traumatic Stress Disorder: An analysis of community and clinical studies. *Journal of Applied Social Psychology, 20*, 1776–1788.

Kessler, R. C., Sonnega, A., Bromet, E., Hughes, M., & Nelson, C. B. (1995). Posttraumatic stress disorder in the national comorbidity study. *Archives of General Psychiatry, 52*, 1048–1060.

Kilpatrick, D. G., Acierno, R., Saunders, B., Resnick, H. S., Best, C. L., & Schnurr, P. P. (2000). Risk factors for adolescent substance abuse and dependence: Data from international sample. *Journal of Consulting and Clinical Psychology, 68,* 19–30.

Kouzis, A. C., & Eaton, W. W. (2000). Psychopathology and the initiation of disability payments. *Psychiatric Services, 51,* 908–913.

Kulka, R. A., Schlenger, W. E., Fairbank, J. A., Hough, R. L., Jordan, B. K., Marmar, C. R., & Weiss, D. S. (1990). *Trauma and the Vietnam war generation: Report of findings from the National Vietnam Veterans Readjustment Study.* New York: Brunner/Mazel.

Lees-Haley, P. R. (1989). Malingering post-traumatic stress disorder on the MMPI. *Forensic Reports, 2,* 89–91.

MacDonald, C., Chamberlain, K., Long, Nigel, & Flett, R. (1999). Posttraumatic stress disorder and interpersonal functioning in Vietnam war veterans: A mediational model. *Journal of Traumatic Stress, 12,* 701–708.

Magruder, K. M., Frueh, B. C., Knapp, R. G., Vaughn, J., Carson, T., Cain, G., & Robert, S. (2002, February). *PTSD symptom severity in VA primary care patients.* Paper presented at the VA Health Services Research 2002 Annual Meeting, Washington, DC.

McGrath, J. M., & Frueh, B. C. (2002). Fraudulent claims of combat status in within the VA? *Psychiatric Services, 53,* 345.

McLellan, T., Luborsky, L., Woody, G., & O'Brien, C. (1980). An improved diagnostic evaluation instrument for substance abuse patients. *Journal of Nervous and Mental Disease, 168,* 26–33.

Mueser, K. T., Goodman, L. B., Trumbetta, S. L., Rosenberg, S. D., Osher, F. C., Vidaver, R., Auciello, P., & Foy, D. W. (1998). Trauma and posttraumatic stress disorder in severe mental illness. *Journal of Consulting and Clinical Psychology, 66,* 493–499.

Newman, E., Kaloupek, D. G., & Keane, T. M. (1996). Assessment of posttraumatic stress disorder in clinical and research settings. In B. A. van der Kolk, A. C. McFarlane, & L. Weisaeth (Eds.), *Traumatic stress: The effects of overwhelming experience on mind, body, and society* (pp. 242–275). New York, NY: Guildford.

Oboler, S. (2000). Disability evaluations under the Department of Veterans Affairs. In R. D. Rondinelli and R. T. Katz (Eds.), *Impairment rating and disability evaluation* (pp. 187–217). Philadelphia, PA: W. B. Saunders.

Orr, S. P., Claiborn, J. M., Altman, B., Forgue, D. F., de Jong, J. B., Pitman, R. K., & Herz L. R. (1990). Psychometric profile of posttraumatic stress disorder, anxious, and healthy Vietnam veterans: Correlations with psychophysiologic responses. *Journal of Consulting and Clinical Psychology, 58,* 329–335.

Petrila, J., & Brink, T. (2001). Mental illness and changing definitions of disability under the Americans with Disabilities Act. *Psychiatric Services, 52,* 626–630.

Rasmusson, A. M., Hauger, R. L., Morgan, C. A., Bremner, J. D., Charney, D. S., & Southwick, S. M. (2000). Low baseline and yohimbine-stimulated plasma neuropeptide Y (NPY) levels in combat-related PTSD. *Biological Psychiatry, 47,* 526–539.

Resnick, H. S. (1996). Psychometric review of Trauma Assessment for Adults (TAA). In B. H. Stamm (Ed.), *Measurement of stress, trauma, and adaptation.* Lutherville, MD: Sidran Press.

Resnick, H. S., Best, C. L., Kilpatrick, D. G., Freedy, J. R., Falsetti, S. A., & Dansky, B. S. (1996). In T. W. Miller (Ed.), *Stressful life events* (2nd ed.). Madison, CT: International Universities Press.

Robins, L. N., Helzer, J. E., Croughan, J. L., & Ratliff, K. S. (1981). National Institute of Mental Health Diagnostic Interview Schedule: Its history, characteristics, and validity. *Archives of General Psychiatry, 38,* 381–389.

Rothke, S. E., Friedman, A. F., Dahlstrom, W. G., Greene, R. L., Arredondo, R., & Mann, A. W. (1994). MMPI-2 normative data for the F–K index: Implications for clinical, neuropsychological, and forensic practice. *Assessment, 1,* 1–15.

Schneider, S. J. (1979). Disability payments for psychiatric patients: Is patient assessment affected? *Journal of Clinical Psychology, 35,* 259–264.

Schnurr, P. P., Spiro, A., & Paris, A. H. (2000). Physician-diagnosed medical disorders in relation to PTSD symptoms in older male military veterans. *Health Psychology, 19,* 91–97.

Sheehan, D. V., Lecrubier, Y., Sheehan, K. H., Amorim, P., Janavs, J., Weiller, E., Hergueta, T., Baker, R., & Dunbar, G. (1998). The Mini-International Neuropsychiatric Interview (MINI): The development and validation of a structured diagnostic psychiatric interview for *DSM-IV* and ICD-10. *Journal of Clinical Psychiatry, 59* (Suppl. 20), 22–33.

Sher, C. D., Stein, M. B., Asmundson, G. J. G., McCreary, D. R., & Forde, D. R. (2001). The Childhood Trauma Questionnaire in a community sample: Psychometric properties and normative data. *Journal of Traumatic Stress, 14,* 843–857.

Smith, D. W., & Frueh, B. C. (1996). Compensation seeking, comorbidity, and apparent exaggeration of PTSD symptoms among Vietnam combat veterans. *Psychological Assessment, 8,* 3–6.

Smith, D. W., Frueh, B. C., Sawchuck, C. N., & Johnson, M. R. (1999). The relationship between symptom overreporting and pre- and post-combat trauma history in veterans evaluated for PTSD. *Depression and Anxiety, 10,* 119–124.

Southwick, S. M., Morgan, C. A., Nicolaou, A. L., & Charney, D. S. (1997). Consistency of memory for combat-related traumatic events in veterans of Operation Desert Storm. *American Journal of Psychiatry, 154,* 173–177.

Southwick, S. M., Paige, S., Morgan, C. A., Bremner, J. D., Krystal, J. H., & Charney, D. S. (1999). Neurotransmitter alterations in PTSD: Catecholamines and serotonin. *Seminars in Clinical Neuropsychiatry, 4,* 242–248.

Spiro, A., Schnurr, P. P., & Aldwin, C. M. (1994). Combat-related posttraumatic stress disorder symptoms in older men. *Psychology of Aging, 9,* 17–26.

Spitzer, R. L., Williams, J. B., Gibbon, M., & First, M. B. (1997). *Structured Clinical Interview for DSM-IV.* Washington, DC: American Psychiatric Press.

Straus, M. A., Hamby, S. L., Boney-McCoy, S., & Sugarman, D. B. (1996). The Revised Conflict Tactics Scale (CTS2): Development and preliminary psychometric data. *Journal of Family Issues, 17,* 283–316.

Sutker, P. B., Winstead, D. K., Galina, Z. H., & Allain, A. N. (1990). Assessment of long term psychosocial sequelae among POW survivors of the Korean conflict. *Journal of Personality Assessment, 54,* 170–180.

Switzer, G. E., Dew, M. A., Thompson, K., Goycoolea, J. M., Derricott, T., & Mullins, S. D. (1999). Posttraumatic stress disorder and service utilization among urban mental health center clients. *Journal of Traumatic Stress, 12,* 25–39.

Wagner, A. W., Wolfe, J., Rotnitsky, A., Proctor, S. P., & Erickson, D. J. (2000). An investigation of the impact of posttraumatic stress disorder on physical health. *Journal of Traumatic Stress, 13,* 41–55.

Wall Street Journal. (1999). Gulf War veterans draw disability compensation at a higher rate than those from any other conflict (p. A1). *Wall Street Journal,* October 27.

Weathers, F. W., Keane, T. M., & Davidson, J. R. (2001). Clinician-administered PTSD scale: A review of the first ten years of research. *Depression and Anxiety, 13,* 132–156.

Weathers, F. W., & Litz, B. (1994). Psychometric properties of the Clinician-Administered PTSD Scale, CAPS-1. *PTSD Research Quarterly, 5,* 2–6.

Weathers, F. W., Ruscio, A. M., & Keane, T. M. (1999). Psychometric properties of nine scoring rules for the Clinician Administered Posttraumatic Stress Disorder Scale. *Psychological Assessment, 11,* 124–133.

Yehuda, R., Boisoneau, D., Lowery, M. T., & Giller, E. L. (1995). Dose-response changes in plasma cortisol and lymphocyte glucocorticoid receptors following dexamethasone administration in combat veterans with and without posttraumatic stress disorder. *Archives of General Psychiatry, 52,* 583–593.

Zatzick, D. F., Marmar, C. R., Weiss, D. S., Browner, W. S., Metzler, T. J., Golding, J. M., Stewart, A., Schlenger, W. E., & Wells, K. B. (1997). Posttraumatic stress disorder and functioning and quality of life outcomes in a nationally representative sample of male Vietnam veterans. *American Journal of Psychiatry, 154,* 1690–1695.

15

Post-Traumatic Stress Disorder (Noncombat)

Alyssa A. Rheingold and Ron Acierno

Description of Noncombat PTSD

Sixty percent of U.S. men and 68% of U.S. women experience a traumatic event at some point during their lives (Kessler, Sonnega, Bromet, Hughes, & Nelson, 1995; Resnick, Kilpatrick, Dansky, Saunders, & Best, 1993). Consequently, these individuals are at significant increased risk for post-traumatic stress disorder (PTSD), a debilitating anxiety disorder originally conceptualized to explain psychiatric symptoms of combat participants. The diagnosis of PTSD requires exposure to a traumatic event depicted by intense fear, helplessness, or horror (Criterion A), followed by symptoms of re-experiencing, avoidance, and hyperarousal enduring for at least one month (*Diagnostic and Statistical Manual for Mental Disorders*, Fourth Edition [*DSM-IV*]; American Psychiatric Association, 1994). Examples of noncombat-related traumatic events include sexual assault, physical assault, natural disaster, serious accident, child sexual abuse, child physical abuse, child neglect, witnessing a traumatic event, and sudden loss of a loved one.

The first subset of PTSD symptoms, reexperiencing symptoms (Criterion B), includes intrusive recollections of the event, flashbacks (where the victim feels as if the event was occurring while awake), nightmares of the event, and exaggerated and intense response to trauma cues. The second set of PTSD symptoms, avoidance and emotional numbing (Criterion C), is indicated by avoidance of thoughts, feeling, activities, places, or people that are reminders of the trauma. In addition, this subset of symptoms includes loss of interest in once pleasurable activities, feelings of detachment from others, inability to recall important aspects of the events, restricted range of emotions, and feelings of a foreshortened future.

Alyssa A. Rheingold and Ron Acierno • National Crime Victims Research and Treatment Center, Medical University of South Carolina, Charleston, South Carolina 29425.

Increased arousal (Criterion D) characterizes the third subset of PTSD symptoms and includes difficulty sleeping, irritability or anger outbursts, difficulty concentrating, hypervigilance, and exaggerated startle response. A diagnosis of PTSD is given when these clusters of symptoms occur more than 1 month in duration. If duration of symptoms is less than 3 months following the event, it is specified as *acute*, and if the duration of symptoms is 3 months or more, it is specified as *chronic*. The disorder can have immediate or delayed onset. PTSD with delayed onset is characterized by symptoms occurring at least 6 months after the trauma.

Epidemiological data confirm that PTSD is common. Lifetime prevalence in the general adult population may be as high as 10% for women (Resnick et al., 1993). Resnick et al. found that 17.9% of women who were exposed to some type of traumatic event met criteria for PTSD at some time in their lives, and 6.7% reported symptoms consistent with current diagnosis of PTSD. Rates of PTSD were significantly higher among crime versus noncrime victims (25.8% vs. 9.4%), with those crime victims who experienced perceived life threat or who were actually injured during the assault at greatest risk.

Women are at a higher risk than men for developing PTSD (Breslau, Davis, Andreski, & Peterson, 1991; Kessler et al., 1995). In women, Breslau et al. (1991) and Resnick et al. (1993) found that assault and rape are the most frequent traumas leading to PTSD. Resnick et al. (1993) reported that the highest rate of both lifetime PTSD (38.5%) and current PTSD (18%) occurred among women with a history of physical assault followed by those with a history of rape (32% lifetime, 12% current). Risk factors for PTSD following rape include history of depression, alcohol abuse, or experienced injury during the rape, and risk factors for PTSD following physical assault include history of depression and lower education (Acierno, Resnick, Kilpatrick, Saunders, & Best,1999).

The Healthcare Maintenance Organization (HMO) population data of Breslau et al. (1991) indicate that those victims with PTSD are over six times as likely as those without PTSD to have some other psychiatric disorder. The national data of Kessler et al. (1995) show that those with PTSD are almost eight times as likely to have three or more disorders as individuals without PTSD. The most frequent PTSD comorbid presentations include depression and panic (Breslau et al., 1991; Falsetti, Resnick, Dansky, Lydiard, & Kilpatrick, 1995; Kessler et al., 1995; Resnick et al., 1993). In summary, PTSD affects roughly one-third of trauma victims, causes serious impairment in daily functioning, and increases the risk for other psychopathology.

Procedures for Gathering Information

As outlined in Table 1, the PTSD interview should begin with a brief description of the interview process along with several statements recognizing possible feelings the client may experience during the interview, particularly when talking about distressing events. Interviewers should make clients aware that information gathered is important for proper assessment and treatment planning, and that a desire to avoid talking about traumatic events and symptomatology, while

TABLE 1. Diagnostic Interview Outline for the Assessment of PTSD

1. Provide brief overview of interview process
2. Address presenting complaint
3. Assess trauma characteristics (Criterion A) while establishing a supportive and nonjudgmental atmosphere
4. Assess lifetime trauma history using behaviorally specific questions and contextually orienting preface statements
5. Assess for the 17 PTSD symptoms (structured interviews can provide reliable and valid assessment)
   (a) Reexperiencing symptoms
   (b) Avoidance behaviors and numbing
   (c) Physiological arousal
6. Assess other Axis I and Axis II diagnoses
   (a) Other anxiety disorders
   (b) Mood disorders
   (c) Substance abuse/dependence
   (d) Borderline personality disorder
7. Assess environmental factors
   (a) PTSD related stimuli
   (b) Other life stressors, poor social support
   (c) Psychosocial and psychiatric history

common, may result in incomplete interventions. The following is an example of opening comments for someone who is being evaluated for treatment:

> Today, I am going to ask you a lot of questions about topics that may be uncomfortable so that I can get a complete picture of what has been going on for you lately. I'm going to ask these questions because it is important for me to recognize all the areas that go into figuring out a plan to help you. I understand that talking about some of the topics may be difficult, and that you may have some feelings of anxiety. Maybe we can also discuss ways of coping with these distressing feelings. I want to assure you that the details of the topics are up to you, and we can go at whatever pace you feel comfortable. O.K.?

This provides the client with some understanding of what is going to happen in the interview; for a PTSD sufferer, this may help to decrease anticipatory anxiety. In addition, normalizing avoidance and anxiety responses is important and helps to establish a supportive environment for clients.

Several open-ended questions are then typically utilized to isolate a client's main concerns and understanding of the problem. Beginning with open-ended questions such as "Please tell me briefly about the most important problem that you are having as a result of the crime" allows a client to describe events and resulting problems in his/her own words. During initial discussions of presenting problems, interviewers should exhibit empathetic listening skills. Those suffering from PTSD very often have difficulty talking about trauma events and resulting symptomatology. Therefore, establishing a supportive, nonjudgmental atmosphere at the beginning of each interview is crucial and allows a client to engage in interview processes, as well as increases motivation for treatment.

Assessment of traumatic events, in addition to symptomatology, is important both for determining whether or not an event meets Criterion A and to identify parameters of the event that will be relevant to treatment. Furthermore, several characteristics of traumatic events, such as perceived life threat, degree of actual physical harm, and chronicity, may be predictive of PTSD symptom severity (Resnick, Kilpatrick, & Lipovsky, 1991). Understanding the specifics of a trauma event may help interviewers to understand an individual's unique experience and perceptions of the event.

After reviewing the details of recent trauma events, assessment efforts should turn to measuring past traumatic experiences. This investigation frequently enhances the understanding of an individual's avoidance, anxiety, and learning history with current functioning. Persons exposed to multiple traumas may display different patterns of PTSD symptomatology and their development of symptoms may be more complex than in persons who experienced only one stressor. Thus, a person with a history of child sexual abuse who is exposed to a recent sexual assault may respond differently from a person without an abuse history.

There is a variety of methods to inquire about traumatic events. Social science research indicates, however, that one approach is far better than the rest. This approach involves using closed-ended behaviorally specific victim screening questions of trauma events to thoroughly assess trauma history. Note that this is in contrast to the supported use of open-ended questions to assess symptomatology. Trauma events are best answered with closed-ended questions, while post-event sequelae are best assessed by open-ended questions.

Behaviorally specific questions are those queries that are well defined and unambiguous in nature, therefore leaving minimal room for differences in interpretation. They utilize operational definitions for each event. Typically, closed-ended questions are to be avoided in diagnostic interviewing; however, assessment of traumatic events is the exception to this rule. This is because many clients find it easier to answer "yes" or "no" to potentially embarrassing and highly personal material. When using closed-ended questions, interviewers must be sure to follow-up acknowledged events comprehensively. Resnick et al. (1993) offer specific victimization screening questions for both noncrime events (e.g., "Have you ever experienced a serious accident at work, car, or somewhere else?"); and crime events such as homicide (e.g., "Has a close friend or family member of yours ever been deliberately killed or murdered by another person or killed by a drunk driver?"); rape (e.g., "Has a man or boy ever made you have sex by using force or threatening to harm you or someone close to you? Just so there is no mistake, by sex we mean putting a penis in your vagina."); contact sexual molestation (e.g., "Not counting the incidents you already told me about, has anybody ever touched your breasts or pubic area or made you touch his penis by using force or threat of force?"); attempted sexual assault (e.g., "Other than the incidents that we've already discussed, have there been situations that did not involve actual sexual contact between you and another person but did involve an attempt by someone to force you to have any kind of unwanted sexual contact?"); and physical assault (e.g., "Has anyone—including family members and friends—ever attacked you without a weapon but with the intent to kill or seriously injure you?"). Some clinicians may feel uncomfortable asking explicit questions either because of their own personal history or because they fear upsetting clients;

however, asking specific, behaviorally oriented trauma questions allows clinicians to reliably assess trauma history. Direct questions also demonstrate to clients that discussion of these topics is accepted by the clinician. Clinicians may require practice in order to comfortably present these questions to clients.

Following positive identification of a Criterion A event, assessment of trauma-related symptom characteristics is warranted. Both closed-ended and open-ended questions may guide the discussion toward evaluating the 17 PTSD symptoms. Structured interviews, such as those listed below, enhance reliability of diagnosis. These interviews involve assessment of all three symptom clusters of PTSD (i.e., reexperiencing symptoms, avoidance behaviors, and physiological arousal symptoms). Note that these PTSD symptoms must be attributed to a specific traumatic event. Assessors should also determine frequency of and impairment due to each symptom to best understand an individual's diagnostic presentation. For example, questions relating to experiencing nightmares may include: "Do you have nightmares about the trauma?...Describe for me briefly what these nightmares are about....How often do you have them each week?...Do the nightmares wake you up at night?...When they wake you up, how quickly are you able to get back to sleep?" As mentioned above, these symptoms need to last for a duration of one month in order to meet criteria for PTSD. Therefore, interviewers should inquire as to the duration of these symptoms.

PTSD is associated with high rates of comorbid disorders (see Keane & Kaloupek, 1997, for review). Proper assessment of other disorders and their relationship to PTSD is advised. Specifically, interviewers should assess for other anxiety disorders such as panic disorder and agoraphobia, as well as depression and substance use disorders. Clinicians should also review symptoms and behaviors associated with various Axis II diagnoses such as histrionic personality disorder or borderline personality disorder. Comprehensive assessment determines conceptualization and subsequent treatment of PTSD in a given individual. For example, exposure-based treatment of PTSD in an individual with severe substance use disorders is typically delayed until the substance disorder is treated. This is because substance abuse is often exacerbated in individuals with PTSD and serves as a maladaptive coping response to reduce anxiety. Treatment of PTSD prior to treatment of the substance abuse may exacerbate symptoms of the latter because PTSD treatment is associated with initial elevations of anxiety during exposure trials.

Several environmental influences relate to development and maintenance of PTSD and should be addressed. First, a review of stimuli that may be conditioned elicitors of PTSD symptoms, including people, places, and other cues in the environment should be completed. When an individual is exposed to a life threatening dangerous situation, aspects of the situation may become conditioned cues, which subsequently take on fear producing properties during future exposure. Individuals then avoid these conditioned cues. These conditioned stimuli cross all senses and could be something the victim sees, hears, smells, tastes, and feels. For example, a young woman who was raped by a man with a beard experiences fear when a friend with a beard comes to visit. She, therefore, may avoid such men. By leaving situations where men with beards are present, her anxiety is reduced (i.e., negatively reinforced), and this avoidance is strengthened. Delineating conditioned fear cues can be accomplished by constructing a fear hierarchy, or a list of feared situations in order of degree of anxiety and avoidance. A scale of 0–10 is typically used for anchor points. Fear hierarchy questions might follow this format:

> On a scale of 0–10, where 0 is no anxiety and 10 is unbearable panic, what rating would you give to the following situations: seeing a man with a beard in the car next to yours as you drive on the highway; being on an elevator with a man with a beard...

A fear hierarchy is especially important as a prelude to behaviorally oriented exposure treatments. In addition, daily monitoring of triggers to anxiety may help individuals to recognize less obvious cues.

Other environmental influences that may prove helpful to address during a PTSD interview include familial factors, other life stressors, and psychiatric history. Poor social support and negative life events may play an important role in determining which victims are most likely to develop chronic PTSD (Brewin, Andrews, & Valentine, 2000). Evaluating how the individual perceives his/her social support network before the trauma, social support since the trauma, psychiatric history, family history of psychopathology, and social and vocational adjustment assist in understanding factors that determine PTSD course and severity (Litz, Penk, Gerardi, & Keane, 1992).

A multi-modal approach should be utilized when gathering information during a diagnostic interview for PTSD. Combining structured interviews (described below) with self-report measures provides convergent validity to the diagnosis. Other assessment techniques such as self-monitoring (of thoughts, anxiety antecedents, and maladaptive behaviors) may also clarify aspects of the diagnostic picture. For example, self-monitoring of thoughts may reveal cognitive distortions developed since the trauma event such as "the world is a dangerous place." The following sections include an illustration of case examples, a review of structured clinical interviews, and suggestions for conducting an appropriate diagnostic interview for PTSD.

CASE ILLUSTRATIONS

Case 1

Dana, a 27-year-old married female, presented with symptoms of fear and avoidance of public places following a robbery at a convenience store where she was employed two months ago. Her husband accompanied her during the interview. Dana reported that she was working alone during the night shift when she was held up at gunpoint by an assailant. The assailant threatened to shoot her if she did not cooperate and turn over the store's cash. Since the robbery, Dana has been unable to return to work, avoids convenience stores as well as all other stores and large crowds, and refuses to leave her home alone. During the interview she commented that she believed she will not live as long as she once expected. She fears that the assailant will find her and kill her. She reported being bothered by vivid images of the robbery on a daily basis and has been going to sleep with the bedside light on. She wakes frequently during the night because of nightmares about the assailant and has difficulty falling back to sleep. She now keeps her window shades and doors shut and locked at all times. She reports that she remains at home most of the day and spends her time watching television. She has been uninterested in completing her usual chores and has been indifferent about visiting her nieces, an activity she used to look forward to doing. When she does venture outside, she feels "on guard" all the time. During the interview, Dana became tearful when discussing the robbery and had difficulty talking about the details. She stated, "I really do not want to talk about it because I get so upset." Dana denied experiencing past traumas. In addition, she denied any drug or alcohol use. She acknowledged smoking a pack of cigarettes daily, a level representing an increase of half a pack a day since the robbery. In terms of social support, she lives with her husband and two children. She noted that her husband has tried to be helpful by accompanying her whenever she leaves the home. Her husband stated that he encouraged Dana to quit her job because he believes it is unsafe. In addition, he acknowledged that he feels more comfortable knowing that someone accompanies Dana whenever she goes out of the house. Financial stressors have increased because Dana has been unable to work, and she fears that they may be evicted from their home soon.

Case 2

Cheryl is a 45-year-old married female who presented with complaints of anxiety, irritability, and difficulty feeling a full range of emotions since she was an adolescent. These symptoms, she stated, are related to sexual abuse she experienced by her father when she was between the ages of 6 and 13. Cheryl reported that her father touched her breasts and vagina on a weekly basis. She denied vaginal or anal penetration. During the assessment of Cheryl's other traumatic experiences, she noted that her father beat her with an extension cord several times during her childhood while he was drunk. In addition, she reported being sexually assaulted when she was 16 years old by a peer. This assault occurred while she was at the peer's house after school, and involved forced vaginal sex. During the assault, the peer stated that he would kill her if she told anyone. Cheryl reported intrusive thoughts about these sexual abuse events, with thoughts about the sexual abuse from her father occurring more frequently. She denied nightmares but stated that she has frequent dreams about someone trying to kill her. She reported daily physical symptoms such as sweaty palms, queasiness, and shaking when reminded of any of these events. She attempted to avoid thoughts, activities, and people that remind her of the assaults. Other PTSD symptoms included feeling distant from others, inability to have "deep loving feelings," difficulty concentrating, and increased irritability. She commented that she experienced panic attacks in the past, with the last one occurring about one year ago. In addition to these anxiety symptoms, Cheryl reported significant depressed mood, lack of interest in activities that she used to enjoy, weight loss, fatigue, feelings of worthlessness, restlessness, and suicidal thoughts. Her anxiety and depressed mood have occurred on and off since adolescence, but recently increased a few months ago upon discovering that her husband was having an affair. She described her relationship with her husband as "rocky," and has caught him having several affairs in the past. She commented that she is planning on remaining with him but that she does not trust him. She reported recurrent use of amphetamines with the last episode being 3 months ago. Cheryl did not have contact with her father at the time of the evaluation. Six months ago, she confided to her sister about the sexual abuse, but her sister called her "crazy" and has not spoken to her since.

These two case examples illustrate the diverse experiences and symptoms of individuals with PTSD. Dana and Cheryl share similar features of the disorder, but differ with regard to stressor event, previous trauma history, psychiatric comorbidity, coping styles, current life stressors, and support network. Even though both women meet criteria for PTSD, these other related factors will play an important role in conceptualizing etiologic and maintaining factors and in selecting treatment.

STANDARDIZED INTERVIEW FORMATS

Unstructured interviews are most commonly used in clinical practice while structured interviews are more often used in research clinics. Awareness of the usefulness of structured interviews in clinical practice is growing, however. Structured interviews offer a template of symptom evaluation and result in more reliable diagnoses. Unstructured interviews often lead to misdiagnosis and uninformed case conceptualizations because of missed information. The following is a brief review of the most frequently used standardized interviews for PTSD. This is not a comprehensive list of all the valid and useful tools available to assess PTSD.

Diagnostic Interview Schedule

The Diagnostic Interview Schedule (DIS; Robins, Cottler, Bucholz, & Compton, 1995) is a highly structured interview that assesses a range of diagnoses. The PTSD module begins with several global preface questions to assess Criterion A events. These are closed-ended questions that range across a variety of traumatic events. The DIS asks about all 17 PTSD symptoms for the trauma that caused the most problems according to the client. The DIS is a convenient interview tool, designed to be administered by trained nonclinicians, therefore, requiring less training than some other structured interviews. It provides clear rules for PTSD assessment; however, some of the trauma assessment questions are not behaviorally specific, resulting in reduced sensitivity. Furthermore, if an individual provides a negative response to the trauma screening question, the PTSD section is not continued. Consequently, it may miss certain trauma events.

The DIS has been used in several major epidemiological studies. Results from the National Vietnam Veterans Readjustment Study (NVVRS; Kulka et al., 1990) indicated that the DIS had high specificity (97.9%) with nonclinicians for a PTSD diagnosis when compared with the Structured Clinical Interview for the *DSM-IV* (SCID) in a veteran population. The DIS, however, exhibited a low rate of sensitivity (21.5%) for the detection of true PTSD cases. Kulka et al. found sensitivity to be higher (82%) when administered by a clinician. Others have found the DIS to exhibit acceptable sensitivity and specificity (Breslau & Davis, 1987).

Structured Clinical Interview for the DSM-IV

The Structured Clinical Interview for the *DSM-IV* (SCID-IV; First, Spitzer, Gibbon, & Williams, 1994) is one of the most frequently used interviews to assess

PTSD. In addition, the SCID covers the full range of *DSM-IV* disorders in specific modules. It is designed to yield diagnoses compatible with *DSM-IV* criteria and actually builds the criteria directly into the interview. The PTSD module of the SCID-IV begins with a preface question that includes a list of different trauma events. Individuals are asked to list as many trauma events that apply. Following Criterion A assessment, the individual is asked to identify the event that has affected him/her the most. Symptom questions are then referred to this "worst" experience. The SCID-IV symptom assessment is similar to the DIS in that each PTSD symptom is queried with closed-ended questions.

Like the DIS, the SCID-IV does not include behaviorally specific questions to determine occurrence of specific types of trauma events and is therefore limited in its sensitivity for certain experiences, such as sexual assault. The SCID-IV does allow for more than three trauma events to be listed in the Criterion A assessment section. However, PTSD symptoms only are asked about in relation to the perceived most distressing event. This restricts the clinician from evaluating complexities of multiple trauma histories in relation to anxiety psychopathology. It also does not adequately measure severity or symptom level.

Ventura, Liberman, Green, Shaner, and Mintz (1998) found excellent interrater reliability on assessments of symptoms across a variety of disorders (overall kappa = 0.85) following extensive training of the interviewers. Specifically, Skre, Onstad, Torgersen, and Kringlen (1991) found good interrater reliability for the PTSD diagnosis for the SCID-III-R version (kappa = 0.77). Hovens et al. (1992) also found the PTSD section of the SCID-III-R version to have good concurrent validity when comparing the SCID with clinical ratings based on the *DSM-III*. The SCID exhibited strong concurrent validity with both the Clinician Administered PTSD Scale (CAPS) and the PTSD Symptom Scale (PSS)—Interview (PSS-I) (Foa & Tolin, 2000).

Anxiety Disorders Interview Schedule for DSM-IV

The Anxiety Disorders Interview Schedule for *DSM-IV* (ADIS-IV; Brown, Dinardo, & Barlow, 1994) is a structured interview that is intended to yield diagnoses compatible with the *DSM-IV*. It is a comprehensive interview specifically assessing *DSM-IV* anxiety and mood disorders. However, revised editions have provided detailed sections on somatoform, psychotic, and substance use disorders. The PTSD section is similar to the other structured interviews discussed thus far. The ADIS-IV begins with a brief assessment of trauma history and then follows with closed-ended questions about each of the 17 PTSD symptoms. Afterward, a series of questions designed to evaluate severity of symptoms is asked. In addition, interviewers assign a 0–8 (0 = none, 8 = very severely disturbing/disabling) global clinical severity rating that indicates their judgment of the degree of distress and impairment associated with the diagnosis.

Several studies have evaluated the psychometric properties of the ADIS-IV and older versions of the ADIS. Blanchard, Kolb, Gerardi, Ryan, & Pallmayer (1986) reported interrater agreement of 93% for PTSD diagnosis on an earlier version. Di Nardo, Moras, Barlow, Rapee, and Brown (1993) also found excellent diagnostic interrater reliability of an earlier version of the ADIS in a sample of 267 anxiety clinic outpatients. Good to excellent interrater reliability (kappas = 0.67–0.86) has also been shown for the ADIS-IV in a study by Brown, Di Nardo, Lehman, and Campbell (2001) with 362 outpatients.

The Clinician Administered PTSD Scale

The CAPS (Blake et al., 1995) is a structured interview specifically designed to assess both lifetime and current PTSD. Its intended users are both clinicians and nonclinicians. The measure presumes a trauma event; therefore, the interview is completed without thorough assessment of Criterion A. It uses both a dimensional and categorical approach to measuring each symptom and assesses both present and lifetime symptomatology. The CAPS explores frequency and intensity of each symptom with a separate 5-point Likert rating scale for each. In addition to the 17 *DSM-IV* symptom items, the CAPS asks an additional eight items that are thought to be associated with PTSD, such as guilt, hopelessness, and feelings of depression. The extra information gathered for each PTSD symptom and the additional items offers a greater depth of clinical data that may be useful for treatment planning. Neal, Busuttil, Herapath, and Stirke (1994) provide a briefer computerized version of the CAPS.

The majority of research investigating the CAPS focuses on combat populations with findings of good interrater reliability, internal consistency, and concurrent validity (Blake et al., 1990). However, some data are available on the reliability and validity of the interview with other clinical populations. The CAPS yielded high to very high reliability coefficients in a civilian population (Blanchard et al., 1995). In addition, in a sample of both combat veterans and civilians, Hovens et al. (1994) found high reliability and moderate validity using a Dutch-language version of the CAPS. In a sample of people who have experienced a traumatic event (noncombat related), the CAPS exhibited good internal consistency and excellent interview-rater reliability (Foa & Tolin, 2000). Foa and Tolin also found the CAPS to have high concurrent validity with the PSS-I and good convergent validity with the SCID.

Self-report instruments may enhance diagnostic efforts with PTSD. These measures also aid in acquiring richer information to better guide diagnosis, treatment planning, and assessment of treatment outcome. Several brief instruments possessing adequate reliability and validity include the PSS (Foa, Riggs, Dancu, & Rothbaum, 1993), the Modified PTSD Symptom Scale (MPSS-SR; Resick, Falsetti, Resnick, & Kilpatrick, 1991; Falsetti, Resick, Resnick, & Kilpatrick, 1992), the Impact of Events Scale (IES; Horowitz, Wilner, & Alvarez, 1979), and the Trauma Symptom Inventory (TSI; Briere, 1995). In addition, there are self-report measures of PTSD for specific traumas such as the Rape Aftermath Symptom Test (RAST; Kilpatrick, 1988) for sexual assault, and the Accident Fear Questionnaire (AFQ; Kuch, Cox, & Direnfeld, 1995) for motor vehicle accidents. For more information on specific instruments, Meichenbaum (1994) offers a comprehensive guide of assessment interviews and self-report measures for assessing and treating PTSD.

Information Critical to Making the Diagnosis

Critical information required for the PTSD diagnosis includes establishing the Criterion A event. Traumatic events, however, are not commonly assessed when patients or clients do not specifically report them. Instead, clinicians may ask overly general or gate-type questions such as "Have you ever been raped?" and do not follow-up with more specific questions if the individual denies this initial question (e.g., the individual may not label it "rape" if her husband did it). This is problematic because trauma history can be grossly underestimated using such nonspecific assessment techniques (Koss, 1993; Weaver, 1998). Behaviorally specific detailed questioning of trauma history allows for more accurate detection of Criterion A events.

Furthermore, with respect to the *DSM-IV* definition of Criterion A, a traumatic event does not include all stressful life events. A stressful situation such as loss of a job or being evicted from a home is not considered a traumatic event. Many clients may describe these types of events as "traumatic." Even though they are distressing, they are not deemed to be life-threatening events, and therefore would not meet Criterion A standards.

Experiencing a traumatic event is a necessary criterion of PTSD, however it is not sufficient. People experience a wide range of normal reactions immediately following exposure to a traumatic event including increased anxiety and depressive symptoms. This does not mean that they automatically qualify as having PTSD. Clinicians need to complete a thorough assessment of the three symptom clusters (reexperiencing, avoidance and numbing, and hyperarousal) before making a diagnosis. All three symptom clusters should be endorsed and should significantly impact the person's daily functioning. For example, a woman who was sexually assaulted in a parking lot may report having occasional thoughts about the assault, feeling "on guard" in several specific situations, and avoiding parking lots at night. These symptoms, however, are not distressing for her and do not affect her ability to perform at her job or cause any difficulties in her personal relationships. She, therefore, would not meet criteria for PTSD because she does not have enough symptoms in each cluster and these symptoms are not impairing. However, in Case Illustration 1, Dana reported several reexperiencing, avoidance, and hyperarousal symptoms, all of which have affected her ability to return to work, her daily pattern of behaviors, and relationships with family members.

In addition to symptom pattern, duration of symptoms is an important aspect in deciding whether a person meets criteria for PTSD. Not only does a person need to report impairment in functioning due to experiencing all three symptom clusters, but also report these symptoms to exist for a duration of 1 month. Subsequently, PTSD cannot be diagnosed until 1 month post event. As mentioned above, many of these symptoms are normal reactions to intense situations and, therefore, may be exhibited for several weeks following a traumatic event. Duration is important in making a diagnosis to establish the difference between a normal reaction and a pathological one.

Obtaining information regarding all of clients' symptoms may be useful in making differential diagnoses when making a diagnosis of PTSD. Clinicians need to be aware of differential diagnoses such as other anxiety disorders as well as psychotic disorders like schizophrenia. For example, reexperiencing and fear symptoms may be mistaken for paranoia or hallucinations or vice versa. Furthermore, clinicians may mislabel trauma-cued panic attacks as panic disorder without a thorough evaluation of the panic attacks.

Moreover, other disorders may accompany PTSD, and their assessment is critical in a complete evaluation of PTSD since diagnostic comorbidity for PTSD is the rule rather than the exception (Kessler et al., 1995; Resnick et al., 1993). Among the most common comorbid diagnoses are major depression, panic disorder, and substance use disorders. It is important to clarify the relationship among these disorders over time. For example, extremely high levels of negative affect produced by trauma exposure may motivate individuals to engage in excessive drinking or drug use to rapidly reduce negative emotions (Kilpatrick, Saunders, Veronen, Best, & Von, 1987). This would suggest that use of a substance is a maladaptive coping response to PTSD symptoms and perhaps could be addressed during treatment. However, discovering that an individual used excessive alcohol and drugs before the trauma event occurred may indicate different treatment options. Therefore, establishing primary diagnoses among comorbid diagnoses during initial diagnostic interviews may aid in case conceptualization and effective treatment planning.

Dos and Don'ts

Do establish a supportive and nonjudgmental environment. The clinical interview is the first contact clients usually have with their therapists. Good rapport is critical. Interviewing individuals with PTSD symptoms presents special challenges. These individuals may be less willing to discuss problems they are currently experiencing due to fear and embarrassment. Building trust allows clients to feel comfortable disclosing traumatic events and post trauma experiences. One hallmark feature of PTSD is avoidance of traumatic memories. By nature of the assessment, the individual is attending to these memories, therefore assessment procedures may temporarily increase anxiety. The pace of the interview often needs to be slowed to allow for more empathetic communication and reassurance as anxiety levels rise. Do acknowledge this increased anxiety, and provide empathy as well as briefly educate clients on ways of coping during interviews.

Do include family members to the extent appropriate. Family members, especially those living with clients, can offer rich data about clients' behaviors and change in functioning. Including family members in the assessment process not only permits clinicians to gather information from family members about a client but also allows direct assessment of a client's support network. Lack of social support is related to increased risk of PTSD (Brewin et al., 2000), therefore proper assessment of a client's support network is helpful. Clinicians may find observing family members' reactions to invitations to join the assessment procedures telling as to the level of support they are offering. In addition, including family members in the evaluation process demonstrates the importance of their involvement in a client's treatment. Do prepare both clients and family members for exacerbation of anxiety and related symptomatology during treatment procedures. With family members present, clinicians can highlight the significance of support provided by family during times of increased arousal. Clinicians can also address family members' behaviors that may enable avoidance or intensify symptoms. For example, Dana's husband's behaviors (from Case Illustration 1), although intended to be supportive, may have assisted the maintenance of Dana's avoidance. Including him in the education about PTSD and treatment planning would maximize Dana's progress by utilizing her support network appropriately.

Do provide an opening statement about the interview process as well as statements defining trauma events. To counter potential barriers to disclosing traumatic events and current problems, be sure to outline information to be covered during the interview at the start. This will assist in establishing a trusting and supportive environment. In addition, providing opening statements for specific trauma questions allows clinicians to orient clients to the nature of the questions to follow, as well as displays sensitivity and knowledge of the frequencies of these events in the population on the part of the interviewer (Resnick, Falsetti, Kilpatrick, & Freedy, 1996). For example, when gathering information about a client's sexual assault history, preface the assessment questions with the following statement, taken from Resnick et al. (1991):

> A type of stressful event that both men and women have experienced is unwanted sexual advances. People do not always report such experiences to the police or discuss them with family or friends. The person making the advances isn't always a stranger, but can be a friend, boyfriend, or even a family member. Such experiences can occur anytime in a person's life—even as a child. These events are sometimes difficult to talk about, but because they can be distressing, they may have an affect on how a person feels. I am going to ask you if you have ever experienced any of these events in your lifetime. (p. 564)

Providing an opening statement to questions about different trauma events informs the client that traumatic experiences are not unusual occurrences. Furthermore, it educates the client that past experiences may relate to current problems that are common in trauma victims. Finally, it clarifies that the assessor needs to know about all traumatic events perpetrated by anyone, not just recent ones perpetrated by strangers.

Do not display discomfort or avoid discussing difficult trauma events. Discussing certain trauma events such as child sexual abuse may be difficult, not only for clients but also for interviewers. Interviewers may either feel uncomfortable using sexual terms or fear upsetting clients. As an interviewer, be aware of your own feelings about these topics and how they may be reflected to your client (Resnick & Newton, 1992). If a clinician avoids discussing his/her client's specific sexual abuse characteristics, his/her behavior may confirm that these events are taboo and not acceptable to discuss. If a clinician is uneasy about discussing these topics, he/she should become familiar with terms and phrases in the structured interviews and measures as well as practice or role-play with colleagues discussing sensitive topics as preparation.

Do ask behaviorally specific questions when assessing trauma events. People may hold stereotypes about the meanings of certain terms (e.g., rape) and therefore may not report a trauma as occurring when it did occur (Resnick et al., 1996). Don't use gate questions such as "Have you ever been sexually abused?" as people may be less likely to provide a positive response even if they were abused. Try to be as specific as possible, such as "Has anyone, including friends or family, ever touched you against your will?" This provides a behaviorally specific definition of the type of situations that you are assessing. In addition, make sure to assess qualitative aspects of trauma, such as perceived life threat and injury, which are associated with increased risk of PTSD (Kilpatrick, Saunders, Amick-McMullan, Best, & Von, 1989).

   Do ask both closed-ended questions and open-ended questions. The interview should not feel like an interrogation. At the same time, much detailed information needs to be assessed. A balance between closed-ended and open-ended questions is necessary for obtaining essential information and allowing clients to explain their feelings in their own words. Closed-ended questions such as "Do you have thoughts about the sexual assault that you cannot get out of your head?" will help to identify specific symptoms of PTSD. Open-ended questions such as "Tell me how the assault has affected your views of yourself or the world" may better assess descriptive data of the affects of the trauma (e.g., self-blame). In addition, using open-ended questions allows clients to tell their story about the trauma and its impact. Overall, closed-ended questions are useful in determining whether or not Criterion A events have occurred, whereas a combination of closed-ended and open-ended questions help delineate symptom presentation.

   Do assess for exposure to other traumas. A variety of potentially relevant traumatic events may occur over a person's lifetime that may contribute in some way to the etiology or maintenance of PTSD (Resnick et al., 1996). It is important to assess multiple stressor events, rather than just the presenting traumatic event. Individuals who experienced multiple traumatic events during their lifetime may exhibit a more complicated symptom presentation, which may require different specialized treatment plans compared to individuals who experienced a single trauma event. If the interviewer for Case Illustration 2 did not ask Cheryl about her trauma history, she may not have obtained information about her exposure to physical abuse and other sexual assault. Knowing about her complete trauma history has significant implications for treatment planning.

   Do fully assess symptom patterns, phobic stimuli, and impairment in functioning. Some structured interviews merely assess whether the 17 symptoms of PTSD are present. A thorough diagnostic interview further assesses characteristics of each symptom. For example, evaluating frequency and distress level of each symptom may provide richer information about the symptom presentation for that individual. This may help guide target symptoms for treatment and provide a reference baseline when reassessing symptoms and diagnosis. Other trauma related variables, such as stimuli that elicit a conditioned fear response, should also be carefully assessed to help determine the antecedents to anxiety. Devising a hierarchy list, as mentioned above, can be useful both to make the client more aware of cues in their environment associated with the traumatic event, as well as to guide treatment planning. In addition, impairment in functioning as a result of PTSD symptoms is important not only to determine whether an individual meets diagnostic criteria for PTSD, but also to inform the interviewer of the extent of distress that the individual is experiencing as a result of the trauma.

Summary

The hallmark of a thorough assessment of PTSD is a multimodal approach. Assessment using a single approach will most likely not provide enough depth or descriptive data. In a clinical setting, a comprehensive clinical interview along with the use of self-report measures will provide adequate information for an appropriate diagnosis as well as the foundation for treatment planning. Further assessment may be warranted throughout treatment to assess treatment progress and target symptoms.

Accurate diagnosis of PTSD is important to appropriate treatment planning. However, there is substantial heterogeneity among PTSD suffers, reflected in different patterns of reexperiencing symptoms, physiological symptoms, behavioral avoidance, stimuli that elicit an anxiety response, and degree of impairment. A good clinical interview reviews each of these areas by means of functional analysis both to generate a comprehensive picture of each individual's syndrome and to identify target areas for treatment.

References

Acierno, R., Resnick, H. S., Kilpatrick, D. G., Saunders, B. E., & Best, C. L. (1999). Risk factors for rape, physical assault, and posttraumatic stress disorder in women: Examination of differential multivariate relationships. *Journal of Anxiety Disorders, 13*, 541–563.

American Psychiatric Association. (1994). *Diagnostic and statistical manual of mental disorders.* (4th ed.). Washington DC: Author.

Blake, D. D., Weathers, F. W., Nagy, L. M., Kaloupek, D. G., Gusman, F. D., Charney, D. S., & Keane, T. M. (1995). The development of a clinician-administered PTSD scale. *Journal of Traumatic Stress, 8*, 75–90.

Blake, D. D., Weathers, F. W., Nagy, L. M., Kaloupek, D. G., Klauminzer, G., Charney, D. S., & Keane, T. M. (1990). A clinician rating scale for assessing current and lifetime PTSD: The CAPS-1. *Behavior Therapist, 13*, 187–188.

Blanchard, E. B., Hickling, E. J., Taylor, A. E., Forneris, C. A., Loos, W., & Jaccard, J. (1995). Effects of varying scoring rules of the Clinician-Administered PTSD Scale (CAPS) for the diagnosis of posttraumatic stress disorder in motor vehicle accident victims. *Behaviour Research and Therapy, 33*, 471–475.

Blanchard, E. B., Kolb, L. C., Gerardi, R. T., Ryan, P., & Pallmayer, T. P. (1986). Cardiac response to relevant stimuli as an adjunctive tool for diagnosing post-traumatic stress disorder in combat veterans. *Behavior Therapy, 17*, 592–606.

Breslau, N., & Davis, G. (1987). Posttraumatic stress disorder: The etiologic specificity of wartime stressors. *American Journal of Psychiatry, 144*, 578–583.

Breslau, N., Davis, G., Andreski, P., & Peterson, E. (1991). Traumatic events and posttraumatic stress disorder in an urban population of young adults. *Archives of General Psychiatry, 48*, 216–222.

Brewin, C. R., Andrews, B., & Valentine, J. D. (2000). Meta-analysis of risk factors for posttraumatic stress disorder in trauma-exposed adults. *Journal of Consulting and Clinical Psychology, 68*, 748–766.

Briere, J. (1995). *Trauma symptom inventory professional manual.* Odessa, FL: Psychological Assessment Resources.

Brown, T. A., DiNardo, P. A., & Barlow, D. H. (1994). *Anxiety Disorders Interview Schedule for DSM-IV (ADIS-IV)*. Albany, NY: Graywind.

Brown, T. A., Di Nardo, P. A., Lehman, C. L., & Campbell, L. A. (2001). Reliability of *DSM-IV* anxiety and mood disorders: Implications for the classification of emotional disorders. *Journal of Abnormal Psychology, 110*, 49–58.

Di Nardo, P. A., Moras, K., Barlow, D. H., Rapee, R. M., & Brown, T. A. (1993). Reliability of *DSM-III-R* anxiety disorder categories using the Anxiety Disorders Interview Schedule-Revised (ADIS-R). *Archives of General Psychiatry, 50*, 251–256.

Falsetti, S. A., Resnick, H. S., Dansky, B. S., Lydiard, R. B., & Kilpatrick, D. G. (1995). The relationship of stress to panic disorder: Cause or effect. In Mazure (Ed.), *Does stress cause psychiatric illness? Progress in psychiatry series* (pp. 111–148). Washington, DC: American Psychiatric Press.

Falsetti, S. A., Resick, P. A., Resnick, H. S., & Kilpatrick, D. G. (1992). *Posttraumatic stress disorder: The assessment of frequency and severity of symptoms in clinical and nonclinical samples*. Paper presented at the 26th Annual Meeting of the Association for the Advancement of Behavior Therapy, Boston.

First, M. B., Spitzer, R. L., Gibbon, M., & Williams, J. B. (1994). *Structured Clinical Interview for Axis I DSM-IV Disorders—Client Edition*. New York: Biometrics Research Department.

Foa, E. B., Riggs, D. S., Dancu, C. V., & Rothbaum, B. O. (1993). Reliability and validity of a brief instrument for assessing posttraumatic stress disorder. *Journal of Traumatic Stress, 6*, 459–473.

Foa, E. B., & Tolin, D. F. (2000). Comparison of the PTSD symptom scale—interview version and the clinician-administered PTSD scale. *Journal of Traumatic Stress, 13*, 181–191.

Horowitz, M., Wilner, N., & Alvarez, W. (1979). Impact of Event scale: Measure of subjective stress. *Psychosomatic Medicine, 41*, 209–218.

Hovens, J. E., Falger, P. R. J., Op Den Velde, W., Schouten, E. G. W., De Groen, J. H. M., & Van Duijn, H. (1992). Occurrence of current posttraumatic stress disorder among Dutch World War II resistance veterans according to the SCID. *Journal of Anxiety Disorders, 6*, 147–157.

Hovens, J. E., van der Ploeg, H. M., Klaarenbeek, M. T. A., Bramsen, I., Schreuder, J. N., & Rivero, V. V. (1994). The assessment of posttraumatic stress disorder with the Clinician Administered PTSD Scale: Dutch results. *Journal of Clinical Psychology, 50*, 325–340.

Keane, T. M., & Kaloupek, D. G. (1997). Comorbidity psychiatric disorders in PTSD: Implications for research. In R. Yehuda & A. McFarlane (Eds.), *Psychobiology of posttraumatic stress disorder*. New York: Annals of the New York Academy of Science.

Kessler, R. C., Sonnega, A., Bromet, E., Hughes, M., & Nelson, C. B. (1995). Posttraumatic stress disorder in the National Comorbidity Study. *Archives of General Psychiatry, 52*, 1048–1060.

Kilpatrick, D. G. (1988). Rape Aftermath Symptoms Test. In M. Hersen & A. S. Bellack (Eds.), *Dictionary of behavioral assessment techniques*. Oxford: Pergamon Press.

Kilpatrick, D. G., Saunders, B. E., Amick-McMullan, A., Best, C. L., & Von, J. M. (1989). Victim and crime factors associated with the development of crime-related post-traumatic stress disorder. *Behavior Therapy, 20*, 199–214.

Kilpatrick, D. G., Saunders, B. E., Veronen, L. J., Best, C. L., & Von, J. M. (1987). Criminal victimization: Lifetime prevalence, reporting to police, and psychological impact. *Crime & Delinquency, 33*, 479–489.

Koss, M. P. (1993). Detecting the scope of rape: A review of prevalence research methods. *Journal of Interpersonal Violence, 8*, 198–222.

Kuch, K., Cox, B. J., & Direnfeld, D. M. (1995). A brief self-rating scale for PTSD after road vehicle accident. *Journal of Anxiety Disorders, 9*, 503–514.

Kulka, R. A., Schlenger, W. E., Fairbank, J. A., Hough, R. L., Jordan, B. K., Marmar, C. R., & Weiss, D. S. (1990). *Trauma and the Vietnam War generation*. New York: Brunner/Mazel.

Litz, B. T., Penk, W. E., Gerardi, R. J., & Keane, T. M. (1992). The assessment of post-traumatic stress disorder. In P. Saigh (Ed.), *Post-Traumatic Stress Disorder: A behavioral approach to assessment and treatment*. New York: Pergamon Press.

Meichenbaum, D. (1994). *A clinical handbook/practical therapist manual for assessing and treating adults with post-traumatic stress disorder (PTSD)*. Ontario: Institute Press.

Neal, L. A., Busuttil, W., Herapath, R., & Stirke, P. W. (1994). Development and validation of the computerized Clinician Administered Posttraumatic Stress Disorder Scale-1—Revised. *Psychological Medicine, 24*, 701–706.

Resnick, H. S., Falsetti, S. A., Kilpatrick, D. G., & Freedy, J. R. (1996). Assessment of rape and other civilian trauma-related PTSD: Emphasis on assessment of potentially traumatic events. In T. W. Miller (Ed.), *Theory of assessment of stressful life events* (pp. 235–271). New York: International Universities Press.

Resnick, H. S., Kilpatrick, D. G., Dansky, B. S., Saunders, B. E., & Best, C. L. (1993). Prevalence of civilian trauma and posttraumatic stress disorder in a representative national sample of women. *Journal of Consulting and Clinical Psychology, 61*, 984–991.

Resnick, H. S., Kilpatrick, D. G., & Lipovsky, J. A. (1991). Assessment of rape-related posttraumatic stress disorder: Stressor and symptom dimensions. *Journal of Consulting and Clinical Psychology, 3*, 561–572.

Resnick, H. S., & Newton, T. (1992). Assessment and treatment of post-traumatic stress disorder in adult survivors of sexual assault. In D. W. Foy (Ed.), *Treating PTSD: cognitive–behavioral strategies. Treatment manuals for practitioners.* (pp. 99–126). New York: Guilford Press.

Resick, P. A., Falsetti, S. A., Resnick, H. S., & Kilpatrick, D. G. (1991). *The Modified PTSD Symptom Scale—Self Report.* St. Louis, MO: University of Missouri & Charleston, SC, Crime Victims Treatment and Research Center, Medical University of South Carolina.

Robins, L. N., Cottler, L., Bucholz, K., & Compton, W. (1995). *Diagnostic Interview Schedule for DSM-IV.* St. Louis: Washington Press.

Skre, I., Onstad, S., Torgensen, S., & Kringlen, E. (1991). High interrater reliability for the Structured Clinical Interview for *DSM-III-R* Axis I (SCID-I). *Acta Psychiatry Scandanavia, 84*, 167–173.

Ventura, J., Liberman, R. P., Green, M. F., Shaner, A., & Mintz, J. (1998). Training and quality assurance with the Structured Clinical Interview for DSM-IV (SCID-I/P). *Psychiatry Research, 79*, 163–173.

Weaver, T. L. (1998). Method variance and sensitivity of screening for traumatic stressors. *Journal of Traumatic Stress, 11*, 181–185.

III

Special Populations

16

Marital Dyads

GARY BIRCHLER, CRISTINA MAGANA, AND
WILLIAM FALS-STEWART

DESCRIPTION OF THE SPECIAL POPULATION

Since the last edition of this book was published, the institution of marriage has remained in a state of significant distress and yet, simultaneously, there has been an impressive pro-marriage effort underway in the United States and in many other countries of the world.

Let us first consider a few prevalent indicators of distress: (1) Although the oft-repeated divorce rate of 50% has improved somewhat over the past several years, the dissolution rate for first-time marriages is still alarming at between 40% and 45% (Goldstein, 1999). (2) Nevertheless, divorced people try again: the rate of first remarriage is approximately 75%, yet the rate of divorce for second marriages is about 60% (Cherlin, 1992). (3) Currently, it has been estimated that nuclear families containing the biological mom, dad, and the kids constitute only about 25% of American households; another 25% of the households contain step-families; and the remaining households do not contain two parents; rather, they are made up of single-parent families, singles in groups, and same-sex adults. (4) Broken marriages result in an increased risk that their children will become divorcees (Amato & DeBoer, 2001) and couples who are parents in stepfamilies have a higher risk for divorce than do adults-only second marriages (McLanahan & Sandefur, 1994). Unfortunately, it appears that these trends serve to perpetuate the divorce cycle indefinitely.

In the context of this geometric progression, or perhaps because of it, during the past decade there has been a pronounced movement to save, improve, and rehabilitate marriage. For example, the Sixth Annual Smart Marriages Conference was held in Washington, DC in July 2002, bringing together over 1,500 marriage educators, therapists, sociological and clinical researchers, who are dedicated to

GARY BIRCHLER AND CRISTINA MAGANA • Department of Veterans Affairs, San Diego Healthcare System, San Diego, California 92108. WILLIAM FALS-STEWART • Research Institute on Addictions, State University of New York at Buffalo, Buffalo, New York.

enhancing the prevalence, the stability, and the quality of marital relationships. As a function of the work of many of these people, the case for marriage becomes more and more compelling. Let us consider a few of the salient findings: (1) In general, women and especially men and children enjoy relatively better mental and physical health benefits being in versus out of the state of marriage (Wallerstein, Lewis, & Blakeslee, 2000). (2) Men and especially women and children benefit socioeconomically from being in versus out of marriage (Gottman & Notarius, 2000; Peterson, 1996). (3) Research indicates that, with the exception of marriages that include high conflict or high abuse, the divorce process itself has negative short- and long-term health consequences for both adults and children, compared to families that stay together (Amato & Booth, 1997). Therefore, it is increasingly clear that there are many positive benefits to staying married and attempting to improve the function and quality of adult intimate relationships. These findings set the stage for the development of primary, secondary, and tertiary interventions designed to promote marital health.

The following chapter will focus on diagnostic interviewing procedures for a tertiary evaluation format designed for clinically distressed couples. Some clarifications and disclaimers are in order at the outset. First, the notion of *diagnostic interviewing* for marital dyads needs some clarification. Unlike the case for individual mental health disorders, the goal is not to reach some definitive research- or clinically based diagnosis, a la the *Diagnostic and Statistical Manual of Mental Disorders* (*DSM IV*; American Psychiatric Association, 1994). Despite significant and ongoing efforts to develop and to define *relational diagnoses* (Kaslow, 1996), to date, good diagnostic interviewing for marital dyads does not result in *the* diagnosis. Rather, the clinician's goal is to obtain a clear definition of personal problems, the internal relationship conflicts, and external stressors faced by a couple, and an analysis of the couple's adaptive processes for coping with these problems.

Second, while the title of the chapter suggests an emphasis on "marital" dyads, the diagnostic procedures are applicable generally to any adult dyad, opposite- or same-sexed, that is attempting to develop and maintain an intimate relationship. Indeed, without prejudice, use of the terms husband, wife, she, he, men, women, spouse, and partner may be used interchangeably.

Third, it should be noted that, in any intimate dyad, so-called relational problems can present in one or more of the following categories (Reiss, 1996): (1) Well-delineated disorders of relationships: In these cases, relationship dysfunction, per se, causes one or both partners sufficient dissatisfaction that the level of distress reaches clinical proportions. These cases present primarily seeking couple therapy. (2) Well-delineated relationship problems that are associated with individual disorders: In clinical practice, there is a tremendous comorbidity of individual and relationship disorders. The question, for diagnostic purposes, is whether relationship therapy may be a necessary and sufficient therapy to remediate the individual's disorder (e.g., certain cases of depression). (3) Disorders that require relational data for their validity (e.g., eating disorders, conduct disorders). (4) Individual disorders whose evocation, course, and treatments are strongly influenced by relationship factors: This category includes disorders where relationship therapy may be indicated, but it is not deemed sufficient alone for the remediation of the individual's problem. The primary concern and methods of diagnosis and intervention are focused on the individual. If the case were determined to be appropriate for relationship analysis, diagnostic interviewing for the couple would be secondary. Categories 1 and 2 will be the focus of this chapter.

Finally, the theoretical orientation for this chapter will be cognitive–behavioral. After more than 30 years of research and clinical practice, Behavioral Marital Therapy (BMT), with the revised name of Behavioral Couple Therapy (BCT) and its closely affiliated renditions of Cognitive–Behavioral Couple Therapy (CBCT), constitutes the most empirically validated and clinically developed form of couple therapy in existence (Baucom, Shoham, Mueser, Daiuto, & Stickle, 1998).

INFORMATION CRITICAL TO MAKING THE DIAGNOSIS: CONCEPTUAL MODELS FOR UNDERSTANDING COUPLE RELATIONSHIPS

Recently, a number of cognitive and behaviorally oriented researchers and theoreticians have offered certain conceptual schemes and heuristic models for understanding the factors that influence and determine the functional status of a couple relationship (Bradbury, 1995; Epstein & Baucom, 1999; Halford, 2001). Taken together, these models suggest that the quality of a couple relationship, at any point in time, is a function of the interaction and adaptation of two individuals. They bring into the relationship their own developmental and personal characteristics, they are significantly influenced by the cultural contexts from which they came and in which they live, and they must cope with life events and environmental factors that demand adjustments.

Birchler, Doumas, and Fals-Stewart (1999) have offered a behavioral–systems framework for evaluating couple dysfunction called "The Seven Cs" (7Cs). During the course of diagnostic interviewing and treatment planning, clinicians may well seek to learn about a given couple's relative strengths and areas for improvement according to these major areas of function: Character features, Cultural and ethnic factors, Contract, Commitment, Caring, Communication, and Conflict resolution (Cole, 1989; Levenson, Carstensen, & Gottman, 1993; Nichols, 1988; Wynne, 1984).

Character Features

From a bio–psycho–social perspective, individuals grow and develop to the point at which each has or has not acquired the essential personal resources necessary to establish and to maintain a healthy interpersonal relationship. These character features may represent personal strengths or constitute what Karney and Bradbury (1995) suggested are *enduring vulnerabilities*. Each partner comes to the marriage with a different developmental history and personality style and, based on a combination of biological, environmental, or experiential factors, some spouses can experience significantly varying levels of character impairments. Note that the term *character* is used in its broadest sense, referring to personal characteristics of the individual that tend to be persistent or that have a major role in defining the individual. For example, a dysthymic disorder, a dependent personality disorder, or a major depressive disorder—all of these conditions would qualify, in our model, as an enduring character feature, whereas, a short-term depressive reaction to a life event would not. Indeed, one's pre-marital character can be influenced adversely by many life experiences (including medical, psychiatric, or substance abuse problems, legal difficulties, traumatic sexual or physical violence experiences). Clearly, one's pre-marital experiences and adaptations to a myriad of developmental challenges can affect marital quality. Additionally, given the prevalence of serial relationships (i.e., multiple marriages) in our contemporary society, it is all the more important to understand what past experiences and expectations each individual brings into the current relationship, and especially whether there are traumatic legacies from one's family of origin or from previous formative relationships (Hazan & Shaver, 1994). There is little doubt that if one or both partners is experiencing a major depression, an anxiety disorder, an active substance abuse problem, a significant personality disorder, or a psychosis, these features of one's *character* can significantly affect marital interaction, satisfaction, and stability (Fals-Stewart, Birchler, Schafer, & Lucent, 1994).

In sum, failure to adequately recognize and treat partners' pathological or self-defeating character features will almost surely result in marital dysfunction. Similarly, failure by the therapist to recognize partners' character strengths may lead to failure to promote such strengths in helping couples to resolve relationship conflicts. The therapist assessing a couple seeking therapy should remember that the relationship between character features and relationship distress is reciprocal; marital conflict often exacerbates or serves to maintain individual dysfunction and vice versa. The treatment of choice in a specific case, that is, individual versus conjoint therapy, is determined importantly by the causal connections and inherent interactions between character features and marital dysfunction.

Cultural and Ethnic Factors

Cultural and ethnic factors in the 7Cs, representing the broadest sense of diversity, refer to the historical and contextual influences on the individuals in the marriage, derived from family, ethnicity, race, gender, religion, class, community, and nationality. It is well known that the influence of these factors can be significant and even dominant in an individual's physical and psychological development (McGoldrick & Giordano, 1996). In our approach, assessment of cultural and ethnic factors includes three primary components: (1) understanding the cultural differences that may exist between the couple and their community, (2) assessment of the cultural differences that may exist between the partners (Falicov, 1995), and (3) the therapist's ability to understand and relate to the couple's cultural identity. All three components are important when exploring contextual influences on couples entering therapy.

When working with a couple, the therapist needs to develop a framework for assessing cultural characteristics (Matthews, 1997). Such a framework should help therapists to ask relevant questions about a couple's culture or differences between the formative cultures of each partner (Loganbill & Stoltenberg, 1983).

On the other hand, although use of a cultural framework is helpful if employed to generate hypotheses, cultural stereotypes should not be used to make assumptions about people based on their cultural identity. Rather, therapists should inquire about how couples view themselves in adhering to the predominant values and behaviors of their particular cultures (Giordano & Giordano, 1995).

Additionally, a therapist must learn about the impact of generalized cultural and family-of-origin differences that may exist between the partners. Beyond race and religion, partners also may have very divergent family traditions, verbal and nonverbal interaction styles, socioeconomic and political standards and expectations, conflicting orientations as to sexual behavior preferences, or the expression of anger and the use of violence in the family. Even gender development can be experienced by partners as a *cultural* difference that causes conflict (Jacobson & Christensen, 1996). Marital discord may be perpetuated by differences in styles of communication and conflict resolution, including how partners celebrate holidays, observe religious ceremonies, cope with losses, express attitudes about parenting, conduct themselves regarding same and opposite-sexed relationships outside the marriage, and maintain different attitudes about separation or divorce. Given the significant potential for conflict regarding all these cultural and ethnic factors, couples need to develop a constructive perspective regarding their differences and similarities (Falicov, 1995). Finally, in a clinical context, effective treatment may require special interventions or consultations that take into account the multitude of cultural factors that may affect family relationships (McGoldrick, Giordano, & Pearce, 1996). In certain complex cases, a referral may need to be made to a therapist better prepared to evaluate and treat cultural- and ethnic-related issues.

Contract

Within the context of relationships and in the view of society, a marriage contract, of course, is an explicit, legally binding agreement with known stipulations. In terms of the relationship-oriented 7Cs, *contract* has been defined as a set of *implicit* expectations that partners have concerning how they will define the relationship and interact with one another. The notion is very similar to the idea that marital *standards* exist for the conduct of the relationship and that there may be congruency or conflict regarding standards held by each partner. Interesting research in this domain has been conducted by Baucom and associates (Baucom, Epstein, Rankin, & Burnett, 1996b). Unlike most other interpersonal contracts, in intimate relationships, members' expectations most frequently are implicit *quid pro quo* arrangements (Sager, 1976).

More recently, in the face of ever-increasing second and third marriages, some partners are developing more explicit marriage contracts. These *pre-nuptial agreements* are usually designed to protect significant assets one partner has acquired prior to the marriage. However, emotional, behavioral, and non-financial security arrangements sometimes are very difficult for people in love to address before or after the wedding. Emotionally laden contract-related issues can develop into significant discrepancies between partners' expectations and their experiences (Baucom et al., 1996a; Strazdins, Galligan, & Scannell, 1997).

Importantly, the stage of a couple's marital life cycle also may affect the relationship contract, as expectations of the marriage and of one's partner can change significantly over time. Couples may negotiate effectively issues relevant to a particular stage in the life cycle, such as whether or not to have children, but they may not be prepared to address other issues, such as when to retire. Couples also may negotiate issues early in their marriage, but as situations change, so may spouses' beliefs or views about a previously functional component of the contract.

Evaluation of the partners' interpersonal contract in the context of marital therapy may take the form of asking partners to articulate their goals and expectations for the relationship regarding behavioral and emotional levels of activity. Therapists also may ask partners to explore their family-of-origin and past relationship experiences to elucidate past influences on current expectations. Once partners' expectations are brought to conscious awareness and articulated, the couple can then explore whether or not these expectations are consistent with the realities experienced in the relationship. Additionally, therapists should look for any changes that have occurred in the couple's original contractual agreement that may be causing discord. If partners' experiences fail significantly to match their expectations, then some couples may choose to renegotiate their marital contracts; others, advisedly, may choose to separate.

Commitment

Commitment is essential for development and maintenance of a quality and durable marriage. Without commitment, there is insufficient trust and faith in the security and stability of the relationship to foster the development of long-term intimacy. Commitment is largely a motivational variable, born of past and present interpersonal experiences. Spouses who develop a collaborative mindset and the desire to meet together whatever challenges they face stand a significantly better chance of avoiding marital dysfunction and dissolution than those partners who may fear abandonment and concurrently threaten relationship dissolution at the first signs of discord and failed expectations (Jacobson & Margolin, 1979). Partners who have or develop the ability and willingness to *commit* to a relationship for the long term and who have or develop the skills that are necessary to resolve the inevitable conflicts, are likely to have the best prognosis for relationship stability and satisfaction (Waite & Gallagher, 2000).

Additionally, commitment becomes a critical variable as couples enter the therapeutic setting to evaluate the quality and viability of the relationship. If the therapeutic goal is to preserve the marriage, there are important early determinations: Are the partners committed to one another in this marriage? Have trust and partner loyalty been damaged by affairs, addictive behaviors, antisocial behaviors, and so forth? If basic commitment to one another has been damaged significantly, then the prognosis for saving or improving the relationship is relatively poor. Indeed, in our experience, if one or both partners have a significant lack of commitment or maintain significant ambivalence toward being in the relationship, this insecure status tends to obstruct other relationship-oriented efforts and inhibits progress toward the development of long-term intimacy. On the positive side, when a strong commitment to the partner and to achieving quality in the relationship are present, often these factors can combine with caring to form the foundation for very effective couple therapy.

In the 7Cs conceptual model, therapists are interested in the presence or absence of three types of commitment: (1) to stability, (2) to quality, and (3) to therapy. The most basic form of relationship commitment is to *stability*. Are both partners planning to stay together over time? However, although many couples manage to stay together for decades, the level of marital quality for some can remain very poor (Lewis & Spanier, 1979). Thus, the second type of relationship commitment is to *quality*. To achieve and maintain a quality relationship, successful partners devote time and energy continually to monitoring and to improving the relationship, to adapting when change is needed, or to accepting certain features of the relationship that are unlikely to change (Christensen & Jacobson, 2000; Doherty, 2001). Finally, whether or not the couple presenting for therapy possesses commitment to relationship stability and quality, in order to gain benefit from treatment, the partners must be committed to the process of *therapy*. Accordingly, even if the relationship is unstable or headed for divorce, conjoint therapy may be beneficial if partners give an honest effort to participate in and to learn from the therapeutic experience.

Caring

Obviously, caring is important to a truly intimate relationship. Caring behaviors derive from both motivational and instrumental (i.e., acquired skills) factors. Expressions of caring encompass not only affection and sex, but also include the development of individual and mutually rewarding activities, quality time together, and a real friendship experience offering interpersonal affirmation, support, understanding, and creativity (Baumeister & Bratlavsky, 1999; Weiss & Heyman, 1997). Marital dissatisfaction often results when partners are *deficient* in the skills of expressing love and affection or, just as likely, when they fail to *maintain* sufficiently formerly expressed caring behaviors (Doherty, 2001; Jacobson & Margolin, 1979; Stuart, 1980). Marital therapy is most successful when the natural exchange of caring behaviors has remained intact or the therapeutic process can facilitate improvement in both the motivational and instrumental determinants of caring. Unfortunately, however, once too much damage has been done to the basic fabric of caring, there seem to be limits to partners' abilities to recover positive, intimate feelings for one another. For some couples, even a solid commitment or practical necessity to stay together, without sufficient caring, can perpetuate an empty and unrewarding relationship.

In a 7Cs analysis, three types or levels of caring behaviors are assessed: Daily caring behaviors, individual and mutually rewarding activities, and affectionate and sexual activities. Marital satisfaction is correlated significantly with the expression of small, positive, repetitive, daily interactional behaviors (Birchler, Weiss, & Vincent, 1975; Gottman, 1990; Wills, Weiss, & Patterson, 1974). Accordingly, daily *caring* and *love* behaviors have been included successfully in the early intervention phases of BMT for nearly two decades (Stuart, 1980; Weiss & Birchler, 1978).

Second, to achieve an optimal balance of self-care, personal independence, and dyadic interdependence, partners also benefit from developing and maintaining a number of individual and mutually rewarding activities, such as recreational social events, personal and joint hobbies, home or family projects, friendship activities, couple day-trips, and vacations. In many cases, distressed couples have to reintroduce these types of positive activities into their personal lives and into their relationships. Moreover, it is unfortunate how often individuals in distressed marriages get caught up in blaming their partners for personal dissatisfaction and, concurrently, they fail to take responsibility for caring for themselves (Halford, 2001). Frequently, distressed partners do not have or have failed to maintain personal friendships and they do not engage in self-rewarding activities.

Finally, one could argue that the most intimate type of caring behaviors is the mutual expression of affection and involvement in sexual activity. Typically, partners in a distressed or dysfunctional relationship have experienced confusion, deterioration, distrust, and perhaps significant damage in these important areas of relating. Usually, and especially in younger couples, demonstrations of affection and specific problems in sexual relating are secondary to other determinants of marital distress (e.g., lack of commitment and caring, poor communication, increased anger, and marital conflict). However, if there is any question about this, the therapist should conduct a functional analysis of the sexual complaints (Derogatis, 1975; Stone, 1987). For example, in older couples, primary sexual dysfunction may result from medical conditions or medications (Crenshaw & Goldberg, 1995). Occasionally, the therapist will encounter a couple whose relationship is suffering because of a primary psychogenic sexual dysfunction that is experienced by one or both partners (e.g., premature ejaculation, inhibited sexual desire, impotence, dyspareunia). If the problem with sex is primary, more formalized sex therapy may be indicated (Leiblum & Rosen, 2000).

Communication

Beyond the basic existence of caring and commitment, effective couple communication is needed to express these values, build the friendship, and allow for identifying and understanding important relationship issues. Although the *will* to communicate certainly is an important motivational variable, the authors believe that the *skill* to communicate significantly affects most couples in their quest for intimacy. Several reports of laboratory marital interaction studies by Levenson, Carstensen, and Gottman, comparing the communication styles and daily activities of younger versus older, satisfied and dissatisfied marriages have demonstrated clearly that mature and successful relationships are characterized by relatively more positive communication and daily interaction patterns. Communication in successful marriages includes positive affect reciprocity, greater use of humor between the partners, less expression of and reciprocal exchanges of negative affect, and less emotional arousal (i.e., physiological tension) when discussing marital conflicts (Levenson, Carstensen, & Gottman, 1994; Carstensen, Gottman, & Levenson, 1995). Moreover, daily interactions of successful marriages were marked by less potential for conflict, greater potential for mutually pleasurable activities, and better overall levels of emotional and physical health (Levenson et al., 1993).

Communication is a nebulous concept to define. In the context of a marriage, effective communication can be defined operationally as: *the message intended and sent by either spouse is exactly the same as the message understood by the other spouse* (Gottman, Notarius, Gonso, & Markman, 1976). Good fidelity in this process requires not only an effective speaker, but also just as importantly there must be an effective listener. Naturally, communication becomes more difficult when the content of the message is confusing or in any way emotionally laden with negative affect, such as blame, criticism, sadness, distress, anger, resentment, or frustration. Distressed partners are known to be selective in their attention to the negative versus the positive components of messages and then to respond with negative behaviors in return (Birchler, Clopton, & Adams, 1984; Gottman, 1979; Jacobson & Holtzworth-Munroe, 1986; Karney & Bradbury, 1995). This self-fulfilling process frequently results in a pattern of reciprocated negative exchanges, including various criticisms and personal attacks. Additionally, many couples seeking therapy also have considerable difficulty sending or receiving positive messages, such as compliments, enjoyment, and expressions of love and affection. Problems in communication represent the most frequent complaints of distressed couples seeking marital therapy. Effective communication is critical for long-term relationship satisfaction. It is the necessary (but not by itself sufficient) requisite for sharing the positive and understanding the negative aspects of couple interaction (Gottman, 1990; Karney & Bradbury, 1995).

Conflict Resolution

Effective communication may help couples to identify and to understand their problems, but often, more than communication and understanding is required for effective resolution of relationship conflict. Because conflict is inevitable in marriage, couples must possess (or soon develop) problem-solving and conflict resolution skills in order to manage their anger and to resolve their disputes. Otherwise, unresolved problems tend to accumulate, and eventually they can damage other important aspects of the relationship (Markman, Stanley, & Blumberg, 2001; Notarius & Markman, 1993). Two fundamental types of conflict resolution are important: (1) joint decision-making and basic problem-solving skills that generally are employed *before* high physiological arousal and conflict are reached and (2) anger management and conflict de-escalation skills which need to be employed *after* high conflict is encountered. Basic problem-solving skills include defining and maintaining focus on the problem at hand, mutual understanding of the issues, and the couple's ability to agree upon and to implement an effective plan to resolve the issue. Anger and conflict management skills include: (1) learning how to identify and anticipate anger arousing situations, (2) recognizing and dampening physiological arousal, (3) developing preventive individual and interpersonal coping mechanisms to avert the anger escalation process, and (4) learning late-stage time-out procedures and, if necessary, negotiating personal safety, antiviolence contracts. Some couples are fortunate to have developed both preventive and remedial types of conflict management skills; some are good at one but not the other. In the clinical setting, when it comes to conflict management, most couples are deficient in both preventive and remedial skills.

Summary of the 7Cs

Most of the ingredients important to a long-term intimate relationship can be accounted for by an analysis of the 7Cs. For many couples these domains of function constitute strengths to build upon or goals to strive for: (1) socially compatible personal values and a healthy personality (i.e., *character*); (2) strong family traditions and compatible or stimulating *cultural and ethnic backgrounds*; (3) a marital *contract* that offers ongoing adaptations and a viable match between partners' expectations and experiences; (4) loyalty to the marriage with a long-term perspective and the desire to work out the inevitable problems (i.e., *commitment*); (5) love, affection, emotional support, and an optimal balance of individual and mutually rewarding activities (i.e., *caring*); (6) open and effective *communication*; and (7) problem-solving and anger management *conflict resolution* skills.

PROCEDURES FOR GATHERING INFORMATION

The social-learning, cognitive–behavioral approach has a fairly distinct tradition of conducting the couple evaluation process. It employs three methods of gathering information in order to understand the problems and strengths of a given relationship and to plan various interventions to accomplish the therapeutic goals. *First*, there is a series of clinical interviews, typically 2–4 sessions, which often include separate interviews with each partner as well as meeting the couple in a conjoint format. In general, the objectives of these so-called *assessment* interviews are to: (1) screen clients for the appropriateness of couple therapy, (2) determine the nature and course of events related to partners' presenting complaints, (3) determine the expectations and goals of the partners for couple therapy, (4) establish an effective therapeutic relationship, and (5) orient the couple to the therapist's orientation and approach to treatment.

Each partner has one or more reasons for initiating couple therapy. Typically, in the first meeting, the therapist will help the partners to develop a problem list, which indicates each person's perception of the problems in the relationship. Problems can be categorized into matters of content and process. Problematic content areas often include specific stress factors that adversely affect the marriage, such as, unemployment, disrupting external events, concerns about finances, sex, in-laws, or child-rearing; annoying personality traits or managing mental or physical illnesses. Process concerns have to do with couple adaptive processes, or *how* the couple interacts. Typical complaints include ineffective ways of communicating with one another and concerns regarding how they attempt to solve problems and manage relationship disputes.

It is also important during the evaluation stage to ascertain the partners' respective goals and expectations for couple therapy. For example, are they both committed to the relationship or is one partner planning separation or divorce? Are the problems identified negotiable for both partners? Are their goals and expectations realistic given partners' levels of competence and motivation? Before making a treatment plan, all these interpersonal competence and motivational issues must be considered. Finally, the initial interviews allow for the therapist to establish a therapeutic relationship with the couple. The therapist must possess sufficient credibility, gain trust, and offer hope that the partners' pain, suffering, dissatisfaction, and distress can be addressed effectively. If this step is not accomplished, the couple may not engage in the therapeutic process. One way to aid in the accomplishment of this preliminary bonding is to explain in advance the purpose and value of the various evaluation and intervention procedures. What is expected from the clients? What is the role and what are the responsibilities of the therapist? How will information be gathered and what is the prognosis for resolving their problems? An open discussion about what will be done and why is another hallmark of the BCT approach.

A *second* fairly unique assessment procedure used in BCT to gather diagnostic information about the couple is the administration of various questionnaires and inventories to learn more about specific strengths and problem areas for each couple. Table 1 presents the 7Cs categories and lists the methods and procedures that may be employed to gather relevant information for each area of interest. The table includes several standardized measures that are designed to assess one or more of the following variables: global relationship satisfaction, communication skills and deficits, areas of change requested by the partners, types of conflict, intensity levels of conflict and styles of conflict resolution, partners' cognitions, expectations, and beliefs about the relationship that may be causing problems,

TABLE 1. Behavioral Couple Therapy: The Seven Cs Assessment Procedures

Domain	Assessment procedures[a]
Character	Interview: psychiatric history, collateral information. Paper-and-pencil instruments: BDI, MCMI-III, MMPI-2, PAI
Culture	Interview: developmental history, family-of-origin history. Observation
Contract	Interview: relationship history. Paper-and-pencil instruments: ACQ, IRA, RBI
Commitment	Interview: relationship history. Paper-and-pencil instruments: DAS, MSI, IRA
Caring	Observation. Paper-and-pencil instruments: DAS, DSFI, IRA
Communication	Observation. Communication sample. Paper-and-pencil instruments: CPQ, CRAC
Conflict resolution	Observation. Communication sample. Paper-and-pencil instruments: CRAC, CTS-R, RTC, ACQ

[a]ACQ is the *Areas of Change Questionnaire* (Weiss & Birchler, 1975). BDI is the Beck Depression Inventory (Beck, Ward, Mendelsohn, Mock, & Erbaugh, 1961). CPQ is the Communication Patterns Questionnaire (Christensen, 1988). CRAC is the *Clinical Rating of Adult Communication* (Basco, Birchler, Kalal, Talbott, & Slater, 1991). CTS-R is the *Conflict Tactics Scale-Revised* (Straus, Hamby, Boney-McCoy, & Sugarman, 1996). DAS is the *Dyadic Adjustment Scale* (Spanier, 1976). DSFI is the *Derogatis Sexual Functioning Inventory* (Derogatis, 1975). IRA is the *Inventory of Rewarding Activities* (Birchler, 1983). PAI is the *Personality Assessment Inventory* (Morey, 1991). MCMI-III is the *Millon Clinical Multiaxial Inventory* (Millon, 1994). MMPI-2 is the *Minnesota Multiphasic Personality Inventory* (Butcher, Dahlstrom, Graham, Tellegren, & Kaemmer, 1989). MSI is the *Marital Status Inventory* (Weiss & Cerreto, 1980). RBI is the *Relationship Beliefs Inventory* (Eidelson & Epstein, 1982). RTC is the *Responses to Conflict Scale* (Birchler & Fals-Stewart, 1994).

sexual function and dissatisfaction, participation in pleasurable events and rewarding social activities, and steps toward divorce. BCT practitioners typically ask the couple to complete a selected set of these instruments either before or at the very beginning of the evaluation process. In most cases feedback and interpretation of the results are given to the couple regarding their responses.

The *third* assessment procedure that is routinely associated with the practice of BCT is observation and analysis of a sample of in vivo marital conflict resolution. That is, couples are helped to identify an existing issue about which they have disagreement. They are asked to spend 10–15 min in the session talking together in a demonstration of just how they go about attempting to resolve the problem. The therapist may or may not leave the room to less obtrusively observe and/or to videotape the communication sample for later review and analysis. The conflict resolution communication sample provides unique information regarding the level of problem-solving skill the couple possesses and the extent to which improvement in communication processes will become treatment goals. Several investigators have developed and employ a simple therapist coding system to quantify a given couple's communication and problem-solving skills (Basco et al., 1991; Markman, Notarius, Stephen, & Smith, 1981).

In summary, the multi-method assessment procedures employed by BCT practitioners provide a solid basis for describing a couple's presenting problems and relationship strengths. The procedures provide both converging and diverging types of information that are used in a systematic manner to conceptualize relationship (dys)function and to formulate a treatment plan.

STANDARDIZED INTERVIEW FORMATS

In this section, we will outline a comprehensive interview format that has been developed and modified in many BCT settings over three decades (Table 2). This basic format has been employed successfully by the senior author for nearly as long (Birchler, 1983). The series of sessions represents a relatively unrestricted approach; managed care considerations notwithstanding. Table 2 is straightforward; selected topics are discussed here for emphasis.

Initial Interview

The initial interview begins with greeting clients and giving them introductory information about the clinic, the therapist(s), discussing any fees or insurance-type issues, defining objectives for the session, and then describing policies about confidentiality. The issue of confidentiality should be covered before getting into the details of the couple's personal lives. In addition to the requirement to break confidentiality based on knowledge of certain threats and risks to self or others (specific laws vary by states), the default ownership of information gained in any manner by the therapist is the individual client. Many couple therapists, present authors included, usually modify this policy so that all members of the therapy group may share information gained by any means. That is, adhering to

TABLE 2. Diagnostic Interviewing for Couples—General Sequence and Content

Session one: Initial interview
  1. Introductions and registration
  2. Discussion of confidentiality issues
  3. Defining objectives of the session
  4. What brings you (each) to the clinic?
  5. Partners' goals and expectations
  6. Identification and analysis of presenting problems
  7. Commitments to complete the evaluation process
     (Couple relationship inventories handed out)

Session two: Second conjoint interview
  8. Collect inventories, debrief partners' experience with intake and inventories
  9. Obtain communication sample of problem-solving abilities
     (with debrief and elaboration of home-based conflict patterns)
  10. Relationship developmental history
  11. Continue assessing status of relationship. Exploration of positive and negative
     features of 7Cs: Character features, cultural and ethnic factors, contract issues,
     commitment by partners to relationship and to therapy, caring behaviors and
     complaints, communication skills issues, and conflict resolution processes

Session three: Individual interviews with each partner
  1. Assessment of individual partners
     (Developmental and prior relationship histories, closer analysis of character
     features, motivational issues, or hidden agendas)
  2. Opportunity to understand and validate the individual partners regarding their
     relationship experiences and perspectives

Session four: Third conjoint interview (Round table)
  1. Interactional summary of multimethod assessment findings
     (Summarize interview data, inventories, and observed problem-solving)
  2. Develop treatment goals and contract, offer referrals, or terminate case

an open confidentiality agreement, there would be no secrets kept from partners by the therapists. In our clinic, partners are told the pros and cons of each policy and the couple has input into the decision. Naturally, in cases where confidentiality may affect personal safety (e.g., domestic violence), open confidentiality may not be appropriate, and strict confidentiality might be required.

We believe that it is important for each partner to have the opportunity (and each should accept the responsibility) to participate in the interview process. Therefore, the couple is informed in advance that the therapist will facilitate the discussion so that each partner can share his or her concerns and offer personal perspectives. Thus, the therapist not only seeks to balance the amount of talk-time, but also may rephrase or reframe partners' complaints into "I" statements versus "You" statements. Partners are encouraged to talk for themselves and not for their partners as discussions ensue about what brings the couple into the clinic, what are members' perceptions of the major problems, and their expectations and goals for counseling.

We strongly encourage both partners to attend the initial session. We are hoping to treat the relationship, and having them together at the outset reinforces the importance of this unit. However, there are rare exceptions. In some cases, one partner insists on being seen alone before their mate is included in the process. While this option is discouraged, we do comply if it is the best or only way to get them started. In cases of the existence or threat of domestic violence, we interview partners separately. The separate interviews may be conducted as the first contact or sometimes, upon learning of the threat during the initial interview, we may break into confidential interviews with separated partners. A third scenario in which individual interviews may be indicated during the first session is in the cases where the partners are so angry, hostile, emotionally upset, or persistent in blaming one another, that the conjoint interview process becomes too destructive or ineffective for gathering the appropriate information. In such cases, Halford (2001) has suggested that the partners be interviewed separately so that the therapist can most efficiently and effectively join with them to learn about their concerns. The couple is brought together later, in the same or in a subsequent meeting, where the therapist can facilitate the development of shared information and common ground for going forward.

Finally, if the primary objectives of the initial interview have been met, the therapist explains exactly what would occur over the following few meetings and the couple is ready to make the decision whether or not to complete the evaluation process. If yes, they are given a package of assessment inventories to complete independently and asked to bring them back for the second interview. In rare instances, for example, in cases where clients have impaired vision, a reading disability, or English as a second language, partners may need assistance to complete the battery.

Session Two

Most couples return for the second evaluation meeting having completed their inventories. These are checked for completion and any missing data are obtained before or after the meeting. On occasion, additional encouragement is needed to get the questionnaires completed before the final assessment session. We have found it useful to ask the couple about their impressions of the intake session and about completing the questionnaires. There is a wide range of potential responses that inform us about motivational, competence, and couple interaction factors. For example, at the low end of the continuum for a good therapy prognosis is the couple that reports no mutual discussion of the first meeting during the entire week, no particularly good impressions of the therapist, and a lack of interest in or appreciation for the purpose of the assessment questionnaires. At the high end, the couple on its own may have initiated serious discussions about the prospects of beginning couple therapy, report good impressions of the competence or likeability of the therapist, and offer hopeful expressions about improving the relationship. In any case, the therapist takes the opportunity to support spouses' participation and frame positively the early efforts of the couple to engage in the therapeutic process.

After debriefing the couple about their experiences in therapy thus far, we give them instructions for conducting the *communication sample*. Based on the

presenting complaints enumerated in session one or from the written questionnaires, the therapist helps the couple to define one or two problems to be discussed for about 10 min. We want an issue that is current, relevant, and worth
discussing, without it being so difficult as to overly upset them. In our setting, the
therapist leaves the room and observes behind a one-way mirror while the discussion is being videotaped. The tape may be used for analysis and/or videotape
feedback to the couple. In settings where observational equipment is not available, the therapist simply instructs the couple to ignore his or her presence and
carry on with the conversation.

With a little experience the therapist can learn much about the couple's
optimal communication skills and factors related to the partners' relationship competence and cohesion. After the sample is completed, we always ask the couple
how representative the discussion was of communication patterns at home. Most
observed communication samples turn out to be fairly representative and therefore
valid for diagnostic purposes. Some clinic displays, however, are reported to be
unique or unusual: they would never talk for 10 min at home, or they would not
be nearly as considerate to one another, etc. Common patterns of dysfunctional
communication observed include couples who avoid conflict (i.e., both are intimi-
dated, mutually withdrawn, or disengaged), those that escalate conflict (i.e., both
partners are defensive and aggressive), or they may display a mixed pattern called
pursuit-distancer or demand/withdraw (Heavey, Christensen, & Malamuth, 1995;
Notarius & Markman, 1993). Employed excessively, none of these styles is constructive and when observed, communication and problem-solving skills may
become targets for intervention. Finally, although infrequent, some couples do
demonstrate good communication skills; in these cases, there is some other reason
for their treatment-seeking behavior.

The activities mentioned above account for about half the time allotted to the
second session. The remainder of the session typically is devoted to two additional tasks: Taking a developmental history of the couple and further exploration
of selected aspects of the 7Cs. The couple is asked to describe how and when they
met, what their early dating was like, and the decisions leading up to marriage (or
engagement, moving in together, etc.). It is believed that the information shared
on this topic and the partners' accompanying positive or negative affect are prognostic of therapy outcome, that is, regarding the early stage of the relationship,
some couples display positive emotion, humor, and ascribe positive attributes to
their partners; others display negative affect and have nothing positive to say
about courtship and marriage, etc. It seems to be something positive to build upon
when partners can access and share warm emotional connections.

Finally, with any time remaining, there are always some aspects of the 7Cs
that benefit from further inquiry. Therapists have heard presenting complaints
from the initial interview or they may be interested in following up on information obtained from the relationship questionnaires. For example, the group can
continue to explore the development and current status of relationship commitment, the change over time in the frequency and types of caring behaviors, the
relationship between the couple and their in-laws, or perhaps how relationship
contract issues have evolved over time. The point is to explore these issues in the

presence of both partners so that each can offer his or her own perspective and get acknowledgement from their partner and the therapist(s).

Session Three

If circumstances noted previously do not dictate an earlier individual history-taking session, we devote the third session to separate interviews for each partner. In our setting, where a co-therapist model prevails, each therapist meets with one of the partners. Alternatively, a solo therapist can split the 60-min hour, perhaps split a 90-min session, or conduct two separate meetings in the same week or over successive weeks. In any case, the purpose of the individual meetings is basically two-fold: First, obtain a thorough developmental history of the individual, including review of topics that might be too sensitive for the conjoint interviews (e.g., history of previous relationships, personal traumas, history and current status of mental illness, and other stressful life events). Second, based in part on previous information, the individual session allows the therapist to probe into critical relationship issues and make an effort to connect and join with the individual at hand. For example, if the issue of personal commitment to the relationship was previously mentioned by either partner, in the private meeting, the therapist may explore in some detail the client's fears, goals, or intentions about committing to this relationship. Hidden agendas may be uncovered (or verified). Ambivalent feelings may be explored and validated. In some instances, the therapist may assist clients in planning how to bring up certain topics to their mates in a constructive manner. The alliance and one–one connection developed during this personal interview often serves the couple well when everyone gets back together. Most contemporary approaches to couple therapy include individual interviews during the diagnostic process.

Session Four

In the present model, the diagnostic interviewing is concluded with the fourth meeting (or the fifth meeting overall if two meetings were scheduled for the individual interviews). We call this meeting the *Round Table* because all parties get together to share information gathered throughout the assessment process and together the group makes a decision whether or not to engage in the intervention stage of treatment.

The Round Table features summaries of the three types of information according to the following sequence: (1) the therapist gives the couple a written summary of the relationship assessment questionnaires, and the basic findings are reviewed, (2) the therapist describes the strengths and areas for improvement based on the observed communication sample, and (3) these data are combined with information obtained in the individual and conjoint interviews, and an overall relationship analysis is offered to the couple based on the 7Cs. In some cases, the therapist simply presents the couple a 7-point rating scale of each of the 7Cs (1 = vulnerability to 7 = strength) and explains the basis for the evaluative scores. Better yet, as an exercise in reaching consensus and defining goals for therapy, the partners are invited to make their own independent ratings after the 7Cs dimensions are defined. These scores are then discussed and compared with the therapist's ratings. Any significant discrepancies are resolved through clarification and discussion.

The final step in the Round Table is for all parties to decide whether couple therapy is indicated, review what the goals, methods, and timeline for interventions would be and give the first homework assignment. The most common variation to this typical plan is a recommendation for concurrent individual or group therapy for one or both partners to work on individual issues. Other outcomes include: (1) one partner wants to enter therapy and the other does not (if so, a referral for individual therapy may be indicated for the interested partner), (2) the therapists recommend couple therapy, but the couple declines (usually issues related to work schedules, insurance coverage/financial problems, lack of desire to work with the particular clinic or therapist, or insufficient motivation to continue work in therapy, and (3) the couple wants couple therapy, but the therapists decline (the couple is perceived at the present time to be unworkable; serious individual problems need to be stabilized or resolved first, or the problems encountered are outside of the therapist's expertise or personal comfort zone).

CASE ILLUSTRATION

A case illustration will be provided to give some life to the diagnostic interviewing process with marital dyads. This is an example of a case where individual psychopathology has resulted in a level of marital distress such that the relationship needs professional attention or else it might not survive. Brad and Shirley were referred for couple therapy by Shirley's individual psychotherapist. Shirley was being treated with antidepressant medications and with cognitive–behavioral therapy (CBT) for major depression, recurrent episodes, severe. During the initial session, Brad, a 43-year-old surgeon, explained that his wife began talking about suicide a few weeks previously and in a serious discussion between them, she indicated that she was not sure she loved him any more and she would just as soon end her miserable life. After 17 years of marriage, this was the first time Shirley, aged 39, said that she might not love him any more. The statement shocked and concerned Brad sufficiently that he requested marital therapy. Shirley, while tearing up several times during the initial interview, admitted that she had reached a point where she believed she could not make her husband happy; indeed that, lifelong, she seemed to refuse to be happy, and that the persistent anxiety and depression that she has battled for years had simply worn her out.

When the couple was asked to outline some of the relationship-based problems, all references were connected to Shirley's battle with depression. She had not worked for several years. She found it almost impossible some days to get out of bed. If she did get up, she was both overwhelmed with the idea of tasks to be accomplished and felt tremendous guilt about not doing them or doing them well enough. Brad claimed that he had run out of strategies to support and motivate his wife to function. With great sorrow, he admitted that out of fear for her well-being, he was anxious to get home each night after work, yet at the same time he dreaded getting there. He never knew whether he would find a morbidly depressed wife, an angry and resentful one, or the occasional one who was more hopeful and in a fairly good mood. Moreover, over recent months, no matter which one he greeted, the dyadic interaction, somehow, soon turned conflictual: they would end up in arguments (if Shirley had the energy) or mutual withdrawal and resentment if she did not. Brad insisted that no matter whether he tried to reach out to support his wife, or he withdrew to give her space, his choice would be the wrong one. Shirley responded that Brad often seemed to be demanding that she be more active or, alternatively, he would simply ignore her. Their social life had bifurcated: Brad, reluctantly, was going to most work- and family-related functions alone; Shirley often stayed home feeling guilty or resentful about being left alone. Their sex life had deteriorated to the point where it had been over six months since the previous encounter. To make matters far worse, the couple recently had purchased a bigger house. It was a "fixer-upper" and the couple was living in the adjacent pool house because a huge remodeling project was underway. Shirley claimed that dealing with all the decisions about remodeling and coping with the inconvenience of living out of suitcases in cramped, rat-infested quarters was simply overwhelming. However, representing the "no win" status of this current relationship, they had decided to purchase the house because the previous home, though familiar, was too small, dark, and dreary. The couple had made a relatively irreversible financial commitment to the new house, but the project had become a daily "monster" for Shirley to face. Throughout the interview each partner's experience and feelings were solicited and validated by the therapist. The initial interview ended with a commendation to the couple for seeking assistance given their challenging problems and encouragement to continue the evaluation with a goal of improving the marriage as an important way to manage Shirley's depression. The couple evidenced some sense of relief and each partner made a strong commitment to participate in the evaluation process. They were given the marital assessment battery to complete before the next session.

At the second session a week later, the couple brought back the completed marital inventories: The DAS, the ACQ, the MSI, the RTC, the IRA, and the BDI (see Table 1 for references). They reported little difficulty completing the questionnaires, although Brad had done them the night before the meeting and Shirley had to work on them over three sittings. They both seemed more hopeful than in the initial interview and reported that it seemed important and a relief to get into couple therapy where they could begin to address some longstanding relationship problems. This collaborative set was good to experience and set the tone for a productive session.

The topic selected for the communication sample was "going out." Brad began the discussion with a monologue concerning how he walks on eggshells anticipating resistance to ideas about going out to socialize. As he talked, Shirley became tearful, but was silent. Eventually, she seemed to get frustrated with his monologue, so she interrupted him and angrily blamed him for pressuring her and using guilt to get her to get out of the house. Brad, in turn, seemed irritated by her display of accusatory negative affect and basically he withdrew from the conversation. Shirley then started crying again, making self- and relationship-depreciating comments. This brief communication sample was a wonderful (if unfortunate) illustration of the maladaptive interaction process that this couple had adopted over time. They reported that the discussion was all too representative of what happens at home.

The remainder of the hour was devoted to learning about the couple's developmental history. They had met at a religion-based college in the Southwest, having grown up in the same western state. Brad was in medical school while Shirley was taking undergraduate courses leading to nursing school. Their religious and social values matched well and they were attracted to one another physically. Brad was confident and outgoing; Shirley was reserved and quiet. She responded well to Brad's leadership in the relationship. They dated steadily for almost 2 years and decided to get married after Brad graduated from medical school and Shirley from undergraduate school. The wedding went very well, but was better attended and supported by Brad's side of the family. The couple moved to the East Coast where Brad began an internship. Soon after the move, as Shirley was trying to get accepted into a nursing school, she had her first episode of major depression since early high school. Brad worked long hours during internship and Shirley, being unemployed and out of school, did not do well by herself. She became so depressed that she saw a psychiatrist for medication. They reported that the medication was only partially helpful; the symptoms of depression somewhat improved. After this first trying year of marriage, Brad had the opportunity to continue his training with a 6-month opportunity in London. The couple hoped the foreign travel would be exciting and enjoyable. However, the same pattern emerged: Brad worked long hours and Shirley was alone without friends, family, or familiar surroundings. She became depressed and was hospitalized for the first time for 2 days with vague suicidal ideation. Her medication was changed, and once again, she improved only somewhat. The couple returned to the United States, completed Brad's training in surgery, and Shirley completed 2 years of nursing school. This period was described as fairly good; they established some friends and the structure of school helped Shirley manage her mood. Then Brad was offered an academic position in a West Coast city, and the couple decided to move. Basically, over the past several years, Brad had been very successful in his work; Shirley had initially worked intermittently as a nurse and not at all for the past 3 years. Her inability to work was attributed to persistent and debilitating depression and anxiety.

It was noted that the couple's description of their relationship history was dominated by their constant preoccupation with anxiety and depression management. Similarly, certain follow-up questions about the quality and level of the 7Cs were reported in this context. For example, the couple professed strong commitment to the marriage, Shirley claiming: "Brad is my best friend and only real support"; Brad saying: "I love this woman and I would never leave her." When asked about caring behaviors, both partners softened as they reported that the expression of affection and sexual interaction was totally dependent on Shirley's mood and whether the couple was getting along. If both situations were positive, a variety of caring behaviors were exchanged and satisfying. Finally, cultural and ethnic factors were a match for these people. From the outset, they decided not to have children. The only problem from a family perspective was that Brad enjoyed frequent contact with his extended family and Shirley was estranged from hers. On many occasions, Brad would participate in activities without her and having people over to their house often was problematic.

Next the individual sessions were conducted. In Brad's case, he grew up as the oldest of four boys in an intact family in Idaho, where his father was a grocery store owner and his mother a stay-at-home mom. He reported no mental illness or conduct disorders among his immediate relatives. His childhood was very positive, and he was an outstanding student and an athlete in high school. He graduated with honors from both undergraduate and medical schools. Before marriage to Shirley, he dated and had casual sexual encounters with two women, but he saw neither for more than a few months. Although he lived in the Southwest, the East, and in London for 6 months, he claimed that his life has been rigidly scripted by his passion for medicine. He was currently the co-director of an Alzheimer Center and said he can maintain a fair balance of academic, personal, and family activities. His parents and all three brothers are married with no broken families. When asked an open question about his relationship with his wife, he admitted that being with her over the 18 years has often been quite a struggle. More recently, he says that he has grown more weary of trying to support her and he is quite concerned about her mortality. His supportive efforts have been less successful, and their interactions more predictable and unsatisfactory over the past 6 months, especially since they purchased the new house. Nevertheless, he had no intention of leaving her, as she sometimes feared.

Compared to Brad, Shirley's childhood and premarital history were much more traumatic. Her father was an alcoholic in a community in Idaho that did not tolerate alcoholism.
There was domestic violence between his parents and she reports that her mother was either
sick or fighting with her husband or children. Shirley now believes her mother's chronic
sickness to be emotionally based, but it was reported as physical illness. Shirley was the
middle of three girls and was anxious and shy all her life. She was either ignored or criticized by both her parents. By junior high school she was spending most of her time at
friends' houses, amazed at how different and how well their families functioned. By high
school, though still shy and reserved, she found solace in getting very good grades ... a
"brain" as schoolmates called her. In retrospect, she believed that her deep-seated problems
with anxiety and depression were caused by her childhood experiences. She could never do
anything right and she was prevented from socializing outside her dysfunctional family
until well into junior high school. With mixed feelings she decided to go away to college in
the Southwest, where she met Brad. He was her first serious boyfriend and the first person
with whom she had sex. She felt that she did not deserve him, that she was making not only
her own, but his life miserable, and she saw no way out ... except possibly suicide. Despite
persistent suicidal ideation and increased references interpersonally, she denied any plan or
significant intent. According to her psychiatrist, and certainly given her personal experience,
her symptoms of depression and anxiety seemed refractory to any combination of antidepressant medications. The next biological treatment that might be considered would be
Electro-Convulsive Shock Therapy, but there were no definite plans at the time of the interview. She remains on medications, however, she still becomes very depressed on almost a
daily basis. She would like her relationship with her husband to endure, but admits that
improvement is critical. Their love is gradually being lost to the battle with depression.

The marital assessment questionnaires were particularly valuable in this case because
so much of the interview time was taken up in describing the relationship history and the
couple's problems dealing with Shirley's depression. The inventories allowed for a broader
review of potential problem areas, strengths, and targets for intervention (see Table 3).

The DAS scores suggested mild marital dissatisfaction for Brad and mild–moderate for
Shirley. These scores confirmed the presence of marital distress, but strengths in the
marriage were suggested as well. The ACQ strongly suggested an "identified patient"

TABLE 3. Pre-treatment Results of Couple Relationship Assessment Battery
for Brad and Shirley

Inventory[a]	Brad	Shirley	Target[b]
Dyadic Adjustment Scale (DAS)	95	85	>100
Areas of Change Questionnaire (ACQ)	5	16	<4
Marital Status Inventory (MSI)	2	2	<4
Responses to Conflict Scale (RTC)	2.4	3.6	<1.4
Beck Depression Inventory (BDI)	5	33	<18
Inventory of Rewarding Activities (IRA)			
% Activities Alone	9	48	26
% Activities Together	30	44	34
% Activities Social	6	2	12
% Activities Family	28	6	20
% Activities Other Adults	27	0	8

[a]Refer to Table 1 for references.
[b]Generally accepted cutoff scores differentiating happy from unhappy clients.

phenomenon, a response pattern that prevailed throughout these data. The couple indicated that the relationship would be improved if Shirley modified 16, compared to Brad's 5 domestic behaviors. A review of specific items implicated Shirley's household duties and social activities outside the home as major problem areas. The MSI suggested that the topic of divorce has come up only in moments of high conflict or desperation. No significant planning for relationship dissolution was endorsed by either partner. The RTC indicated that both partners engaged in significant levels of maladaptive responses to marital conflict. However, an inspection of items suggested that Brad's style was more passive-withdrawal and Shirley expressed a mixed style of passive-withdrawal and active-aggressive behaviors. A BDI score of five confirmed that Brad denied any significant depressive symptomatology, while Shirley, as expected, endorsed very high levels (a score of 33). Finally, the IRA displayed a pattern of engagement in rewarding activities that was out of balance for one partner compared to the other and compared to happy couples. Shirley engaged in a disproportionate amount of four out of five categories: excessive activities alone, and too few adult couple social, family, or activities with other adults (without husband). In contrast, Brad had three of five categories with skewed data: proportionately too few activities alone, adult couple social, and too much activity with other adults, excluding his wife. In summary, the inventories strongly confirmed that Shirley, related to her experience with major depression and anxiety, was seen by both partners as the major dysfunctional partner. The fact that Brad had learned and was practicing maladaptive coping behaviors within the relationship had escaped the couple's awareness. Additionally, the extent that the couple's adaptive processes had become compromised was not something they could well comprehend at the beginning of treatment.

The couple entered the Round Table session with some normal anticipatory anxiety, even though, to their credit, and unlike many couples, they brought and had maintained a strong collaborative set. The data obtained from the relationship assessment inventories and from the communication sample were shared with the couple in a way to acknowledge that not only Shirley, but also the couple was struggling significantly with major depression. It was as if an unwelcome intruder had entered their home from the outset and presented them a near overwhelming challenge. However, once everyone acknowledged the depression issue up front, the main emphasis during the remainder of the feedback session was on the malfunctioning of the couple's adaptive processes to cope optimally with the problems in the relationship. To make this point, the therapist highlighted and interpreted data gathered from all three assessment methods (as discussed above). The 7Cs were explored to impress upon the couple that the quality of their adaptive behaviors is a function of both partners. This couple benefited from having the 7Cs defined and then they independently rated the level of function for the couple as a unit. These scores were then compared with the therapist's ratings. The empathically oriented group discussion served as an opportunity to reach consensus and to outline treatment goals. For the sake of brevity, the 7Cs consensus scores reached by the group for Brad and Shirley, on the 1–7 point scale were: Character features = 2 (coping with severe major depression; somewhat incompatible desires for social engagement), Cultural and ethnic factors = 6 (many similar values and cultural traditions), Contract = 4 (mixed, some major expectations for the marriage not matched by experience, for both partners), Commitment = 6 (basically no desire to leave the marriage by either partner, entering therapy to improve quality), Caring = 4 (mixed, despite deterioration in sex and affection, strong underlying respect, affirmation, and support for one another), Communication and Conflict resolution = 2 (both of these adaptive processes malfunctioning significantly).

Thus, based on the findings of the entire diagnostic interviewing process, the treatment goals negotiated and endorsed by the couple included: (1) enhanced coordination of care and management of Shirley's symptoms of anxiety and depression. The plan was for the psychiatrist, the individual CBT therapist, and the couple therapist to collaborate on a master plan to integrate the concurrent therapies. Unless the vegetative behaviors, comorbid anxieties, the hopelessness, pervasive negative thinking, and intermittent suicidal ideation could be addressed, there would be little improvement in either partner's lives or in their relationship. Shirley was still in the process of trial and error with atypical mood stabilizing medications. The plan for CBT was to intensify an independent program of enhanced cognitive restructuring and behavioral activation. Whereas Brad previously had been self-nominated as the person primarily responsible for Shirley's engagement in personal and social activities, the primary responsibility would now be turned over to Shirley and her CBT therapist. In this context, the couple therapy would be designed to analyze and to rehabilitate the couple's caring behaviors and their communication and problem-solving skills. Primarily, we wanted to help the couple replace walking on eggshells, multiple levels of guilt in both partners, unspoken reciprocal resentments, making erroneous assumptions, and conflict-avoidant tendencies with much more open, assertive, and direct communications. In the context of enhancing their existing commitment and fundamental respect and caring for one another, teaching them how to listen to and empathize with their partner, while being fully responsible for self satisfaction in life, seemed appropriate. Some additional work in the areas of caring and contract would result in a successful therapy outcome. The caring improvements would include recovering previous expressions of affection and sexual activity. The contract work would include some combination of change and acceptance: each partner verbalizing and behaviorally being responsible for getting more of what they expect from self and partner, or alternatively, learning to accept certain aspects of their self and partner with less concern and pressure for change.

This book does not concern itself with the formal intervention stages of treatments. However, the reader may note that traditional BCT (Jacobson & Margolin, 1979), CBCT (Baucom & Epstein, 1990), and the more recent versions of Integrative Behavioral Couple Therapy (IBCT) (Jacobson & Christensen, 1996) and Self-regulatory Couple Therapy (SRCT) (Halford, 2001) all would serve well as approaches to be employed to help this couple.

DOS AND DON'TS

This short list of Dos and Don'ts applies to the orientation and formats discussed above, using a cognitive–behavioral approach for diagnostic interviewing with distressed couples. Additionally, based on experience and opinion, not on science and facts, the following are offered for consideration.

Dos

Do treat the relationship as your client. Work to establish a collaborative set and take every opportunity to frame the couple's strengths and problems in interactional terms. Helping couples to perceive themselves as being on the same team, versus being adversaries, is half the battle toward success in couple therapy.

Do grab onto as many parts of the elephant (i.e., the distressed couple) as possible. Extra work is involved in obtaining information using more than one assessment method. Interviewing is a necessary, but not a sufficient, procedure for gathering diagnostic information. Standardized assessment inventories offer more extensive, specific, objective, quantitative, within- and across-couple comparative information than interviewing alone. Observed samples of problem-solving communication can provide more objective, skill-related information than do interviews or inventories.

Do use a straightforward psycho-educational approach with couples. We advocate informing the couple honestly and completely about what you are planning, thinking, and assuming about them. We assume that people are doing the best that they can to lead a satisfactory life and make a satisfying relationship. We explain our assessment methods, their purposes, their findings, and offer the couple an honest appraisal of the health of their relationship. There are no unexplained, hidden, or strategic manipulations for the benefit of the couple or the therapist.

Don'ts

Don't keep secrets that would jeopardize your moral, ethical, legal, therapeutic, or relationship advocate standing. Apart from laws relating to confidentiality and apart from safety issues involving domestic violence, we encourage clients to be open and honest with their partners. Insignificant personal and appropriately private issues notwithstanding, we do not keep secrets regarding affairs, substance abuse, hidden agendas, etc. that contradict pro-relationship goals (when the treatment contract is to maintain and improve the marriage). If the perpetrator does not elect to disclose such critical information, we usually will not divulge the secret ourselves, but we will terminate the couple therapy.

Don't establish alliances with individuals that will compromise the effectiveness of the conjoint therapy. Again, legal and personal safety imperatives aside, it is tempting to ally with partners whom we like, for whom we feel sorry, or with partners who have the power in the dyad. However, we suggest that therapists be aware of this tendency. It is better to assume that partners make a 50–50 contribution to the status of the relationship. Make alliances only in the interest of helping the partner and the couple to reach appropriate goals.

Don't make assumptions about the book by reading its cover, that is, couples present for evaluation in many states of (dys)function. It is tempting to note partners' psychiatric diagnoses, their active and recovering status regarding substance abuse, their poor premorbid childhoods and adulthood relationship histories, and other factors that sometimes correlate with poor prognosis for change (e.g., old age, certain ethnic and religious factors, socioeconomic status, employment status, etc.) and conclude prematurely that a couple is unworkable or does not deserve the expenditure of therapeutic resources. This natural tendency is a mistake. It is not possible to determine, in advance of careful evaluation and a trial of appropriate interventions, which couple is and which couple is not a good candidate for treatment. Some of the most awful-sounding cases can indeed be the most rewarding. If people show up, they deserve to give therapy at least a trial. The real data about motivation and competence come in fast enough once interventions are underway.

Summary

Diagnostic interviewing with distressed marital dyads is composed of part art, part science. To date, the BCT approach is one of only two empirically validated treatment approaches. Traditionally, practitioners employ three methods to gather diagnostic information: conjoint and individual interviews for learning about the partners' presenting complaints, individual and relationship developmental histories, and reports of their adaptive processes employed to maintain the relationship. Standardized relationship assessment questionnaires are administered to increase the breadth and efficiency of information gathered and to allow for within- and across-couple quantifiable comparisons. Finally, couples are asked to provide in vivo samples of problem-solving communication so that the provider can observe directly the conflict resolution abilities of the couple. Taken together, these data provide a wealth of information that can be used to learn about individual and couple resources and vulnerabilities, life events and related stressors that may affect the couple, and the quality of adaptive processes developed by the dyad to influence relationship outcomes. Following a series of evaluation sessions, the couple and the therapist decide whether couple therapy is indicated and, if so, relationship treatment goals are defined. The 7Cs heuristic model is described as a useful way to summarize domains of function that are critical for the maintenance of long-term relationship intimacy.

References

Amato, P. R., & Booth, A. (1997). A generation at risk. Cambridge, MA: Harvard University Press.

Amato, P. R., & DeBoer, D. D. (2001). The transmission of marital instability across generations: Relationship skills or commitment to marriage? Journal of Marriage & the Family, 63, 1038–1051.

American Psychiatric Association. (1994). Diagnostic and statistical manual of mental disorders (4th ed.). Washington, DC: Author.

Basco, M. A., Birchler, G. R., Kalal, B., Talbott, R., & Slater, M. A. (1991). The clinician rating of adult communication (CRAC): A clinician's guide to the assessment of interpersonal communication skill. Journal of Clinical Psychology, 47, 368–380.

Baucom, D. H., & Epstein, N. (1990). Cognitive–behavioral marital therapy. New York: Brunner/Mazel.

Baucom, D. H., Epstein, N., Daiuto, A. D., Carels, R. A., Rankin, L. A., & Burnett, C. K. (1996a). Cognitions in marriage: The relationship between standards and attributions. Journal of Family Psychology, 10, 209–222.

Baucom, D. H., Epstein, N., Rankin, L. A., & Burnett, C. K. (1996b). Assessing relationship standards: The Inventory of Specific Relationship Standards. Journal of Family Psychology, 10, 72–88.

Baucom, D. H., Shoham, V., Mueser, K., Daiuto, A. D., & Stickle, T. R. (1998). Empirically supported couple and family interventions for marital distress and adult mental health problems. Journal of Consulting and Clinical Psychology, 66, 53–88.

Baumeister, R. F., & Bratlavsky, E. (1999). Passion, intimacy, and time: Passionate love as a function of change in intimacy. Personality and Social Psychology Bulletin, 3, 49–67.

Beck, A. T., Ward, C. H., Mendelsohn, M., Mock, J., & Erbaugh, J. (1961). An inventory for measuring depression. Archives of General Psychiatry, 4, 561–571.

Birchler, G. R. (1983). Marital dysfunction. In M. Hersen (Ed.), Outpatient behavioral therapy: A clinical guide (pp. 229–269). New York: Grune & Stratton.

Birchler, G. R., Clopton, P. L., & Adams, N. L. (1984). Marital conflict resolution: Factors influencing concordance between partners and trained coders. American Journal of Family Therapy, 12, 15–28.

Birchler, G. R., Doumas, D. M., & Fals-Stewart, W. S. (1999). The Seven Cs: A behavioral systems framework for evaluating marital distress. *The Family Journal, 7*, 253–264.

Birchler, G. R., & Fals-Stewart, W. (1994). The Response to Conflict Scale: Psychometric properties. *Assessment, 1*, 335–344.

Birchler, G. R., Weiss, R. L., & Vincent, J. P. (1975). Multimethod analysis of reinforcement exchange between maritally distressed and nondistressed spouse and stranger dyads. *Journal of Personality and Social Psychology, 31*, 349–360.

Bradbury, T. N. (1995). Assessing the four fundamental domains of marriage. *Family Relations, 44*, 459–468.

Butcher, J. N., Dahlstrom, W. G., Graham, J. R., Tellegren, A., & Kaemmer, B. (1989). *Minnesota Multiphasic Personality Inventory (MMPI-2): Manual for administration and scoring.* Minneapolis: University of Minnesota Press.

Carstensen, L. L., Gottman, J. M., & Levenson, R. W. (1995). Emotional behavior in long-term marriage. *Psychology & Aging, 10*, 140–149.

Cherlin, A. (1992). *Marriage, divorce, remarriage.* Cambridge, MA: Harvard University Press.

Christensen, A. (1988). Dysfunctional interaction patterns in couples. In P. Noller & M. A. Fitzpatrick (Eds.), *Perspectives on marital interaction* (pp. 31–52). Clevedon, UK: Multilingual Matters.

Christensen, A., & Jacobson, N. S. (2000). *Reconcilable differences.* New York: Guilford.

Cole, C. L. (1989). Relationship quality in long-term marriages: A comparison of high-quality and low-quality marriages. In L. Ade-Ridder & C. B. Hennon (Eds.), *Lifestyles of the elderly* (pp. 61–70). Oxford, OH: Human Sciences Press.

Crenshaw, T. L., & Goldberg, J. P. (1995). *Sexual pharmacology.* New York: Norton.

Derogatis, L. R. (1975). *Derogatis sexual functioning inventory.* Baltimore: Clinical Psychometrics Research.

Doherty, W. J. (2001). *Take back your marriage.* New York: Guilford.

Eidelson, R. J., & Epstein, N. (1982). Cognition and relationship maladjustment: Development of a measure of dysfunctional relationship beliefs. *Journal of Consulting and Clinical Psychology, 50*, 715–720.

Epstein, N., & Baucom, D. H. (1999, November). Advances in cognitive–behavioral couple therapy: Assessment and intervention with behavioral patterns and cognitive themes. Workshop presented at the Association for Advancement of Behavior Therapy. Toronto, Canada.

Falicov, C. J. (1995). Cross-cultural marriages. In N. S. Jacobson & A. S. Gurman (Eds.), *Clinical handbook of couple therapy* (pp. 231–246). New York: Guilford.

Fals-Stewart, W., Birchler, G. R., Schafer, J. C., & Lucent, S. (1994). The personality of marital distress: An empirical typology. *Journal of Personality Assessment, 62*(2), 223–241.

Giordano, J., & Giordano, M. A. (1995). Ethnic dimensions in family therapy. In R. Mikesell, D. Lusterman, & S. McDaniel (Eds.), *Integrating family therapy.* Washington, DC: American Psychological Association.

Goldstein, J. R. (1999). The leveling of divorce in the United States. *Demography, 36*, 409–414.

Gottman, J. M. (1979). *Marital interaction: Experimental investigations.* New York: Academic Press.

Gottman, J. M. (1990). How marriages change. In G. R. Patterson (Ed.), *Depression and aggression in family interaction* (pp. 75–101). Hillsdale, NJ: Erlbaum.

Gottman, J. M., & Notarius, C. I. (2000). Decade review: Observing marital interaction. *Journal of Marriage & the Family, 62*, 927–947.

Gottman, J. M., Notarius, C., Gonso, J., & Markman, H. (1976). *A couple's guide to communication.* Champaign, IL: Research Press.

Halford, W. K. (2001). *Brief therapy for couples.* New York: Guilford.

Hazan, C., & Shaver, P. R. (1994). Attachment as an organizational framework for research on close relationships. *Psychological Inquiry, 5*, 1–22.

Heavey, C. L., Christensen, A., & Malamuth, N. M. (1995). The longitudinal impact of demand and withdrawal during marital conflict. *Journal of Consulting and Clinical Psychology, 63*, 797–801.

Jacobson, N. S., & Christensen, A. (1996). *Integrative couple therapy.* New York: Norton.

Jacobson, N. S., & Holtzworth-Munroe, A. (1986). Marital therapy: A social learning/cognitive perspective. In N. S. Jacobson & A. S. Gurman (Eds.), *Clinical handbook of marital therapy* (pp. 29–70). New York: Guilford.

Jacobson, N. S., & Margolin, G. (1979). *Marital therapy: Strategies based on social learning and behavior-exchange principles*. New York: Brunner/Mazel.

Karney, B. R., & Bradbury, T. N. (1995). The longitudinal course of marital quality and stability: A review of theory, method, and research. *Psychological Bulletin, 118*, 3–34.

Kaslow, F. W. (1996). *Handbook of relational diagnosis*. New York: Wiley.

Leiblum, S. R., & Rosen, R. C. (2000). *Principles and practice of sex therapy* (3rd ed.). New York: Guilford.

Levenson, R. W., Carstensen, L. L., & Gottman, J. M. (1993). Long-term marriage: Age, gender, and satisfaction. *Psychology & Aging, 8*, 301–313.

Levenson, R. W., Carstensen, L. L., & Gottman, J. M. (1994). The influence of age and gender on affect, physiology, and their interrelations: A study of long-term marriage. *Journal of Personality and Social Psychology, 67*, 56–68.

Lewis, R. A., & Spanier, G. B. (1979). Theorizing about the quality and stability of marriage. In W. R. Burr, R. Hill, F. I. Nye, & I. L. Reiss (Eds.), *Contemporary theories about the family: Research-based theories* (pp. 268–294). New York: Free Press.

Loganbill, C., & Stoltenberg, C. (1983). The case conceptualization format: A training device for practicum. *Counselor Education and Supervision, 22*, 237–238.

Markman, H. J., Notarius, C., Stephen, T., & Smith, R. (1981). Behavioral observation systems for couples: The current status. In E. Filsinger & R. Lewis (Eds.), *Observing marriage: New behavioral approaches*. Beverly Hills, CA: Sage.

Markman, H. J., Stanley, S. M., & Blumberg, S. L. (2001). *Fighting for your marriage*. San Francisco, CA: Jossey-Bass.

Matthews, A. K. (1997). A guide to case conceptualization and treatment planning with minority group clients. *The Behavior Therapist, 20*(3), 35–39.

McLanahan, S., & Sandefur, G. (1994). *Growing up with a single parent*. Cambridge, MA: Harvard University Press.

McGoldrick, M., & Giordano, J. (1996). Overview: Ethnicity and family therapy. In M. McGoldrick, J. Giordano, & J. Pearce (Eds.), *Ethnicity and family therapy* (pp. 1–30). New York: Guilford.

McGoldrick, M., Giordano, J., & Pearce, J. (1996). *Ethnicity and family therapy*. New York: Guilford.

Millon, T. (1994). *Millon clinical multiaxial inventory III: Manual for the MCMI-III*. Minneapolis, MN: National Computer Systems.

Morey, L. C. (1991). *Personality assessment inventory: Professional manual*. Tampa, FL: Psychological Assessment Resources.

Nichols, W. C. (1988). *Marital therapy*. New York: Guilford Press.

Notarius, C. I., & Markman, H. (1993). *We can work it out: Making sense of marital conflict*. New York: Putnam's Sons.

Peterson, R. R. (1996). A re-evaluation of the economic consequences of divorce. *American Sociological Review, 61*, 528–536.

Reiss, D. (1996). Foreward. In F. W. Kaslow (Ed.), *Handbook of relational diagnosis* (pp ix–xv). New York: Wiley.

Sager, C. J. (1976). *Marriage contracts and couple therapy: Hidden forces in intimate relationships*. New York: Brunner/Mazel.

Spanier, G. B. (1976). Measuring dyadic adjustment: New scales for assessing the quality of marriage and similar dyads. *Journal of Marriage and the Family, 38*, 15–28.

Stone, J. D. (1987). Marital and sexual counseling of elderly couples. In G. R. Weeks & L. Hof (Eds.), *Integrating sex and marital therapy: A clinical guide* (pp. 221–244). New York: Brunner/Mazel.

Straus, M. A., Hamby, S. L., Boney-McCoy, S., & Sugarman, D. B. (1996). The revised Conflict Tactics Scales (CTS2): Development and preliminary psychometric data. *Journal of Family Issues, 17*, 283–316.

Strazdins, L. M., Galligan, R. F., & Scannell, E. D. (1997). Gender and depressive symptoms: Parents' sharing of instrumental and expressive tasks when their children are young. *Journal of Family Psychology, 11*, 222–233.

Stuart, R. B. (1980). *Helping couples change*. New York: Guilford Press.

Waite, L. J., & Gallagher, M. (2000). *The case for marriage*. New York: Doubleday.

Wallerstein, J., Lewis, J. M., & Blakeslee, S. (2000). *The unexpected legacy of divorce*. New York: Hyperion.

Weiss, R. L., & Birchler, G. R. (1975). *Areas of Change Questionnaire*. Unpublished manuscript, University of Oregon at Eugene.

Weiss, R. L., & Birchler, G. R. (1978). Adults with marital dysfunction. In M. Hersen & A. S. Bellack (Eds.), *Behavior therapy in the psychiatric setting* (pp. 331–364). Baltimore: Williams and Wilkins.

Weiss, R. L., & Cerreto, M. (1980). The Marital Status Inventory: Development of a measure of dissolution potential. *American Journal of Family Therapy, 8,* 80–86.

Weiss, R. L., & Heyman, R. E. (1997). A clinical-research overview of couples interactions. In W. K. Halford & H. J. Markman (Eds.), *Clinical handbook of marriage and couples intervention* (pp. 13–41). Chichester, UK: Wiley.

Wills, T. A., Weiss, R. L., & Patterson, G. R. (1974). A behavioral analysis of the determinants of marital satisfaction. *Journal of Consulting and Clinical Psychology, 42,* 802–811.

Wynne, L. C. (1984). The epigenisis of relational systems: A model for understanding family development. *Family Process, 23,* 297–318.

17

Children

KOREN M. BOGGS, REBECCA S. GRIFFIN, AND
ALAN M. GROSS

DESCRIPTION OF POPULATION

The foundation of diagnostic interviewing involves obtaining all relevant information pertaining to a presenting problem in order to support sound clinical judgments. Diagnosis is frequently the first step in problem conceptualization and the determination of an appropriate course of treatment. Diagnosis also serves as a communication tool between the clinician and other individuals involved in carrying out subsequent intervention strategies. Because of its pivotal role in the treatment process, diagnostic interviewing should be approached with prudence, thoroughness, and a constant focus on the client's best interest. When children are the focus of a diagnostic evaluation, special considerations arise and must be taken into account. This chapter will review the fundamental aspects of diagnostic interviewing as it pertains to children.

Importance of the Developmental Process

The normative developmental process is an important frame of reference necessary for the assessment of childhood disorders. Without knowing what milestones are accomplished by most children of a given age, a clinician might not easily recognize deviations from typical childhood growth and development. Although a clear understanding of normal developmental processes is essential, it is also important to remember that there can be a great degree of variability within which a child reaches various milestones. Ages by which children learn to walk, talk, toilet, or read are offered simply as norms, and failure to acquire these skills by a certain age is not necessarily cause for alarm. For example, a child experiencing difficulties with toilet training at age three is not uncommon. There would

---

KOREN M. BOGGS, REBECCA S. GRIFFIN, AND ALAN M. GROSS • Department of Psychology, University of Mississippi, University, Mississippi 38677.

be greater cause for concern if significant difficulties persisted at age four or five. Unless the behavior is significantly problematic or causing unnecessary distress to the child, the best strategy in many cases is to simply wait and continue monitoring development.

Clinicians working within a child population may frequently be called upon to alleviate parent anxiety regarding whether their child is "normal" if milestones are not met easily or in a timely fashion. It is important to become familiar with normal progression and attainment of physical, cognitive, and emotional abilities. Sattler (1998) offers a helpful review of appropriate developmental considerations, as well as possible indicators of abnormal development from birth to eighteen years. By remaining familiar with what is normal, you can be more confident in reassuring parents that slight deviations along the development timeline are not necessarily causes for alarm.

Sattler also provides useful appendices for quick reference of common trends in cognitive development, language acquisition, concept of self, person perception, moral judgment, temporal concepts, and recognition of emotion. Since the clinical interview should necessarily be tailored to a child's current developmental level (e.g., verbal communication skills, ability to discuss abstract ideas), it is helpful to know what a child's peer group typically attains. To become familiar with normal activities during any developmental stage, it can be quite helpful simply to observe a regular school classroom and take note of social and academic abilities possessed by most children. Through informal observations of children playing, a clinician can acquire vast and useful knowledge that can later serve as a frame of reference in analyzing interactions with children of the same development phase.

Varying Presentations of Symptoms

Another vital point to keep in mind is that clinical disorders have varying presentations during childhood. The *Diagnostic and Statistical Manual of Mental Disorders*, Fourth Edition, Text Revision (*DSM-IV-TR*; American Psychiatric Association [APA], 2000) contains a section focusing entirely on disorders usually first diagnosed in childhood (e.g., learning disorders, developmental disorders, Oppositional Defiant Disorder [ODD], Attention-Deficit/Hyperactivity Disorder [ADHD]). However, the child can potentially be diagnosed with almost any mental disorder currently identified in the *DSM-IV-TR*. The *DSM-IV-TR* recommends that, when evaluating a child, "the clinician should consider the diagnoses included in this section but also should refer to the disorders described elsewhere in this manual" (p. 39). Across available diagnostic categories, the *DSM-IV-TR* does seem to recognize that childhood presentation of many disorders differs from typical adult presentation. In many cases, specific child symptoms are required in order for a child to meet diagnostic criteria as compared to an adult. For example, with Specific Phobia, it is not necessary for children to recognize that their fears are excessive or unreasonable, or with Generalized Anxiety Disorder, only one of six symptoms of anxiety is required in order for a child to receive the diagnosis. A general familiarity with *DSM-IV-TR* diagnostic categories is not enough; the clinician must be on the lookout for these unique distinctions in childhood presentations of symptoms.

Although the *DSM-IV-TR* does make these adjustments, it is important to recognize that symptomatology can also vary among children and between different age groups. Depression or anxiety does not necessarily present the same in children as it would in adults. Presentation may also vary by age. For example, children with somatic complaints may actually be experiencing anxiety or depression, and children with externalizing behavior problems are frequently struggling with depression or learning difficulties, or are simply responding to stressors that might appear unrelated at first glance.

Even the same disorder can have varying clinical pictures. For example, Schwartz, Gladstone, and Kaslow (1998) note that symptom presentation of childhood depression is closely tied to current developmental phase. Depression in infancy may present in the form of feeding or sleep problems, sad or frowning faces, or decreased attentiveness or curiosity. Preschoolers may seem irritable, have somatic complaints or sleep disturbance, experience separation anxiety, or have temper tantrums. Symptoms during later childhood include unhappiness, irritability, academic difficulties, phobias, and verbalizations of helplessness or self-deprecation. Depression during adolescence may involve social withdrawal, apathy, substance abuse, eating disorders, or suicidal ideation. Because of these varying presentations across developmental stages, it is simply not enough to know that childhood depression is "different" from adulthood depression. These issues stress the importance of understanding a child's current developmental level as well as what is normal for same-age peers.

Furthermore, as with adults, many children present with symptoms that overlap across several possible diagnoses, leaving clinicians to struggle with handling the issue of comorbidity. As a result of comorbidity of symptoms, it is often difficult to determine what diagnosis is primary and should be the focus of treatment. When symptom presentation is unclear, it can also be difficult to decide which disorders to rule out. Diagnostic categories with vague guidelines certainly do not make this task an easy one. When this issue comes up, it seems most prudent to make the best possible judgment regarding which diagnoses to assign or rule out, and then continue to monitor and reassess symptom presentations as treatment proceeds. In many cases, the decision about what to label a cluster of behaviors seems less important than identifying which symptoms are most distressing and attempting to alleviate them.

All of these concerns can easily put the clinician in a precarious position when assigning the correct diagnosis to a pattern of symptoms. There can often be serious repercussions if the diagnosis is inaccurate (e.g., a change in educational programming, qualifications for special services or funding). However, whether we would like to or not, we certainly cannot do away with the task of diagnosing and sharing that diagnosis with relevant others. Because of the issues discussed heretofore, it seems most vital that clinicians should not put too much emphasis on the diagnosis itself in guiding the treatment process. Assigning the initial diagnostic label does not end the task of evaluating the presenting problem. Assessing symptom presentation should be an ongoing process.

Special Issues

Unlike adults who often seek treatment voluntarily, children are commonly referred for treatment by parents or teachers. Children may not possess an awareness of problematic behaviors that are occurring or may not have an understanding of the assessment and therapeutic process. For these reasons, the clinician may encounter a unique resistance that must be handled carefully in order to elicit cooperation during the interview so that diagnosis and treatment can proceed accurately.

If the child is extremely resistant or hostile during the interview, information may not be fully obtained during the initial session. The interviewer's best course of action under these circumstances would be to maintain a nonjudgmental stance and to avoid both verbal and nonverbal cues of disapproval or criticism of the respondent's uncooperativeness. Sattler (1998) suggests explaining that you as the interviewer respect the respondent's privacy and understand that some topics can be difficult to share with another person at the first meeting. Instead, try focusing on obtaining more factual information and save sensitive topics for the end of the session or even for a different meeting. It is also helpful to remember that many children have difficulty expressing feelings verbally, and sometimes much can be gained from interacting informally with the child. Be flexible in dealing with apprehensive or resistant children, and do not assume that they will be ready to provide information immediately when called upon to do so.

PROCEDURES FOR GATHERING INFORMATION

Interviewing Guidelines

One of the major components of a child assessment will be an unstructured or semistructured interview conducted with the child, parents, teachers, and other family members. It is important to obtain information from as many sources as possible in order to formulate a comprehensive understanding of the problem at hand. The goal of the interview should be to gain a clear picture of what problematic behaviors are occurring and what personal or environmental variables exist that seem to be contributing to or maintaining the behaviors. Questions should address duration, frequency, and intensity or severity of the behaviors. The interviewer should attempt to discover the settings in which the behaviors are present and absent and how behavior patterns vary across contexts or environments.

Interviewing the parents first will usually be the easiest way to obtain important factual information which children may find difficult to report themselves. Parents may initially benefit from reassurance that their child's problems or reactions are common and not beyond assistance. Refrain from any insinuation that parents or teachers are to blame for the child's behavior. Encourage respondents to be complete in their descriptions of their child's behavior and assist them in identifying positive aspects of the child's behavior or tactics that have worked to alleviate the behavior in the past.

In addition to interviewing parents alone, it can be useful to talk to the parents and child together. This allows the clinician to explain the purpose of the interview to the child and may help alleviate anxiety the child may be experiencing. Also, talking with the child and parents together can provide a brief opportunity to observe directly typical interactions or communication patterns. It can be useful to see first-hand how disagreements are handled and how parents respond to the child's requests.

Interviewing the child alone can provide additional opportunity for the clinician to ask specific questions and observe behavior informally. The approach taken during the interview of a child will certainly differ from an interview with an adult. When interviewing a child, take age and developmental level into account and keep in mind the referral question when formulating questions. For example, a child referred for hyperactivity would not be suited to a lengthy question-and-answer session. Time spent building rapport will be important since many children may be suspicious or reluctant to talk about what is bothering them. Asking direct, simple questions and making efforts to alleviate any anxiety surrounding the interview will be likely to improve the quality of information you receive from the child.

As in any therapeutic interaction, qualities such as warmth, openness, and empathy can enhance the interview experience for those involved. As a clinician, developing a consistent style of interviewing can ensure that you consistently gather as much information as possible during this stage of the assessment process. Sattler (1998) provides a thorough discussion of tips for interviewing children and involved adults, as well as sample open-ended questions for probing specific areas. Sattler also offers suggestions for tailoring interviews to specific referral questions (e.g., child maltreatment, custody evaluations, medical illness). Approach the interview as you would any therapeutic interaction, maintaining a supportive atmosphere and conveying interest and empathy throughout the session.

Information to Be Obtained

Interviews conducted should evaluate several key areas, which are relevant to almost any referral question. A comprehensive developmental and family history should be obtained through specific questioning of parents. This would include asking about any complications during pregnancy or birth of the child, inquiring about when the child achieved significant developmental milestones, and assessing any significant social changes or losses in the child's family or support system. The child's medical and educational history should also be discussed. The clinician should ask about parenting style, how behavior is typically managed in the home, and what has been effective in coping with the behavior thus far.

Throughout the interview and the entire diagnostic process, it is useful for the clinician to seek an understanding of contingencies that are supporting the child's current behavior patterns. This requires identification of all possible antecedents and consequences that are influencing the behavior in some way. Questioning how the child's behavior varies by context or in response to various disciplinary styles or specific individuals can be extremely important. Having an understanding of when the behavior occurs, does not occur, or is exacerbated can help determine whether the child's behavior is simply a function of a particular environment or set of task demands.

Direct Observation

When feasible for the clinician, a direct observation of the child can be extremely helpful. Seeing a child in a more natural environment (e.g., a classroom, interacting with parents or peers during unstructured play) can allow for assessment of typical response patterns and coping skills. As an objective observer, the clinician may detect things that are sometimes difficult for involved others to perceive. Useful data can be obtained during this phase of assessment through collection of interval, frequency, and contextual data. Ascertaining antecedents and consequences that are governing the actions within a given context can become part of an intervention plan to restructure the environment itself in order to change the child's behavior.

Standardized Rating Scales

The use of standardized self-report or behavior assessment measures can be quite useful to the clinician. Rating scales are usually normed on a representative sample of children and standardized according to age group and gender in order to present a clear picture of "normal" behavior in the general population. For most rating scales, there is a cutoff point beyond which a child is considered to have scored in the clinically significant range, suggesting that there may be something atypical about a child's behavior within a given domain. The data obtained from such scales are not intended to support solely a diagnosis, but can be used as evidence to further investigate behavior that appears to be problematic. Rating scales can serve as indicators for behavior that is significantly outside the normal range for a child's age and can lead the clinician to form hypotheses to be pursued later during the interview.

Standardized rating scales can be administered to several individuals familiar with the child's behavior, and then results can be compared to determine the degree of consistency in a child's behavior across various contexts. It is usually helpful to obtain ratings from a child's teachers, parents, and from any other relevant adult. Information obtained from multiple informants can provide a clearer understanding of how a child's environment is contributing to his or her behavior. When multiple informants disagree greatly, this can also offer clues as to what might be governing the child's presenting problems (e.g., parents' lack of awareness of a problem, poor classroom management skills on the teacher's part). Commonly used rating scales include the Child Behavior Checklist (CBCL; Achenbach, 1991), the Conners' Rating Scales—Revised (CRS-R; Conners, 1997), and the Behavior Assessment System for Children (BASC; Reynolds & Kamphaus, 1992). It is useful to consider the referral question of an evaluation in order to select the most appropriate scale to use. Reitman, Hummel, Franz and Gross (1998) provide an informative review of available rating scales, including evaluations of ease of use and treatment utility.

Additional Assessment

Additional assessment techniques may be helpful if the clinician deems it necessary based on parental or teacher reports or apparent deficits are observed through interactions with the child. This could include further medical testing to rule out health problems, cognitive testing to determine intellectual abilities or identify specific deficits, or academic testing to evaluate a child's ability to achieve in school. Further assessment may be conducted by the clinician when possible, or may require referral to a different agency or physician.

CASE ILLUSTRATION

Consider the following case illustration as an example of how one might proceed using the strategies described previously in this chapter. Rufus P was an eight-year-old Caucasian male referred by his teachers for difficulties in school. Rufus was accompanied by his 35-year-old mother, Mrs. P. His father was not present. Rufus' two siblings, an older sister, age ten, and a younger brother, age two, were not present. Mrs. P presented recent notes sent home by his teachers describing Rufus as having a problem focusing at school, being chronically unorganized, late, not completing work, being inattentive, and being fidgety or seeming to run on a motor. Mrs. P appeared to be distressed by these reports and claimed that Rufus' behavior was also problematic at home.

In the initial meeting with his mother, the clinician attempted to obtain a description of the problem along with historical and developmental data:

CLINICIAN: Mrs. P, please begin by telling me about your concerns regarding Rufus' behavior.

MRS. P: Well, he is having trouble at school. And he is difficult at home, also.

CLINICIAN: Please explain what is happening at school.

MRS. P: His teachers tell me that he is having trouble finishing his assignments and following directions. They also tell me that he seems to move around a lot, like he can't stop moving and fidgeting at his desk.

CLINICIAN: Tell me more about the trouble he has finishing assignments.

MRS. P: It's not that he cannot do the work, Rufus is smart. He knows how to do the work, but he can't pay attention. It's like he gets distracted by the littlest things, someone dropping their books, or kids talking in the hall.

The initial clinical hypothesis was that Rufus' behavior patterns may be consistent with the criteria for ADHD put forth in the *DSM-IV-TR*. In this, a child must display six or more predefined behaviors (e.g., easily distractible, fidgety, blurts out) under one of two categories: inattention or hyperactivity–impulsivity. If the child meets criteria for both categories, the clinician may render a diagnosis of ADHD-Combined Type. In addition to the behavioral criteria, there are a number of qualifying conditions that must be met as well. For example, it is necessary for some of the behaviors to have appeared before age 7.

The symptoms present must cause "clinically significant impairment in social, academic, or occupational functioning" (APA, 2000, p. 93). Moreover, symptoms must interfere with functioning across two or more settings.

The clinician attempted to determine how closely the child's behavior pattern matched this definition of ADHD:

CLINICIAN: Do you see the same behaviors at home that you described to me before?

MRS. P: Yes, he also has trouble finishing chores and sitting still.

CLINICIAN: Describe some of these instances.

MRS. P: For example, he is supposed to clear the table and load the dishwasher after dinner. He'll start taking the dishes to the sink, and if he hears something going on in the living room, he just stops and goes in there. It's like he can't do one thing for more than a minute. Except watch Pokemon.

CLINICIAN: How do you handle these behaviors?

MRS. P: Usually, I get aggravated and tell him to get back to it. Sometimes I have to remind him three or four times to finish.

CLINICIAN: How does Rufus react to your reminders?

MRS. P: He always apologizes and doesn't argue with me. It just gets tiring for me, and I want him to be more independent.

CLINICIAN: Does Rufus seem to be overactive at home, as well?

MRS. P: He is always on the go. As soon as he gets up, he is running around the house playing. Even when the other children are worn out, he never seems to get tired.

CLINICIAN: How long has this been going on? At home? At school?

MRS. P: I remember Rufus having troubles like these even before he was five. His teachers started noticing problems when he started last year in first grade.

CLINICIAN: Other than the problems you mentioned, did Rufus begin walking and talking as expected? Tell me about his development.

MRS. P: His development was normal. We didn't notice anything out of the ordinary.

Additional questions gathered information regarding duration, frequency, intensity, and severity of the behavior. Especially important to this case, the interviewer attempted to discover the situations in which Rufus' behaviors were present or absent. In the interest of rapport and to facilitate accurate and open reporting on the part of the parent, the clinician did not insinuate blame toward Mrs. P or Rufus' teachers. The clinician also observed casual interactions between Rufus and Mrs. P and took note of how conflicts were resolved. She also encouraged Rufus to share opinions and ideas about his current situation.

Using a child version of a structured clinical interview can provide a format for interacting with the child. In this example, the clinician used the Schedule for Affective Disorders and Schizophrenia for School Aged Children (K-SADS), Present and Lifetime Version (K-SADS-PL; Kaufman, Birmaher, Brent, Rao, & Ryan, 1996). Since the entire administration of the K-SADS-PL can be quite lengthy, an excerpt from only the ADHD supplement to the core instrument is provided. To ensure an accurate representation of administration, the questions are provided nearly verbatim from the original instrument. Per the instructions of the instrument's developers, the clinician altered the questions to match the child's developmental level. For additional information and a comprehensive overview of the K-SADS, please refer to the section entitled Standardized Interview Formats.

After having met with Mrs. P, the clinician then met with Rufus. After a brief conversation to establish rapport, the clinician administered the K-SADS-PL. This structured clinical interview was employed in order to efficiently rule out possible comorbid diagnoses, to gather necessary information regarding symptom characteristics (i.e., duration, severity, frequency, onset, etc.), and to provide an opportunity for behavioral observation of Rufus during interaction with the clinician:

CLINICIAN: Rufus, do you ever get in trouble for talking too much in class?

RUFUS: Um, yeah. Pretty much every day my teacher puts my name on the board.

CLINICIAN: Do people often tell you to be still?

RUFUS: Yes.

CLINICIAN: Do you have trouble staying still?

RUFUS: Sometimes even when people like my teachers and my mom tell me to be still, I feel like I can't.

CLINICIAN: Do you get in trouble for talking out of turn?

RUFUS: I get in trouble a lot. People say that I interrupt them.

The relatively formal and rigid questioning follows the format prescribed by most structured interview formats. In an unstructured interview, the clinician may spend more time building rapport with the child and asking more open-ended questions. In this respect, the information gathered is limited by the particular instrument being used. Additional discussion of the comparison between structured and unstructured interviewing can be found in the subsequent section.

After meeting with Rufus, the clinician again met with Mrs. P and asked her to complete a behavioral rating scale, the—CRS-R (parent form). It was suggested that this instrument would provide additional data concerning specific behaviors associated with ADHD and related diagnoses (e.g., ODD). The clinician also requested that Rufus' teachers and his father complete behavior rating scales in order to obtain information about Rufus' behaviors in many contexts. The clinician asked that they complete a CRS-R, teacher form and parent form, respectively:

CLINICIAN: Mrs. P, it would help me understand Rufus and his behavior better if you were to fill out a rating form for me. This is called the Connors' Rating Scale and consists of several questions about behaviors sometimes seen in children with problems similar to Rufus'.

MRS. P: Okay.

CLINICIAN: It would also help if Rufus' teachers could fill these out. I will give some to you before you leave today. I would also like for Rufus' father to fill out a parent form of the Connors'.

MRS. P: Thank you. I will bring these to you at our next appointment.

Obtaining information from multiple informants broadened the scope of understanding of Rufus' behavior across situations and environments. In this example, Mrs. P and his teachers rated Rufus' behaviors within the clinically significant range, suggesting that they may be consistent with symptoms of ADHD.

It was important that the clinician conduct direct observation of Rufus in session and in school. Observation of Rufus in multiple environments provided an opportunity to corroborate the reports of parents and teachers, particularly since there were a few expected discrepancies (e.g., between some ratings of severity of behaviors across teachers). In this example, the clinician noticed that Rufus had difficulty sitting still in the interview room, was unable to attend to tasks or questions for longer than a few minutes, and seemed distracted by extraneous stimuli. Upon observation in the school setting (via videotape), Rufus was observed to engage in the same types of behaviors (e.g., constantly fidgeting, talked out of turn). The reported discrepancies across teachers seemed to be attributed to the amount of extraneous stimuli in the room. For example, it was reported that Rufus was less severely impaired by his behaviors in a classroom where only four other children were present. Furthermore, the level of noise observed in the classroom was significantly lower than in other classrooms. The clinician also noted that the room appeared to be more organized, with less visual distractions.

Before making a clinical decision regarding final diagnosis, the clinician considered all data obtained through interviews, rating scales, and observation. Based on the interview with Mrs. P, it was determined that Rufus' problems were present both at school and at home. Furthermore, it was determined that symptoms of ADHD were present before Rufus was 7 years old and had persisted for at least 6 months. Moreover, Rufus' developmental history appeared to be within the normal range. In the excerpt of the child interview, it was apparent that Rufus demonstrated difficulties consistent with the *DSM-IV-TR* definition of ADHD, Combined Type. In the entire administration of the K-SADS-PL, it was determined that no comorbid diagnoses were warranted. The rating scales completed by Mrs. P and Rufus' teachers substantiated the initial hypothesis of the clinician. Refer to the section below entitled Information Critical to Making the Diagnosis for further considerations in arriving at a diagnosis.

STANDARDIZED INTERVIEW FORMATS

Behavioral interviews are an integral part of the diagnostic process. It is imperative that clinical data be collected regarding symptom history, development, and the context surrounding behaviors seen as problematic. A spectrum of diagnostic interviews exists for this purpose, ranging from unstructured formats that allow for greater flexibility in question presentation and data collection, to highly structured formats which provide a predetermined set of questions and probes designed to be administered in a rigid format. Refer to Table 1 for a condensed overview of the interview schedules presented in this section.

All of the structured interviews follow the same paradigm in terms of scoring and output, that is, although the schedules differ in format and structure, they are all designed to mimic what a clinician does when using a diagnostic system: systematically rule out or accept criteria based on the client's report of

TABLE 1. Structured Interview Formats: Characteristics

	DISC-IV	CAPA	ChIPS	CAS	ISCA	K-SADS	DICA-R
Age range	6–17	9–17	6–18[a]	7–adol.	8–17	6–18	6–17
Administration time	70–120 min.	1–2 hr	21–49 min.	1 hr	2.5–3.5 hr	1–2 hr	1–2 hr
Interviewer qualifications	Minimally trained	Highly trained[b]	Moderately trained	Highly trained	Moderately trained	Highly trained	Highly trained
Forms	Parent Child	Parent Child	Parent Child	Child	Child Follow-up	Parent Child	Parent Child Adolescent
Primary Diagnostic Categories	Anxiety Behavior Mood Schizophrenia Substance Miscellaneous	Behavior Mood Anxiety Eating Sleep Elimination Substance Tic	Externalizing Substance Eating Mood Elimination Schizophrenia	Mood Somatic Psychotic Externalizing Anxiety	*Core:* Mood Anxiety Elimination Externalizing *Addenda:* Childhood Anxiety Eating Substance Personality	Affective Psychotic Anxiety Behavioral Substance	Externalizing Substance Mood Anxiety Eating Elimination Gender Identity Somatization

[a]With a previously-assessed IQ of 70 or above.
[b]CAPA certification recommended.

symptom presence, duration, and severity, and determine if the constellation of symptoms is in accord with a predetermined diagnostic category. Most of the schedules accomplish this by asking a series of "stem" questions that probe broad areas of psychological distress. Following endorsement of a "stem" question, the client is then asked a number of "contingent" questions that collect data on symptom features (e.g., severity, duration). Fundamentally, these interview schedules are the diagnostic systems in question form.

The degree to which a particular interview is structured relates directly to its diagnostic reliability. That is, the more highly structured the interview, the greater the diagnostic reliability. This is perhaps the greatest strength of the highly structured interview and the greatest weakness of the unstructured interview. However, the unstructured interview lends itself to functional analysis of behavior, an advantage that greatly aids in effective treatment planning. Moreover, the unstructured interview allows for idiographic assessment in an environment designed by the clinician, contributing to the establishment of rapport.

Several structured and semistructured interviews exist for use by clinicians in determining diagnoses. Sattler (1992) suggests that although highly structured interviews minimize the need for clinical inference, provide for greater interrater agreement, and can be administered by a range of professionals, there are a number of weaknesses inherent in their administrative process. The rigid format of question presentation seems somewhat artificial and may hinder natural communication between clinician and client. Moreover, the narrow range of topics covered in a highly structured interview may limit interviewees' responses. This can impede the development of therapeutic rapport. This limitation can be particularly problematic in the assessment of children, as it is important that the child feel comfortable in order to facilitate accurate self-report. Other researchers note that children's immature cognitive abilities, restricted understanding of the interview process (e.g., consequences of endorsing questions), propensity to acquiesce out of a desire to please the interviewer, and lack of awareness of symptom presence, duration, and onset may also attenuate symptom reporting (Bidaut-Russell et al., 1995; Lucas et al., 1999).

The formats presented below all cover a wide range of diagnostic categories and can be used in cases where comorbid disorders are suspected, or where symptom presentation is unclear or could be classified in multiple categories (e.g., symptom overlap exists between depression and anxiety). There also exist interview formats for more specialized use (e.g., the Anxiety Disorders Interview Schedule for Children [ADIS-C], Silverman & Nelles, 1988, and the Autism Diagnostic Interview [ADI], Le Couteur et al., 1989). The number of these instruments far exceeds the space in this chapter. However, most of the instruments are indexed in online and intralibrary databases, and may be available in clinics that serve specialized populations (e.g., Pervasive Developmental Disorders Clinics, etc.).

Structured Interview Formats

DISC-IV

The highly structured format of the Diagnostic Interview Schedule for Children (DISC) enables both clinicians and nonclinicians to use this instrument in research and clinical settings. In development through the National Institute of Mental Health (NIMH) since 1979, the DISC has undergone several revisions concurrent with modifications in the popular classification systems on which it is based. Specifically, these revisions paralleled changes in diagnostic criteria put forth in the *DSM-IV* (APA, 1994) and in the International Classification of Diseases, 10th edition (ICD-10; World Health Organization, 1993). The resulting current version, the *DISC-IV*, was made available for use in 1997 and is based on the *DSM-IV* and the ICD-10 classification systems. In addition to changing unreliable questions from previous versions, the authors also added sections for assessing substance use and schizophrenia making the *DISC-IV* more compatible with some adult interviews (Shaffer, Fisher, Lucas, Dulcan, & Schwab-Stone, 2000).

The *DISC-IV* can be used to assess for over 30 psychological disorders (e.g., anxiety disorders, disruptive behavior disorders, mood disorders) in children from 6 to 17 years old. It is designed to detect diagnoses occurring in both the past 4 weeks and the past 12 months. The longer time frame aids in the assessment of disorders that may be related to school (e.g., ADHD, separation anxiety disorder). Two analogous forms of the *DISC-IV* exist: the DISC-P for parents or knowledgeable caretakers of children aged 6–17 years, and the DISC-Y, intended for direct administration to children from 9 to 17 years old. Both forms are designed to gather the same information regarding behaviors and symptomatology. Their questions are virtually the same, differing primarily in their phrasing (i.e., "Did *you* feel..." vs. "Did *he* feel..."). In totality, the *DISC-IV* contains nearly 3,000 questions, although it is unlikely that all of the questions would be administered given that many of the questions are contingent upon endorsement of previous items. Administration time can range from 70 to 120 min depending on several factors including informant characteristics (e.g., parent vs. child self-report) and on number of diagnostic modules administered, as some interviewers may choose to omit particular sections based on setting or purpose of the interview. For example, researchers interested in screening for participants with anxiety disorders may not administer the schizophrenia module. Questions on the *DISC-IV* follow a "stem/contingent structure" (Shaffer et al., 2000, p. 30) in which 358 stem questions are asked of all informants. If a respondent endorses a stem question, a series of contingent questions are asked in an attempt to gain information regarding duration, frequency, and severity of the behavior to determine if it meets diagnostic criteria for a symptom as stated in the DSM or ICD (Shaffer et al., 2000; Reitman et al., 1998). If interviewers are interested in lifetime prevalence of diagnoses, they may choose to administer the "whole-life" module included at the end of the *DISC-IV*.

Scoring of the paper-and-pencil form of the *DISC-IV* is relatively simple when using the computer scoring procedure, but can be a tedious and error-prone task if scored manually. A single computer-assisted administration and scoring system that can minimize interviewer error and increases consistency across administrations is available (Shaffer et al., 2000). Extensive psychometric data on the *DISC-IV* is not yet available, although its developers state that "the current standard NIMH *DISC-IV* compares favorably with earlier versions" (Shaffer et al., 2000, p. 35) and data from early versions are provided in their review of the *DISC-IV*. Reitman et al. (1998) noted that "combinations of both parent and child reports seem to produce the highest reliabilities" (p. 558). Shaffer and colleagues (2000) provide an overview of past and current versions of the DISC and include information on other versions in development (e.g., Teacher DISC, DISC Predictive Scales, Present State DISC, Quick DISC).

CAPA

The Child and Adolescent Psychiatric Assessment (CAPA; Angold et al., 1995) is a structured interview schedule appropriate for use with children aged nine to seventeen years. It provides the interviewer with a format for collecting data on the onset, duration, frequency, and intensity of symptoms in order to assign a diagnosis based on criteria from the *DSM-IV* (APA, 1994), *DSM-III-R* (APA, 1987), and the ICD-10 (World Health Organization, 1993). The CAPA assesses a time frame of three months prior to the interview. In addition to providing a diagnostic script, it includes questions regarding sociodemographic data, family structure and functioning, peer and adult relationships, and ratings of psychosocial impairment that may result from psychiatric symptomatology. Parallel forms of the instrument are available for either child self-report or parent report. Diagnostic categories covered in the CAPA include disruptive behavior disorders, mood disorders, anxiety disorders, eating disorders, sleep disorders, elimination disorders, substance disorders, tic disorders, and other disorders such as schizophrenia and posttraumatic stress disorder. Like the *DISC-IV*, the CAPA is modular in form and can be administered in part or in whole at the interviewer's discretion. For example, if a clinician suspects a diagnosis in the mood disorders category, but not the eating disorders or substance disorders categories, he or she may choose to omit those particular modules in the interest of time, and maintenance of interest and rapport on the part of the client. A feature unique to the CAPA is the inclusion of the CAPA Glossary, which provides operational definitions of terms used in the interview with the goal being to minimize subjectivity in the administration and scoring of the instrument. Moreover, it reduces interviewer confusion over the exact definition of a particular symptom (Angold & Costello, 2000).

Average administration time for the parent report version is approximately 1 hr. An additional hour is required for administration of the child self-report version. Developers of the CAPA recommend that administrators have at least a bachelor's degree, but need not be experienced clinicians. They do suggest that prospective administrators complete a four-week training curriculum and become certified by a CAPA trainer prior to independently conducting the interview. Scoring of the CAPA is done by computer and utilizes algorithms derived from the *DSM-III*, *DSM-IV*, and the ICD-10. Psychometric data on the CAPA have been relatively favorable, with test-retest reliability coefficient (κ) values reported to range from 0.55 for Conduct Disorder to 1.0 for substance abuse/dependence (Angold & Costello, 1995 as cited in Angold & Costello, 2000). Angold and Costello (2000) provide an extensive review of the CAPA including information on additional reliability and validity studies as well as descriptions of "CAPAs for special purposes" (p. 47) such as the Young Adult Psychiatric Assessment (YAPA) and the Preschool-Age Psychiatric Assessment (PAPA).

ChIPS

The Children's Interview for Psychiatric Syndromes (ChIPS; Weller, Weller, Teare, & Fristad, 1999) is a structured interview appropriate for use with children aged six to eighteen years with a previously assessed IQ of 70 or above. Two parallel versions of this instrument exist, the ChIPS for administration to the child, and the P-ChIPS designed for administration to the parent. The two versions are virtually identical, differing only in pronoun usage in the questions (e.g., ChIPS questions ask "Do *you* ...," where the P-ChIPS questions ask "Does *he/she* ..."), and in presence of questions regarding psychotic symptoms and schizophrenia (i.e., the ChIPS includes such questions). The ChIPS consists of seventeen sections divided into two parts: fifteen sections that assess for twenty Axis-I disorders (e.g., ADHD, depression, anxiety, oppositional defiant disorder) as defined in the *DSM-IV* (APA, 1994), and two sections that gather information regarding psychosocial stressors (e.g., neglect and abuse). Apart from the twenty Axis-I disorders, the ChIPS cannot be used to assess mental retardation or learning disabilities. Administration time averages 35 minutes and can range from 21 to 49 minutes depending on number of symptoms present, or items endorsed. The developers of the ChIPS report that trained lay interviewers can administer the interview, provided they are supervised by a clinician extensively familiar with the *DSM-IV* (1994) (Weller, Weller, Fristad, Rooney, & Schechter, 2000).

Like the highly structured *DISC-IV*, the questions on the ChIPS are organized in a "branching" or stem and contingent question format. In other words, interviewers ask a series of stem questions that broadly assess across the twenty diagnostic categories included on the ChIPS. If an interviewee endorses a stem question, a series of branch questions are asked relative to symptom impairment, duration, and onset (Weller et al., 2000). Early studies investigating the psychometric properties of this rather new instrument show the ChIPS to have at least adequate concurrent, content, and predictive validity, and at least adequate test–retest and interrater reliability. A review of the five studies to date on the psychometric properties of the ChIPS can be found in Weller et al., 2000.

Semistructured Interview Formats

CAS

The Child Assessment Schedule (CAS; Hodges, Stern, Cytryn, & McKnew, 1981, as cited in Hodges, Kline, Stern, Cytyrn, & McKnew, 1982) is primarily a semistructured interview suitable for use with children from age 7 through adolescence. It is composed of two parts: a semistructured interview of the child consisting of approximately 75 questions pertaining to eleven content areas, including self-image, mood, anxiety, behavior, school, activities, friends, family, and thought disorder, and a set of 53 items regarding specific observations made by the examiner. *DSM* criteria are included within these content areas. Hodges and Saunders (1989) found moderate to high internal consistency for each of these eleven content scales.

The second section of the CAS surveys the interviewer with reference to her perceptions of the child's cognitive ability, quality of verbal communication and nonverbal expression of emotions, insight, motor coordination and activity level, grooming, and several other domains, all of which provide information valuable to construction of the clinical picture of the child. The average administration time for the CAS is approximately one hour. Reitman et al. (1998) note "the use of the CAS requires a considerable degree of clinical judgment" (p. 558). Furthermore, Hodges et al. (1982) assert that it is imperative that the person administering the interview have a great deal of experience with children and a large knowledge base in the area of child development. In a study by Hodges, Cools, and McKnew (1989) the CAS was found to have good test–retest reliability with respect to three variables: symptom scores ($r = 0.89$, $p < 0.001$), item endorsement ($r = 0.60$, $p < 0.001$), and diagnostic presence or absence (r ranging from 0.38 to 1.00).

ISCA

Originally named the Interview Schedule for Children (ISC; Kovacs, 1985), the Interview Schedule for Children and Adolescents (ISCA; Kovacs, 1997) is a semistructured interview designed to assess for psychiatric diagnoses in children aged eight to seventeen years. Two versions of the instrument exist, the ISCA and the Follow-up Interview Schedule for Adults (FISA). The FISA is used primarily in the collection of longitudinal data from adults and young adults previously diagnosed using the ISCA. The core instrument yields diagnoses in the categories of mood disorders, anxiety disorders, elimination disorders, externalizing disorders, and other single-diagnosis categories found in the *DSM-IV* (APA, 1994). Addenda to the core instrument contain questions designed to generate diagnoses from the categories of childhood disorders, other anxiety disorders not previously assessed, eating disorders, substance disorders, and personality disorders (Sherrill & Kovacs, 2000). Administration time is around 2.5 hr for a parent and 1 hr for a child. It is recommended that administrators should be clinicians trained in semistructured interviewing and especially familiar with diagnostic systems such as the *DSM-IV* (APA, 1994).

The ISCA consists of five sections totaling around 70 questions and a single question concerning the "global functioning and degree of impairment across social roles" (Sherrill & Kovacs, 2000, p. 67) that reportedly measures the *Severity of the Current Condition*. These section titles include symptoms and signs, behavioral observations, mental status, the clinician's impressions of the child's social maturity, and developmental milestones. Unlike the highly structured DISC-IV, there are no stem questions on the ISCA. The ISCA does provide uniform queries (e.g., "Do things bother you, 'get on your nerves'? Have you been feeling cranky/crabby?" [Sherrill & Kovacs, 2000, p. 69]) for initial screening and supplies additional questions (e.g., "Do you 'snap' at your parents/siblings/friends? a lot? many times? Once in a while?" [Sherrill & Kovacs, 2000, p. 69]) for more in depth symptom assessment. The interviewer then rates responses from the parent and child individually, followed by an overall rating based on responses from both informants. To arrive at a diagnostic decision, the interviewer then "weighs and combines data from multiple informants in order to arrive at summary ratings that reflect the best estimate of 'reality'" (Sherrill & Kovacs, 2000, p. 69).

Kovacs (1985) reports that the reliability of symptom ratings using the ICSA was examined through calculation of interrater agreement statistics such as the intraclass correlation coefficient (ICC), Cohen's κ, and uncorrected percent agreement. Mean ICC values across content areas ranged from 0.77 to 1.00. Mean κ values across content areas ranged from 0.90 to 1.00, and mean percent agreement values ranged from 99 to 100%. Additional details, psychometric data, and explanations of other statistical calculations can be found in Sherrill and Kovacs' (2000) review of the ISCA.

K-SADS

The K-SADS (Puig-Antich & Chambers, 1978) is also referred to as the "Kiddie SADS." The K-SADS is a semistructured interview for children ages six to eighteen years, with both children and parents serving as informants. This instrument provides diagnoses for affective, eating, tic, psychotic, and behavioral disorders. There are currently three versions of the K-SADS available, which are consistent with *DSM-IV* diagnostic criteria. Each version typically takes between one and two hours to administer. Both the K-SADS-E (with an "epidemiological" focus) and the K-SADS-PL (with a "present" and "lifetime" focus) are intended to provide a current and lifetime psychiatric diagnosis. The K-SADS-P IVR (with a "present state" focus) assesses current symptoms as well as those present during the year prior to the interview (Ambrosini, 2000). The most commonly used form is the most recent version of the instrument, the K-SADS-PL (Kaufman et al., 1997). This instrument is also modular in form, beginning first with an unstructured section in which information is garnered regarding presenting complaints and client and family history. Following this is the *Screen Interview*, a section essentially the same as the "probe" or "stem" questions in other interview formats in that information is obtained on broad presenting symptoms. Based on responses provided in the *Screen Interview*, the clinician determines which of five modules (affective, psychotic, anxiety, behavioral, and substance abuse) to administer or omit, and in what order the modules should be presented (e.g., if it is reported that the onset of a child's depressive symptomatology preceded the onset of his anxious symptomatology, administer the affective disorders module first, then the anxiety disorders module).

Contributing to the K-SADS-PL's *semistructured* status is the direction to clinicians that it is not necessary to present the "probe" questions verbatim. Instead, administrators are urged to tailor question presentation to characteristics of the child being interviewed. For example, consider the cognitive abilities and overall maturity of the child, and use examples from the parent and child's self-report when asking follow-up questions (Kaufman et al., 1996). Ambrosini (2000) provides a review of how the K-SADS was developed, its psychometric properties (which appear so far to be acceptable, even good in some instances), and what areas are specifically addressed by each of the three available versions.

DICA-R

The Diagnostic Interview for Children and Adolescents—Revised (DICA-R; Reich & Welner, 1998) is a semistructured interview for children ages six to seventeen years. There are separate interview sections for parents, children, and adolescents. Administration time usually falls between one and two hours, although a computerized version is also available and can be quicker to administer. The aim of the DICA-R is to arrive at a lifetime diagnosis within *DSM-IV* or ICD-10 criteria. Reich (2000) notes that although the DICA-R is often "referred to as structured and classified with the DISC" (p. 61), it is actually a semistructured interview. She notes that there are standardized administration procedures requiring specific wording and presentation of questions, but that there are also allowances for deviating from the protocol. The interviewer must make judgments about when deviations should be made, and specific probes can be used to investigate an area further. Reich also notes that when interviewers must deviate completely from standard questions, they should rely on their DICA-R training to offer alternative presentations of the questions. In addition to offering a psychiatric diagnosis, the DICA-R also contains sections to assess stressors in psychosocial areas as well as perinatal and early development.

INFORMATION CRITICAL TO MAKING THE DIAGNOSIS

It is not simply enough to conduct interviews and direct observation of the child in his or her environment. Rather, the clinician must consider a number of factors when synthesizing and making sense of the information gathered. First, it is important to evaluate the quality of the information gathered. Reflect upon your interactions with the child, the parents, and others you interviewed. Are all of the informants qualified to contribute to the pool of information? Perhaps one of the child's teachers filled out a rating scale, but only sees the child for 1 hr every other day. It is also important at this point to assess the informants' capacity to give accurate information regarding context and behavior. If you interviewed the child, did he or she demonstrate an understanding of the questions you asked? Evaluate each informant's level of awareness, insight, and general stability.

When you have multiple informants, it is likely that there will be some level of disagreement between their reports. It is common, even, for parental reports to differ. In this case, it may be useful to further question the parents on the topic(s) on which they differed. It would be important to know the reason for the discrepancy. For example, parents may disagree on appropriate discipline methods, or on the frequency or severity of a behavior. The differing reports could be due to family characteristics (e.g., mother stays home, father works and has less exposure to children).

Current family dynamics can impact or exacerbate problematic behavior in children. For example, an impending divorce, birth of a sibling, death of a family member or pet, or family relocation can have some bearing on presenting problematic behaviors. Be aware that parents may not readily offer this type of information, and it may take encouragement and probing after the establishment of rapport to elicit this crucial data.

It is imperative that information be gathered regarding medication history (including current medication), medical history (i.e., current or past illnesses, family medical history), and developmental history (including when developmental milestones were met). In some cases, it may be appropriate to refer the child for a medical evaluation to rule out biological conditions known to affect behavior.

Finally, keep in mind all relevant ethical considerations. These include, but are not limited to, responsibilities to the client (the parents *and* the child), explaining confidentiality and its limits, and including the child in the process as much as possible. When working with a family, it is sometimes difficult to delineate to whom your primary ethical obligations lie. Although the child is minor and the parents are technically the "client," always remember that the principal motive should be protecting the best interest of the child.

DOS AND DON'TS

Do be supportive and establish rapport, focus on the best interest of the child, make the child aware of the process, and allow him or her to participate as much as possible in the assessment process. Maintain confidentiality to a reasonable extent. Identify the child's strengths and understand normal developmental progression so you can recognize deviations.

Do not communicate in a condescending or judgmental manner with the child. Do not be too abrupt in questions or interactions with the child or be too playful and lose focus of the interview. Do not ask only closed-ended questions, ask leading questions or allow the child to respond in an attempt to gain approval. Do not base diagnosis on one source of information, and most importantly, do not force a diagnosis.

SUMMARY

The intention was to provide a comprehensive overview of the child diagnostic process with particular attention to the diagnostic interview. The chapter began with an overview of factors to be considered when conducting a diagnostic evaluation of a child. These included the importance of understanding the developmental process as well as being aware of varying presentations of symptoms across age groups. Following this introduction to the population, guidelines for interviewing both the child and relevant others (e.g., parents) were presented. In this section, the importance of direct observation and obtaining information from multiple sources was highlighted. The importance of understanding the developmental process, as well as being aware of varying presentations of symptoms across age groups were also discussed. To illustrate principles of interviewing a child, a case example was provided. This example offered a broad picture of the diagnostic endeavor, beginning with an unstructured interview with the parent, including a structured interview with the child, and ending with an explanation of the decision-making process employed by the clinician. This also illustrated the importance of collecting additional data through behavior rating scales and multiple informants.

The second half of the chapter provided a review of the most frequently used comprehensive standardized clinical interviews, including descriptions of several structured interviews (e.g., DISC-IV, CAPA) and semistructured interviews (e.g., CAS, K-SADS). Discussion of the advantages and weaknesses of using these instruments was offered. Additional evaluation of their utility in comparison to unstructured interviews led to the conclusion that if a structured or semistructured interview is used, it should be accompanied by a thorough functional assessment of the problematic behaviors.

In conclusion, the diagnostic process is best viewed as an ongoing evaluation of the context surrounding behavior. The process does not end with the assignment of a diagnostic code. Rather, the initial evaluation serves as a beginning point for treatment planning, as the objective of any assessment should be to gather meaningful information that will aid in the improvement of the presenting condition.

REFERENCES

Achenbach, T. M. (1991). *Integrative guide for the 1991 CBCL/4-18, YSR, and TRF profiles*. Burlington, VT: University of Vermont Department of Psychiatry.

Ambrosini, P. J. (2000). Historical development and present status of the schedule for affective disorders and schizophrenia for school-age children (K-SADS). *Journal of the American Academy of Child and Adolescent Psychiatry, 39*(1), 49–58.

American Psychiatric Association. (1987). *Diagnostic and statistical manual of mental disorders* (3rd ed.). Washington, DC: Author.

American Psychiatric Association. (1994). *Diagnostic and statistical manual of mental disorders* (4th ed.). Washington, DC: Author.

American Psychiatric Association. (2000). *Diagnostic and statistical manual of mental disorders* (4th ed., text revision). Washington, DC: Author.

Angold, A., & Costello, E. J. (2000). The child and adolescent psychiatric assessment (CAPA). *Journal of the American Academy of Child and Adolescent Psychiatry, 39*(1), 39–48.

Angold, A., Prendergast, M., Cox, A., Harrington, R., Simonoff, E., & Rutter, M. (1995). The child and adolescent psychiatric assessment. *Psychological Medicine, 25*, 739–753.

Bidaut-Russell, M., Reich, W., Cottler, L. B., Robins, L. N., Compton, W.M., & Mattison, R.E. (1995). The diagnostic interview schedule for children (PC-DISC v3.0): Parents and adolescents suggest reasons for expecting discrepant answers. *Journal of Abnormal Child Psychology, 23*(5), 641–659.

Conners, C. K. (1997). *Manual for Conners' Rating Scales—Revised*. North Tonawanda, NY: Multi-Health Systems.

Hodges, K., Cools, J., & McKnew, D. (1989). Test–retest reliability of a clinical research interview for children: The child assessment schedule. *Journal of consulting and clinical psychology, 1*(4), 317–322.

Hodges, K., Kline, J., Stern, L., Cytryn, L., & McKnew, D. (1982). The development of a child assessment interview for research and clinical use. *Journal of Abnormal Child Psychology, 10*(2), 173–189.

Hodges, K., & Saunders, W. (1989). Internal consistency of a diagnostic interview for children: The child and assessment schedule. *Journal of abnormal child psychology, 17*(6), 691–701.

Kaufman, J., Birmaher, B., Brent, D., Rao, U., & Ryan, N. (1996). *Kiddie-Sads—Present and Lifetime Version (K-SADS-PL)*. Retrieved July 5, 2001, from http://www.wpic.pitt.edu/ksads.

Kaufman, J., Birmaher, B., Brent, D., Rao, U., Flynn, C., Moreci, P., Williamson, D., & Ryan, N. (1997). Schedule for affective disorders and schizophrenia for school-age children—present and lifetime version (K-SADS-PL): Initial reliability and validity data. *Journal of the American Academy of Child and Adolescent Psychiatry, 36*(7), 980–988.

Kovacs, M. (1985). The interview schedule for children (ISC). *Psychopharmacology Bulletin, 21*, 991–994.

Kovacs, M. (1997). *The interview schedule for children and adolescents (ISCA): Current and lifetime (ISCA—C & L) and current and interim (ISCA—C & I) versions.* Pittsburgh: Western Psychiatric Institute and Clinic.

Le Couteur, A., Rutter, M., Lord, C., Rios, P., Robertson, S., Holdgrafer, M., & McLennan, J. (1989). Autism diagnostic interview: A standardized investigator-based instrument. *Journal of Autism and Developmental Disorders, 19*(3), 363–387.

Lucas, C.P., Fisher, P., Piacentini, J., Zhang, H., Jenson, P.S., Shaffer, D., Dulcan, M., Schwab-Stone, M., Regier, D., & Canino, G. (1999). Features of interview questions associated with attenuation of symptom reports. *Journal of Abnormal Child Psychology, 27*(6), 429–437.

Puig-Antich, J., & Chambers, W. (1978). *The schedule for affective disorders and schizophrenia for school-age children (Kiddie-SADS).* New York: New York State Psychiatric Institute.

Reich, W. (2000). Diagnostic interview for children and adolescents (DICA). *Journal of American Academy of Child and Adolescent Psychiatry, 39*(1), 59–66.

Reich, W., & Welner, Z. (1998). *Revised version of the Diagnostic Interview Schedule for Children and Adolescents (DICA-R).* St. Louis: Washington University School of Medicine, Department of Psychiatry.

Reitman, D., Hummel, R., Franz, D. Z., & Gross, A. M. (1998). A review of methods and instruments for assessing externalizing disorders: Theoretical and practical considerations in rendering a diagnosis. *Clinical Psychology Review, 18*(5), 555–584.

Reynolds, C. R., & Kamphaus, R. W. (1992). *Manual: Behavior assessment system for children.* Circle Pines, MN: American Guidance Service.

Sattler, J. M. (1992). *Assessment of children* (3rd ed.). San Diego, CA: Jerome M. Sattler.

Sattler, J. M. (1998). *Clinical and forensic interviewing of children and families.* San Diego, CA: Jerome M. Sattler.

Schwartz, J. A., Gladstone, T. R. G., & Kaslow, N. J. (1998). Depressive disorders. In Ollendick, T. H., & Herson, M. (Eds.), *Handbook of child psychopathology* (pp. 269–289). New York: Plenum Press.

Shaffer, D., Fisher, P., Lucas, C. P., Dulcan, M. K., & Schwab-Stone, M. E. (2000). NIMH diagnostic interview schedule for children version IV (NIMH DISC-IV): Description, differences from previous versions, and reliability of some common diagnoses. *Journal of the American Academy of Child and Adolescent Psychiatry, 39*(1), 28–38.

Sherrill, J. T., & Kovacs, M. (2000). Interview schedule for children and adolescents (ISCA). *Journal of the American Academy of Child and Adolescent Psychiatry, 39*(1), 67–75.

Silverman, W. K., & Nelles, W. B. (1988). The anxiety disorders interview schedule for children. *Journal of the American Academy of Child and Adolescent Psychiatry, 27*(6), 772–778.

Weller, E. B., Weller, R. A., Fristad, M. A., Rooney, M. T., & Schechter, J. (2000). Children's interview for psychiatric syndromes (ChIPS). *Journal of the American Academy of Child and Adolescent Psychiatry, 39*(1), 76–84.

Weller, E. B., Weller, R. A., Teare, M., & Fristad, M. A. (1999). *Children's interview for psychiatric syndromes (ChIPS).* Washington, DC: American Psychiatric Press.

World Health Organization. (1993). *The ICD-10 classification of mental and behavioural disorders: Diagnostic criteria for research.* Geneva: Author.

18

Sexually and Physically
Abused Children

ANTHONY P. MANNARINO AND
JUDITH A. COHEN

DESCRIPTION OF THE PROBLEM

Sexual and physical abuse are not psychiatric disorders but are traumatic events to which children may be exposed. Accordingly, there is not a constellation of traits or symptoms which characterize sexually or physically abused children. In fact, research has demonstrated that sexually and physically abused children exhibit a diverse array of emotional and behavioral difficulties (Einbender & Friedrich, 1989; Mannarino, Cohen, & Gregor, 1989) and that a substantial minority of abused children is apparently asymptomatic (Finkelhor, 1990).

There are at least two distinct roles that mental health professionals may have when interviewing children who allegedly have been sexually or physically abused. One would be that of a clinical evaluator whose primary task is to determine the nature and extent of psychological problems that exist secondary the abuse. In this role, the interviewer would be assessing psychiatric symptomatology as reported by both the child and parent(s) in order to generate a psychiatric diagnosis and systematic plan for treatment. This professional role would be similar to that of other mental health professionals who routinely interview children who present with a variety of complaints, including anxiety and depressive symptoms, attentional problems, and other behavioral difficulties.

The second major role would be that of a forensic or investigative interviewer. In this capacity, the professional would attempt to determine the likelihood that a child has been abused. Over the past 15 years, mental health professionals have been actively involved in the investigative interviewing process in many jurisdictions around the country. Their role has typically been to assist a legal entity such

ANTHONY P. MANNARINO AND JUDITH A. COHEN • Department of Psychiatry, Allegheny General Hospital, Pittsburgh, Pennsylvania 15212.

as the local child protective service system (CPS) or juvenile or family court in making an official abuse determination. Unfortunately, this role has come under intense scrutiny and professionals have been sharply criticized, in part, because of their involvement in a number of highly publicized cases in which questionable interview techniques were used. These cases have raised general concerns in the child abuse literature about what is the appropriate investigative interview format for alleged victims (Myers, 1992) and the potential suggestibility of children as witnesses (Ceci & Bruck, 1995).

This chapter will focus primarily on the role of the investigative interviewer. Moreover, it will largely focus on sexually abused children. Since there is no medical evidence to substantiate sexual abuse in the majority of cases (Muram, 1989), verbal disclosures by the child are key in documenting that something inappropriate has occurred. These disclosures are frequently obtained during an investigative interview. In contrast, documentation of physical abuse has been based largely on medical evidence. In this regard, presence of unexplained physical injuries that could not have resulted from an accident is the standard employed in most states to substantiate physical abuse. Although alleged victims of physical abuse may be interviewed whenever possible, they are typically very young (three and under) and not capable of providing extensive verbal disclosures.

It should be noted that throughout this chapter the female pronoun will be used for simplicity when referring to victims of child abuse. However, this in no way suggests that boys are not frequently victims of either sexual or physical abuse or that the problems that they manifest secondary to the victimization experience are not significant.

Prior to discussing specific procedures for gathering information, several matters will be addressed which have important implications for the interviewing process. These include professional issues (e.g., role definition and boundaries, confidentiality, and neutrality), practice guidelines that have been promulgated by professional organizations regarding the evaluation of sexually and physically abused children, and recent empirical research related to investigative interviewing.

PROFESSIONAL ISSUES

Mental health professionals who conduct investigative interviews with children who allegedly have been sexually or physically abused must be aware of a number of professional issues that have significant implications for the quality of their work. These include role definition and boundaries, confidentiality, and neutrality.

Role Definition and Boundaries

It is extremely important that the role boundaries of an investigative interviewer be defined prior to an evaluation. For example, the purpose of the interview(s), limits of confidentiality, and who will be informed of the interview findings must be clarified with all parties. It is particularly essential that the interviewer clarify that the interview process is not treatment and that a different professional would offer therapeutic services if these are necessary. Clarification of one's professional role should also occur with attorneys if they represent any of the parties (e.g., child; nonabusive parent or other relative; alleged perpetrator). In some cases, a court order or other written document may specify the nature of the interviewer's role. In other instances, meeting with parents, other relevant parties, or both prior to interviewing the child may be sufficient. Regardless of how it is achieved, clarification of the interviewer's role can potentially help the professional avoid later confusion and misunderstandings. More importantly, it can reduce the probability that an abused child will be subjected to additional interviews by multiple investigators, which can be a particularly traumatic outcome.

Confidentiality

With limited exceptions, based on the ethical principles of mental health professionals, they are required to keep confidential the information provided to them during diagnostic interviewing and treatment. This ethical principle applies to children as well, except if there is potential danger to the child (i.e., self-injurious behaviors; suicidality) or serious threats made against other individuals. When professionals conduct investigative interviews with alleged victims of child abuse, this principle is no longer true. In all 50 states, there are mandated reporting requirements for mental health professionals if there is suspicion of child abuse (Kalichman, 1993). Moreover, in forensic evaluations/investigative interviews, there is typically no confidentiality as there is an expectation that the information gathered will be reported to the court, CPS, or other third party.

Given these legal reporting requirements and the unique nature of a forensic evaluation, it is essential that the interviewer inform an alleged abuse victim of the limits of confidentiality. This task may be particularly difficult with very young children who have limited verbal understanding and perhaps some confusion about the purpose of the interview. Nonetheless, the interviewer should attempt to clarify confidentiality in a manner consistent with the child's developmental level. Such an open discussion may cause a child initially to feel reticent to talk about possible abuse, particularly if there have been threats related to disclosure. However, directly addressing the issue of confidentiality will decrease the likelihood that the child will feel betrayed if she discloses abusive episodes and this information is subsequently brought to the attention of a caseworker or the court. For sexual abuse victims in particular, a sense of betrayal is an issue to which they are already acutely sensitive in many instances.

Neutrality

Gathering information objectively is essential to the interview process, but may not be easily achieved in the area of child abuse. Alleged victims tend to elicit our sympathy and compassion. Moreover, investigative interviewers who have had extensive experience in treating abused children may believe that they rarely lie or are not easily coached to make false allegations. In contrast, investigative interviewers who have also conducted many custody evaluations may be inherently suspicious of any type of allegation, particularly if it is made by an angry parent. Either type of subjective bias can reduce the objectivity of the interview process.

The investigative interviewer who assesses alleged victims of child abuse must remain neutral. The goal is to conduct as impartial an interview as possible and to provide objective information to an outside party as to the likelihood that the abuse did or did not occur. Interviewers need to be aware of their biases and the impact of previous clinical experience, so that they can proceed with interview protocols without unwarranted assumptions or compromised neutrality.

PRACTICE GUIDELINES

During the past several years, a number of professional organizations have published practice guidelines regarding the evaluation of alleged victims of sexual or physical abuse. There is little doubt that these guidelines have emanated, in part, from concerns about how child abuse evaluations were being conducted and criticisms of mental health professionals for unsound and questionable interview techniques. The scope of this chapter does not permit an extensive discussion of these guidelines, although a few relevant issues will be highlighted.

Published guidelines are now available from the American Academy of Child and Adolescent Psychiatry (AACAP) ("Practice parameters for the forensic evaluation of children and adolescents who may have been physically or sexually abused" [AACAP, 1997]), the American Psychological Association (APA) (*Guidelines for Psychological Evaluations in Child Protection Matters* [APA, 1998]), and the American Professional Society on the Abuse of Children (APSAC) (*Guidelines for Psychosocial Evaluation of Suspected Sexual Abuse in Children* [APSAC, 1996]). Although these guidelines are very different from each other (e.g., the AACAP provides extensive information about how to conduct an evaluation, whereas the APA focuses more on relevant ethical principles), they all offer reasonable and acceptable standards for professionals to follow when evaluating alleged child abuse victims. For instance, all of the documents address issues related to objectivity and neutrality, defining the limits of confidentiality, and clarifying role boundaries.

These practice guidelines were not intended to be mandatory codes of conduct for professionals who evaluate alleged victims of child abuse. Instead, they provide guiding principles as to how to proceed with these evaluations in the most rigorous and clinically sound manner. Nonetheless, given the current scrutiny and skepticism that surrounds the investigative interviewing process, it is essential that mental health professionals be familiar with these guidelines and try to incorporate them into their overall plan as to how to competently interview this vulnerable population of children.

EMPIRICAL RESEARCH RELATED TO INVESTIGATIVE INTERVIEWING

Due to the controversies that have arisen with respect to interviewing alleged victims of child abuse, research on this and related topics has gained increased prominence during the past decade. In particular, empirical studies have focused on children's suggestibility, trauma and memory, children as witnesses in the courtroom, and interview techniques. Again it is beyond the scope of this chapter to discuss any of these areas at great length, but there is an excellent, comprehensive review recently provided by Saywitz, Goodman, and Lyon (2002).

A few of the findings from this literature have direct relevance to the current discussion about investigative interviewing. First, studies have demonstrated that children can be suggestible and that younger children are more suggestible than older children (Ceci & Bruck, 1993). Also, suggestibility typically increases in response to repeated questioning. Additionally, decreased accuracy in recall increases as interview questions become more specific and focused. Of particular concern are questions that require a "yes/no" response or questions in which a child must choose from two possible options. The latter types of questions are most prone to inaccurate recall (Orbach & Lamb, 2000; Saywitz et al., 2002).

As reviewed by Saywitz et al. (2002), research has demonstrated that free recall in response to open-ended questions is the best interview technique to obtain accurate memory of previous events. However, young children may not provide extensive information in response to open-ended questions and may leave out critical details. Thus, the interviewer may be faced with the dilemma of asking more focused questions at the risk of increased inaccuracy. Moreover, much of the research on children's suggestibility and memory has taken place in analog studies that have not actually involved a true investigation of alleged abuse. Therefore, it is not clear how easily the findings from these studies generalize to real cases of child abuse investigation.

There are obviously a number of issues related to children's memory and suggestibility that will continue to be debated in the literature. Nonetheless, a growing consensus among both researchers and clinicians suggests that investigative interviewers should at least begin the interview process with open-ended questions that provide the opportunity for the child to provide any information that she remembers. Moreover, even in later stages of the interview process, open-ended questions are still best, although if more focused questions become necessary, the interviewer should try to use the previous information provided by the child as the appropriate cue or context. Recently, there have been some attempts to develop structured interview protocols that rely on free recall to open-ended questions (Orbach et al., 2000) or interview strategies that encourage elaboration without the use of suggestive or leading questions (Saywitz & Snyder, 1996). These are important developments which will enhance the quality of the investigative interviewing process.

PROCEDURES FOR GATHERING INFORMATION

As mentioned previously, this section on specific data gathering procedures will pertain primarily to sexually abused children.

General Issues

Number of Interviews

The manner in which an interviewer proceeds in obtaining information about possible sexual abuse is a function, at least in part of the child's age and developmental status. Although there may be pressure from the legal system to gather the relevant data in one interview, this may not be possible. Particularly for younger children with limited verbal and cognitive skills, several interviews may be required. Moreover, gaining the child's trust and establishing an atmosphere of warmth and encouragement are critical. Achieving these goals may take multiple sessions. Accordingly, an interviewer needs to proceed slowly and cautiously. It is important to note that not all interview sessions will necessarily include questions about the alleged abuse. This is particularly true for the early sessions (APSAC, 1996). Also, as repeated questioning will increase the inaccuracy of recall (Ceci & Bruck, 1993), this strategy should clearly be avoided.

Interviewing Child without Alleged Perpetrator

If a child has allegedly been sexually abused by a parent, it is certainly not appropriate for that parent to be present during any of the investigative interviews. In fact, the alleged perpetrator should not even accompany the child to the interviewer's office. In many sexual abuse cases, the victim has been threatened with some type of harm if there is any disclosure. Accordingly, the presence of the alleged perpetrator during an interview would be highly intimidating for the child.

In addition, many abuse victims maintain positive feelings toward the perpetrator, especially when the abuser is a parent. Often children are afraid that the perpetrator will be punished or that they will not be permitted any contact with this individual. These are significant reasons for a child not to provide information about possible sexual abuse. Presence of the alleged perpetrator during the interview would only serve to reinforce these issues and make it extremely difficult for a child to be truthful. It should also be noted that the APSAC practice guidelines (1996) specifically indicate that it is not necessary to interview the alleged perpetrator to determine whether or not sexual abuse has occurred.

Interviewing Child without Nonabusive Parent

In the majority of cases of either intra- or extrafamilial abuse, the child is brought to the examiner's office by the nonabusive parent. Nonetheless, every attempt should be made to interview the child on an individual basis. This may be difficult for younger children who would experience much anxiety if asked to separate from their parent. Such anxiety can be alleviated by permitting the parent to remain in the office for 10–15 min so that the child can become more comfortable. Moreover, having a parent wait just outside the office or keeping the door ajar for a few minutes can be reassuring.

There are at least two reasons for interviewing a child in the absence of the nonabusive parent. First, if a parent is present, a child may feel compelled to say what she believes the parent wants to hear, although this may not necessarily reflect what actually occurred. For example, if a child knows that the parent does not believe that any abuse occurred, she may be highly reticent to make any disclosure in that parent's presence. Alternatively, a child may feel obliged to agree with an angry parent who is alleging abuse by an ex-spouse, even if there has not been any type of maltreatment. In either scenario, a child can be influenced regarding what is disclosed in order to obtain a parent's approval or, at least, avoid disapproval. Accordingly, the truth about the alleged abuse may not be revealed.

The second major reason for interviewing a child on an individual basis is related to legal issues. If charges are being pressed against the alleged perpetrator or if the case is being reviewed in juvenile or family court, the presence of a parent during the interview may be perceived as a contaminating factor. Although an interviewer may feel that a parent can help a child feel more relaxed and comfortable, the attorney representing the alleged perpetrator will no doubt suggest that the parent influenced the content of the child's statements. In a criminal proceeding, this could result in charges being dismissed; in family or juvenile court, the child might be forced to have unsupervised contact with an abusive parent because the allegations are determined to be unfounded. Given the potential for such highly negative and potentially traumatic outcomes, an interviewer should make every attempt to interview a child alone, so that findings will be deemed more acceptable to the legal/judicial system.

Essential Data to Be Gathered

Questioning a child about inappropriate touching or possible involvement in sexual activities is a very difficult and sensitive part of the interview process. In this regard, it cannot be overemphasized how critical it is that the child supply the information about any alleged abuse in response to open-ended questions. Leading or suggestive questions are almost always inappropriate, although an inexperienced interviewer may not be aware when a specific question has that quality. (More extensive discussion of leading questions will take place in the "Dos and Don'ts" section of this chapter.)

Details about the Abuse

In addition to obtaining information about the identity of the alleged perpetrator and the specific nature of the sexual acts perpetrated against the child, other details need to be explored. These would include the number of abusive episodes, where the abuse occurred, whereabouts of the child's primary caretaker (if different from abuser) when the abuse occurred, and the child's feelings about the incident(s). Moreover, the following issues should be addressed: threats or promise of rewards made by the perpetrator, reasons for delaying disclosure if this has occurred, and whether the alleged perpetrator told the child to keep the abuse a "secret." It is also important to ascertain the child's feelings as to who is responsible for the abuse, whether she has felt emotional support since the disclosure, and what she believes are the consequences for the alleged perpetrator and herself, now that the abuse has been disclosed. Again, as much as possible, every attempt should be made to gather information about the details of the victimization experience through open-ended questions in which the child provides the information about what allegedly occurred.

Children will, of course, vary in the amount of information that they can provide as a function of age, level of trust, etc. Moreover, disclosure may occur on a gradual basis, with more details being given over time. Nonetheless, even children as young as 3 years old can provide some basic details about what may have occurred. This information is critical in helping the interviewer eventually determine the likelihood that a child may have been sexually abused.

Interviewer's Reaction to Disclosures

The interviewer's reaction to the information provided by the child can be a critical determinant regarding how much additional information is disclosed. An interviewer who is judgmental of the alleged perpetrator or who reacts strongly to horrible details may make the child feel scared, guilty, embarrassed, or responsible for what happened. Any of these feelings will inevitably result in a child being reluctant to talk further about any alleged abuse. It is essential, therefore, that an interviewer be calm and nonjudgmental when details are being provided.

It may take extensive experience in interviewing sexually abused children to achieve this type of emotional reaction. Professionals are human and prone to strong and judgmental responses to the disclosure of sexual abuse as are other members of society. Being aware of one's own feelings about sexual abuse and monitoring one's emotional reactivity to this issue can help professionals to respond to the information provided by alleged victims in an encouraging but objective, neutral, and nonjudgmental manner.

Use of Anatomically Correct Dolls

Anatomically correct (AC) dolls were originally designed as a diagnostic tool to assist interviewers in assessing young children or older children with limited verbal skills. It was hoped that children who could not use words to describe any alleged sexual abuse could demonstrate with the dolls what was perpetrated against them. Unfortunately, a great controversy has evolved about the appropriate use of AC dolls in interviewing alleged abuse victims (Boat & Everson, 1994; White & Santilli, 1988).

One of the greatest concerns about utilization of AC dolls has been that they are suggestive to young children and that this could result in explicit sexual play even in the absence of previous sexual abuse. However, empirical studies have failed to support such a contention. For example, Sivan, Schor, Koeppel, and Noble (1988) found no demonstrations of simulated sexual intercourse in their sample of 144 3–8-year-old nonsexually abused children observed in free play with AC dolls.

Similarly, Everson and Boat (1990) reported that only 6% of their nonsexually abused 2–5-year-old subjects demonstrated behavior clearly suggestive of sexual intercourse during a doll interview. Thus, there is little empirical support for the notion that AC dolls elicit explicit sexual behavior in "normal," nonabused children.

APSAC recently (1995) published a set of practice guidelines for the "Use of anatomical dolls in child sexual abuse assessments." This document identifies several "appropriate uses" for AC dolls, including assessing the child's labels for body parts and for the child to use to demonstrate any alleged abusive activities. The latter may be particularly important for very young alleged victims with limited verbal skills. Despite these potential uses for AC dolls, it should be noted that no experts on investigative interviewing have advocated their use as part of the interview process (AACAP, 1997). Moreover, using AC dolls as a diagnostic test to determine whether or not abuse has occurred has no empirical support (APSAC, 1995).

CASE ILLUSTRATIONS

Two cases will be discussed below which illustrate some of the data gathering procedures described in the previous section. In both cases, names and other factual details have been changed to protect the identity of the victims. The interview format used in these case illustrations has some parallels to what has been developed by Orbach et al. (2000) and Sternberg et al. (1997) in that there is a strong emphasis on open-ended questions.

Case 1

This case involved a 4-year-old boy named Billy who was allegedly sexually abused by his father during visits. The parents were divorced and the father had partial custody of Billy every other weekend. The mother had become suspicious of possible sexual abuse because of Billy's use of precocious sexual terms and excessive masturbation immediately after visits with the father. When she asked her son about possible inappropriate touching, he responded that "daddy" had been touching him "down there." Prior to this child being interviewed, the attorneys for both parents agreed that an evaluation could be performed by a court appointed professional. The following dialogue demonstrates interview questions and techniques that are appropriate with a very young child.

During the first interview with Billy which lasted about 45 min, there were a series of warm-up questions about preschool, play interests, etc. Then Billy was asked about the reason for the interview.

INTERVIEWER: Billy, do you know why your Mommy brought you to see me today?
BILLY: I don't know. (Long pause.) I think it's about Daddy.
INTERVIEWER: I see. What about Daddy?
BILLY: I visit with Daddy on Saturdays. Sometimes we go to the toy store.
INTERVIEWER: Wow! Sounds like fun. Can you tell me more about your visits with Daddy?

BILLY: He bought me a fire truck. I saw a fire one time.

INTERVIEWER: You did.

BILLY: But that wasn't with my Daddy.

INTERVIEWER: Oh, I see. What else happens when you see your Daddy?

BILLY: We go to grandma's. She lets me bake cookies with her.

INTERVIEWER: That sounds like fun.

BILLY: Daddy's not nice sometimes.

INTERVIEWER: Can you tell me about that?

BILLY: (Looks somewhat scared and just shrugs his shoulders.)

The above set of questions illustrate that very young children typically give brief answers, that they can quickly change the topic, and that they may become quiet and withdrawn when they are feeling uncomfortable. The interviewer decided to allow Billy to play for a few minutes. By the end of the interview, Billy seemed relaxed and happy when the interviewer suggested that Billy return to his office for another session the following week. At the next interview, Billy was able to talk more about what happened with his father. Again the interview started with some warm-up questions prior to the following inquiry.

INTERVIEWER: Last time you were telling me about visits with your Daddy. Do you remember?

BILLY: Yeah, we have fun. But sometimes he's not nice.

INTERVIEWER: Oh, I see. Can you tell me everything about when Daddy's not nice?

BILLY: He touched me.

INTERVIEWER: Who touched you?

BILLY: (Glancing downward and looking sullen.) Daddy.

INTERVIEWER: Can you tell me about when Daddy touched you?

BILLY: (No response. Still looking sad. Then pointing to a game on a shelf). What's that? Can we play with it?

INTERVIEWER: It's hard to talk about when Daddy touched you, isn't it?

BILLY: (Nods head affirmatively.)

INTERVIEWER: I understand. Let's try again. Just tell me about everything that happened when Daddy touched you.

BILLY: He touched my pee-pee.

INTERVIEWER: Tell me more about what happened.

BILLY: (Rubbing his genital area.) He touched me like this.

INTERVIEWER: Can you tell me what happened next?

BILLY: I sucked his pee-pee. Stuff came out. I drank it until it was all gone.

This disclosure made Billy quite anxious. He became very distracted and indicated that he wanted to be reunited with his mother. (The interviewer decided to discontinue this line of questioning until the third and final interview at which time additional details were gathered. Space does not permit a discussion of the third interview.) Billy was again given the opportunity to play. He seemed to cheer up considerably and was having a good time when the interview session ended. It was also important to convey to Billy that he had not done anything wrong and that it was okay for having talked about what happened. This type of encouragement is totally acceptable and particularly significant for young children.

It is important to emphasize, though, that a child should receive words of encouragement and positive feedback no matter what she discloses, even if there is a denial of abuse or if there are inconsistencies in her statements. Also, as this case illustrates, several interviews may be required with very young children.

Case 2

This second case involved a 9-year-old girl named Laura who was allegedly sexually abused by her father over several years. This was an intact family with two younger siblings. Laura had initially disclosed the abuse to her mother who did not believe her. She subsequently told her maternal grandmother who called the local CPS. Laura and her siblings were then placed into temporary foster care because her father would not leave the house. Soon afterward, a local juvenile court judge ordered an evaluation to assess Laura's credibility about abuse allegations. The excerpts which follow illustrate procedures for alleviating a child's anxiety, gathering details in a nonleading manner, and obtaining information about a child's feelings about the alleged perpetrator and/or abuse.

INTERVIEWER: You seem to be kind of nervous.

LAURA: (Shaking head affirmatively.) I am.

INTERVIEWER: Do you know why you're here?

LAURA: Yes, but I don't want to talk. Can you ask my caseworker what happened? She knows about everything that happened with my father.

INTERVIEWER: I understand why you feel nervous or afraid. It's okay if you feel this way.

LAURA: I just can't talk about it. It's too embarrassing. Please ask my caseworker.

INTERVIEWER: I understand. This is a hard situation to be in.

The above exchange did seem to help Laura to become more comfortable. The interviewer then provided Laura with the opportunity to tell what happened.

INTERVIEWER: You mentioned when we started about everything that happened with your father. Can you tell me about everything that happened as best as you can remember?

LAURA: You know, that's why I'm here. Please ask my caseworker.

INTERVIEWER: I could but it's important that I hear from you, too. Can you tell me about what happened?

LAURA: Well, it was my father. I'm too shy to talk about it.

INTERVIEWER: I understand. Please go ahead with what you were going to say.

LAURA: (After a few seconds.) My father, he touched me.

INTERVIEWER: Can you tell me about all that happened?

LAURA: He touched me on my bottom. He put his pee-pee in my bottom.

INTERVIEWER: Tell me what happened next.

LAURA: He made me touch it with my mouth.

INTERVIEWER: Touch what?

LAURA: His pee-pee.

INTERVIEWER: Where did this happen?

LAURA: In the bathroom.

INTERVIEWER: Where was the bathroom?

LAURA: In our house.

INTERVIEWER: I'm not sure how often this happened.

LAURA: Lots of times.

INTERVIEWER: Can you tell me how often that means?

LAURA: Every week. Sometimes more.

Laura did a good job providing details about the alleged abuse. Encouragement was offered as well as positive feedback that she was trying very hard to remember what happened despite her embarrassment and anxiety. General nonsuggestive questions were used so that Laura could provide the information about what had occurred. This is important, even if questions have to be repeated or if the interviewer appears to the child to be a bit "dumb" or "slow." Again, leading questions should be avoided, wherever possible.

After more information about details was gathered, questions were asked about Laura's feelings about what had happened.

INTERVIEWER: How did you feel when your father did those things to you?

LAURA: I felt bad.

INTERVIEWER: Can you tell me more about your feelings?

LAURA: I was mad. How could a father do this stuff? I told my mother but she didn't believe me.

INTERVIEWER: Does she believe you now?

LAURA: I think so.

INTERVIEWER: How do you feel toward your father now?

LAURA: I love him. But I'm still mad. He has to go to some kind of doctor to get help.

INTERVIEWER: How do you feel about being away from home?

LAURA: Sad. Maybe it's my fault. Maybe I shouldn't have said anything. He could get into trouble.

INTERVIEWER: What kind?

LAURA: Go to jail.

INTERVIEWER: How would you feel about that?

LAURA: A little happy and a little sad. He did some nice things with me, too.

The above excerpt illustrates the kinds of feelings which are commonly found in sexually abused children, such as their sense of betrayal, ambivalence toward the perpetrator, and their feelings of responsibility for the abuse. Questioning a child about her feelings is important not only for investigative purposes but also for clinical reasons. Resolving these kinds of feelings is typically a critical component of treatment for most child victims.

CRITICAL INFORMATION TO MAKE DIAGNOSIS

General Concerns

Although interviewing a child with regard to possible sexual abuse is a critical part of the diagnostic process, other assessment procedures are also necessary.

In this regard, a medical examination is typically suggested despite the absence of physical findings in the large majority of cases (Muram, 1989). Nonetheless, a physician can rule out sexually transmitted diseases and also provide reassurance to the child and/or parents that she is not "damaged." In addition, interviewing the nonabusive parent to obtain background information and history (APSAC, 1996), interviewing the alleged abusive parent when allegations arise during custody disputes (Benedek & Schetky, 1987), and gathering data from collateral sources are important diagnostic procedures. Use of abuse-related assessment instruments such as the Child Sexual Behavior Inventory (Friedrich et al., 1992) or the Trauma Symptom Checklist for Children (Briere, 1995) may be very helpful in determining symptomatology secondary to the alleged abuse. However, it should be remembered that the presence of specific symptoms is not pathognomonic of sexual abuse.

In drawing conclusions as to the likelihood that the child has been abused, interview findings clearly must be evaluated in the context of other sources of data. Nonetheless, there are a number of criteria that can be used in examining interview results which may relate to a child's credibility. (Please see Myers et al., [1989] and AACAP [1997] for parallel discussions.) It must be strongly emphasized, though, that there are no empirical data which demonstrate that the presence or absence of any of these factors confirms or disconfirms abuse and that there are many exceptions to the broad guidelines suggested below.

SPECIFIC CRITERIA

Convincing Details

Children will vary widely in the amount of information that they can provide about alleged abuse based on their chronological age, developmental level, anxiety, level of trust, etc. Also, disclosure may occur gradually, with more details discussed over time. Nonetheless, children who can provide convincing details are likely to be perceived as more credible than those who only give minimal information such as "daddy touched my pee-pee." Generally, it has been our clinical experience that even preschool children can specify where the abuse occurred, whether anyone else was present, and some details about the exact nature of the inappropriate touching.

Age-Appropriate Terminology

It is common for abuse victims to use their own terminology to describe the private parts of the body and sexual acts with which they may have been forced to engage. Accordingly, interviewers can expect to hear words like "pee-pee," "stick," "peachy," etc. to describe the private parts and statements like "daddy put his thing in my bum" or "he made me rub it" to describe the actual sexual experience. Of course, some children will use adult terms, especially if they have been in therapy related to possible abuse, have participated in sexual abuse prevention programs, or live in a family in which their parents have taught them adult terminology. Generally, though, most actual abuse victims will use words and descriptions which are consistent with their age and overall developmental status.

Consistency

It is inevitable that alleged child sexual abuse victims will not be totally consistent from one interview to the next or across interviewers with regard to the information that they provide. Again, age, developmental level, etc. will be important influences. In addition, inconsistencies can result because different questions are asked by different interviewers. Gradual disclosure of more details over time may also result in apparent inconsistencies. Nonetheless, if a child's statements are generally consistent, this would enhance her credibility.

Affect Consistent with Allegations

In our clinical experience, when a child has truly been sexually abused, her affect is usually consistent with the allegations. Thus, embarrassment, anxiety, shame, and fear are commonly found when a victim is providing information about the abuse. However, there are numerous exceptions to this general guideline. Children who have been interviewed several times or have been in therapy related to the alleged abuse may present details in a relatively straightforward manner without significant distress. Also, children who have received much emotional support from parents after disclosure may feel reasonably comfortable in talking about what occurred. Accordingly, this factor has to be carefully considered. Absence of anxiety or other signs of emotional distress when discussing the allegations does not necessarily diminish a child's credibility.

Other Factors

There are other factors that merit some attention. The interviewer must try to assess whether a child has been coached or influenced with regard to the information that she provides. Again, however, caution must be exercised. Sometimes even in legitimate abuse cases, a parent instructs a child "to tell the doctor the truth" or "just say what happened." Also, it is important to evaluate whether an alleged victim has any motivation to make a false allegation. With older children or adolescents who have more advanced sexual knowledge and possible sexual experience, they are more capable of fabricating abuse. This may occur out of anger, a desire to seek retaliation for perceived rejection, or to gain attention.

Again, it cannot be emphasized enough that the above criteria are very broad guidelines and that many children who have actually been abused will meet one or more criteria but not the others. Determining whether a child has been sexually abused is a very serious and complex task, which requires the integration of interview findings with data from other assessment procedures and from additional sources other than the child. Unfortunately, in some cases, the information gathered may be inconsistent or conflictual and leave the interviewer feeling very uncertain about the possibility of abuse. In these situations, it is strongly recommended that the interviewer not hesitate to express this uncertainty in any written report that is prepared.

Dos and Don'ts

Suggestive Questions

Interview procedures for abused children have come under attack in the past decade because of a concern that leading or suggestive questions are frequently used. Particularly with regard to sexually abused children, there have been reported cases in which criminal convictions have been overturned, in part, because the interview process was suggestive and/or coercive (Myers, 1996). This issue becomes an even greater concern when investigators are not adequately trained in interviewing abused children. Although an inexperienced interviewer may generally understand that suggestive questions are inappropriate, he/she may not be aware when a specific question has that quality.

During the interview process, it is essential that the child provide information about any alleged abuse to which she has been subjected. Leading or suggestive questions are generally not acceptable, although more focused questions (e.g., "Can we talk about Jennifer, your babysitter, now?" may be necessary if the child has not responded to open-ended questions. To illustrate, asking a child, "Did daddy touch your pee-pee?", particularly if it is an initial question, is leading in at least three ways. Specifically, this type of question makes the assumptions that the child has been touched inappropriately, that the father is the perpetrator, and that genital fondling was the type of sexual activity which occurred. It is worth adding that young children may have a propensity to respond affirmatively to yes/no type questions, particularly in an attempt to gain the interviewer's approval. Leading or suggestive questions can therefore result in a child being guided or influenced to provide a specific response which may or may not reflect the reality of what actually happened.

The following dialogue illustrates how leading questions can contaminate interview findings.

INTERVIEWER: Do you know why you're here today?
CHILD: (Nods affirmatively.)
INTERVIEWER: Good. Can you tell me how your daddy touched you?
CHILD: He touched me in a yucky way.
INTERVIEWER: Did he touch your pee-pee?
CHILD: Yes.
INTERVIEWER: Did he make you touch his pee-pee?
CHILD: I think so.

In contrast, the following dialogue illustrates more appropriate general questions to which the child supplies the information about what happened.

INTERVIEWER: Have you ever had any problems with touching or someone bothering you?
CHILD: Yes.
INTERVIEWER: Can you tell me about that?
CHILD: My daddy touched my pee-pee.
INTERVIEWER: Can you tell me everything that happened?
CHILD: He touched my pee-pee with his pee-pee.
INTERVIEWER: How did he do that?
CHILD: He put it inside me.

As mentioned above, an interview replete with leading or suggestive questions may be challenged in court and perceived as contaminated. A judge could order a new evaluation which is inherently more stressful for the child. Furthermore, the court proceedings in such a case may become even more prolonged. It is therefore critical to avoid leading or suggestive questions not only to insure that valid, reliable information is obtained but also to increase the likelihood that one's findings are perceived as objective within the legal system. Again, more focused questions may become necessary if the child has not responded to open-ended questions but focused questions should not imply that the interviewer is attempting to obtain only certain types of information (i.e., "Can we talk about school?" would be acceptable but "Can we talk about touching problems at school?" would not be okay.)

Interviewer Response to Child's Statements

In a previous section of this chapter, it was briefly discussed how the interviewer's reactions to a child's disclosures may affect the remainder of the interview process. This issue will be more fully elaborated here. Many children who have been sexually abused have kept this a secret for an extended period of time. Disclosure of what occurred may be very upsetting and can be accompanied by anxiety, shame, or embarrassment. An interviewer who responds in a negative way to a child's presentation of details will likely make her feel even more uncomfortable. Further disclosures would then be improbable. This type of inappropriate emotional reaction is illustrated below.

INTERVIEWER: Can you tell me more about what happened?
CHILD: He made me put it in my mouth. He made me lick it.
INTERVIEWER: How horrible!
CHILD: (No response, appearing sad.)
INTERVIEWER: It was disgusting what he did. No wonder you have a hard time talking about it.

In a similar vein, being judgmental of the alleged perpetrator may result in an exacerbation of a child's fear that her disclosure may cause something bad to happen to him. Again, this can have a dampening effect on the likelihood of additional statements.

INTERVIEWER: How do you feel about what your daddy did to you?
CHILD: Bad. I'm very angry at him.
INTERVIEWER: You should be! He's a wicked man. How would you feel if he goes to jail?
CHILD: Half and half. Happy but a little sad, too.
INTERVIEWER: I understand but he deserves to go for what he did.

More appropriately, the interviewer needs to respond to a child's disclosures in a relatively benign and straightforward but supportive manner. This will lessen her anxiety and not make her feel that she has done anything wrong or that she is bad. Furthermore, a neutral perspective should be maintained toward the alleged perpetrator, with a focus on the child's feelings, not the interviewer's. In this regard, it may take many interviews with abused children for a professional to learn to achieve this type of constructive emotional response.

Professionals who interview allegedly abused children face a difficult and complex task. Proceeding in a cautious manner is essential as the stakes are too high to do otherwise. Using biased interview procedures lacking in objectivity or deriving conclusions which are not supported by the data may potentially result in greater stress for a child victim who has already been subjected to a traumatic life event.

SUMMARY

This chapter has focused on investigative interviewing with physically and sexually abused children, although most of the discussion has been geared toward the latter group. General professional issues have been addressed, as well as practice guidelines and relevant research on investigative interviewing. In addition, case illustrations have been used to highlight specific interviewing techniques and to demonstrate how certain procedures are inappropriate. It has been emphasized throughout the chapter that determining that a child has been abused is a difficult and complex task. Although broad guidelines were suggested in order to make such a determination, cases will vary tremendously and many abused children will not meet one or more of these criteria. Interviewers must therefore proceed in a cautious manner and draw conclusions based on an integration of interview findings with data from other assessment procedures and from additional sources other than the child.

REFERENCES

American Academy of Child and Adolescent Psychiatry. (1997). Practice parameters for the forensic evaluation of children and adolescents who may have been physically or sexually abused. *Journal of the American Academy of Child and Adolescent Psychiatry, 36,* 423–442.

American Professional Society on the Abuse of Children. (1993). *Use of anatomical dolls in child sexual abuse assessments.* Chicago: Author.

American Professional Society on the Abuse of Children. (1996). *Guidelines for psychosocial evaluation of suspected sexual abuse in children.* Chicago: Author.

American Psychological Association. (1998). *Guidelines for psychological evaluations in child protection matters*. Washington, DC: Author.

Benedek, E. P., & Schetky, D. H. (1987). Problems in validating allegations of sexual abuse. Part 2: Clinical evaluation. *Journal of the American Academy of Child and Adolescent Psychiatry, 26*, 916–921.

Boat, B. W., & Everson, M. D. (1994). Anatomical doll exploration among non-referred children: Comparisons by age, gender, race, and socioeconomic status. *Child Abuse and Neglect, 18*, 139–153.

Briere, J. (1995). *The Trauma Symptom Checklist for Children (TSC-C) manual*. Odesa, FL: Psychological Assessment Resources, Inc.

Ceci, S. J., & Bruck, M. (1993). Suggestibility of the child witness: A historical review and synthesis. *Psychological Bulletin, 113*, 403–439.

Ceci, S. J., & Bruck, M. (1995). *Jeopardy in the courtroom: A scientific analysis of children's testimony*. Washington, DC: American Psychological Association.

Einbender, A., & Friedrich, W. N. (1989). The psychological functioning and behavior of sexually abused girls. *Journal of Consulting and Clinical Psychology, 57*, 155–157.

Everson, M. D., & Boat, B. W. (1990). Sexualized doll play among young children. Implications for the use of anatomical dolls in sexual abuse evaluations. *Journal of the American Academy of Child and Adolescent Psychiatry, 29*, 736–742.

Finkelhor, D. (1990). Early and long-term effects of child sexual abuse: An update. *Professional Psychology: Research and Practice, 21*, 325–330.

Friedrich, W. N., Grambsch, P., Damon, L., Hewitt, S. K., Koverola, C., Lang, R., Wolfe, V., & Broughton, D. (1992). The Child Sexual Behavior Inventory: Normative and clinical comparisons. *Psychological Assessment, 4*, 303–311.

Kalichman, S. C. (1993). *Mandated reporting of suspected child abuse: Ethics, law and policy*. Washington, DC: American Psychological Association.

Mannarino, A. P., Cohen, J. A., & Gregor, M. (1989). Emotional and behavioral difficulties in sexually abused girls. *Journal of Interpersonal Violence, 4*, 437–451.

Muram, D. (1989). Child sexual abuse: Relationship between sexual acts and genital findings. *Child Abuse and Neglect, 13*, 211–216.

Myers, J. E. B. (1992). *Legal issues in child abuse and neglect*. Newbury Park, CA: Sage.

Myers, J. E. B. (1996). Joint hearings to attack investigative interviews: A further assault on children's credibility. *Child Maltreatment, 1*, 213–222.

Myers, J. E. B., Bays, J., Becker, J., Berliner, L., Corwin, D. L., & Saywitz, K. J. (1989). Expert testimony in child sexual abuse litigation. *Nebraska Law Review, 68*, 1–145.

Orbach, Y., & Lamb, M. (2000). Enhancing children's narratives in investigative interviews. *Child Abuse and Neglect, 24*, 1631–1648.

Orbach, Y., Hershkowitz, I., Lamb, M., Sternberg, K. J., Esplin, P. W., & Horowitz, D. (2000). Assessing the value of structural protocols for forensic interviews of alleged child abuse victims. *Child Abuse and Neglect, 24*, 733–752.

Saywitz, K., & Snyder, L. (1996). Narrative elaboration: Test of a new procedure for interviewing children. *Journal of Consulting and Clinical Psychology, 64*, 1347–1357.

Saywitz, K. J., Goodman, G. S., & Lyon, T. D. (2002). Interviewing children in and out of court. In J. E. B. Myers, L. Berliner, J. Briere, C. T. Hendrix, C. Jenny, & T. A. Reid (Eds.), *The APSAC handbook on child maltreatment* (pp. 349–377). Thousand Oaks, CA: Sage.

Sivan, A. B., Schor, D. P., Koeppel, G. K., & Noble, L. D. (1988). Interaction of normal children with anatomical dolls. *Child Abuse and Neglect, 12*, 295–304.

Sternberg, K. J., Lamb, M. E., Hershkowitz, I., Yudilevitch, L., Orbach, Y., Esplin, P. W., & Hovav, M. (1997). Effects of introductory style on children's abilities to describe experiences of sexual abuse. *Child Abuse and Neglect, 21*, 1133–1146.

White, S., & Santilli, G. (1988). A review of clinical practices and research data on anatomical dolls. *Journal of Interpersonal Violence, 3*, 430–442.

19

Older Adults

Barry Edelstein, Lesley Koven,
Adam Spira, and Andrea Shreve-Neiger

In 1999 there were 34.5 million adults aged 65 years or older in the United States (Administration on Aging, 2000). This group constituted 12.7% of the entire U.S. population. Older adults are also getting older, with individuals having a life expectancy of an additional 17.8 years once they reach the age of 65. The number of older adults is increasing at a higher rate than individuals under the age of 65. By 2030 we will have twice the number of older adults as we did in 1999, and they will represent 20% of the U.S. population.

In 1998 most community dwelling older adults (67%) lived in a family setting, although this figure diminishes with the age of the individual. Approximately 45% of these individuals who were 85 years of age and older lived in family settings. Approximately 31% of the community dwelling older adults lived alone in 1998 (Administration on Aging, 2000). Only about 4.3% of older adults lived in nursing homes in 1997, although the percentage increases substantially with age. Only 1.1% of individuals who were 65–74 years of age lived in nursing homes, whereas 19% who were 85 years and older lived in nursing homes (National Center for Health Statistics, 1997).

In 1996, 27% of older adults rated their health as fair or poor, compared with 9.2% for all individuals (Administration on Aging, 2000). Among individuals aged 65–74 in 1997, 30% reported a limitation due to a chronic condition, whereas among those 75 years and older, 50.2% reported such limitations. Over 14% of older adults in 1994 experienced difficulties performing activities of daily living (e.g., bathing, dressing, eating), and 21% experienced difficulties with independent activities of daily living (e.g., preparing meals, shopping, managing money). Among the most frequently occurring chronic conditions are arthritis, hypertension, hearing impairments, heart disease, cataracts, orthopedic impairments, and diabetes.

BARRY EDELSTEIN, LESLEY KOVEN, ADAM SPIRA, AND ANDREA SHREVE-NEIGER • Department of Psychology, West Virginia University, Morgantown, West Virginia 26506.

Reports of the prevalence of mental disorders among older adults have ranged from 20% (U.S. Department of Health and Human Services, 1999) to 25% (Gatz, Kasl-Godley, & Karel, 1996). Unfortunately, mental disorders of older adults are less likely than those of younger adults to be diagnosed (U.S. Department of Health and Human Services, 1999; Valenstein et al., 1998). The prevalence, nature, and course of mental disorders can be quite different from that of disorders of younger adults. These age-related differences can substantially affect the assessment and diagnosis process and outcome, as the reader will soon learn.

The purpose of this chapter is to offer the reader a concise discussion of diagnostic assessment issues that are important to consider when undertaking the assessment of older adults. We begin with a brief introduction that describes the epidemiology of aging and the psychopathology of older adults. We then turn to procedures for gathering information, with an emphasis on multi-method assessment. A case study illustrating some of the complexity of differential diagnoses with older adults follows. We then move to a discussion of structured interviews with an eye to instruments used with or developed for older adults. A relatively detailed discussion of age relevant factors to consider when entertaining diagnoses for older adults is then offered, followed by some very practical "dos" and "don'ts" in the context of age-related changes one must anticipate and consider in the conduct of diagnostic assessment.

PROCEDURES FOR GATHERING INFORMATION

Multimethod Assessment: Minimizing Threats to Validity

Several variables (e.g., halo effect, social demands) threaten the validity of information gathered through the clinical interview, no matter the age of the interviewee (Groth-Marnat, 1997). However, when conducting diagnostic interviews with older adults, the clinician should be aware of additional threats that may compromise the validity of data collected via interview (Edelstein, Northrop, Staats, & Packard, 1996). For example, older adults may suffer from cognitive deficits from a variety of sources, including dementia, medical illness, and side-effects of medications, that may influence the amount and accuracy of information gathered during assessment (Edelstein & Semenchuk, 1996). In addition, cognitively unimpaired older adults may have difficulty providing accurate information regarding particular aspects of their histories relevant to the diagnostic process. Furthermore, older adults, as a function of cohort and cultural background, may minimize or deny symptoms (Blazer, 1996; Wong & Baden, 2001). Taken together, these factors recommend that the clinician supplement information gathered through older adults' self-report with information from other sources (i.e., multimethod assessment). Thus, in addition to the clinical interview, additional procedures for gathering information will be discussed, including behavioral observation, interviewing informants, and a review of medical records.

Clinical Interview

A successful diagnostic interview requires the client to disclose a considerable amount of information concerning mental and emotional health (Kanfer & Schefft, 1988). Thus, the clinician should take steps to maximize the likelihood that clients will disclose by taking time to develop rapport prior to the discussion of sensitive subject matter (Kaplan & Sadock, 1998; Zarit & Zarit, 1998). This is particularly important with today's older adults, who were raised within a society reluctant to discuss issues related to mental health (MacDonald & Schnur, 1987). Once rapport has been sufficiently established, the clinician can begin the essential component of the interview, the mental status examination.

Mental Status Examination.   The mental status examination (MSE) can be a very useful tool for the diagnosis of individuals from a range of clinical populations (Akiskal & Akiskal, 1994; Robinson, 2000), including older adults. Although the content of the MSE varies from clinician to clinician and from case to case, general statements can be made regarding the exam. The MSE is usually a semistructured interview during which the clinician investigates aspects of the client's cognitive and psychodiagnostic status through the examination of the three response systems (i.e., cognitive, motor, and physiological behavior; Lang, 1968). Specific aspects of the client's functioning that are commonly examined during the MSE, include appearance, psychomotor activity, attitude toward the examiner, mood, suicidal and homicidal ideation, affect, speech, perceptual experiences (e.g., hallucinations), thought content, cognitive status (e.g., orientation, memory, concentration), impulsivity, judgment, insight, and reliability (Kaplan & Sadock, 1998; Silver & Herrmann, 1991). In addition, the examiner should be sure to screen for suicidal and homicidal ideation.

The length of the MSE can vary widely and is dictated by the purpose of the evaluation, the ability of the examinee to communicate with the examiner, and the complexity of the symptom picture yielded by the interview. For example, a 15-min interview may be sufficient to determine that a stroke victim's memory and language ability have been significantly impaired, and that a diagnosis of multi-infarct dementia is appropriate. However, a case that requires a particularly fine-grained evaluation of mental and diagnostic status may take significantly longer. For example, extensive assessment may be required to determine whether mild cognitive and functional deficits are best accounted for by a long history of schizophrenia, a traumatic brain injury, or by dementia due to a more recently developed organic brain disorder. Further details regarding the content and conduct of the MSE are discussed in Chapter 2.

Functional Assessment.   The behavioral approach to psychopathology emphasizes that overt behavior is controlled by its antecedents and consequences (Martin & Pear, 1999; Skinner, 1974). Given this proposition, it follows that knowledge of the historical antecedents to, and consequences of a given behavior are critical to the manipulation of that behavior. When clinicians are aware of the learning history that has produced a given response, they are able to make statements regarding the function of that behavior (i.e., the environmental contingencies that maintain it). The A–B–C model, (i.e., antecedent–behavior–consequence) has been used to describe the relation between behavior and environmental contingencies (Martin & Pear, 1999). Although elaborate and formal functional assessment procedures have been developed (e.g., functional analysis; Iwata et al., 1994), an informal functional assessment can be conducted during the clinical interview. For example, when a client describes a given behavior (B), such as social withdrawal, it is not necessarily clear whether this behavior is a symptom of depression, anxiety, schizophrenia, or some other factor. Functional assessment can assist in this process of differential diagnosis. The examiner can inquire regarding the antecedents (A) to and consequences (C) of withdrawal. For example, a client might report feeling anxious in social situations (A) before withdrawing (B). In addition, he or she might report feeling a reduction in anxiety after withdrawing (C). The results of this informal functional assessment would indicate that the client's social withdrawal is negatively reinforced (i.e., maintained) by the subsequent avoidance of social anxiety. In other words, the client's social withdrawal functions to avoid anxiety elicited by social contact. Although this functional approach is not usually thought of as a diagnostic tool, it can be especially practical in this enterprise; it points not only to diagnosis—in this case, social phobia— but also to treatment, by elucidating the variables that control the behavior in question.

Behavioral Observation. During the clinical interview, the examiner can gather important diagnostic information from direct observation of the client's overt motor behavior. Data collected through behavioral observation can enrich the diagnostic impressions resulting from the verbal exchange with the examinee by providing additional evidence for these impressions. For example, the observation of psychomotor agitation following the older adult's report of constant tension and worrying would provide additional evidence for a diagnosis of generalized anxiety disorder. On the other hand, behavioral observation can yield evidence of clinical phenomena that the client denied, misrepresented, or failed to report. Normal aging involves changes (e.g., reduced speed of information processing, working memory and sensory deficits) that can impact older adults' self-reports (Park, 1999). In light of this, and the other threats to validity described above, data collected through behavioral observation is especially important to the process of diagnostic interviewing when working with this population.

In addition to providing information regarding the structural, or topographical nature of a client's problems, behavioral observations made in the context of the clinical interview can inform diagnosis by contributing to functional assessment. Over the course of the interview, the clinician has the opportunity to directly observe antecedents to problematic behaviors that might emerge (e.g., agitation, anxiety, crying), and the effects that his or her own behaviors (i.e., the consequences of the client's behaviors) have on the client's subsequent behavior. Thus, behavioral observations within the interview can be used to supplement the functional assessment performed on the basis of the client's self-report.

Interviewing Informants. The clinician can also obtain valuable information by interviewing individuals familiar with the client's behavioral and diagnostic history. Although the self-reports of informants are vulnerable to the same threats to validity as the self-reports of informants (Edelstein & Semenchuk, 1996), these individuals can provide information that older clients either cannot remember (e.g., previous diagnoses, changes in functional status), or are reluctant to disclose (e.g., sexual issues, urinary incontinence, other behavioral disturbances). In addition, informants are often in control of the environmental contingencies within which the client operates. Thus, they can be especially helpful in the enterprise of functional assessment and the implementation of subsequent behavioral interventions.

Review of Records

Psychosocial History. A review of older clients' psychological and medical records can provide information valuable to the diagnostic process. For example, reports from past psychological and psychiatric evaluations may contain detailed psychosocial histories that can be particularly useful in determining whether the client's current functional status and symptom picture represents a change from previous levels of functioning. Because criteria for several disorders require that the symptoms noted represent a change (i.e., in functional status, mood, etc.), such information can be useful in the diagnostic process (American Psychiatric Association, 1994). In addition, prior records of psychological disturbances might indicate whether the individual has exhibited symptoms of the disorder for a period sufficient to warrant a given diagnosis (e.g., more than 6 months for schizophrenia). Furthermore, prior reports can assist in differential diagnosis. For example, clients with long-standing symptoms of schizophrenia may also have a history of concurrent mood disturbances that they are unable to report due to cognitive impairment. A review of medical records might yield evidence of these episodes that would indicate a diagnosis of schizoaffective disorder, rather than schizophrenia. Although past reports can be helpful in the diagnostic process, the clinician should be wary of the means by which past examiners arrived at diagnoses. For example, before endorsing a prior report's diagnosis of mental retardation, the clinician should ensure that formal intelligence testing was conducted before the client was 18 years old (American Psychiatric Association, 1994).

Medical History and Laboratory Results. Older adults exhibit relatively high medical morbidity rates (Frazer, Leicht, & Baker, 1996). In light of the elevated incidence of medical disorders in this population, the clinician should consider that psychological symptoms (e.g., depression, anxiety, cognitive impairment, psychosis) might best be accounted for by medical conditions. For example, hypothyroidism can present as depression, hyperthyroidism can produce manic symptoms, and cardiopulmonary disorders can present as anxiety (Carmin, Pollard, & Gillock, 1999; Frazer et al., 1996). A review of an individual's medical history can help determine whether a constellation of symptoms is due to a psychological diagnosis, a pre-existing medical condition, or a combination of medical and psychological disorders.

If an individual's medical history is positive for diagnoses that might present as psychological problems, recent laboratory reports can assist the clinician in determining whether medical variables are responsible for a patient's psychological complaints. For example, a thyrotropin-releasing hormone (TRH) stimulation test can indicate whether a client's depressive symptoms are best explained by a thyroid disorder (Blazer, Busse, Craighead, & Evans, 1996). Laboratory test results can also assist in differential diagnosis. The results of an MRI, for instance, may be used to determine whether cognitive deficits are best accounted for by cerebral atrophy related to a brain disease (e.g., Alzheimer's disease, multi-infarct dementia) a depressive disorder, or a combination of the two (Blazer et al., 1996; Riley, 1994).

CASE ILLUSTRATION

One of the more commonly asked assessment questions encountered by clinicians who assess older adult clients, is whether a client is suffering from depression, dementia, or both. The following case illustrates the challenges of arriving at a differential diagnosis when faced with this diagnostic question.

Lynn is an 83-year-old Caucasian woman who has resided in a nursing home for several months following injuries suffered in a fall. You are seeing her at the request of the Director of Nursing, who is concerned about changes in Lynn's behavior over the past few weeks. Lynn is accompanied by her daughter, Natalie. Natalie is concerned that Lynn appears apathetic at times and no longer attends social activities. Lynn complains of difficulties with concentration and memory, and has experienced difficulty remembering the subject of conversations. She is also disoriented at times and becomes frustrated and angry when this occurs. Last night, Lynn walked into the bedroom of a male patient and climbed into his bed. When the patient explained to Lynn that she was in the wrong room and tried to move her, Lynn struggled with him and then began crying. Natalie reports that Lynn seems unhappy and withdrawn most of the time. Natalie explains that she has never seen Lynn like this before.

You peruse Lynn's chart and find that she has a family history of Alzheimer's disease, but she has no known history of mental illness. She has not had any recent changes in her medication. She has lost 8 lb. in the past three weeks, putting her just under her ideal weight range.

After speaking with staff, you learn that 4 weeks ago, Lynn was given a new roommate after her roommate of 9 months died. Lynn's new roommate is bedridden and non-communicative. Lynn's daughter tells you that she has not been able to visit as often because she is going through a custody battle with her ex-husband. She further reports that each time she has visited in recent weeks, she has noticed a decline in Lynn's cognitive abilities and a change in Lynn's affect and mood.

When you interview Lynn, you notice that her gait is slow and unsteady. She is still wearing her bedclothes and her hair is uncombed at 3 PM. She has forgotten her glasses. She seems to hesitate and look around the room between steps. As you interview her, she is polite, but tearful. She reports that she is not interested in activities that she formerly enjoyed, she sleeps much more often, her appetite is almost non-existent, and she worries constantly about her daughter and grandchildren. Her memory and concentration are markedly impaired, a source of great distress for her, and she reports feeling worthless and unhappy. Lynn frequently needs to be prompted to complete sentences because her sentences trail off as she stares out the window. She asks you to repeat questions several times because she reports having forgotten the question. In light of Lynn's symptoms (e.g., memory and concentration deficits and reports of depressed mood) you are uncertain whether Lynn is experiencing depression or dementia.

You interview nursing staff about Lynn's behavior at various times during the day and find that she leaves her room only for meals, has difficulty finding her room when she returns, and becomes agitated and tearful when trying to locate her room. When other residents approach her, she either complains or does not respond at all; they quickly leave her alone.

You orally administer a self-report measure of depression (Geriatric Depression Scale [GDS]; Yesavage et al., 1983). Lynn endorses 12 out of 15 items on the brief version of the GDS. The GDS is chosen rather than a lengthy, time consuming, structured interview because of Lynn's apparent depression and cognitive deficits. You then assess her memory using a few simple working, primary and secondary memory tasks to evaluate the extent of her cognitive impairment. When you assess Lynn's memory using the Hopkins Verbal Learning Test (HVLT—Revised; Shapiro, Benedict, Schretlen, & Brandt, 1999), you find that her performance is inconsistent, sometimes within normal limits, other times far below. Although she cries throughout the interview process and reports feeling frustrated and worthless, you find that Lynn's memory is not as bad as she reports it to be. When you tell this to Lynn, she shakes her head and tells you that the reason she has done well on some of the memory items is that the tasks were easy. Lynn performs well on simple tests of short-term memory (e.g., recalling a series of numbers), but performs poorly on tests that require greater concentration and working memory (e.g., digits backward). To further assess for possible dementia, the Boston Naming Test (Goodglass & Kaplan, 1983), a test of language and word finding ability, is administered in which Lynn performs within normal limits. On follow-up tests, her rate of forgetting is within normal limits. Lynn endorses 12 out of 15 depression items on the GDS. In light of this high score, specific questions regarding possible depression are asked to flesh out the clinical impression yielded by the GDS and to determine whether Lynn meets the *Diagnostic and Statistical Manual of Mental Disorders, Fourth Edition (DSM-IV)* criteria for an affective disorder.

Based upon Lynn's reports, her performance, your observations, and reports from staff and family, you conclude that Lynn is probably experiencing a major depressive episode. This conclusion is based on Lynn's rate of decline (moderately rapid; more rapid might have suggested a stroke), complaints of deficits (abundant), emotional reaction to deficits (marked distress), evaluation of accomplishments (minimized), and poor performance on memory tasks requiring concentration, but not simpler memory tasks. These symptoms are all indicators of depression. Had Lynn been experiencing dementia, the rate of decline would have been slower and her complaints about her decline, as well as her emotional reaction to them, would probably have been inconsistent (sometimes complaining, other times not reporting any distress related to her decline). A stroke or transient ischemic attack probably would have produced a more rapid decline in cognitive functioning. It is possible that Lynn's recent experiences (new roommate, concern for daughter) may have resulted in depression, which impacts concentration abilities, mood, and memory.

Structured Interviews

In an era when health maintenance organizations and other third-party payers require empirically based methods of assessment, structured interviews provide an effective way of standardizing evaluations and demonstrating diagnostic validity. Structured interviews provide a systematic evaluation by standardizing (1) the wording of clinical inquiries, (2) the sequencing of inquiries, and

(3) the quantification of responses (Rogers, 2001). This systematic evaluation of relevant symptoms and standardized coverage leads to a smaller probability of misdiagnosis and missed diagnoses (Rogers, 2001).

Semistructured interview schedules provide fewer rules for conducting the interview but include statements, probes, or outlines for questioning at the option of the interviewer. Some interviews were developed to be used by nonclinicians and require little skill, while others require extensive clinical experience which should be administered only by mental health professionals. Typically, interviews that involve less structure tend to require more skill and clinical inference on the part of the interviewer (Edelstein & Semenchuk, 1996).

We lack sufficient space to discuss all available structured interviews of relevance to older adults, therefore a few representative interviews will be discussed briefly for illustrative purposes. The Structured Clinical Interview for *DSM-IV* (SCID-I) is a semistructured interview designed to assist in determining a *DSM-IV* Axis I diagnosis (First, Gibbon, Spitzer, & Williams, 1996). The original SCID was developed to maximize validity of diagnostic assessments by allowing the interviewer to rephrase questions, ask further questions for clarification, challenge inconsistencies, and use clinical judgment in making a diagnosis (Blanchard & Brown, 1998). Separate versions of the SCID-I have been developed for research and clinical uses. The clinical version, the SCID-I-CV, is briefer than the research version and focuses primarily on core diagnostic information and on the most common diagnoses (First et al., 1996). Further, the SCID-P (Patient) is used with adult psychiatric patients and the SCID-NP (Non-patient) is used with individuals who have not been identified as psychiatric patients. Few studies have examined the psychometric properties of the SCID with an older adult sample. However, in a study examining the interrater reliability of the SCID-III-R with inpatient and outpatient old adults, respective percentage agreement was 85% for major depression, 94% for anxiety disorders, and 100% for somatoform disorders. Overall percentage agreement for all diagnoses was 91% (Segal et al., 1993).

The Geriatric Mental State Schedule (GMS; Copeland et al., 1976) is a semistructured interview for examining the mental state of older adults. The GMS is based on items from the eighth edition of the Present State Examination (Wing, Birley, Cooper, Graham, & Isaacs, 1967) and the Present Status Schedule (Spitzer, Fleiss, Burdock, & Hardesty, 1964). The GMS Schedule—Depression Scale (Ravindran, Welburn, & Copeland, 1994) is a 33-item semistructured interview that is comprised of items drawn from the GMS based on their ability to discriminate between depressed and non-depressed older adults and their sensitivity to change following pharmacological treatment.

The Comprehensive Assessment and Referral Evaluation (CARE; Gurland et al., 1977) is focused on assessing cognitive health, including items related to memory and orientation; psychiatric health, which includes questions about depression and anxiety, and physical health; and social status, including items related to degree of isolation, housing, and income. The CARE is administered in a semistructured fashion, takes approximately 1–2 hr to administer and score, and requires extensive training in administration. A short version of the CARE, the

SHORT-CARE measures depression, dementia, and disability exclusively (Gurland, Goldon, Teresi, & Challop, 1984).

The Cambridge Mental Disorders of the Elderly Examination (CAMDEX; Roth et al., 1986) is a multi-element assessment instrument that focuses on the diagnosis of dementia. It includes diagnostic interviews, collateral interviews, medical procedures, and a structured interview for cognitive dysfunctions referred to as the CAMCOG. The CAMCOG incorporated 11 items from the Mini Mental Status Exam (MMSE; Folstein, Folstein, & McHugh, 1975), with an additional 43 items to address other areas of cognitive dysfunction, such as language, abstract thinking, and calculation. In reliability studies of the CAMCOG, interrater reliability coefficients ranged from 0.50 to 1.00, with most (78.3%) of individual items exceeding 0.75 (Hendrie et al., 1988). In validity studies, the CAMCOG has been found to be effective in distinguishing dementia from depression with 92% sensitivity and 96% specificity (Hendrie et al., 1988).

Factors to Consider before Arriving at a Diagnosis

In addition to information gained from interviews, direct observations, and review of records, the following factors should be considered before arriving at a diagnosis.

Consideration of Medical Conditions

Many of the most common medical conditions diagnosed in older adults have numerous psychological symptoms (Frazer et al., 1996). However, medical professionals are often insufficiently prepared to assess the psychological manifestations of physical illness. Similarly, many physical disorders, when undetected, can appear as psychological symptoms, and mental health practitioners are often unaware of the possible underlying medical conditions.

Depression is a common psychological symptom associated with many chronic medical conditions. For example, Starkstein and Robinson (1989) reported a 41% rate of depression among outpatients with Parkinson's disease, and rates of major depression in cancer patients vary from 6% to 42% (Rodin, Craven, & Littlefield, 1993). Depression is also the most common psychological feature associated with chronic obstructive pulmonary disease (COPD); approximately one-quarter to one-half of individuals with COPD experience some form of depressive symptomatology (Murrell, Himmelfarb, & Wright, 1983). Patients with chronic heart disease also experience depressive symptomatology at a rate of between 10% and 20% (Cohen-Cole, 1989). Finally, depression is a common psychological manifestation of diabetes. Lustman, Griffith, Clouse, and Cryer (1986) estimated a lifetime prevalence of major depression among diabetes patients at 32.5% and point prevalence rates at 14%. Anxiety is also common in patients with Parkinson's disease (Schiffer, Kurlan, Rubin, & Boer, 1988), COPD (Frazer et al., 1996), and cardiovascular disease (Cohen-Cole, 1989).

Clinicians must be knowledgeable of the frequent comorbidity of medical and mental disorders, especially when the psychological symptoms are the initial presentation of the disease. Psychological symptoms may be reduced with successful treatment of the physical illness; therefore, it is crucial that clinicians consider medical illnesses as possible causes for psychological symptoms.

Consideration of Medication Effects

Approximately 80% of older adults suffer from at least one chronic health problem (Knight, Santos, Teri, & Lawton, 1995). As a result of these high rates of chronic illnesses, older adults consume more medications than any other age group (Ferrini & Ferrini, 1993). However, older adults are also at higher risk of adverse drug reactions than any other age group because of age-related changes in physiology and increased use of multiple medications, both prescribed and over-the-counter.

Some of the psychological symptoms presented by older adults may be the result of medications. For example, levodopa and carbidopa, the most commonly used pharmacological agents to treat Parkinson's disease, can result in central nervous system effects, such as confusion, hallucinations, and nightmares. Other medications, such as bromocriptine, pergolide, and selegiline, used as adjuncts to levodopa–carbidopa, may also increase the risk of confusion and hallucinations (Smith & Reynard, 1992). Medications used to treat COPD have numerous psychological side-effects. For example, theophylline, a commonly used bronchodilator, can cause cognitive impairment, anxiety, agitation, and insomnia. Similarly, oral corticosteroids, such as prednisone, used to treat COPD can cause a wide range of mental disturbances such as anxiety, euphoria, depression, and psychosis (Frazer et al., 1996). Side-effects of many cardiovascular drugs, such as propanol, a beta-blocker, include depression, confusion, delusions, paranoia, disorientation, agitation, and fatigue (Salzman, 1992). Further, nifedipine, a calcium channel blocker anti-hypertensive has nervousness and mood changes among its side-effects. Finally, delusions, forgetfulness, illogical thoughts, paranoid delusions, and sleep disturbances may be associated with antidepressant use (Salzman, 1992). In light of these potential side-effects, clinicians should thoroughly assess their clients' medication use to rule out drug side-effects when conceptualizing psychological symptoms.

Unique Presentations of Axis I Disorders in Older Adults

The presentation of Axis I disorders may vary greatly between younger and older adults. The most frequent differences between older and younger adults in the presentation of depression include lower prevalence of dysphoria, fewer ideational symptoms (e.g., guilt, suicidal ideation), and increases in selected somatic complaints (Fiske, Kasl-Godley, & Gatz, 1998). Gatz and Hurwicz (1990) hypothesized that depressed older adults may be more likely to experience a lack of positive feelings rather than active negative feelings. Loss of interest, lack of energy, sleep disturbance, suicidal thoughts, and feeling blue have all been found to best distinguish depressed from non-depressed older adults (Koenig, Cohen, Blazer, Krishnan, & Sibert, 1993; Norris, Snow-Turek, & Blankenship, 1995).

Fatigue and changes in appetite and sexual activity did not distinguish, and may reflect medical conditions or normal aging. Fiske et al. (1998) describe several subtypes of depression common in older adults, such as melancholic depression, which includes symptoms such as extreme loss of pleasure in most activities and lack of reactivity to pleasurable stimuli. Masked depression involves differential reports of physical rather than psychological symptoms, such as gastrointestinal disorders, poor health, musculoskeletal problems, or cardiovascular problems. Depletion syndrome involves primarily somatic and vegetative symptoms in depressed older adults who have had good premorbid psychosocial functioning and no evidence of psychosis.

Whereas little research exists on age differences in anxiety disorders, preliminary evidence suggests that the prevalence and content of older adults' fears and worries is different from that of younger adults. For example, Liddel, Locker, and Burman (1991) noted a significant decrease in fears with advancing age and Person and Borkovec found that older adults worried more about health, whereas younger adults worried more about family and finances (as cited in Stanley & Beck, 2000). Thus, the content of worry may reflect developmentally appropriate themes across the life span (Kogan, Edelstein, & McKee, 2000; Stanley & Beck, 2000).

In studies of age-differences in Generalized Anxiety Disorder and Panic Disorder, considerable similarity was found in the clinical characteristics of younger and older adults (Beck, Stanley, & Zebb, 1996; Raj, Corvea, & Dagon, 1993). Thus, although the prevalence and overall frequency of anxiety symptoms appear to decrease with age, the characteristics of anxiety disorders appear to remain consistent with advancing age.

Unique Presentations of Axis II Disorders in Older Adults

Personality disorders are defined within the *DSM-IV* (American Psychiatric Association, 1994) as rigid and inflexible personality traits that lead to functional problems and intra-psychic conflict. These disorders usually arise during adolescence or early adulthood. Therefore, older adults with personality disorders have likely had symptoms for several decades. Several theories exist regarding the impact of aging on personality disorders. The predisposition hypothesis states that middle-aged and older adults with personality disorders are more vulnerable to age-related stressors such as loss, physical illness, and dependency. When confronted with such events, they cope poorly, and experience increased psychopathology with age (Sadavoy & Leszcz, 1987). The maturation hypothesis holds that immature personality types such as histrionic, narcissistic, antisocial, and borderline, improve with age, whereas the mature personality disorder types such as obsessive, schizoid, and paranoid, worsen with age (Kernberg, 1984; Tryer, 1988). The improvement of personality disorders, such as borderline, may be related to normal decreases in activity level associated with aging. For example, a frail elderly patient may not have the same ability to engage in behaviors characteristic of borderline personality disorder, such as promiscuous sex or reckless driving (Abrams, 1990).

There is virtually no longitudinal research studying the course of personality disorders into old age. However, preliminary findings suggest that individuals with borderline personality disorder continue to experience high levels of comorbid Axis I disorders and increased suicide risk (Zweig & Hillman, 1999). Further, research indicates that the prevalence of borderline and antisocial personality disorder dramatically decreases with age (Perry, 1993).

Interaction of Cognitive Impairment and Mental Disorder

A diagnostic challenge that is more common among older than younger adults arises from the interaction of cognitive impairment and mental disorders. Requests for clinicians to differentiate between various mental disorders and dementia are relatively common, particularly when the disorders share several symptoms. The task of differentiating among these disorders oftentimes goes beyond a dichotomous choice. Individuals can experience a combination of several disorders (e.g., dementia, depression, anxiety) or even a single disorder with symptoms of others. For example, it is not uncommon for individuals to become depressed and anxious as they attempt to deal with the initial realization that they are experiencing dementia, and later as they begin to find even simple daily activities to be increasingly difficult. The prospect of further decline is often anxiety arousing and depressing.

To illustrate the problem of differential diagnosis, one need only consider the potential shared symptoms of depression and Alzheimer's disease, as illustrated in the case above. Poor concentration or attention associated with depression can lead to poor performance on tests of immediate or short-term memory, a characteristic of dementia. Other symptoms in common can include disruptions in the sleep cycle, apathy, greater dependence on others, fatigue, and changes in psychomotor activity. The formal differentiation of depression and dementia is beyond the scope of this chapter. The interested reader is referred to Kaszniak and Christenson (1994) for an excellent discussion regarding the differentiation of dementia and depression.

Older Adult Diagnostic Issues

As previously noted, the diagnosis of mental disorders among older adults can be particularly challenging due to the differences in symptom experience and clinical presentation of older adults, in comparison to younger adults. For example, depressed older adults are less likely to report dysphoria (Gallo, Anthony, & Muthen, 1994) than younger adults with the same level of overall depression. Older adults are also less likely to report ideational symptoms (e.g., guilt) than younger adults, and more likely to report somatic symptoms (Fiske et al., 1998). These age-related differences not only complicate the diagnostic process, but also call into question the validity of current *DSM-IV* criteria when applied to older adults. Moreover, there is some evidence that symptom levels and patterns that would not currently meet *DSM-IV* criteria for major disorders, are nevertheless problematic for older adults. The most recent *Surgeon General's Report on Mental Health* (U.S. Department of Health and Human Services, 1999) noted that "many older individuals present with somatic complaints and experience symptoms of depression and anxiety that do not meet the full criteria for depressive or anxiety disorders. The consequences of these subsyndromal conditions may be just as deleterious as the syndromes themselves" (p. 340). Indeed, though the prevalence of major depression among community dwelling older adults is similar to that of younger adults (approximately 1–2%; Blazer & Williams, 1980), the prevalence of clinically significant subsyndromal or minor depression is much higher (approximately 5–10%; Blazer & Williams, 1980; Mulsant & Ganguli, 1999).

In an attempt to address the high prevalence and clinical impact of minor depression, Kumar and Lavretsky (2001) have proposed a set of criteria for what they term sustained minor depression, which involves a modification of the *DSM-IV* criteria for minor depression. What is particularly interesting and supportive of this effort are the preliminary MRI findings reported by Kumar and colleagues that reveal structural changes in patients with late-onset minor depression that are comparable to those found with Major Depressive Disorder (Kumar & Lavretsky, 2001). Moreover, Kumar and Lavretsky (2001) also note that polysomnographic studies have revealed that biological markers of Major Depressive Disorder are found among patients who do not meet criteria for this disorder. Such findings suggest that, at least for older adults, depression may best be conceptualized along a continuum rather than categorically (cf. Caine, Lyness, King, & Connors, 1994).

Anxiety presents a similar diagnostic criterion problem for older adults. Though little research has addressed the nature and presentation of anxiety disorders among older adults, recent work by Kogan and Edelstein (in press) suggests that, in contrast to younger adults, older adults who experience even low levels of fears, find these fears disruptive in their daily lives. Though no research has addressed the potential reasons for this finding, a recent study of psychophysiological responses of older adults to stressful or anxiety-arousing stimuli may offer some insight into what may be contributing to these findings. Lau et al. (2001) found that, in response to stress induced by a Stroop task, older adults exhibited longer recovery of skin conductance levels than younger adults. Moreover, younger adults exhibited a steeper slope in the recovery of skin conductance levels over repeated presentations of the stressful task. Older adults also exhibited slower recovery of baseline systolic blood pressure following the presentation of stressful stimuli. Interestingly, this delayed recovery was obtained only among older adults reporting low levels of fear. Overall, these findings might be interpreted to suggest that older adults, in contrast to younger adults, experience the effects of stressful or anxiety arousing stimuli for longer periods due to the slower recovery and habituation.

The foregoing age-related differences regarding depressive and anxiety symptoms suggest that the current *DSM-IV* criteria may be insufficient for fully capturing the range, magnitude, and characteristics of older adult psychopathology. At the very least, clinicians should consider the possibility that subsyndromal levels of psychopathology may be clinically significant for older adults.

One approach to the older adult diagnostic problem is to retain the *DSM-IV* criteria and adopt a symptom severity approach that is consistent with the depressive continuum noted above (cf., Nease, Volk, & Cass, 1999). Research by these authors addressing mood and anxiety symptoms yielded valid clusters of symptom severity (e.g., low severity, high severity) that permitted the establishment of relations among the clusters and various outcome variables (e.g., health-related quality of life). This approach could be particularly appealing with older adults who may exhibit subsyndromal symptoms that are sufficiently disturbing to warrant intervention, as suggested by the examples of depression and fears described above.

Another approach to the *DSM-IV* criteria problem is the abandonment of syndromal classification in favor of a functional approach (e.g., Hayes, Wilson, Gifford, Follette, & Stroshal, 1996). With such an approach (i.e., functional analysis), one would organize problematic behaviors according to the functional processes that are hypothesized to have produced and maintained them. This approach could have considerable appeal to behaviorally oriented clinicians whose interventions are often focused on the functions of problem behaviors. Regardless of how the field addresses these diagnostic issues, the clinician is cautioned to be circumspect when considering the presenting symptoms of older adults and when assigning diagnoses.

DOS AND DON'TS

Ageism

The interviewer's and client's own biases can greatly affect the client's attitude during the interview, the therapist's interpretation of responses, and the final diagnosis. The interviewer and client may have preconceived beliefs as to what is considered "normal aging." These assumptions may be erroneous, but often result from socially accepted negative attitudes regarding older adults.

Butler (1980) defines ageism as a system of negative attitudes and false beliefs, discriminatory behaviors, and institutional norms and policies that perpetuate stereotypes about older adults, reduce their opportunities for a satisfactory life, and undermine their personal dignity. As such, ageism pervades society and thus can affect both the client and the interviewer.

The client may arrive at the interview with the ageist belief that mental illness is an inevitable part of normal aging. The client may also have labeled his or her problem as senility, considering it normal to become a bit senile with old age, and may mistakenly feel that there is no recourse for it as a result. The interviewer may succumb to ageism by dominating the interview, and thus being less respectful and patient. In addition, the interviewer, based on a client's age, may be more likely to assume that a disturbance has an organic or biological basis, and may recommend prescription drugs as a result. Older women are frequently the victims of both ageism and sexism due to society's stereotypic views of them as sick and alone (Edelstein & Semenchuk, 1996). In these cases, ageism may result in a poorer prognosis.

The interviewer can guard against ageist practice by becoming more aware of the normal aging process and having increased exposure to older adults, especially those who are high functioning and thus dispel ageist stereotypes.

Interviewers should examine their biases prior to the interview and become particularly vigilant for any bias that may emerge during the interview. If it becomes clear during the interview that the client has adopted many ageist beliefs about him or herself, the interviewer can dispute the beliefs and offer more realistic alternative explanations. Knowing that a problem is not inevitable, and that it may be addressed and ultimately resolved can give the client a great sense of relief and newfound control.

Sensory Considerations

Physiological changes, especially within the sensory system, are common occurrences in normal aging (Winogrond, 1984). Sensory deficits can influence information processing, mobility, independence, social behavior, and self-concept (Edelstein, Martin, & Goodie, 2000), and thus can influence or alter the assessment outcome. As a result, it is critical to assess for any possible sensory deficits, so that the most accurate diagnosis and appropriate treatment goals are established for the client. Several visual changes commonly occur as part of normal aging. Examples include increased lens density and inflexibility, which result in greater susceptibility to glare and problems with changes in light intensity, and yellowing of the lens, which decreases one's ability to discriminate among colors within the blue–violet color spectrum (Kline & Scialfa, 1996). In addition, loss of lens elasticity may result in reduced visual acuity, and liquification of the vitreous humor may lead to retinal detachment (Garzia & Trick, 1992; Kline & Scialfa, 1996). These changes can affect the older adult's performance during assessment, which may result in an inaccurate portrayal of the client's true abilities or may mask more critical underlying problems. The interviewer can, however, improvise and accommodate the client with poor vision in a number of ways.

The interviewer should ask the client at the start of the interview if he or she has any visual deficits and if he or she normally wears corrective lenses. If the client wears lenses but is not wearing them for the interview, ask the client to put them on if he or she has them. Reading glasses and a magnifying glass may be kept in the office in case the client has forgotten his or hers. The font size of any textual information should be larger than normal (14 or 16 font), but not too large (greater than 16 font), which may further impair reading (Edelstein et al., 2000).

In order to reduce glare during the assessment, the interviewer can utilize antiglare computer monitor screens, seat the client so he or she is not facing a window, and use dull or darker shades of paper rather than high-gloss paper for any self-report measures (Edelstein et al., 2000). The lighting in the room should be bright but not glaring, and should primarily illuminate the interviewer's face. If the client continues to have difficulty seeing the interviewer's face, avoid nonverbal directions or cues. It is crucial to remember that because a client is visually impaired, it does not mean that he or she is hard of hearing. Speak in a normal tone unless you have reason to believe that the client cannot hear well. Ask the client what the specific visual deficits are, and how the interview environment can be modified to better suit his or her individual needs.

Deficits in hearing rank second only to arthritis among chronic health conditions affecting older adults (Maurer & Rupp, 1979). Older adults, especially males, with hearing loss may have difficulty understanding conversational speech due to an inability to detect high frequency tones, such as consonant sounds (Kline & Scialfa, 1996). If the interviewer is female, this may also cause problems due to the female's voice being characteristically higher in pitch than that of a male. In addition, background noise may make hearing difficult for the client with hearing loss. Hearing loss can affect an older adult's psychological well-being in a number of ways, such as increasing paranoia, hostility, and depression (Winogrond, 1984). As a result, to ensure optimal assessment performance, it is crucial for the interviewer to assess and compensate for hearing deficits in the following ways.

The interviewer should ask at the outset if the client has any hearing loss and if he or she wears a corrective device, such as a hearing aid. If the client wears or has a hearing aid, he or she should be encouraged to wear it throughout the interview. To assess for hearing difficulty indirectly, the interviewer can look for behavioral cues during the interview such as the client tilting or turning his or her head to one side while moving forward, or asking for statements to be repeated frequently. The interviewer can accommodate the hearing-impaired client by first eliminating any source of background noise. The interviewer should also speak slowly and distinctly in short, simple sentences, and then check with the client for comprehension. Because some clients will rely on lip reading, it is important not to over-enunciate words which causes facial distortion and makes it more difficult for the client to understand (Edelstein et al., 2000). Again, good lighting on the interviewer's face can aid in effective communication, and sitting close to the client will also make lip reading and hearing easier. If the client is becoming frustrated or fatigued, take frequent breaks. If communication is greatly disrupted due to the client's hearing loss, nonverbal forms of communication may be employed, such as providing the questions in written form.

Regardless of the type of sensory impairment, communication with the client, through direct questioning or indirect observation, is vital when accommodating for each client's individual needs. Assessment and compensation for any sensory deficit should occur before or near the beginning of the interview. Addressing sensory impairment at the outset will ensure the client's optimal assessment performance and consequently increase the validity of diagnostic impressions.

Memory and Cognition

Although declines in memory and cognitive abilities are not inevitable with age, some aspects of memory and cognition change characteristically over the life span (Howe, 1988) and may affect the older adult's assessment performance. Changes in memory with aging can consist of poor encoding as well as difficulty retrieving already encoded information (Howe, 1988). In addition, it appears that older adults have difficulty integrating memory context, which aids as a retrieval cue (Craik & Jennings, 1992; Smith, 1996). As a result, older adults may have greater difficulty retrieving information without environmental cues, or may have difficulty with working memory even when contextual cues are present.

Working memory involves holding information in memory while simultaneously using that information. Working memory may be used to solve a problem, make a decision, or learn new information (Craik & Jennings, 1992). Deficits in working memory result in older adults having difficulty retaining or acting on complex information that is conveyed during the interview. Older adults may also have difficulty inhibiting task-irrelevant thoughts when trying to utilize working memory (Smith, 1996).

The interviewer can encourage the client to bring documents or records to the interview to aid with recall when discussing medical and psychiatric histories. To accommodate for working memory difficulties, the interviewer can break complex information into smaller elements and be sure the client has retained previous elements before moving on to more information. The interviewer can also encourage the client to take notes during the interview if a question seems especially salient or if the client is afraid he or she may forget something that has been discussed. Finally, to keep the client from getting side-tracked by irrelevant information, the interviewer can ask short questions without any tangential or irrelevant content that may cause unnecessary confusion for the older adult.

Changes in cognition that may occur with age include declines in processing speed, discourse comprehension, attention, mental flexibility, and inductive reasoning, and maintenance or improvement of crystallized intelligence, language ability, and creativity (Park, 1999). The interviewer should capitalize on the cognitive strengths of the client and minimize tasks that would require the use of weaker cognitive skills.

The interviewer should repeat new information or questions, or allow extra response time for the client with slowed attention or information processing. It is also helpful to give the client a copy of the questions that will be asked so he or she can refer to them whenever necessary. To accommodate for deficits in flexibility, the interviewer should avoid abrupt transitions and speak in concrete terms (Edelstein et al., 2000). If the client is having trouble making inferences or utilizing inductive reasoning, the interviewer can ask the client to describe how he or she arrives at a decision and what aspects are especially important to consider during problem-solving (Edelstein et al., 2000). Many older adults have extensive language ability, factual knowledge, and creativity. These are valuable skills to note during an interview as they may be beneficial later when establishing goals and implementing a treatment.

Circadian Issues

There is growing evidence to suggest that cognitive processes follow similar rhythms as biological functioning, with peak cognitive performance coinciding with peak physiological performance (May, Hasher, & Stoltzfus, 1993). In addition, the time of peak performance during the day seems to vary by age, with older adults peaking cognitively in the morning as opposed to younger adults, who peak in the evening (Yoon, May, & Hasher, 1997). Inhibitory processes, which filter or prevent irrelevant information from entering working memory, also are most active during circadian peak time.

In order to obtain optimal assessment performance, the interviewer should try to assess the older adult client earlier in the day rather than later in order to maximize cognitive functioning and inhibitory processing. If the interview cannot occur at what is suspected to be the client's optimal circadian peak time, the interviewer should record the time of the interview so it can be taken into account when diagnosis is considered.

Cohort Issues

The final consideration to be made when interviewing the older adult is sensitivity to age cohort issues. The cohort to which the client belongs may have preconceived ideas regarding mental health treatment and individuals who seek treatment. The client may feel stigmatized for needing an assessment. In addition, the client may have specific religious values or beliefs about privacy, gender roles, and sexuality that may surface during the interview. The interviewer must be careful not to offend the client and also be sensitive to any stigma the client may feel. The interviewer should convey warmth and acknowledge the discomfort that can be associated with an initial assessment. The interviewer should also start with demographic information and medical history and then ease into more personal questions later in the interview after rapport has been established. It is ultimately through communication and sensitivity that the interviewer can elicit the older client's trust and optimal assessment performance.

SUMMARY

We have presented information regarding the interviewing of older adults that should at least enable clinicians to avoid most of the more common pitfalls one encounters in working with older adults, whose normative and non-normative development offer significant challenges in the assessment process. In addition, we have suggested many practical considerations that will hopefully benefit the clinician who is faced with the complicated task of sorting out the many intertwined contributions of biological, social, and environmental factors that so often contribute to the clinical presentations of older adults.

REFERENCES

Abrams, R. (1990). Personality disorders in the elderly. In D. Binenfeld (Ed.), *Verwoerdt's clinical geropsychiatry* (pp. 151–163). Baltimore: Williams & Wilkins.

Administration on Aging. (2000). A profile of older Americans: 2000. U.S. Department of Health and Human Services.

Akiskal, H. S., & Akiskal, K. (1994). Mental status examination: The art and science of the clinical interview. In M. Hersen & S. M. Turner (Eds.), *Diagnostic interviewing* (2nd ed., pp. 25–51). New York: Plenum.

American Psychiatric Association. (1994). *Diagnostic and statistical manual of mental disorders* (4th ed.). Washington, DC: Author.

Beck, J. G., Stanley, M. A., & Zebb, B. J. (1996) Characteristics of Generalized Anxiety Disorder in older adults: A descriptive study. *Behaviour Research and Therapy, 34*, 225–234.

Blanchard, J. J., & Brown, S. H. (1998). Structured diagnostic interview schedules. In C. R. Reynolds (Ed.), *Assessment* Vol. 4 (pp. 97–130). Oxford: Elsevier Science.

Blazer, D. G. (1996). The psychiatric interview of the geriatric patient. In E. W. Busse & D. G. Blazer (Eds.), *Textbook of geriatric psychiatry* (pp. 175–189). Washington, DC: American Psychiatric Press.

Blazer, D. G., Busse, E. W., Craighead, W. E., & Evans, D. (1996). Use of the laboratory in the diagnostic workup of older adults. In E. W. Busse & D. G. Blazer (Eds.), *Textbook of geriatric psychiatry* (pp. 191–209). Washington, DC: American Psychiatric Press.

Blazer, D., & Williams, C. D. (1980). Epidemiology of dysphoria and depression in an elderly population. *American Journal of Psychiatry, 137*, 439–444.

Butler, R. N. (1980). Ageism: A foreword. *Journal of Social Issues, 36*, 8–11.

Caine, E. D., Lyness, J. M., King, D. A., & Connors, B. A. (1994). Clinical and etiological heterogeneity of mood disorders in elderly patients. In L. S. Schneider, C. F. Reynolds III, B. D. Lebowitz, & A. J. Friedhoff (Eds.), *Diagnosis and treatment of depression in late lie: Results of the NIH Consensus Development Conference* (pp. 23–53). Washington, DC: American Psychiatric Press.

Carmin, C. N., Pollard, C. A., & Gillock, K. L. (1999). Assessment of anxiety disorders in the elderly. In P. A. Lichtenberg (Ed.), *Handbook of assessment in clinical gerontology* (pp. 59–90). New York: Wiley.

Cohen-Cole, S. A. (1989). Depression in heart disease. In R. G. Robinson & P. V. Rabins (Eds.), *Depression in coexisting disease* (pp. 27–39). New York: Igaku-Shoin.

Copeland, J. R., Kelleher, M. J., Kellett, J. M., Gourlay, A. J., Gurland, B. J., Fleiss, J. L., & Sharpe, L. (1976). A semistructured clinical interview for the assessment of diagnosis and mental state in the elderly: The Geriatric Mental State Schedule: 1. Development and reliability. *Psychological Medicine, 6*, 439–449.

Craik, F. I. M., & Jennings, J. M. (1992). Human memory. In F. I. M. Craik & T. A. Salthouse (Eds.), *The handbook of aging and cognition* (pp. 51–110). Hillsdale, NJ: Erlbaum.

Edelstein, B. A., & Semenchuk, E. M. (1996). Interviewing older adults. In L. L. Carstensen, B. A. Edelstein, & L. Dornbrand (Eds.) *The practical handbook of clinical gerontology* (pp. 153–173). Thousand Oaks, CA: Sage.

Edelstein, B., Northrop, L., Staats, N., & Packard, N. (1996). Assessment of older adults. In M. Hersen & V. Van Hasselt (Eds.), *Psychological treatment of older adults: An introductory textbook*. New York: Plenum.

Edelstein, B., Alberts, G., & Estill, S. (1988). Adult diagnostic interview schedules. In M. Hersen & A. S. Bellack (Eds.), *Dictionary of behavioral assessment techniques* (pp. 16–17). New York: Pergamon.

Edelstein, B. A., Martin, R. R., & Goodie, J. L. (2000). Considerations for older adults. In M. Hersen & M. Biaggio (Eds.), *Effective brief therapies: A clinician's guide* (pp. 433–448). San Diego, CA: Academic Press.

Ferrini, A. F., & Ferrini, R. L. (1993). *Health in the later years* (2nd ed.). Dubuque, IA: Wm C. Brown Communications.

First, M. B., Gibbon, M., Spitzer, R. L., & Williams, J. B. W. (1996). *User's guide for the Structured Clinical Interview for DSM-IV Axis I Disorders B Research Version (SCID-I, version 2.0, February 1996 Final Version)*. New York: Biometrics Research Department, New York State Psychiatric Institute.

Fiske, A., Kasl-Godley, J. E., & Gatz, M. (1998). Mood disorders in late life. In B. Edelstein (Ed.), *Comprehensive clinical psychology, Vol. 7: Clinical geropsychology* (pp. 193–229). Oxford: Elsevier Science.

Folstein, M. F., Folstein, S. E., & McHugh, P. R. (1975). Mini-mental state: A practical method of grading cognitive state of patients for the clinician. *Journal of Psychiatric Research, 12*, 189–198.

Frazer, D. W., Leicht, M. L., & Baker, M. D. (1996). Psychological manifestations of physical disease in the elderly. In L. L. Carstensen, B. A. Edelstein, & L. Dornbrand (Eds.), *The practical handbook of clinical gerontology*. Thousand Oaks, CA: Sage.

Gallo, J. J., Anthony, J. C., & Muthen, B. O. (1994). Age differences in the symptoms of depression: A latent trait analysis. *Journal of Gerontology: Psychological Sciences, 49*, P251–P264.

Garzia, R. P., & Trick, L. R. (1992). Vision in the 90's: The aging eye. *Journal of Optometric Vision Development, 23*, 4–41.

Gatz, M., & Hurwicz, M. (1990). Are old people more depressed? Cross-sectional data on Center for Epidemiological studies depression scale factors. *Psychology and Aging, 5*, 284–290.

Gatz, M., Kasl-Godley, J. E., & Karel, M. J. (1996). Aging and mental disorders. In J. Birren & K. W. Schaie (Eds.), *Handbook of the psychology of aging* (4th ed., pp. 365–382). New York: Academic Press.

Goodglass, H., & Kaplan, E. (1983). *The assessment of aphasia and related disorders*. Philadelphia: Lea & Febiger.

Groth-Marnat, G. (1997). *Handbook of psychological assessment* (3rd ed.). New York: Wiley.

Gurland, B. J., Kuriansky, J., Sharpe, L., Simon, R., Stiller, P., & Birkelt, P. (1977). The Comprehensive Assessment and Referral Evaluation (CARE) B rational, development, and reliability. *International Journal of Aging and Human Development, 8*, 9–42.

Gurland, B., Goldon, R. R., Teresi, J. A., & Challop, J. (1984). The SHORT-CARE: An efficient instrument for the assessment of depression, dementia, and disability. *Journal of Gerontology, 36*, 166–169.

Hayes, S., Wilson, K., Gifford, E., Follette, V., & Strosahl, K. (1996). Experimental avoidance and behavioral disorders: A functional dimensional approach to diagnosis and treatment. *Journal of Consulting and Clinical Psychology, 64*, 1152–1168.

Hendrie, H. C., Hall, K. S., Brittain, H. M., Austrom, A. G., Farlow, M., Parker, J., & Kane, M. (1988). The CAMDEX: A standardized instrument for the diagnosis of mental disorders in the elderly— a replication with a US sample. *Journal of the American Geriatrics Society, 36*, 402–408.

Howe, M. L. (1988). Measuring memory development in adulthood: A model-based approach to disentangling storage–retrieval contributions. In M. L. Howe & C. J. Brainerd (Eds.), *Cognitive development in adulthood* (pp. 39–64). New York: Springer-Verlag.

Iwata, B. A., Pace, G. M., Dorsey, M. F., Zarcone, J. R., Vollmer, T. R., Smith, R. G., Rodgers, T. A., Lerman, D. C., Shore, B. A., Mazaleski, J. L., Goh, H., Cowdery, G. E., Kalsher, M. J., McCosh, K. C., & Willis, K. D. (1994). The functions of self-injurious behavior: An experimental-epidemiological analysis. *Journal of Applied Behavior Analysis, 27*, 215–240.

Kanfer, F., & Schefft, B. (1988). *Guiding the process of therapeutic change*. Champaign, IL: Research Press.

Kaplan, H. I., & Sadock, B. J. (1998). *Kaplan and Sadock's synopsis of psychiatry* (8th ed.). Baltimore, MD: Williams & Wilkins.

Kaszniak, A. W., & Christenson, G. D. (1994). Differential diagnosis of dementia and depression. In M. Storandt & G. R. Vanden Bos (Eds.), *Neuropsychological assessment of dementia and depression in older adults: A clinician's guide* (pp. 81–117). Washington, DC: American Psychological Association.

Kernberg, O. (1984). *Severe personality disorders: Psychotherapeutic strategies*. New Haven, CT: Yale University Press.

Kline, D. W. & Scialfa, C. T. (1996). Visual and auditory aging, ch. 10. In J. E. Birren & K. W. Schaie (Eds.), *Handbook of the psychology of aging* (4th ed., pp. 181–203). New York: Academic Press.

Knight, B. G., Santos, J., Teri, L., & Lawton, M. P. (1995). The development of training in clinical geropsychology. In B. G. Knight, L. Teri, P. Wohlford, & J. Santos (Eds.), *Mental health services for older adults: Implications for training and practice in geropsychology* (pp. 1–8). Washington, DC: American Psychological Association.

Koenig, H. G., Cohen, H. J., Blazer, D. G., Krishnan, K. R. R., & Sibert, T. E. (1993). Profile of depressive symptoms in younger and older medical inpatients with major depression. *Journal of the American Geriatrics Society, 41*, 1116–1176.

Kogan, J. N., & Edelstein, B. A. (in press). Modification and psychometric examination of a self-report measure of fear in older adults (in press). *Journal of Anxiety Disorders*.

Kogan, J., Edelstein, B., & McKee, D. (2000). Assessment of anxiety in older adults: Current status. *Journal of Anxiety Disorders, 14*, 109–132.

Kumar, A., & Lavretsky, H. (2001). Clinically significant non-major depression in the elderly: Clinical impact versus diagnostic uncertainty. *Clinical Geriatrics, 9*, 13–15.

Lang, P. J. (1968). Fear reduction and fear behavior: Problems in treating a construct. In J. M. Shilieu (Ed.), *Research in psychotherapy* (Vol. 3, pp. 90–102). Washington, DC: American Psychological Association.

Lau, A., Edelstein, B., & Larkin, K. (2001). Psychophysiological responses of older adults: A critical review with implications for assessment of anxiety disorders. *Clinical Psychology Review, 21*, 609–630.

Lau, A. W., Larkin, K. T., Edelstein, B. A., Scotti, J. R., Rankin, E. D., & Parker, R. K. (2001, August). *Psychophysiological responses of older adults to stressful stimuli*. Paper presented at the meeting of the American Psychological Association, San Francisco, CA.

Liddell, A., Locker, D., & Burman, D. (1991). Self-reported fears (FSS-II) of subjects aged 50 years and older. *Behaviour Research and Therapy, 29,* 205–212.

Lustman, P. J., Griffith, L. S., Clouse, R. E., & Cryer, P. E. (1986). Psychiatric illness in diabetes mellitus: Relationship to symptoms and glucose control. *Journal of Nervous and Mental Disease, 174,* 736–742.

MacDonald, M. L., & Schnur, R. E. (1987). Anxieties and American elders: Proposals for assessment and treatment. In L. Michelson & L. M. Ascher (Eds.), *Anxiety and stress disorders: Cognitive–behavioral assessment and treatment* (pp. 395–423). New York: Guilford.

Martin, G., & Pear, J. (1999). *Behavior modification: What it is and how to do it.* Upper Saddle River, NJ: Simon & Schuster.

Maurer, J. F., & Rupp, R. R. (1979). *Hearing and aging: Tactics for intervention.* New York: Grune & Stratton.

May, C. P., Hasher, L., & Stoltzfus, E. R. (1993). Optimal time of day and the magnitude of age differences in memory. *Psychological Science, 4,* 326–330.

Mental health: Report of the Surgeon General. (1999). Http://www.surgeongeneral.gov/library/mentalhealth/toc.html

Mulsant, B. H., & Ganguli, M. (1999). Epidemiology and diagnosis of depression in late life. *Journal of Clinical Psychiatry, 60*(Suppl. 20), 9–15.

Murrell, S. A., Himmelfarb, S., & Wright, K. (1983). Prevalence of depression and its correlates in older adults. *American Journal of Epidemiology, 117,* 173–185.

National Center for Health Statistics. (1997). An overview of nursing home facilities: Data from the 1997 National Nursing Home Survey, Advance Data No. 311, March 1, 2000.

Nease, D., Volk, R., & Cass, A. (1999). Investigation of a severity based classification of mood and anxiety symptoms in primary care patients. *Journal of American Board of Family Pratice, 12,* 21–31.

Norris, M. P., Snow-Turek, A. L., & Blankenship, L. (1995). Somatic depressive symptoms in the elderly: Contribution or confound? *Journal of Clinical Geropsychology, 1,* 5–17.

Park, D. C. (1992). Applied cognitive aging research, ch. 9. In F. I. M. Craik & T. A. Salthouse (Eds.), *Handbook of aging and cognition* (pp. 449–493). Hillsdale, NJ: Erlbaum.

Park, D. C. (1999). Cognitive aging, processing resources, and self-report. In N. Schwarz, D. Park, B. Knauper, & S. Sudman (Eds.), *Cognition, aging, and self-reports* (pp. 45–69). Philadelphia: Taylor & Francis.

Perry, J. C. (1993). Longitudinal studies of personality disorders. *Journal of Personality Disorders, 7*(Suppl.), 63–85.

Raj, B. A., Corvea, M. H., & Dagon, E. M. (1993). The clinical characteristics of Panic Disorder in the elderly: A retrospective study. *Journal of Clinical Psychiatry, 54,* 150–155.

Ravindran, A. V., Welburn, K., & Copeland, J. R. M. (1994). Semi-structured depression scale sensitive to change with treatment for use in the elderly. *British Journal of Psychiatry, 164,* 522–527.

Riley, K. P. (1994). Depression in older adults: Detection, dysfunction, and treatment. In B. R. Bonder & M. B. Wagner (Eds.), *Functional performance in older adults* (pp. 256–268). New York: F. A. Davis Company.

Robinson, D. J. (2000). *The psychiatric interview—explained.* Port Huron, MI: Rapid Psychler Press.

Rodin, G., Craven, J., & Littlefield, C. (1993). *Depression in the medically ill.* New York: Brunner/Mazel.

Rogers, R. (2001). *Handbook of diagnostic and structured interviewing.* New York: Guilford Press.

Roth, M., Tym, E., Mountjoy, C. Q., Huppert, F. A., Hendrie, F. A., Verma, S., & Goddard, R. (1986). A standardized instrument for the diagnosis of mental disorder in the elderly with special reference to the early detection of dementia. *British Journal of Psychiatry, 149,* 698–709.

Sadavoy, J., & Leszcz, M. (1987). *Treating the elderly with psychotherapy: The scope for change in late life.* Madison, CT: International Universities Press.

Salzman, C. (1992). *Clinical geriatric psychopharmacology* (2nd ed.). Baltimore: Williams & Wilkins.

Schiffer, R. B., Kurlan, R., Rubin, A., & Boer, S. (1988). Evidence for atypical depression in Parkinson's disease. *American Journal of Psychiatry, 145,* 1020–1022.

Segal, D., Hersen, M., Van-Hasselt, V., Kabacoff, V. B., Kabacoff, R. I., & Roth, L. (1993). Reliability of diagnosis in older psychiatric patients using the Structured Clinical Interview for DSM-III-R. *Journal of Psychopathology and Behavioral Assessment, 15,* 347–356.

Shapiro, A. M., Benedict, R. H.-B., Schretlen, D., & Brandt, J. (1999). Construct and concurrent validity of the Hopkins Verbal Learning Test—Revised. *Clinical Neuropsychologist, 13,* 348–358.

Silver, I. L., & Herrmann, N. (1991). History and mental status exam. In J. Sadavoy, L. W. Lazarus, & L. F. Jarvik (Eds.), *Comprehensive review of geriatric psychiatry* (pp. 149–169). Washington, DC: American Psychiatric Press.

Skinner, B. F. (1974). *About behaviorism*. New York: Random House.

Smith, A. D. (1996). Memory, ch. 13. In J. E. Birren & K. W. Schaie (Eds.), *Handbook of the psychology of aging* (4th ed., pp. 236–250). New York: Academic Press.

Smith, C. M., & Reynard, A. M. (1992). *Textbook of pharmacology*. Philadelphia: W. B. Saunders.

Spitzer, R. L., Fleiss, J. L., Burdock, E. I., & Hardesty, A. S. (1964). The Mental Status Schedule: Rationale, reliability, and validity. *Comprehensive Psychiatry, 5*, 384–395.

Stanley, M. A., & Beck, J. G. (2000). Anxiety disorders. *Clinical Psychology Review, 20*, 731–754.

Starkstein, S. E., & Robinson, R. G. (1989) Depression and Parkinson's disease. *Journal of Nervous and Mental Disorders, 178*, 27–31.

Strorandt, M., & VandenBos, G. R. (Eds.). (1995). *Neuropsychological assessment of dementia and depression in older adults: A clinician's guide*. Washington, DC: American Psychological Association.

Tryer, P. (Ed.). (1988). *Personality disorder: Diagnosis, management, and course*. London: Wright.

U.S. Department of Health and Human Services. (1999). *Mental Health: A report of the Surgeon General*. Rockville, MD: Author.

Valenstein, M., Kales, H., Mellow, A., Dalack, G., Figueroa, S., Barry, K., & Blow, F. C. (1998). Psychiatric diagnosis and intervention in older and younger patients in a primary care clinic: Effect of a screening and diagnostic instrument. *Journal of the American Geriatric Society, 46*, 1499–1505.

Wing, J. L., Birley, J. L. T., Cooper, J. W., Graham, P., & Isaacs, A. (1967). Reliability of a procedure for measuring and classifying present psychiatric state. *British Journal of Psychiatry, 113*, 499–515.

Winogrond, I. R. (1984). Sensory changes with age-impact on psychological well-being. *Psychiatric Medicine, 2*, 1–23.

Wong, G., & Baden, A. L. (2001). Multiculturally sensitive assessment with older adults: Recommendations and areas for additional study. In L. A. Suzuki, J. G. Ponterotto, & P. J. Meller (Eds.), *Handbook of multicultural assessment: Clinical, psychological, and educational applications* (pp. 497–522). San Francisco: Jossey-Bass.

Yesavage, J. A., Brink, T. L., Rose, T. L., Lum, O., Huang, V., Adey, M., & Leirer, O. (1983). Development and validation of a geriatric depression screening scale: A preliminary report. *Journal of Psychiatric Research, 17*, 37–49.

Yoon, C., May, C. P., & Hasher, L. (1997). Age differences in consumers' processing strategies: An investigation of moderating influences. *Journal of Consumer Research, 24*, 329–342.

Zarit, S. H., & Zarit, J. M. (1998). *Mental disorders in older adults: Fundamentals of assessment and treatment* New York: Guilford.

Zweig, R. A., & Hillman, J. (1999). Personality disorders in adults: A review. In E. Rosowsky, R. C. Abrams, & R. A. Zweig (Eds.), *Personality disorders in older adults: Emerging issues in diagnosis and treatment* (pp. 31–54). Mahwah, NJ: Lawrence Erlbaum Associates.

Index